ROBERT N. BERK, M.D.

Professor and Chairman, Department of Radiology,
University of California, San Diego, School of Medicine; and
Chief, Department of Radiology, University Hospital,
San Diego, California

JOSEPH T. FERRUCCI, Jr., M.D.

Professor, Department of Radiology, Harvard Medical School and
Chief, Division of Gastrointestinal Radiology,
Massachusetts General Hospital, Boston, Massachusetts

GEORGE R. LEOPOLD, M.D.

Professor and Vice-Chairman, Department of Radiology,
University of California, San Diego, School of Medicine;
and Chief, Division of Ultrasonography, University Hospital,
San Diego, California

Radiology of the GALLBLADDER and BILE DUCTS
Diagnosis and Intervention

1983

W. B. SAUNDERS COMPANY

Philadelphia □ London □ Toronto
Mexico City □ Rio de Janeiro □ Sydney □ Tokyo

W. B. Saunders Company: West Washington Square
Philadelphia, PA 19105

1 St. Anne's Road
Eastbourne, East Sussex BN21 3UN, England

1 Goldthorne Avenue
Toronto, Ontario M8Z 5T9, Canada

Apartado 26370—Cedro 512
Mexico 4, D.F., Mexico

Rua Coronel Cabrita, 8
Sao Cristovao Caixa Postal 21176
Rio de Janeiro, Brazil

9 Waltham Street
Artarmon, N.S.W. 2064, Australia

Ichibancho, Central Bldg., 22-1 Ichibancho
Chiyoda-Ku, Tokyo 102, Japan

Library of Congress Cataloging in Publication Data

Berk, Robert N.

Radiology of the gallbladder and bile ducts.

Includes bibliographical references and index.

1. Gallbladder—Radiography.   2. Bile ducts—Radiography.
3. Radiology, Interventional.   I. Ferrucci, Joseph T.
II. Leopold, George R.   III. Title. [DNLM: 1. Cholangiography.   2. Cholecystography. WI 750 R1297]

RC849.B44 1982   616.3′6507572   82–40186

ISBN 0–7216–1728–X   AACR2

Radiology of the Gallbladder and Bile Ducts
Diagnosis and Intervention   ISBN 0–7216–1728–X

Last digit is the print number: 9   8   7   6   5   4   3   2   1

To SONDRA, BRENDA, and PATSY

CONTRIBUTORS

George Berci, M.D., F.A.C.S.
Associate Clinical Professor, Department of Surgery, University of California, Los Angeles, School of Medicine; Associate Director, Department of Surgery, Cedars-Sinai Medical Center, Los Angeles, California

H. Joachim Burhenne, M.D., F.R.C.P.(C)
Professor and Chairman, Department of Radiology, University of British Columbia, British Columbia, Canada

Morton I. Burrell, M.D.
Professor, Department of Radiology, Yale University School of Medicine; Chief, Division of Gastrointestinal Radiology, Yale-New Haven Hospital, New Haven, Connecticut

Joseph E. Geenen, M.D.
Clinical Professor of Medicine, The Medical College of Wisconsin, Milwaukee; Director, Digestive Disease Center, St. Luke's Hospital, Racine, Wisconsin

J. Andrew Hamlin, M.D.
Staff Radiologist, Department of Radiology, Cedars-Sinai Medical Center, Los Angeles, California

Robert E. Koehler, M.D.
Professor, Department of Radiology, University of Alabama School of Medicine, Birmingham, Alabama; Attending Radiologist, University of Alabama Hospitals, Birmingham, Alabama

George R. Leopold, M.D.
Professor of Radiology, University of California, San Diego, California

Peter M. Loeb, M.D.
Clinical Professor, Department of Medicine, University of Texas Southwestern Medical School, Dallas, Texas

Peter R. Mueller, M.D.
Associate Professor, Department of Radiology, Harvard University School of Medicine, Boston, Massachusetts

Edward B. Singleton, M.D.
Professor of Radiology, Baylor College of Medicine; Clinical Professor of Radiology, University of Texas Medical School at Houston; Director of Radiology, St. Luke's Episcopal Hospital, Texas Children's Hospital and Heart Institute, Houston, Texas

Howard M. Spiro, M.D.
Professor, Department of Medicine, Yale University School of Medicine; Chief, Division of Gastroenterology, Yale-New Haven Hospital, New Haven, Connecticut

Robert J. Stanley, M.D.
Professor and Chairman, Department of Radiology, University of Alabama School of Medicine; Chief Radiologist, University of Alabama Hospitals, Birmingham, Alabama

Edward T. Stewart, M.D.
Professor, Department of Radiology, The Medical College of Wisconsin; Chief, Gastrointestinal Radiology, Milwaukee County Medical Complex and Froedtert Memorial Lutheran Hospital, Milwaukee, Wisconsin

Eric vanSonnenberg, M.D.
Assistant Professor, Department of Radiology, University of California, San Diego, School of Medicine, San Diego, California

Heidi S. Weissman, M.D.
Assistant Professor of Radiology and Nuclear Medicine, Albert Einstein College of Medicine, Bronx, New York; Adjunct Attending Physician of Radiology and Nuclear Medicine, Montefiore Hospital and Medical Center, New York, New York

Robert K. Zeman, M.D.
Assistant Professor of Radiology, Georgetown University School of Medicine, Washington, D.C.; Director, Abdominal Imaging Division, Department of Radiology, Georgetown University Hospital, Washington, D.C.

PREFACE

The first five chapters of this book are an extension and update of material that originally appeared in a monograph on radiology of the gallbladder and bile ducts by Robert Berk and Arthur Clemett published in 1977. In the preface to that book the authors wrote, "A cynic once said that writing a monograph is like moving old bones from one graveyard to another. This may often be true, but it does not apply when the subject is the radiology of the biliary tree and the year is 1977. Despite all the previous publications on the topic, the radiologic diagnosis of diseases of the gallbladder and bile ducts is a more dynamic subject at the present time than ever in the past." Little did these authors suspect that the progress they recognized was only the beginning of an astonishing renaissance in the field. They could not have known that accelerated advances in diagnosis and treatment of diseases of the gallbladder and bile duct would warrant an expanded monograph on the subject just five years later.

Clearly, the most significant event since the publication of the first monograph has been the burgeoning use of sonography for the evaluation of the gallbladder and bile ducts. Simple to perform, independent of liver and gallbladder function, quick, noninvasive, and accurate, it offers numerous advantages over oral cholecystography, which has been held sacrosanct by nearly everyone for so long. Computed tomography, although valuable in many circumstances for the detection of biliary tract disease, has not had nearly the impact of sonography.

The introduction of new radionuclides for the evaluation of the gallbladder has been an important advance in gallbladder imaging that was not even mentioned in the 1977 monograph. This technique, along with methods for the direct visualization of the bile ducts by percutaneous transhepatic cholangiography and endoscopic retrograde cholangiography, has rendered the intravenous cholangiogram nearly obsolete.

Most remarkable of all has been the introduction and widespread use of interventional techniques. Nonoperative, radiologically guided manipulations of the biliary tract can now be performed via the transhepatic catheter, through the T-tube fistula tract, or after endoscopic papillotomy. Procedures such as stone removal, biliary drainage, stricture dilatation, endoprostheses insertion, and biopsy are becoming commonplace. Indeed, they seem to occupy more and more of the radiologist's day, and the end isn't yet in sight. Who would be so presumptuous as to predict what might be the content of a third book published five years hence?

There are inherent difficulties in planning a book that is intended to serve multiple functions. Most radiologists still use oral cholecystography as the primary diagnostic test for cholelithiasis, and for them a chapter on oral cholecystography and the biliary contrast materials is of the utmost value. Yet, for others who have progressed more rapidly in the evolution from oral cholecystography to sonography, information on oral cholecystography is archaic and a chapter on sonography is of greatest interest. Nearly everyone agrees that intravenous cholangiography is presently of marginal value, yet there is still a need for the procedure when sonography is not available and even sometimes when it is. Hence, a chapter on intravenous cholangiography, which is of no interest to many, must be included. Consequently, writing a book for radiologists whose needs differ widely requires the inclusion of information that is not of the same interest and importance to all.

Another difficulty is that for some, a monograph describing the radiographic manifestations of diseases of the gallbladder and bile ducts might best be organized according to pathology and so would include chapters on congenital, inflammatory, and neoplastic disease. However, in practice the various pathologic entities are evaluated in the light of the radiologic modalities employed. Consequently, to be of maximal value for most physicians, residents, and students, chapters prepared according to the radiographic examination (e.g., oral cholecystography, sonography, transhepatic cholangiography) are more appropriate. This format, however, makes a certain amount of duplication inevitable and requires that specific entities be discussed in different parts of the book. We hope this inconvenience will be excused, if, on the other hand, the book's organization serves the practical needs of readers to maximum advantage.

We have tried to make the book comprehensive, yet we recognize that it is virtually impossible to achieve this goal. Also, we understand that our own personal bias and that of our contributors, which inevitably stems from individual experiences and interests, require that certain aspects of the subject be emphasized more than others.

Despite these limitations, we hope the reader will find the contents of this monograph suitably organized, properly balanced, and reasonably complete and that the book will serve as an update on this rapidly evolving subject.

ROBERT N. BERK, M.D.
JOSEPH T. FERRUCCI, JR., M.D.
GEORGE R. LEOPOLD, M.D.

CONTENTS

ix

THE PLAIN ABDOMINAL RADIOGRAPH

by Robert N. Berk, M.D.

1

The oldest and simplest radiologic procedure for the detection of diseases of the gallbladder and bile ducts is plain radiography of the abdomen. The examination requires no special preparation of the patient, and the results are known immediately. Scrupulous attention to proper radiographic technique is essential if the examination is to provide maximum diagnostic information. Most commonly, gallstones are evident, which establishes the diagnosis of cholelithiasis. Acute diseases of the biliary tree can be detected, such as acute cholecystitis, empyema of the gallbladder, and gallstone ileus. Except for emphysematous cholecystitis, the radiographic features of acute cholecystitis are nonspecific, and correlation of the clinical data with the x-ray findings is usually necessary to confirm the radiologic diagnosis. Chronic diseases of the gallbladder, such as chronic cholecystitis with porcelain gallbladder or milk of calcium bile, produce classic radiologic manifestations that are readily discernible on the plain abdominal radiograph.

CHOLELITHIASIS

The solubility of cholesterol in bile depends on the relative concentrations of cholesterol, bile salts, and lecithin in bile.[1] When these proportions are disturbed for any reason, the bile becomes lithogenic, and cholesterol precipitates, forming gallstones. Cholesterol is not radiopaque, and consequently most gallstones,

in the U.S. at least, are not visible on plain abdominal radiographs. Some gallstones are composed of calcium bilirubinate or have a mixed composition and contain sufficient calcium to be detectable (Figs. 1–1 and 1–2). The concentration of calcium is sufficient to make the calculi radiopaque on plain abdominal radiographs in only 10 to 15 per cent of patients,[2, 3] so that the plain radiograph is of relatively little value in detection of cholelithiasis as compared with cholecystography. However, because of the high incidence of cholelithiasis in the population, it is still common to find radiopaque gallstones on plain abdominal radiographs or, incidentally, in patients having radiographic studies of the stomach, colon, urinary tract, or chest (Fig. 1–3). It is estimated that, in the U.S., 10 per cent of men and 20 per cent of women between the ages of 55 and 65 have gallstones.[4]

In diseases associated with an increased incidence of cholelithiasis, such as hemolytic anemias, Crohn's disease, cirrhosis, diabetes mellitus, and hyperparathyroidism,[5-7] it may be possible to establish the diagnosis of the primary disease as well as detect the gallstones on the plain abdominal radiograph. In patients with sickle cell anemia, the thickened trabecular architecture of the skeleton may be visible as well as the gallstones (Fig. 1–4). Abnormal loops of intestine may be apparent in patients with Crohn's disease; ascites may be visible in those with cirrhosis; severe vascular calcification may be present in diabetics; and pan-

1

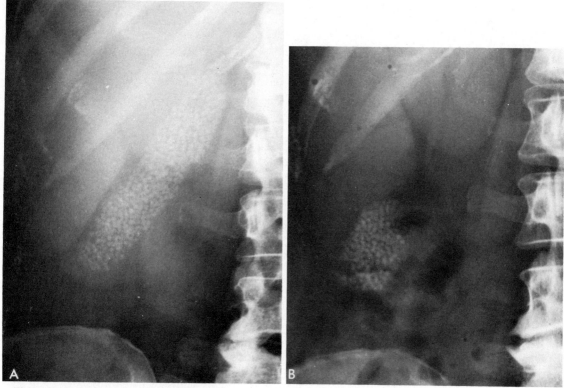

Figure 1–1. Supine *(A)* right posterior oblique and *(B)* plain abdominal radiographs showing innumerable small radiopaque gallstones shifting in position in the gallbladder.

creatic calcification may be identified in those with hyperparathyroidism.

Not all round or oval calcifications in the right upper quadrant are due to gallstones.[2] An oral cholecystogram or sonogram should be performed to confirm the diagnosis of cholelithiasis prior to surgery. Careful consideration must be given to calcification in the kidney from a wide variety of renal diseases including tuberculosis, kidney stones, renal cysts and tumors, nephrocalcinosis, and calculi in calyceal diverticula (Figs. 1–5 and 1–6). Rarely, Pantopaque instilled in a renal cyst may simulate cholelithiasis (Fig. 1–7A). A calculus in the appendix may resemble a gallstone when the appendix is in an abnormal location or when the appendix has been perforated and the appendicolith is free in the peritoneal cavity (Fig. 1–7B). Contrast material in colonic diverticula may be mistaken for gallstones when the diverticula involve the hepatic flexure (Fig. 1–8). Calcifications in the liver, adrenal gland, costal cartilages, lymph nodes, arteries, and veins and even cutaneous lesions such as neurofibromas and lipomas may have the appearance of gallstones (Fig. 1–9).

Occasionally, gallstones can be recognized on plain abdominal radiographs by the appearance of distinctive stellate radiolucencies in the right upper quadrant (Fig. 1–10).[8] The radiolucencies are due to gas-containing fissures or faults within the gallstones. This phenomenon has been aptly referred to as the "Mercedes-Benz" sign, since the radiolucent cracks have a tri-radiate pattern similar to the symbol of the German automobile. Recognition of this sign makes the diagnosis of cholelithiasis possible in the absence of calcification. Most authors agree that nitrogen fills the faults created by shrinkage of cholesterol crystals composing the gallstones.[8, 9] In a cogent review of the subject, Meyers and O'Donohue suggest that cases of spontaneous disappearance of gallstones may be due to the crumbling of the stones that occurs when gallstones split along the fissures.[9] The fragments are then small enough to pass through the cystic and common ducts. These authors also speculate that, because of the low specific gravity of gas-containing gallstones, the stones have a propensity to float in bile, which increases their likelihood of reaching the cystic duct and predisposes them to passage through the ducts even before the autofragmentation stage.

Text continued on page 10

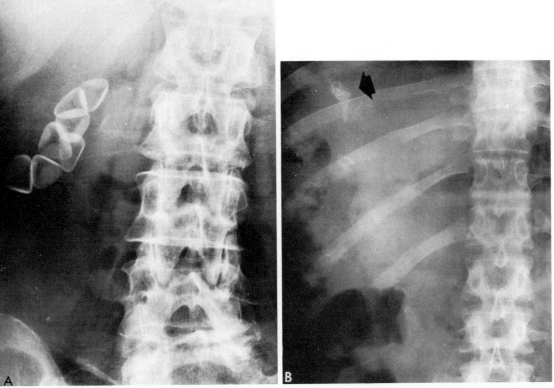

Figure 1–2. *A,* Plain abdominal radiograph showing multiple, faceted gallstones in the gallbladder. *B,* Plain abdominal radiograph from another patient showing radiopaque gallstones in an unusual location owing to severe atrophy of the liver secondary to hepatitis (arrow).

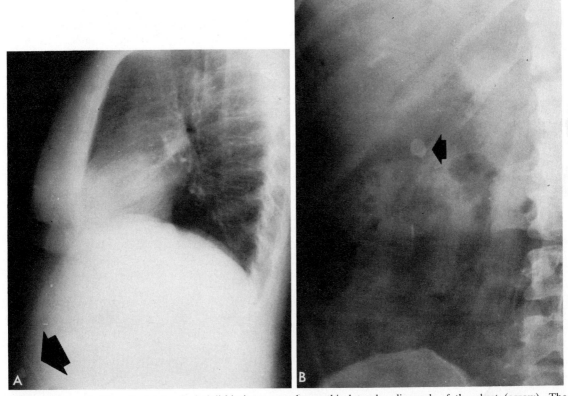

Figure 1–3. *A,* The diagnosis of cholelithiasis was made on this lateral radiograph of the chest (arrow). The gallstone was seen on a plain abdominal radiograph *(B)* and confirmed on oral cholecystography.

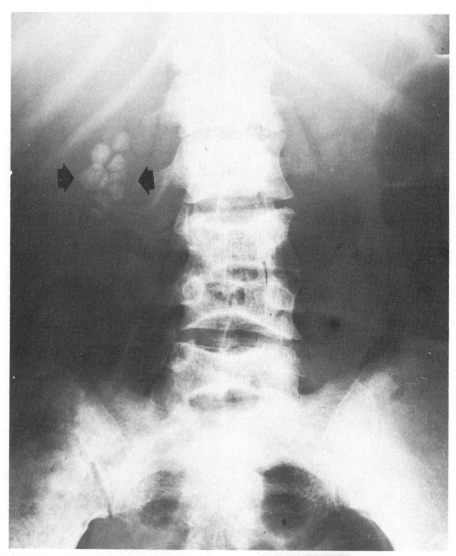

Figure 1–4. Plain abdominal radiograph of a patient with sickle cell anemia and cholelithiasis (arrows). The thickened trabecular architecture of the bones and changes in the vertebral bodies, typical of sickle cell anemia, are apparent.

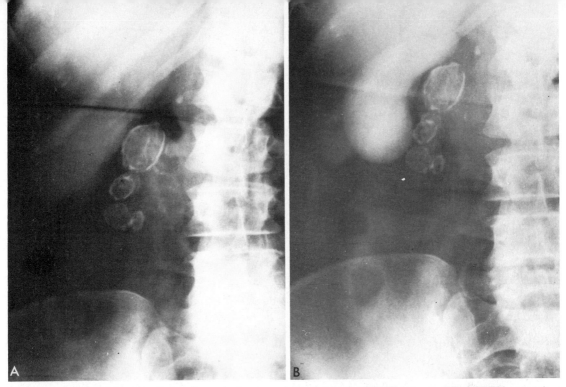

Figure 1–5. *A*, Plain abdominal radiograph showing calcification in the kidney owing to tuberculosis (autonephrectomy) that simulates gallstones. *B*, Oral cholecystogram shows that the calcifications are outside of the gallbladder.

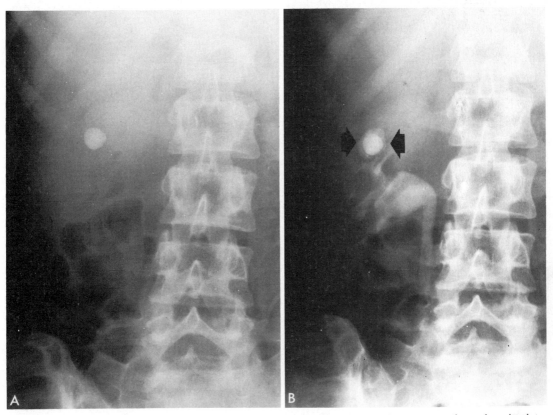

Figure 1–6. *A*, Plain abdominal radiograph showing a calcification in the right upper quadrant that simulates a gallstone. *B*, Radiograph from an intravenous pyelogram shows that the calculus is in a calyceal diverticulum in the right kidney (arrows).

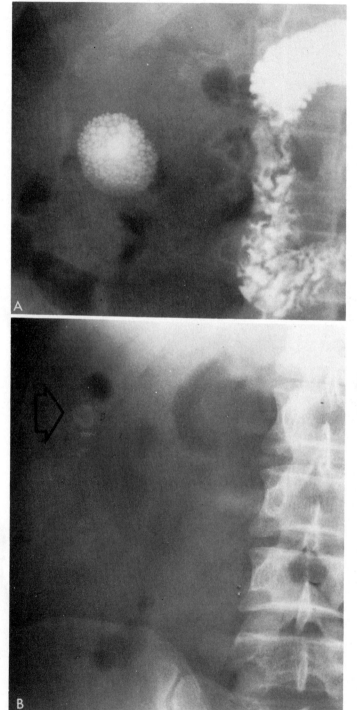

Figure 1–7. *A,* Radiograph showing Pantopaque in a right renal cyst. Barium is visible in the duodenum. An oral cholecystogram performed later was normal. *B,* Plain abdominal radiograph showing a calcified fecalith in a patient with acute perforated appendicitis with an appendicolith lying free in the abdomen (arrow). The calcification simulates a calcified gallstone in the gallbladder.

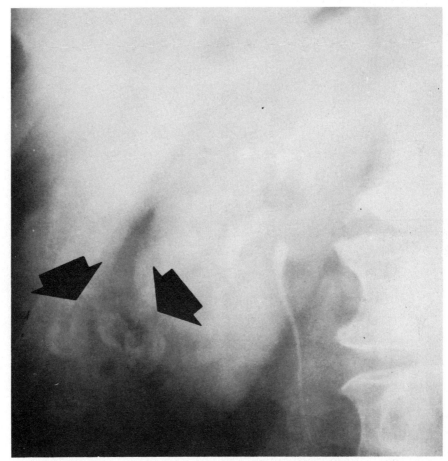

Figure 1–8. Radiograph made during an intravenous pyelogram showing contrast material in the right ureter. The densities (arrows) are due to contrast material from an intravenous cholangiogram done one day earlier. The contrast material that simulates radiopaque gallstones is in the diverticula of the hepatic flexure of the colon.

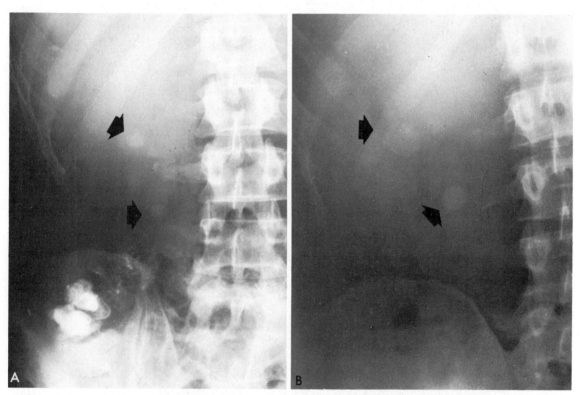

Figure 1–9. *A, B,* Plain abdominal radiographs of two patients with neurofibromatosis. The neurofibromas in the skin of the abdomen may be confused with radiopaque gallstones (arrows). *C, D,* Radiographs of the chest showing a subcutaneous lipoma that simulates an opacified gallbladder in an ectopic location (arrows).

Illustration continued on opposite page

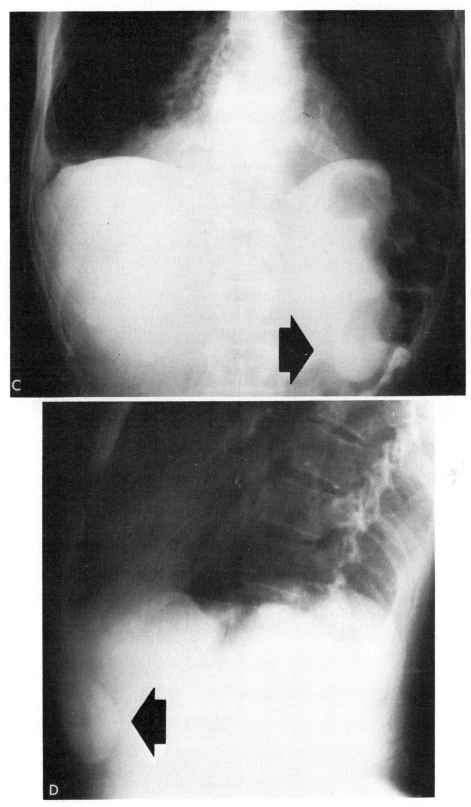

Figure 1–9. *Continued*

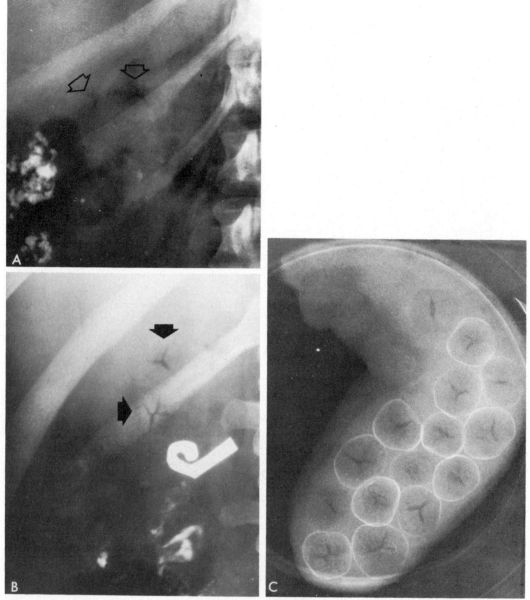

Figure 1–10. *A, B,* Radiographs of the abdomen from two different patients showing tri-radiate radiolucencies, indicating the presence of gallstones (Mercedes-Benz sign) (arrows). *C,* Radiograph of the gallbladder after cholecystectomy in the patient shown in *A.* The calcified surface of the gallstones visible on the radiograph of the specimen was not apparent *in vivo.*

ACUTE CHOLECYSTITIS

Acute cholecystitis nearly always is the result of obstruction of the cystic duct by a gallstone.[10] Hyperemia and edema of the gallbladder wall follow and lead to an acute inflammatory infiltrate, hemorrhage, and necrosis. The gallbladder usually distends with pus and blood mixed with bile and gallstones. The bile, which is sterile initially, becomes infected as the disease progresses. If the calculus disimpacts, as it does in 85 per cent of patients, the acute inflammatory process rapidly subsides.[11] However, if the obstruction persists, the disease may progress to empyema and perforation of the gallbladder, with a localized abscess in the right upper quadrant or generalized peritonitis.

The findings on the abdominal radiograph depend on the stage and severity of the dis-

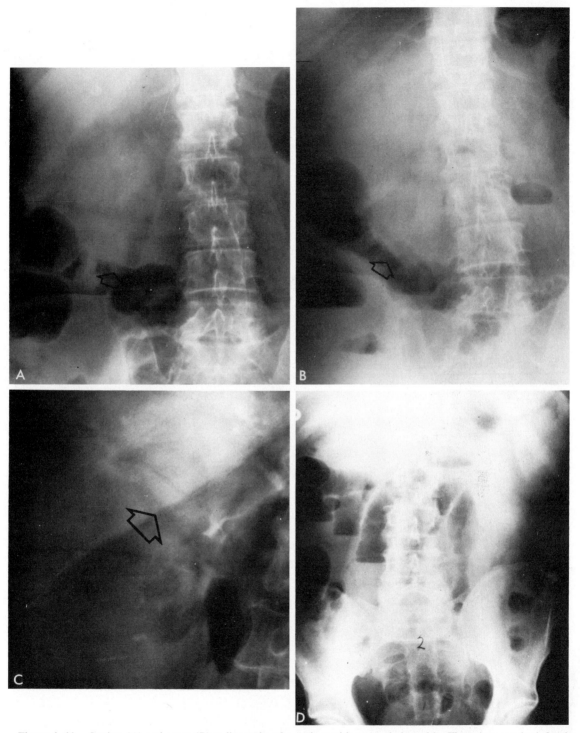

Figure 1–11. Supine *(A)* and erect *(B)* radiographs of a patient with acute cholecystitis. There is a poorly defined mass displacing the right portion of the transverse colon (arrow). Several air-fluid levels are visible on the upright projection. *C,* Four-hour radiographs from an intravenous cholangiogram showing opacification of the common bile duct (arrow) and visualization of the right kidney. Failure of the gallbladder to opacify by four hours after injection of Cholografin indicates the presence of cystic duct obstruction and confirms the diagnosis of cholecystitis in this case. *D,* Upright abdominal radiograph from another patient with acute cholecystitis, showing dilated loops of small bowel with air-fluid levels.

ease. If the inflammatory reaction is mild, the radiograph may be normal or may reveal only the presence of gallstones. Progression of the disease in the gallbladder and extension of the inflammatory process to adjacent peritoneal surfaces cause a reflex inhibition of motility in adjacent segments of the intestine (sentinel ileus).[12, 13] The abdominal radiograph shows paralytic ileus with distended, air-filled loops of bowel and multiple air-fluid levels localized in the right upper quadrant of the abdomen. The distended gallbladder may be visible as a mass adjacent to the liver (Fig. 1–11). Initially, short segments of the small intestine are involved, but as the inflammatory reaction extends to involve more of the peritoneum, motility in longer segments of the small intestine and colon is disturbed. At this stage, the abdominal radiograph shows marked small bowel distention and numerous air-fluid levels. If the colon does not participate in the paralytic ileus, the radiographic findings may simulate a mechanical small bowel obstruction. Rarely, the inflammatory process produces dilatation of the colon without concomitant changes in the small intestine (colon ileus). When empyema of the gallbladder develops, a mass adjacent to the liver may be apparent on the abdominal radiograph (Fig. 1–12). Occasionally, the radiologic diagnosis of perforation of the gallbladder can be made if gallstones are identified free in the peritoneal cavity remote from the gallbladder.[14] If the inflammatory process subsides despite the persistence of cystic duct obstruction, the gallbladder may distend with mucus-producing hydrops.[10] In this circumstance, the enlarged gallbladder is usually visible on the abdominal radiograph (Fig. 1–13).[3]

Emphysematous cholecystitis is an uncommon variant of acute cholecystitis in which gas is present in the gallbladder wall and in the lumen.[15] The gas is caused by infection with gas-forming organisms of the *Clostridium* species, although some cases are due to anaerobic streptococci, *Escherichia coli,* and staphylococci.[16] Gangrene is a common pathologic feature.[16] As distinct from ordinary acute cholecystitis, 20 per cent of patients with emphysematous cholecystitis have diabetes.[10] In addition, the incidence of emphysematous cholecystitis is three times greater in men than in women.[10] A substantial number of patients do not have associated cholelithiasis.[16]

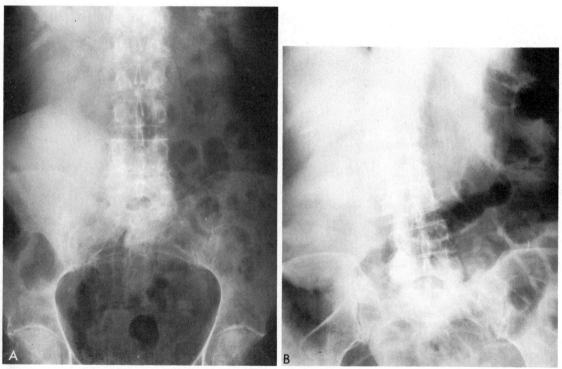

Figure 1–12. Supine *(A)* and erect *(B)* plain abdominal radiographs in a patient with a perforated gallbladder and a right upper quadrant abscess. A large mass is present in the right upper quadrant. Gallstones were found free in the peritoneal cavity at surgery.

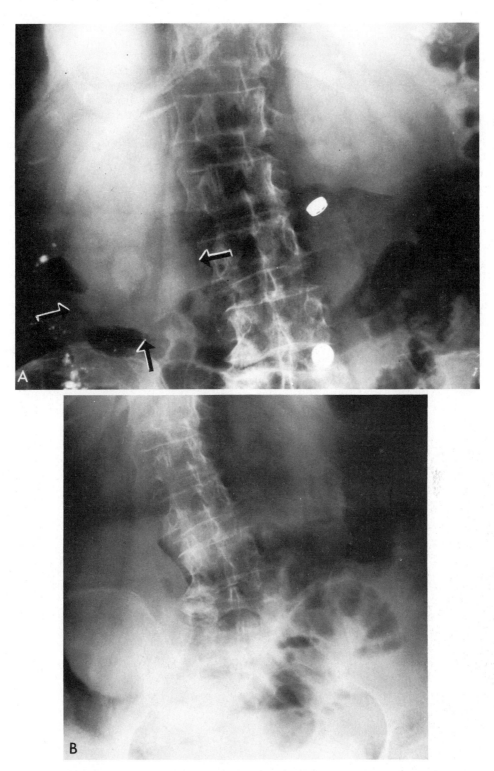

Figure 1–13. Supine *(A)* and erect *(B)* plain abdominal radiographs in a patient with hydrops of the gallbladder. The distended gallbladder and a faintly calcified gallstone (arrows) are apparent.

Hence, emphysematous cholecystitis is quite distinct from typical acute cholecystitis. The pathogenesis of this form of cholecystitis is probably occlusion of the cystic artery with subsequent ischemia, necrosis, and infection of the gallbladder.[16-18] Because of the high incidence of gangrene, it is not surprising that the diagnosis implies a risk of gallbladder perforation five times that expected from ordinary acute cholecystitis.[16]

Gas usually is not visible until at least 24 to 48 hours after the onset of the cholecystitis.[19] Radiographs made after this interval show gas in the lumen of the gallbladder, in the gallbladder wall, and occasionally in the tissues adjacent to the gallbladder (Figs. 1–14, 1–15, and 1–16). Erect or decubitus radiographs of the abdomen may disclose a gas-bile interface in the gallbladder. When air is present in the biliary tree owing to a cholecysto-enteric fistula, it does not occur in the wall of the gallbladder and usually is evident in the common duct.

PORCELAIN GALLBLADDER

Extensive calcification in the wall of the gallbladder has been named calcifying cholecystitis, cholecystopathia chronica calcerea, or simply calcified gallbladder.[20] The term "porcelain gallbladder" has been used to emphasize the blue discoloration and brittle consistency of the gallbladder wall.[21] Since most cases of gallbladder calcification are not reported, the incidence of the disease is difficult to determine; however, various studies of postoperative gallbladder specimens show a 0.06 to 0.8 per cent occurrence of extensive mural calcification.[20] The disease is five times more frequent in women than in men.[22] The mean age of these patients is 54 years, with a range of 38 to 70 years.[22] A paucity of symptoms is characteristic, so that the diagnosis frequently is made by the detection of a palpable mass in the right upper quadrant or by the discovery of typical gallbladder calcification on abdominal radiographs.[22]

Pathologically, the calcification occurs in two forms.[23] In one variety, there is a broad continuous band of calcification in the muscularis; in the other form, the calcifications are multiple and punctate and occur in the glandular spaces of the mucosa. Gallstones are present in nearly all instances of gallbladder calcification, and usually a stone obstructs the cystic duct with hydrops of the gallbladder.[24] The gallbladder wall is thickened by chronic inflam-

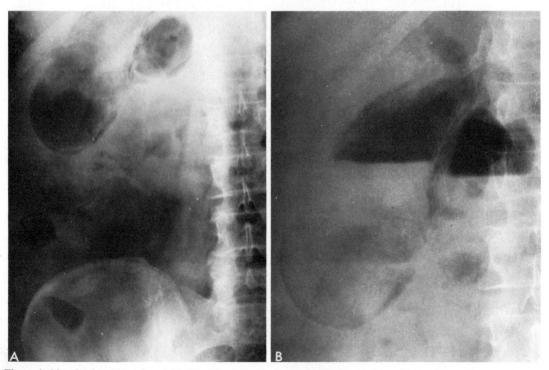

Figure 1–14. Supine *(A)* and upright *(B)* plain abdominal radiographs in a patient with emphysematous cholecystitis. Gas is present in the gallbladder lumen and in the gallbladder wall. A bile-gas interface is visible in the body and neck of the gallbladder in *B*.

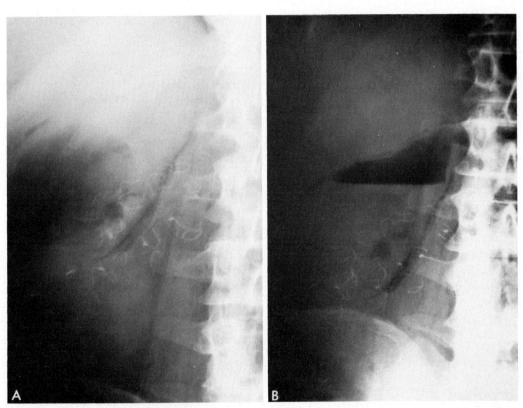

Figure 1–15. *A, B,* Supine plain abdominal radiographs in two patients with emphysematous cholecystitis. Gas is visible in the gallbladder wall as well as in the lumen.

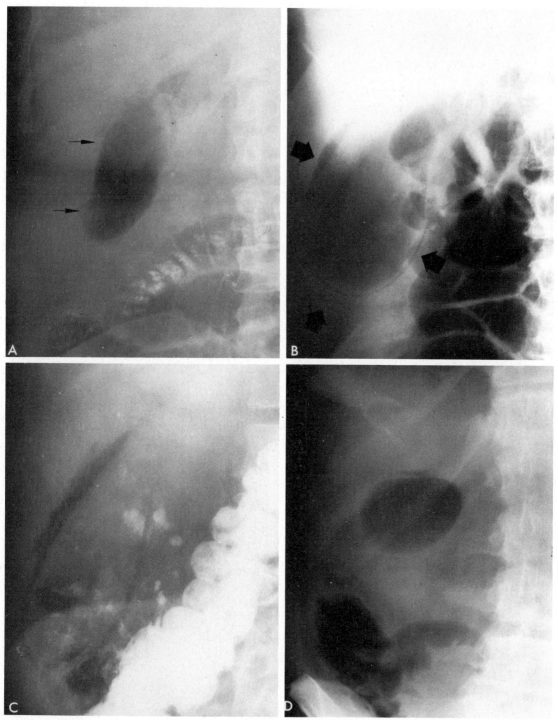

Figure 1–16. *A, B,* Abdominal radiographs of two patients with emphysematous cholecystitis in which gas is visible in the gallbladder wall (arrows) as well as in the lumen. *C,* Abdominal radiograph of another patient with emphysematous cholecystitis showing gas in the wall of the gallbladder. A small amount is also visible in tissues adjacent to the gallbladder wall. *D,* Another case of emphysematous cholecystitis with gas in the wall and lumen of the gallbladder.

mation, and the mucosa is often denuded. The contents usually are sterile.[25]

Most authors consider the calcification to be a sequela of a low-grade chronic inflammation, but others have emphasized the possibility that the calcification may be secondary to intramural hemorrhage or an imbalance in calcium metabolism.[21, 22, 26]

The plain abdominal radiograph shows a characteristic ring of calcification that conforms to the shape and location of the gallbladder (Figs. 1–17 and 1–18). The thickness of the calcification varies, and the distribution often is uneven and discontinuous. The gallbladder usually is large, although there is considerable variation. Porcelain gallbladder must be distinguished from a single, large, calcified gallstone. Solitary gallstones are rarely as large as a porcelain gallbladder, but exceptions to the rule make a definite diagnosis difficult (Fig. 1–19). Visualization of the gallbladder during oral cholecystography and sonography is unlikely in either case.

Review of the literature reveals 26 examples of carcinoma occurring in the presence of a porcelain gallbladder (Figs. 1–20 and 1–21). The tumors are predominantly diffusely infiltrating adenocarcinoma, although squamous cell carcinoma has been described.[27] Most of the cases were reported by Etala, who found 16 patients with porcelain gallbladder in 78 cases of carcinoma of the gallbladder in a series of 1,786 cholecystectomies.[26] Among the 1,786 cases, there were 26 instances of porcelain gallbladder, so that 16 of the 26 patients (61 per cent) with porcelain gallbladder had carcinoma. That the tumors were invasive and not merely focal abnormalities of the mucosa is apparent from the fact that only two of the 78 patients survived five years. In a review of 45 cholecystectomies, Cornell and Clarke found 16 patients with porcelain gallbladder, two of whom (12.5 per cent) had adenocarcinoma.[22] Six other cases of carcinoma occurring in a porcelain gallbladder were reported,[23, 27, 28] the first case described by Brown in 1932.[29] Two additional cases reported in 1973 by Berk, Armbuster, and Saltzstein bring the total number recorded to 26.[30]

Since not all cases of porcelain gallbladder, carcinoma of the gallbladder, and porcelain gallbladder associated with carcinoma are reported, it is impossible to determine the frequency with which the two diseases occur

Text continued on page 22

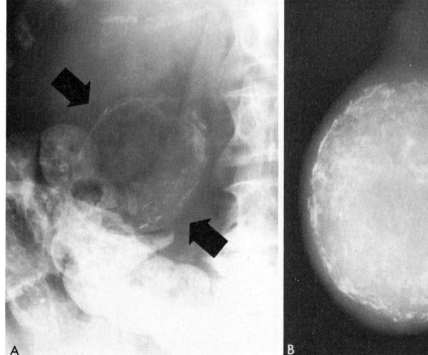
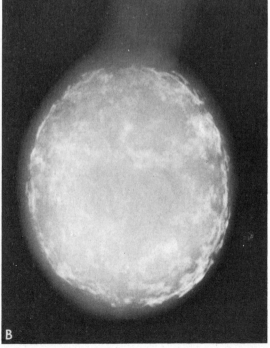

Figure 1–17. *A,* Plain abdominal radiograph of a patient with a porcelain gallbladder, showing a large, heavily calcified gallbladder (arrows). Barium is in the colon from a previous barium enema. *B,* Radiograph of the surgical specimen showing the calcium in the wall of the gallbladder.

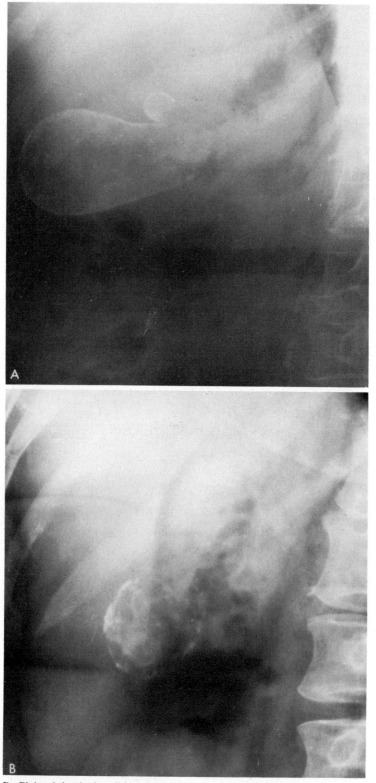

Figure 1–18. *A–D,* Plain abdominal radiographs from four patients with porcelain gallbladder, illustrating the various types of calcification that can occur.

Illustration continued on opposite page

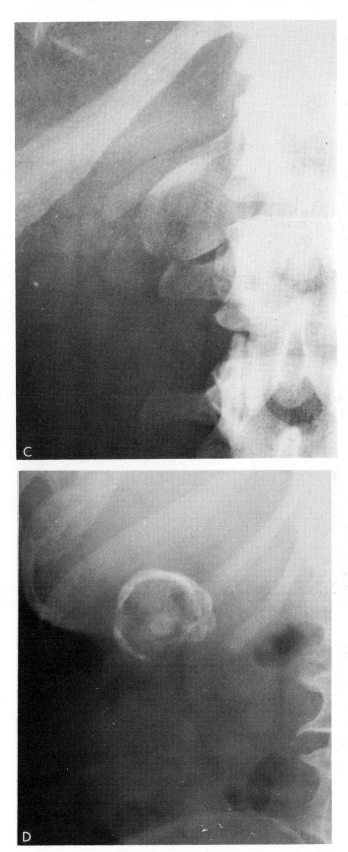

Figure 1–18. *Continued*

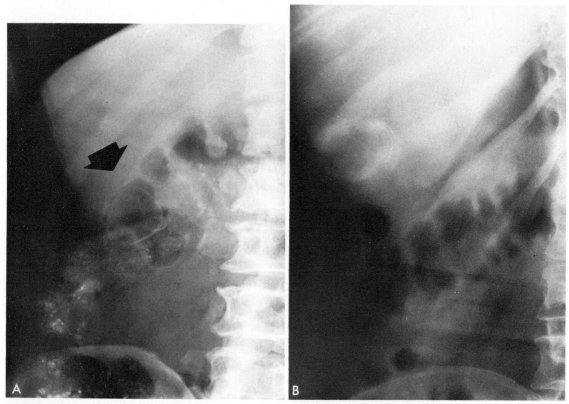

Figure 1–19. *A, B,* Plain abdominal radiographs in two patients, each with a single large calcified gallstone (arrow). Differentiation from porcelain gallbladder is impossible. The gallstone in the first patient was palpable on abdominal examination. Unabsorbed Telepaque is present in the colon in *A.*

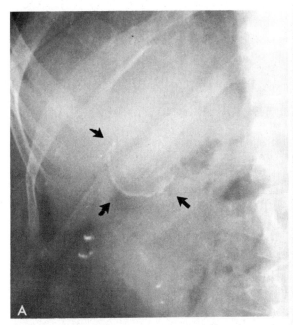

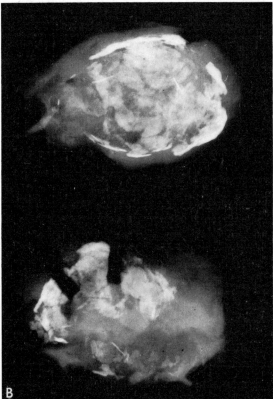

Figure 1–20. *A,* Plain abdominal radiograph showing calcification in the porcelain gallbladder. *B,* Radiograph of the gallbladder made after cholecystectomy, showing the calcification of the gallbladder wall. *C,* Photograph of the gallbladder made after the specimen had been divided in half, showing necrotic tumor in the lumen and marked thickening of the gallbladder wall. *D,* Histologic section of the gallbladder wall made after decalcification, showing islands of adenocarcinoma. (From Berk, R. N., Armbuster, T. G., and Saltstein, S. L.: Radiology *106*:29, 1973.)

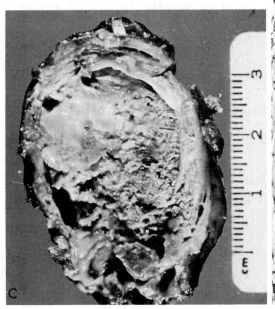

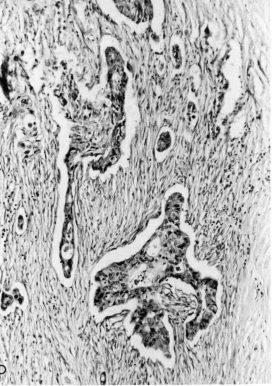

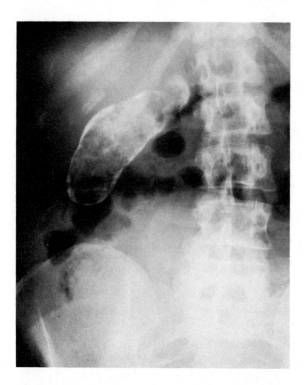

Figure 1–21. Plain abdominal radiograph in a second patient with porcelain gallbladder associated with adenocarcinoma of the gallbladder. Calcification in the gallbladder is evident.

together. It is clear that porcelain gallbladder is uncommon in cases of carcinoma of the gallbladder, but the frequency of carcinoma in porcelain gallbladder is striking. Polk estimated the frequency to be 22 per cent.[27] Kazmierski emphasized the high frequency of malignant transformation in porcelain gallbladder.[25] Most authors agree that carcinoma occurs in the porcelain gallbladder with sufficient frequency to warrant prophylactic cholecystectomy for patients with a porcelain gallbladder, even when the disease is asymptomatic.[30]

Little is known about the mechanism by which carcinoma develops in porcelain gallbladder. Both carcinoma and calcification may result from a chronic inflammatory process in the gallbladder wall. Petrov and Krotkina were able to produce gallbladder carcinoma by introducing hard foreign bodies into the gallbladder wall.[31] The carcinogenic stimulus may be secondary to degeneration and regeneration of the epithelium caused by the inflammatory changes in the gallbladder wall or may be related to a chemical carcinogen formed in the stagnant bile.

MILK OF CALCIUM BILE

Milk of calcium bile, or the limy bile syndrome, is characterized by the presence of radiopaque material in the gallbladder sufficient to produce opacification of the gallbladder on plain abdominal radiographs. The putty-like material in the gallbladder lumen is composed of calcium carbonate and less often of calcium phosphate or calcium bilirubinate.[32] The cystic duct is obstructed by a gallstone, and the gallbladder is chronically inflamed. Holden and Turner reported six cases in which passage of the limy bile and associated gallstones occurred spontaneously.[33]

Milk of calcium bile may simulate the findings of a normally opacified gallbladder following oral cholecystography (Fig. 1–22). Differentiation requires knowledge of whether the patient was given cholecystographic contrast material. In other cases, the limy bile has a granular pattern that suggests the correct diagnosis (Figs. 1–22 and 1–23).

SPONTANEOUS BILIARY-ENTERIC FISTULA

Spontaneous communication between the biliary tract and the intestine is the result of erosion of a gallstone in 90 per cent of cases, although 6 per cent develop because of penetration of a peptic ulcer into the common duct and the remaining 4 per cent are the result of tumor or trauma.[34] In 80 to 90 per cent of cases the gallstone passes spontaneously with-

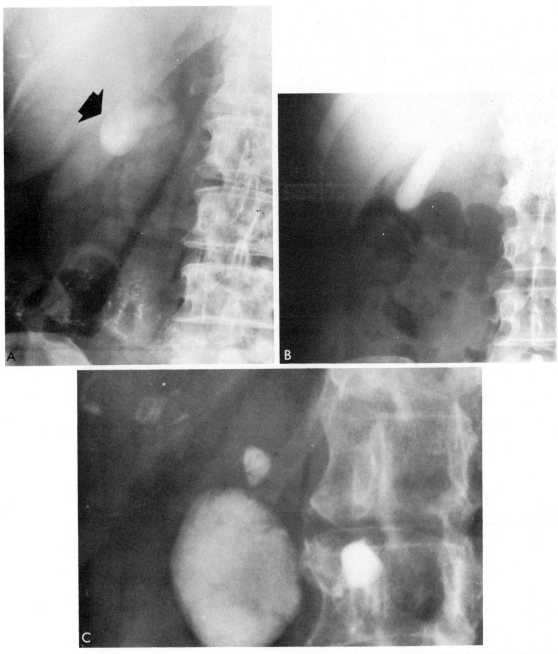

Figure 1-22. *A–C,* Plain abdominal radiographs of three patients with milk of calcium bile. The limy bile in the gallbladder simulates a normal bladder following a cholecystogram. Radiopaque gallstones are visible in the cystic duct in *C.*

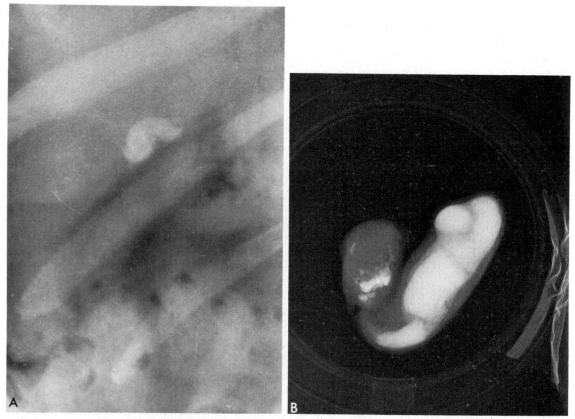

Figure 1–23. A, Plain abdominal radiograph showing milk of calcium bile. B, Radiograph of the gallbladder after cholecystectomy. A granular pattern of calcification may help to distinguish milk of calcium bile from contrast material in the gallbladder.

out causing symptoms.[35] However, if the gallstone is larger than 2.5 cm, it may cause an obturation type of intestinal obstruction (gallstone ileus).[36]

Spontaneous biliary-enteric fistula due to passage of a gallstone between the gallbladder and intestine is preceded by recurrent episodes of acute cholecystitis. The inflammatory response in the gallbladder extends to involve the adjacent bowel.[37] A gallstone may then erode by pressure to form a fistula through which the gallstone passes into the intestine. Wakefield, Vickers, and Walters reported a series of 176 fistulas in which 57 per cent involved the duodenum, 18 per cent were into the colon, and the remainder were multiple or involved the stomach.[38] Gallstones may also erode into a bronchus, the pleural cavity, portal vein, renal pelvis, urinary bladder, or aorta.[39-41]

Of all intestinal obstruction, gallstone ileus is the most insidious and difficult to diagnose clinically.[37] The mortality of the disease is five times that of any other small bowel obstruc-tion. The average age of these patients is 69 years. Although gallstone ileus accounts for only 2 per cent of all cases of intestinal obstruction, it causes 20 per cent of the obstruction in patients over 65 and 24 per cent in patients over 70.[37] Eighty-one per cent of instances of gallstone ileus occur in women.[42]

The intestinal obstruction may be constant or intermittent and usually occurs in the terminal ileum where the stone is unable to pass through the ileocecal valve (60 per cent).[43-45] The next most common locations are the proximal ileum (24 per cent) and distal jejunum (9 per cent), where spasm or simple diameter disproportion is the cause of obstruction.[37] Erosion into the colon occurs in less than 5 per cent of cases. In these patients, obstruction usually occurs in the sigmoid colon where the bowel is often narrowed by diverticulosis. A cholecysto-colonic fistula may cause diarrhea because of the effect of bile salts on the colonic mucosa (cholerrheic enteropathy).[46-48] Erosion of the gallstone into the stomach may cause pyloric obstruction.[49]

The radiologist is in a unique position to establish the diagnosis of gallstone ileus because of the classic features of the disease on the plain abdominal radiograph. First described by Rigler in 1941, the cardinal plain film radiographic findings are hoop-shaped, dilated loops of small bowel; air in the biliary tree; and a gallstone in an ectopic location in the abdomen (Figs. 1–24, 1–25, and 1–26).[50] Barium studies are often useful and are discussed in the next chapter.

Eisenman, Finck, and O'Loughlin suggested that there is a characteristic appearance of the small bowel on supine plain abdominal radio-

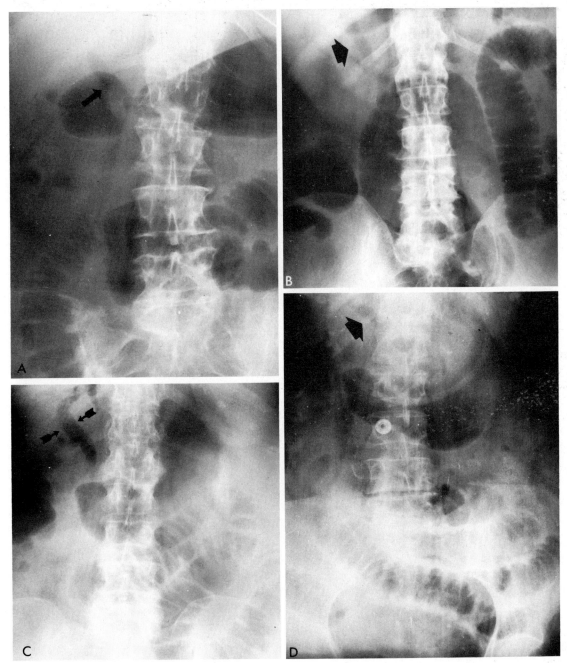

Figure 1–24. *A–D,* Plain abdominal radiographs in four patients with gallstone ileus. Loops of dilated small bowel and air in the biliary tree (arrows) are apparent.

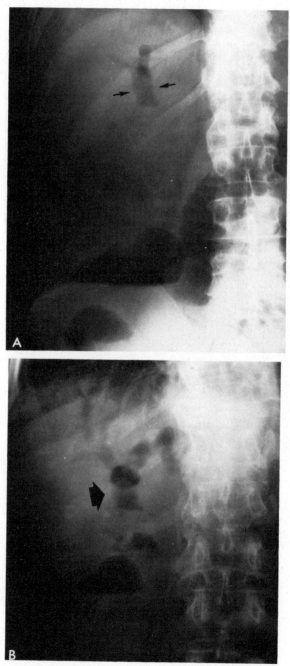

Figure 1–25. *A–D,* Plain abdominal radiographs in four patients with gallstone ileus showing air in the biliary tree (arrows).

Illustration continued on opposite page

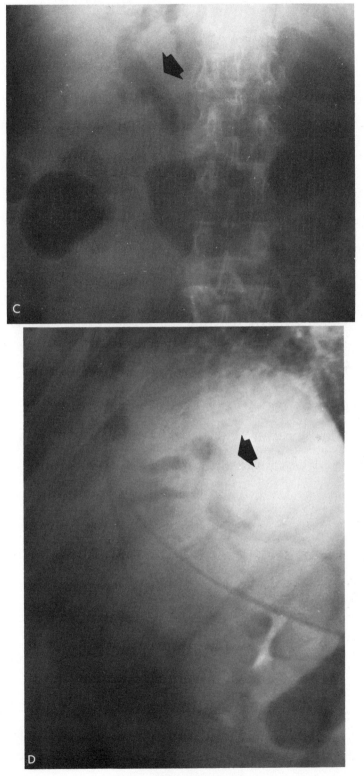

Figure 1–25. *Continued*

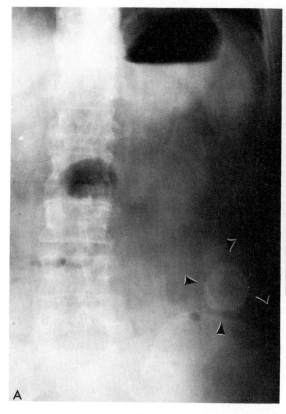

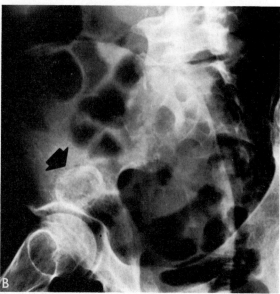

Figure 1–26. Upright plain abdominal radiograph *(A)* and right posterior oblique radiograph of the pelvis *(B)* in two patients, showing a large gallstone in an ectopic location (arrows). In both cases, the gallstones had passed into the intestine through a cholecysto-duodenal fistula. The calculus passed spontaneously and did not cause intestinal obstruction in either patient.

graphs in cases of gallstone ileus, which they termed the "loop obturation pattern."[51] In this pattern there is minimal to moderate gaseous distention of the small bowel; prominent valvulae conniventes that do not show extreme degrees of effacement; clear delineation of the fluid-containing loops of bowel; and frequently a radial configuration of the loops of bowel. Essentially, the sign pertains to the characteristics of obstructed small bowel in which there is a small amount of gas associated with moderately distended, fluid-filled, obstructed small intestine. The exceptionally well-delineated loops of small bowel typically contain a moderate amount of gas and assume a radial configuration. This characteristic loop obturation pattern was present in 86 per cent of the patients in the series of Eisenman, Finck, and O'Loughlin.[51]

Gas in the gallbladder or biliary tree is visible in nearly two-thirds of patients with gallstone ileus (Fig. 1–25).[51] A suspicion of gallstone ileus or the finding of gas in the biliary tree is sufficient indication to perform a barium examination of the upper gastrointestinal tract if additional studies are necessary to establish the diagnosis. Gas in the biliary tree may be due to previous surgery including a choledochoduodenostomy, a cholecystojejunostomy, or a sphincterotomy. Rarely, gas may be caused by ascending cholangitis due to a gas-forming organism or may result from reflux of air through a patulous sphincter of Oddi in aged patients.[52] Gas in the portal venous system usually collects toward the periphery of the liver, whereas gas in the bile ducts is more prominent in the region of the porta hepatis.[13] Occasionally, fat surrounding the common bile duct may simulate gas within the duct. However, the fat is not as radiolucent as gas in the bile duct and does not involve intrahepatic portions of the biliary tree.

The third radiographic finding in the classic triad associated with gallstone ileus is the presence of a gallstone in an ectopic location in the abdomen. This can be detected in between one-fourth and one-half of patients with the disease (Fig. 1–26).[13, 50, 51]

Gallstone ileus should be treated by emergency surgery in which the obstructing stone is removed through a small enterotomy incision.[37, 44] Surgical treatment of the cholecystoduodenal fistula is almost never indicated acutely.

References

1. Admirand, W. H., and Small, D. M.: The physico-chemical basis of cholesterol gallstone formation in man. J. Clin. Invest. 47:1043, 1968.
2. Donner, M. W., and Weiner, S.: Diagnostic evaluation of abdominal calcifications in acute abdominal disorders. Radiol. Clin. North Am. 2:145, 1964.
3. Berk, R. N.: Radiology of the gallbladder and bile ducts. Surg. Clin. North Am. 53:973, 1973.
4. Friedman, D. K., Kannel, W. B., and Dawber, T. R.: Epidemiology of gallbladder disease: observations in Framingham study. J. Chronic Dis. 19:273, 1966.
5. Flye, M. W., and Silver, D.: Biliary tract disorders and sickle cell disease. Surgery 72:361, 1972.
6. Cohen, S., et al.: Liver disease and gallstones in regional enteritis. Gastroenterology 60:237, 1971.
7. Selle, J. G., et al.: Cholelithiasis in hyperparathyroidism, a neglected manifestation. Arch. Surg. 105:369, 1972.
8. Stoney, R. J., Combs, R. C., and Obata, W. G.: Gas-containing gallstones. Ann. Surg. 155:212, 1962.
9. Meyers, M. A., and O'Donohue, N.: The Mercedes-Benz sign: insight into the dynamics of formation and disappearance of gallstones. Am. J. Roentgenol. 119:63, 1973.
10. Way, L. W., and Sleisenger, M. H.: Acute Cholecystitis. In Sleisenger, M. H., and Fordtran, J. H. (eds.): Gastrointestinal Diseases. Philadelphia: W. B. Saunders Co., 1973, pp. 1120–25.
11. duPlessis, D. J., and Jersky, J.: Management of acute cholecystitis. Surg. Clin. North Am. 53:1071, 1973.
12. Weens, H. S., and Walker, L. A.: The radiologic diagnosis of acute cholecystitis and pancreatitis. Radiol. Clin. North Am. 2:89, 1964.
13. Friman-Dahl, J.: Roentgen Examinations in Acute Abdominal Diseases, 2nd ed. Springfield: Charles C Thomas, 1960, pp. 34–333.
14. Isch, J. H., Finneran, J. C., and Nahrwold, D. L.: Perforation of the gallbladder. Am. J. Gastroenterol. 55:451, 1971.
15. Nelson, S. W.: Extraluminal gas collections due to diseases of the gastrointestinal tract. Am. J. Roentgenol. 115:225, 1972.
16. Mentzer, R. M., et al.: A comparative appraisal of emphysematous cholecystitis. Am. J. Surg. 129:10, 1975.
17. Holgersen, L. L., White, J. L., and West, J. P.: Emphysematous cholecystitis, a report of five cases. Surgery 69:102, 1971.
18. Campbell, E. W., and Rogers, C. L.: Submucosal gallbladder emphysema. J.A.M.A. 227:790, 1974.
19. McCorkle, H., and Fong, E. E.: Clinical significance of gas in the gallbladder. Surgery 11:851, 1942.
20. Buckstein, J.: The Digestive Tract in Roentgenology, Vol. 2, 2nd ed. Philadelphia: J. B. Lippincott Co., 1953, p. 988.
21. Osler, W.: The Principles and Practice of Medicine, 10th ed. New York: Appleton, 1925.
22. Cornell, C. M., and Clarke, R.: Vicarious calcification involving the gallbladder. Ann. Surg. 149:267, 1959.
23. Oschner, S. F., and Carrera, G. M.: Calcification of the gallbladder (porcelain gallbladder). Am. J. Roentgenol. 89:847, 1963.
24. Phemister, D. B., Rewbridge, A. G., and Rusisill, H.: Calcium carbonate gallstones and calcification of the gallbladder following cystic duct obstruction. Ann. Surg. 94:493, 1931.
25. Kazmierski, R. H.: Primary adenocarcinoma of gallbladder with intramural calcification. Am. J. Surg. 82:248, 1951.
26. Etala, E.: Cancer de la vesicular biliar. Prensa Med. Argent. 49:2283, 1962.
27. Polk, H. C.: Carcinoma and the calcified gallbladder. Gastroenterology 50:582, 1966.
28. Fahim, R. B., et al.: Carcinoma of the gallbladder: a study of its modes of spread. Ann. Surg. 156:114, 1962.
29. Brown, R.: Calcification of gallbladder. West. J. Surg. 40:70, 1932.
30. Berk, R. N., Armbuster, T. G., and Saltzstein, S. L.: Carcinoma in the porcelain gallbladder. Radiology 106:29, 1973.
31. Petrov, N. N., and Krotkina, N. A.: Experimental carcinoma of the gallbladder. Supplementary data. Ann. Surg. 125:241, 1947.
32. Besic, L. R., Krawzoff, G., and Tiesenga, M. F.: Limy bile syndrome. J.A.M.A. 193:145, 1965.
33. Holden, W. S., and Turner, M. J.: Disappearing limy bile. Clin. Radiol. 23:500, 1972.
34. Hicken, N. F., and Coray, Q. B.: Spontaneous gastrointestinal biliary fistulas. Surg. Gynecol. Obstet. 82:723, 1946.
35. Railford, T. S.: Intestinal obstruction due to gallstones (gallstone ileus). Ann. Surg. 153:830, 1961.
36. Fox, P. F.: Planning the operation for cholecystoenteric fistula with gallstone ileus. Surg. Clin. North Am. 50:93, 1970.
37. Hudspeth, A. S., and McGuirt, W. F.: Gallstone ileus, a continuing surgical problem. Arch. Surg. 100:668, 1970.
38. Wakefield, E. G., Vicker, P. M., and Walters, W.: Cholecystoenteric fistulas. Surgery 5:674, 1939.
39. Powers, J. H.: Acute intestinal obstruction due to impacted gallstones. Surg. Gynecol. Obstet. 47:416, 1928.
40. Schwegler, N., and Endrei, E.: Gallstone in the lung. Radjology 115:541, 1975.
41. Broadbent, N. R. G., and Taylor, D. E. M.: Gallstone erosion of the aorta. Aust. N.Z. J. Surg. 45:207, 1975.
42. Brochis, J. G., and Gilberg, M. C.: Intestinal obstruction by gallstones. Br. J. Surg. 44:461, 1956.
43. Foss, H. L., and Summers, J. D.: Intestinal obstruction from gallstones. Ann. Surg. 115:721, 1942.
44. Way, L. W., and Sleisenger, M. H.: Gallstone Ileus. In Sleisenger, M. H., and Fordtran, J. H. (eds.): Gastrointestinal Diseases. Philadelphia: W. B. Saunders Co., 1973, p. 1126.
45. Piedad, O. H., and Wels, P. B.: Spontaneous internal biliary fistula, obstructive and nonobstructive types. Ann. Surg. 175:75, 1972.
46. Shocket, E., Evans, J., and Jonas, S.: Cholecysto-duodenocholic fistula. Arch. Surg. 101:523, 1970.
47. Grossman, E. T.: Cholecystocolic fistula—an unusual cause of diarrhea. Am. J. Gastroenterol. 55:277, 1971.
48. Hofman, A. F.: The syndrome of ileal disease and the broken enterohepatic circulation. Gastroenterology 52:752, 1967.
49. Redding, M. E., Anagnostopoulos, C. E., and Wright, H. K.: Cholecystopyloric fistula with gastric outlet obstruction. Ann. Surg. 176:210, 1972.
50. Rigler, L. G., Bormen, C. N., and Noble, J. F.: Gallstone obstruction pathogenesis and roentgen manifestations. J.A.M.A. 77:1753, 1941.
51. Eisenman, J. I., Finck, E. J., and O'Loughlin, B. J.: Gallstone ileus. A review of the roentgenographic findings and report of a new roentgen sign. Am. J. Roentgenol. 101:361, 1967.
52. Scott, M. G., Pygott, F., and Murphy, L.: Significance of gas or barium in the biliary tract. Br. J. Radiol. 27:253, 1954.

BARIUM STUDIES OF THE GASTROINTESTINAL TRACT

2

by Robert N. Berk, M.D.

Prior to the introduction of cholecystography by Graham and Cole in 1923, radiologists relied heavily on the detection of radiographic abnormalities in the stomach, duodenum, and colon for the diagnosis of gallbladder disease. Indeed, according to Cole, some radiologists were so enthusiastic about these indirect findings that they were blinded to the great importance of cholecystography and were hesitant to accept the new technique.[1]

Lodged on the undersurface of the right lobe of the liver, the gallbladder usually lies anteriorly and laterally to the first and second portions of the duodenum (Fig. 2–1). The fundus of the gallbladder is in close proximity to the superior aspect of the right side of the transverse colon. The neck of the gallbladder and the cystic duct cross in front of the duodenum, where they serve as the anatomic boundary between the first and second portions of the duodenum.[2] The common bile duct descends behind the duodenal cap, in a groove between the pancreas and duodenum, before it joins the pancreatic duct and inserts into the papilla of Vater in the posteromedial wall of the second portion of the duodenum.

These intimate anatomic relationships account for the fact that an impression by the gallbladder, cystic duct, or common duct can often be seen radiographically on the barium-filled duodenum in normal patients (Figs. 2–2 and 2–3). Similarly, propinquity of these struc-

tures accounts for the pathologic changes in the duodenum and colon that can occur in association with inflammatory and neoplastic diseases of the biliary tract.

ACUTE CHOLECYSTITIS

The acute inflammatory reaction of the gallbladder that occurs in acute cholecystitis may produce displacement, edema, and/or disordered motility in the adjacent portions of the duodenum. Barium studies of the duodenum typically show narrowing of the lumen, thickening of the mucosal folds, spasm, and irritability (Fig. 2–4).[3] The postbulbar segment and proximal part of the second portion of the duodenum are affected, particularly along the superior and lateral aspects. Eccentric inflammatory changes in these locations are characteristic. Chronic cholecystitis is less likely to result in radiographic abnormalities, but adhesions occur that may angulate and kink the duodenal wall. Carcinoma of the gallbladder frequently infiltrates locally, and when the duodenum is involved the radiographic distinction between tumor and cholecystitis is usually impossible to make on the basis of radiologic changes in the duodenum.[4]

Since the gallbladder usually lies near the hepatic flexure of the colon, acute cholecystitis can produce an abnormality of the colon that

30

Text continued on page 40

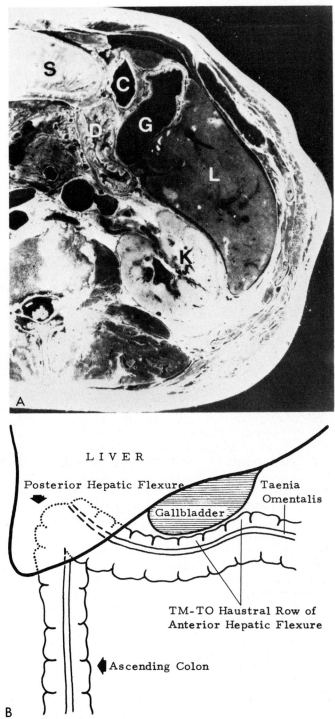

Figure 2–1. *A*, Transverse section of the right upper quadrant of the abdomen at the midplane of the right kidney (K), showing intimate relationships of the gallbladder (G) to the hepatic flexure of the colon (C) and the liver (L). (D) duodenal bulb and proximal descending duodenum. (S) stomach. *B*, Schematic drawing of the frontal gallbladder-colon relations.

Illustration continued on following page

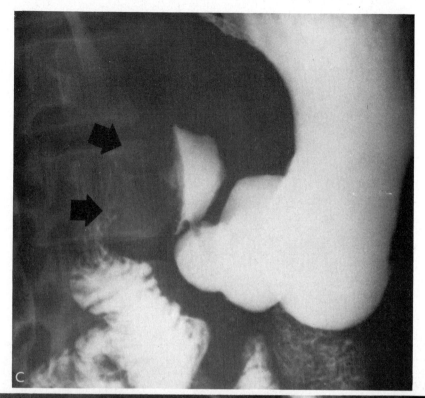

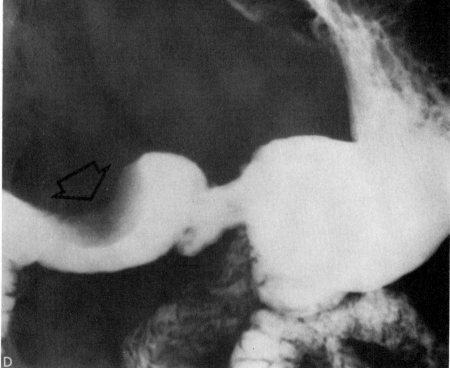

Figure 2–1. *Continued.* *C–E,* Radiographs from the upper gastrointestinal examination in three patients, showing the normal impression of the gallbladder on the duodenum *(C, D)* and on the gastric antrum *(E).* (*A* and *B* from Ghahremani, G. G., and Meyers, M. A.: Am. J. Roentgenol. *125*:21, 1975.)

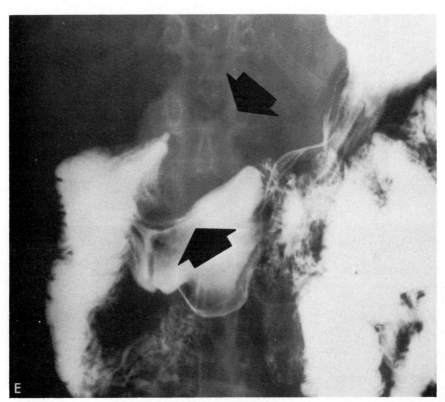

Figure 2–1. *Continued*

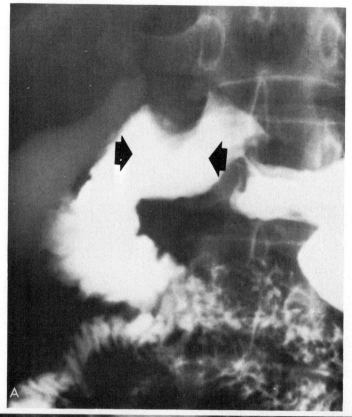

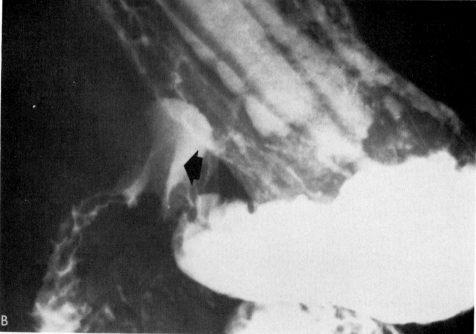

Figure 2–2. *A–D,* Radiographs from the upper gastrointestinal examination showing an impression on the duodenum produced by a normal common duct in three patients (arrows). The impression in *D* is exaggerated because of hepatomegaly.

Illustration continued on opposite page

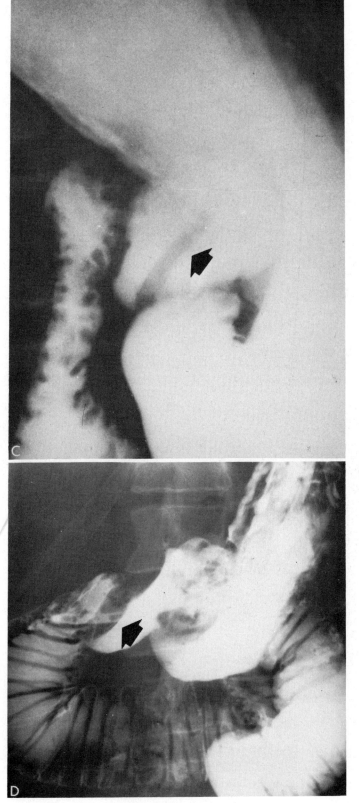

Figure 2–2. *Continued*

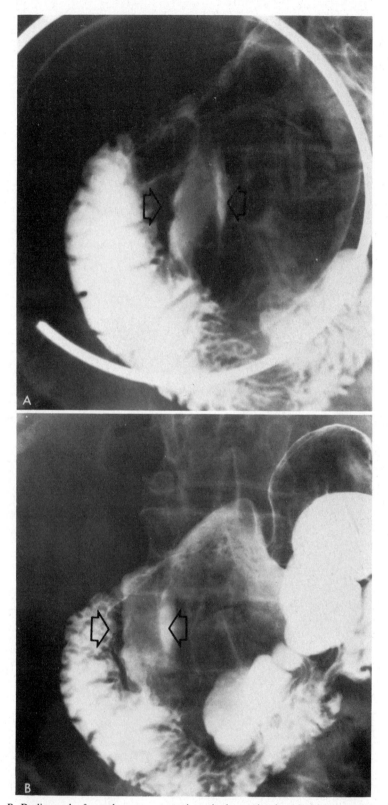

Figure 2–3. *A, B,* Radiographs from the upper gastrointestinal examination showing an impression on a duodenal diverticulum produced by a normal common duct (arrows). *C,* Radiograph from a T-tube cholangiogram in the same patient, showing the relation between the diverticulum and the common duct. The duct inserts into the neck of the diverticulum.

Illustration continued on opposite page

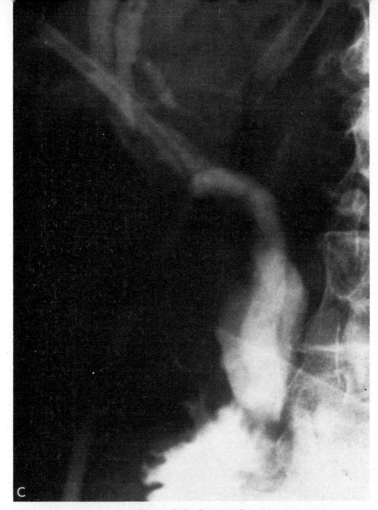

Figure 2–3. *Continued*

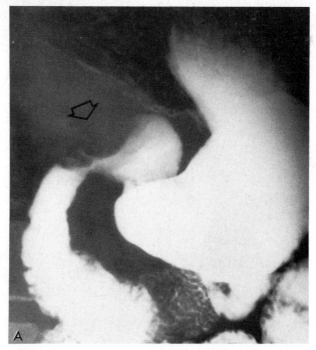

Figure 2–4. *A–E,* Radiographs from the upper gastrointestinal examination in five patients with acute cholecystitis showing characteristic inflammatory changes in the duodenum (arrows).

Illustration continued on following page

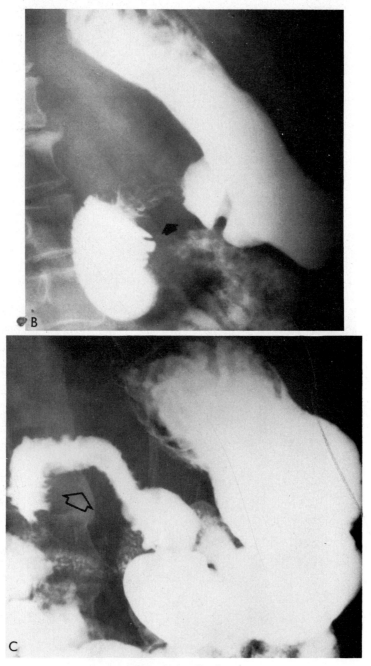

Figure 2–4. *Continued*

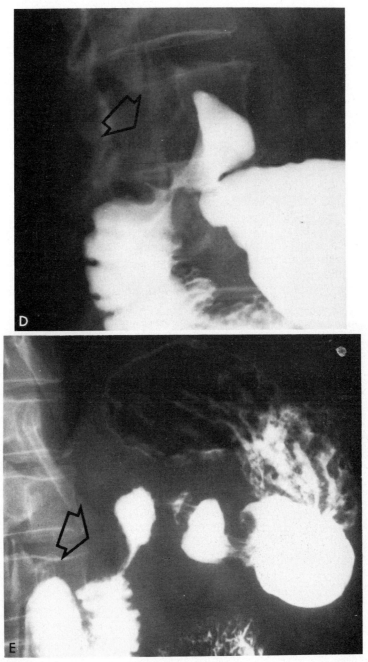

Figure 2–4. *Continued*

is visible on barium enema examination. There may be a smooth extrinsic impression along the superior margin of the colon or there may be more marked changes consisting of edema, spasm, stricture, or obstruction (Fig. 2–5).[5, 6] The radiographic findings may simulate segmental inflammatory disease of the colon such as acute diverticulitis, primary or metastatic carcinoma of the colon, or a colonic abnormality secondary to acute pancreatitis and pancreatic carcinoma. The administration of glucagon is useful to distinguish spasm from organic stricture, but either may occur in acute cholecystitis.

DILATATION OF THE COMMON BILE DUCT

Since the gallbladder and common duct lie in close anatomic relation to the duodenum, barium studies of the upper gastrointestinal tract in patients with obstructive jaundice may show indirect evidence of dilatation of the common duct and gallbladder. The distended duct produces a tubular impression on the duodenum, usually in the postbulbar segment (Fig. 2–6). The broad, radiolucent defect courses from above downward and to the right behind the barium-filled duodenum. In cases of obstructive jaundice, a distended gallbladder often produces a smooth impression on the lateral wall of the duodenal bulb.

Enlargement of the papilla of Vater may be present in patients with obstructive jaundice when the obstruction is due to carcinoma of the papilla, choledocholithiasis with a gallstone impacted at the papilla, or compression of the common duct in association with pancreatitis.[7] Differentiation among these diagnostic possibilities is not always precise on a radiologic basis alone, even when hypotonic duodenography is used. However, carcinoma of the papilla typically produces an irregular nodular or ulcerated polypoid mass, whereas, in cases with edema of the papilla from an impacted

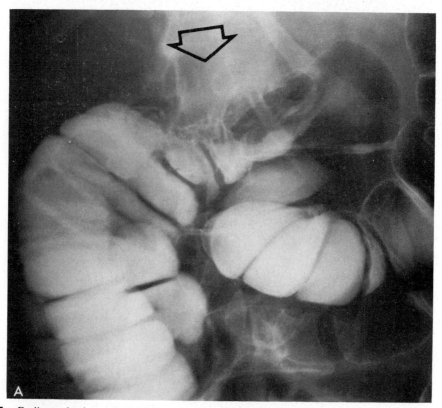

Figure 2–5. Radiographs from the barium enema examination in three patients with cholecystitis. *A,* There is extrinsic impression along the superior aspect of the hepatic flexure of the colon (arrow). *B,* There is localized displacement of the transverse colon due to distended gallbladder (arrows). *C,* There is spasm, irritability, and deformity of the transverse colon due to the adjacent inflammation involving the gallbladder (arrow).

Illustration continued on opposite page

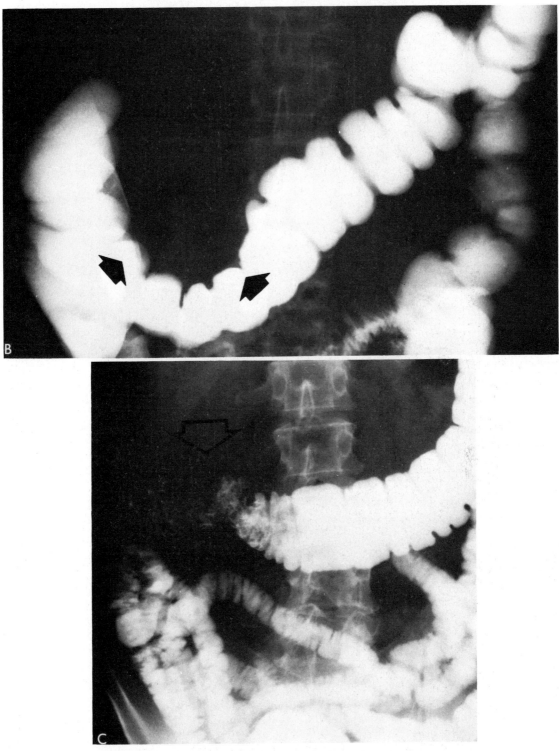

Figure 2–5. *Continued*

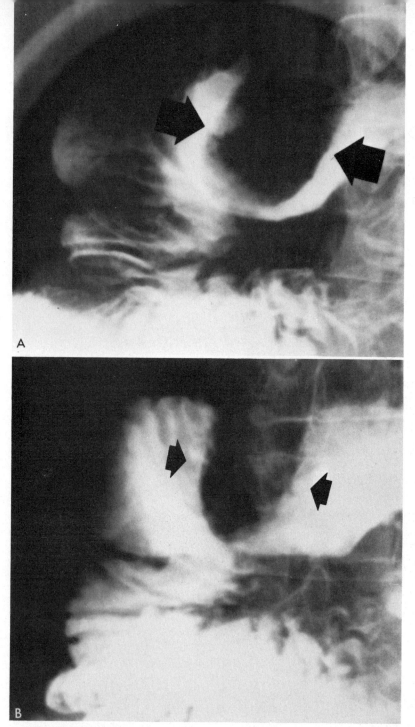

Figure 2–6. *A, B,* Radiographs from an upper gastrointestinal examination in a patient with obstructive jaundice due to carcinoma of the papilla of Vater. There is a tubular impression on the first portion of the duodenum owing to a markedly dilated common duct (arrows).

gallstone or from pancreatitis, the enlarged papilla is usually smooth and round, with the appearance of an intramural benign tumor (Figs. 2–7, 2–8, and 2–9).[8] When the papilla is edematous owing to pancreatitis (Poppel's sign),[9] other effects of the pancreatitis on the duodenum generally are apparent. These include effacement, spiculation, nodularity and flattening of the mucosal folds, and stretching of the duodenal loop.

Dilatation of the common bile duct due to a choledochal cyst may cause a mass in the region of the common duct on barium studies of the upper gastrointestinal tract.[10] Depending on the size of the cyst, the antrum of the stomach may be displaced upward and the

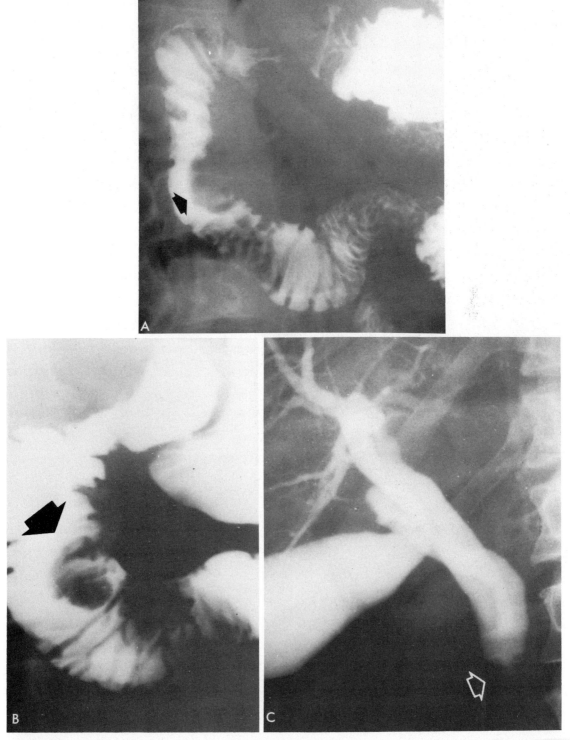

Figure 2–7. *A, B,* Radiographs from the upper gastrointestinal examination in two patients with adenocarcinoma of the papilla of Vater. In each case a polypoid mass with an irregular surface is visible at the papilla of Vater (arrows). *C,* Transhepatic cholangiogram in the patient shown in *B.* There is dilatation of the common duct, with an abrupt termination due to tumor extending from the papilla into the bile duct (arrow).

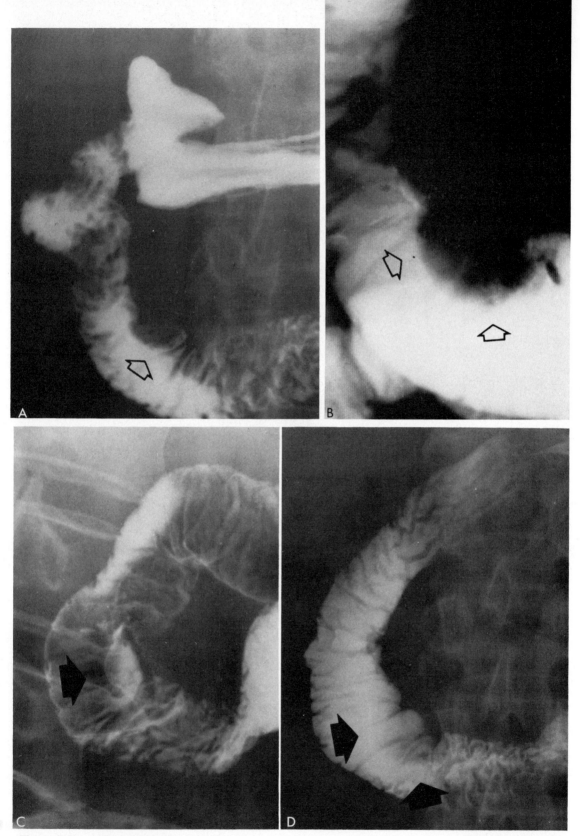

Figure 2–8. *A–D,* Radiographs from the upper gastrointestinal examination in four patients with obstructive jaundice due to a gallstone impacted at the papilla of Vater (arrows). The papilla is enlarged in each case owing to edema caused by the gallstone.

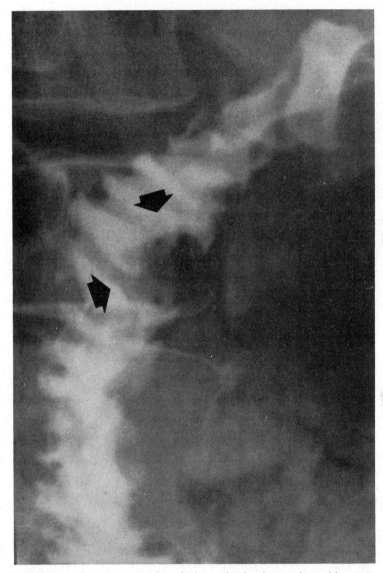

Figure 2–9. Radiograph from the upper gastrointestinal examination in a patient with acute pancreatitis, showing the descending portion of the duodenum. There is edema of the papilla of Vater (arrows), effacement of the mucosal folds, and widening of the duodenal loop.

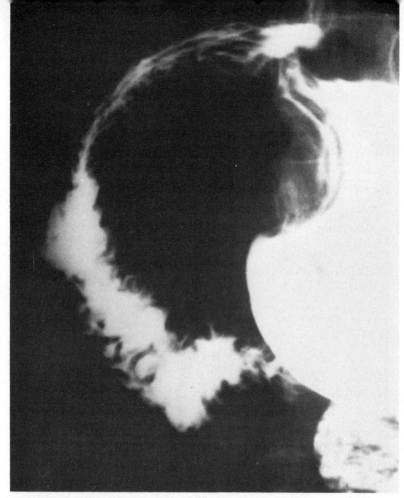

Figure 2–10. Radiograph from the upper gastrointestinal tract in a patient with a choledochocele. There is widening and stretching of the duodenal loop and displacement of the gastric antrum.

duodenal loop may be widened (Fig. 2–10). A choledochocele causes a polypoid defect in the second portion of the duodenum, producing radiologic features indistinguishable from those of carcinoma of the papilla of Vater or edema of the papilla due to an impacted gallstone or pancreatitis.[11]

BILIARY-ENTERIC FISTULA

Barium examination of the upper gastrointestinal tract is often useful in the detection and evaluation of biliary-enteric fistulas. In such cases, barium usually flows through the fistula and outlines the biliary tree. The fistula may be the result of previous surgery performed to relieve actual or potential obstruction of the common duct. A number of operations are used for this purpose including sphincterotomy, choledochoduodenostomy, cholecystoduodenostomy, and cholecystojejunostomy (Fig. 2–11).

As described in detail in the preceding chapter, spontaneous biliary-enteric fistulas most often are due to erosion of a gallstone from the gallbladder into the intestinal tract but also may occur secondary to erosion by a peptic ulcer or tumor. When gallstone ileus occurs, the findings on the plain abdominal radiograph are often characteristic. However, when they are not, barium given by mouth usually establishes the diagnosis by demonstrating an obturation-type small bowel obstruction. As shown in Figure 2–12, the obstructing gallstone can be seen in the barium column at the point of obstruction. However, most gallstones fail to produce intestinal obstruction. In such cases the gallstone may be demonstrated in otherwise normal small intestines or colon as it passes harmlessly through the bowel (Fig. 2–13). Barium may fill the biliary tree during barium studies with or without other radiologic findings (Fig. 2–14).

The gallstone may erode into the stomach, creating pyloric obstruction or a gastric bezoar[12] (Fig. 2–15). Similarly, the stone may erode into the duodenum and cause duodenal obstruction or a duodenal bezoar (Bouveret's syndrome)[13] (Fig. 2–16). Figure 2–17 illustrates a case in which gallstones caused partial obstruction of a colostomy stoma in a patient

46

Text continued on page 54

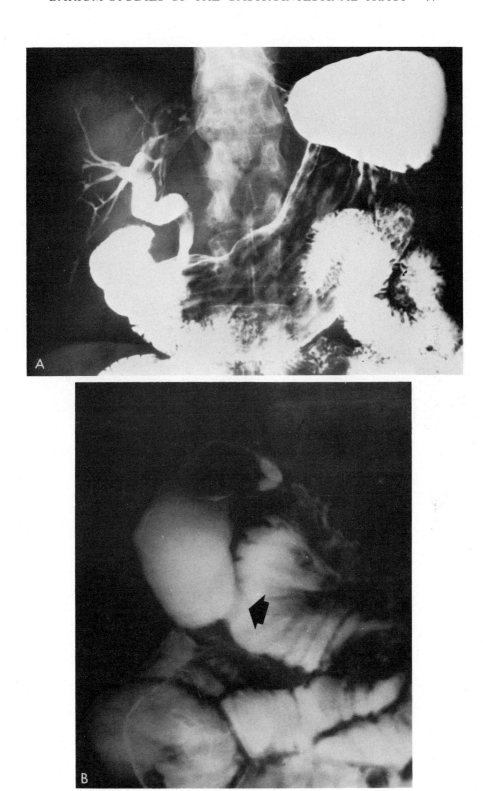

Figure 2–11. Radiographs from the upper gastrointestinal examination of a patient who had a sphincterotomy *(A)* and of a second patient who had a cholecystoduodenostomy (arrow) *(B)*. *A,* Barium is visible in the biliary tree. *B,* Barium is visible in the gallbladder.

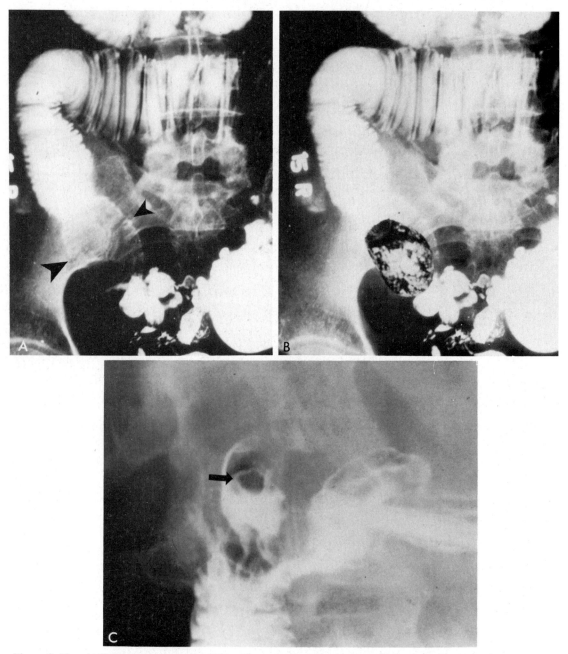

Figure 2–12. *A,* Radiograph from a small bowel examination showing obstruction of the proximal jejunum caused by a large gallstone (arrows). Barium is present in the colon from a previous barium enema study. *B,* After surgical removal, the stone was superimposed on the original radiograph. *C,* Radiograph of the duodenum in the same patient showing the cholecysto-duodenal fistula with barium in the collapsed gallbladder. A small gallstone is evident in the gallbladder (arrow).

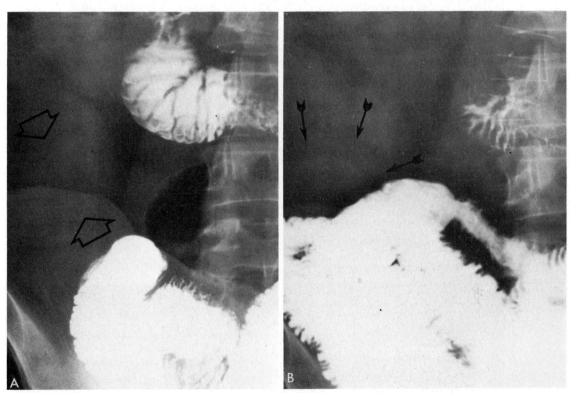

Figure 2–13. *A, B,* Radiographs from the small intestine examination in a patient with a spontaneous cholecysto-duodenal fistula, showing a large gallstone in the intestine that was not producing obstruction (arrows). The patient passed the stone spontaneously the following day. No air was visible in the biliary tree.

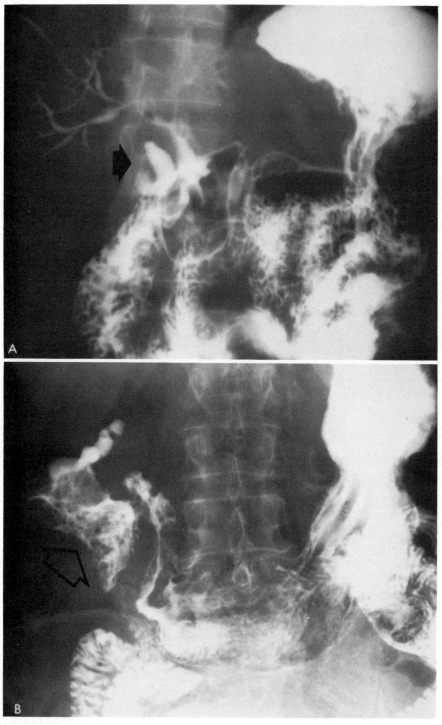

Figure 2–14. *A,* Radiograph from a patient with a spontaneous cholecysto-duodenal fistula due to cholelithiasis and cholecystitis with barium visible in the gallbladder (arrow). *B,* Radiograph from a second patient with spontaneous cholecysto-duodenal fistula due to cholecystitis and cholelithiasis, with barium visible in a necrotic gallbladder (arrow). In both cases no ectopic gallstone was identified and there was no intestinal obstruction.

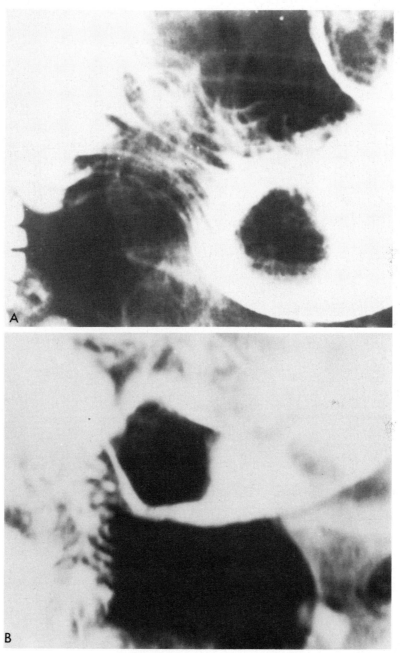

Figure 2–15. *A, B,* Upper gastrointestinal examination showing gallstones in the stomach in a patient who had a cholecysto-gastric fistula due to acute cholecystitis.

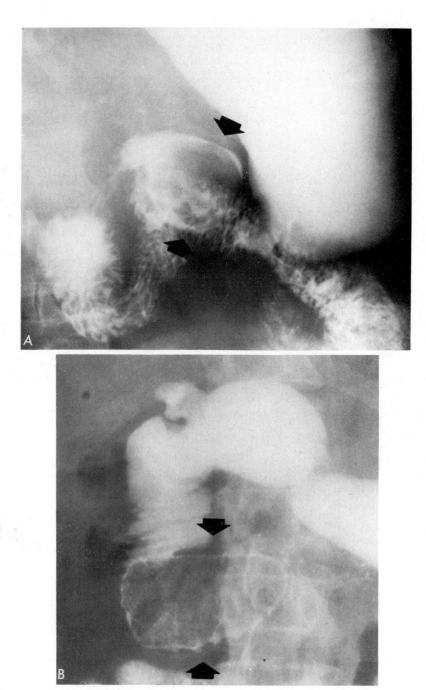

Figure 2–16. *A,* Radiograph from the upper gastrointestinal examination of a patient with a spontaneous cholecysto-duodenal fistula, showing a large gallstone in the duodenal bulb (arrows). *B,* Radiograph from the upper gastrointestinal examination in a patient with a spontaneous cholecysto-duodenal fistula, showing an obstructing gallstone in the third portion of the duodenum (arrows). An irregularity in the duodenum at the site of the fistula is apparent.

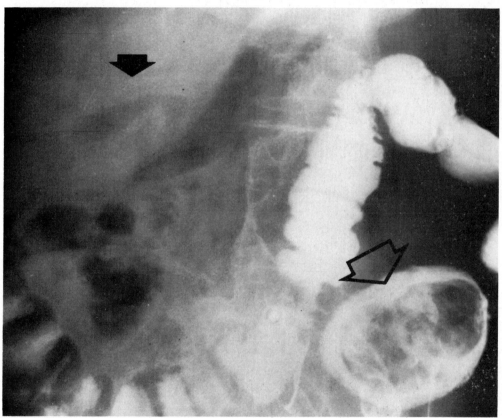

Figure 2–17. Radiograph from the barium enema examination in a patient with a cholecystocolic fistula, showing two large gallstones (open arrow) proximal to a colostomy in the descending colon. Air is visible in the biliary tree (closed arrow).

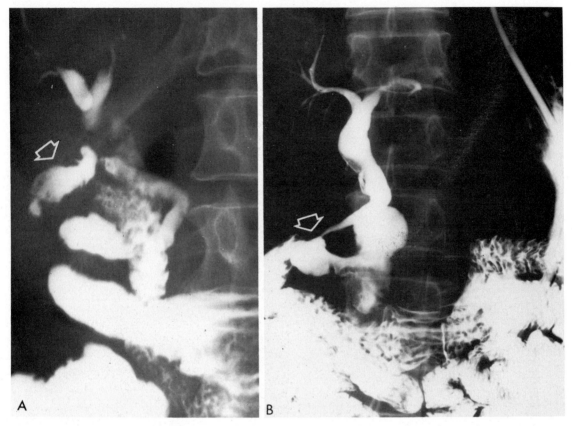

Figure 2–18. *A,* Radiograph from the upper gastrointestinal examination in a patient with cholecysto-duodenal fistula due to carcinoma of the gallbladder, showing barium in the biliary tree. Barium outlines the lumen of the gallbladder (arrow). *B,* Radiograph from another patient with a spontaneous choledochoduodenal fistula due to penetration of a duodenal ulcer (arrow) into the common duct. There is marked deformity of the duodenal bulb.

who had had a previous left hemicolectomy for carcinoma of the sigmoid colon. The gallstone entered the transverse colon through a cholecysto-colonic fistula. Barium enema examination showed the gallstone in the colon proximal to the colostomy and air (but not barium) in the biliary tree. The patient had no symptoms, except for those related to prolapse of the colostomy stoma.

Rarely, direct extension of carcinoma of the gallbladder into the duodenum or penetration of a peptic ulcer of the duodenum into the biliary tree may lead to a cholecysto-duodenal fistula indistinguishable from a communication secondary to cholecystitis and cholelithiasis (Fig. 2–18).

References

1. Cole, W. H.: Historical features of cholecystography: the Carman Lecture. Radiology 76:354, 1961.
2. Gray, H.: *In* Goss, C. M. (ed.): Anatomy of the Human Body, 27th ed. Philadelphia: Lea & Febiger, 1959, p. 1279.
3. Berk, R. N.: Radiology of the gallbladder and bile ducts. Surg. Clin. North Am. 53:973, 1973.
4. Khilnani, M. T., Wolf, B. S., and Finkel, M.: Roentgen features of carcinoma of the gallbladder on barium-meal examination. Radiology 79:264, 1962.
5. Crawford, A.: An "irregularity" in transverse colon diagnosis. Aust. N.Z. J. Surg. 41:50, 1971.
6. Ghahremani, G. G., and Meyers, M. A.: The cholecysto-colic relationships: a roentgen-anatomic study of the colonic manifestations of gallbladder disorders. Am. J. Roentgenol. 125:21, 1975.
7. Eaton, S. B., and Ferrucci, J. T.: Radiology of the Pancreas and Duodenum. Philadelphia: W. B. Saunders Co., 1973, p. 174.
8. Eaton, S. B., et al.: Diagnosis of choledocholithiasis by barium duodenal examination. Radiology 102:267, 1972.
9. Poppel, M. H.: The roentgen manifestations of relapsing pancreatitis. Radiology 62:514, 1954.
10. Han, S. Y., Collins, L. C., and Wright, R. M.: Choledochal cyst: report of five cases. Clin. Radiol. 20:332, 1969.
11. Alden, J. F., and Sterner, E. R.: Choledochocele. Ann. Surg. 145:269, 1957.
12. Braxton, M., and Jacobson, G.: Intragastric gallstone. Am. J. Roentgenol. 78:631, 1957.
13. Halaz, N. A.: Gallstone obstruction of the duodenal bulb (Bouveret's syndrome). Am. J. Dig. Dis. 9:856, 1963.

BILIARY CONTRAST MATERIALS

by Robert N. Berk, M.D.,
and Peter M. Loeb, M.D.

3

INTRODUCTION AND HISTORICAL REVIEW

Successful radiographic visualization of the biliary tree is achieved by taking advantage of the liver's capacity to eliminate organic compounds into the bile.[1-4] When selected organic compounds are made radiopaque by iodination, they are suitable for use as contrast materials for opacification of the biliary tree. The development of oral and intravenous biliary contrast agents evolved from an ingenious application of a fortuitous finding.[5] In 1909, Abel and Rowntree were searching for a long-acting intravenous cathartic and noted that tetrachlorphenolphthalein was almost entirely excreted by the liver into bile.[6] Graham, in 1924, was aware of their work and also of the report by Rous and McMaster[7] that showed that bile is concentrated in the gallbladder.[8] He theorized that an iodine or bromine derivative of phenolphthalein, by virtue of the high atomic number of the halogen, would be radiographically visible in the gallbladder once it had been excreted by the liver and concentrated in the gallbladder. Subsequently, Graham and Cole obtained successful cholecystograms in dogs and humans by the injection of tetrabromophenolphthalein.[9] Tetraiodophenolphthalein was then made commercially available as Iodeikon, which was used for cholecystography but was limited in its effectiveness by a high incidence of side effects including nausea, vomiting, diarrhea, and hypotension.[10] In 1940, iodoalphionic acid (Priodax) was introduced as an oral agent and was found to be associated with a decreased incidence of side effects and an improvement in the radiologic visualization of the gallbladder.[5]

In 1951, Hoppe and Archer developed iopanoic acid (Telepaque) by testing a series of aromatic tri-iodo-alkanoic acid derivatives.[11-13]

This compound had greater efficiency and was safer than agents used previously. It has been estimated that more than 40 million doses of iopanoic acid have been administered since 1952.[1] The basic structure of the molecule has been altered only slightly to produce other compounds now available for use in oral cholecystography (Fig. 3–1A). All of these compounds are of limited value for visualization of the bile ducts. However, in 1953, sodium iodipamide (Biligrafin), a dimer of iodinated tri-iodobenzoic acid, was introduced; this could be administered intravenously and produced radiographic visualization of the common bile duct.[5] In 1955, sodium iodipamide was replaced by the methylglucamine salt (Cholografin). Other compounds developed for intravenous cholangiography differ only slightly from iodipamide (Fig. 3–1B).[4]

It has become apparent that the radiographic contrast materials currently used for oral and intravenous administration have, to a large extent, different physicochemical properties. An oral cholecystographic agent must have properties that allow absorption from the intestinal tract as well as preferential excretion by the liver into bile. Oral cholecystography is unique in this regard, since no other radiographic contrast procedures that depend on excretion of a contrast material can achieve success by oral administration of the agent. The primary goal of oral cholecystography is opacification of the gallbladder, which requires not only hepatic excretion but concentration of the contrast agent by the gallbladder. Visualization of the bile ducts is a secondary, often fortuitous, achievement with this technique.

Intravenous cholangiographic contrast agents are utilized to obtain radiographic opacification of the bile ducts and to determine patency of the cystic duct.[4] Therefore, an intravenous contrast agent must have physico-

IOPANOIC ACID (Telepaque)

$$CH_2\text{-}\underset{\underset{C_2H_5}{|}}{CH}\text{-}COOH$$

IOCETAMIC ACID (Cholebrine)

$$CH_3\text{-}\underset{\underset{O}{\|}}{C}\text{-}N\text{-}CH_2\text{-}\underset{\underset{CH_3}{|}}{CH}\text{-}COOH$$

SODIUM TYROPANOATE (Bilopaque)

$$CH_2\text{-}\underset{\underset{C_2H_5}{|}}{CH}\text{-}COONa$$

A

SODIUM IPODATE (Oragrafin)

$$CH_2\text{-}CH_2\text{-}COONa$$

IODIPAMIDE (Cholografin)

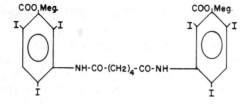

IOGLYCAMIDE (Biligram)

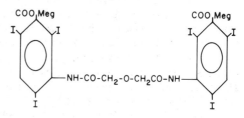

IODOXAMATE (Cholevue)

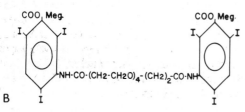

B

IOTROXAMIDE

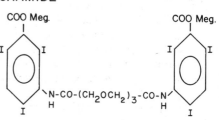

Figure 3–1. Chemical formulae. *A,* Oral cholecystographic contrast materials. *B,* Intravenous cholangiographic contrast materials.

chemical properties that allow intravenous administration and hepatic excretion of the compound in sufficient quantities and concentrations to permit direct radiographic visualization of the bile ducts.

In this chapter, some of the complex physicochemical and pharmacokinetic interactions of the oral and intravenous biliary contrast

agents that determine and affect intestinal absorption and/or biliary excretion will be described. An understanding of the pharmacokinetics of oral and intravenous contrast materials will provide a basis to enable the physician to use these agents more rationally to ensure maximum efficiency, accuracy, and safety.

Table 3–1. ORAL CHOLECYSTOGRAPHIC CONTRAST AGENTS

		Molecular Weight	Organic Bound Iodine (%)	Preparation (gm)
Iopanoic acid	Telepaque (Winthrop)	571	66.7	0.5 tablet
Sodium tyropanoate	Bilopaque (Winthrop)	641	57.4	0.75 capsule
Calcium ipodate	Oragrafin Calcium (Squibb)	1234	61.7	3.0 granules
Sodium ipodate	Oragrafin Sodium (Squibb)	620	61.4	0.5 capsule
Iocetamic acid	Cholebrine (Mallinckrodt)	614	62.0	0.75 tablet

PHYSICOCHEMICAL PROPERTIES

There are several fundamental similarities in the chemical structure of the oral cholecystographic agents and the intravenous cholangiographic agents. Both the oral and intravenous agents are aromatic tri-iodo-alkanoic acid derivatives (Fig. 3–1). The oral cholecystographic agents consist of a single tri-iodinated benzene ring with a prosthetic group at the number one position and an amino group at the number three position.[11-14] The intravenous contrast agents are all dimers of tri-iodobenzoic acid and differ only in the length and composition of the polymethylene chain that connects the two iodinated benzene rings. The oral and intravenous biliary contrast agents do not contain a prosthetic group at the number five position of the benzene ring. This appears to be an important structural feature that permits predominantly biliary, rather than renal, excretion of the compounds.[15]

The oral cholecystographic agents differ from one another in the prosthetic group attached to the benzene ring and/or substitution on the amino group.[16, 17] They are all polar lipids with a balance between hydrophilic and lipophilic groups that allows dissolution in the intestinal lumen, absorption, and hepatic ex-

cretion. There are marked differences in the water solubility of the oral cholecystographic agents, which is determined by variations in these two substituted groups (Fig. 3–1).[18] Iopanoic acid (Telepaque) is the least water soluble of the available oral cholecystographic agents. Subsequently, sodium tyropanoate (Bilopaque), the sodium and calcium salts of ipodate (Oragrafin), and iocetamic acid (Cholebrine) have been introduced for clinical use.[3, 16, 19-25] These compounds are more soluble in water but less lipid soluble than iopanoic acid. The oral agents all contain approximately 60 per cent iodine per molecule, and the recommended dose is 3.0 gm (Table 3–1).

The four intravenous contrast agents are relatively strong dibasic acids compared with the oral agents, and at the pH of body fluids they are almost completely ionized, highly soluble in water, and poorly soluble in lipids.[2, 17, 26] Iodipamide (Cholografin, Biligrafin) and ioglycamide (Biligram) contain 50 per cent iodine per molecule and have similar molecular weights (Table 3–2).[27, 28] The longer polymethylene chain of iodoxamate (Cholevue) accounts for its lower percentage of iodine (45 per cent) and its higher molecular weight (1678). Only iodipamide is presently available for use in the U.S. Ioglycamide is widely used

Table 3–2. INTRAVENOUS CHOLANGIOGRAPHIC CONTRAST AGENTS

		Molecular Weight	Organic Bound Iodine (%)	Preparation (% solution)
Methylglucamine iodipamide	Cholografin (Squibb) Biligrafin (Schering)	1530	50	52.0
Methylglucamine ioglycamide	Biligram, Bilivistin (Schering)	1518	50	52.0
Methylglucamine iodoxamate*	Cholevue (Winthrop)	1678	45	40.3
Methylglucamine iotroxamide*	— (Schering)	1606	47.3	38.0

*Under investigation.

in Europe.[28-32] Iodoxamate and iotroxamide are new contrast agents currently being investigated.[33-36]

INTESTINAL ABSORPTION

For intestinal absorption of an oral cholecystographic agent to occur, the contrast agent must first dissolve in the bulk water phase of the gastrointestinal lumen and diffuse across the poorly mixed layer of water (unstirred water layer) between the bulk water phase and the intestinal mucosa.[15, 17-18, 37-39] The oral cholecystographic agent then diffuses in a passive process across the lipid membrane of the gastrointestinal mucosa. Therefore, ultimate absorption requires dissolution of the contrast material in both water and lipid.[39] Even though the intravenous contrast agents are highly soluble in water, they are not absorbed since they are largely insoluble in lipid.

Solubility of the oral cholecystographic agents in the intestinal lumen is affected by the physical form of the contrast material, the pH of the intestinal fluid, and the presence of biologic detergents, i.e., bile salts.[1, 18, 37, 38] Studies have clearly demonstrated that the physical state of the contrast materials in the intestine has a profound influence on the rate of intestinal absorption.[40-42] The crystals of the commercial tablet of Telepaque (iopanoic acid) appear to be larger and have a smaller surface area–to–weight ratio than the crystals formed by the acid precipitation of the sodium salt of iopanoate (Fig. 3–2).[41] This probably explains why the acid precipitate of the sodium salt of iopanoate is more soluble in water at physiologic pH than the commercial tablet of iopanoic acid. The acid precipitate of iopanoate forms when sodium iopanoate is administered orally and passes through the acid environment of the stomach. Studies in animals and man reveal that the iopanoate is absorbed more rapidly when administered as a sodium salt than as an acid.[41, 43, 44] Sodium iopanoate is used in Europe, but only the acid, Telepaque, is approved for use in the U.S.

The hydrogen ion concentration of the gastrointestinal lumen profoundly influences the ionization and solubility of the oral cholecystographic agents.[41, 45, 46] The oral cholecystographic agents are all weak acids with relatively wide ranges of aqueous solubility at the pH of the proximal small intestine (pH 6.5) (Fig. 3–2).[47] The ionized form of the compounds is more soluble in aqueous solutions than the unionized form, and, in accordance with the Henderson-Hasselbalch equation, the concentration of the ionized form depends on the pH of the gastrointestinal contents. Hence, a weak acid, such as iopanoic acid (pKa 5.9), is almost completely un-ionized and virtually insoluble in water at the low pH of the stomach. Likewise, the ionization and solubility of the other oral contrast agents are also reduced at the pH of the stomach.[18] As an oral contrast agent enters the more alkaline pH of the small intestine, the ionization and solubility of the compound increase. Nelson and associates solubilized iopanoate in a highly alkaline solution and instilled the solution directly into the duodenum of dogs. These investigators concluded that increased solubility of iopanoate resulted in an increased rate of absorption, since 50 per cent of the dose was excreted in bile within two hours.[46] However, at the pH of the proximal small intestine, iopanoic acid is poorly soluble in aqueous solutions. At a pH of 7.4, the solubility of tyropanoate is fifty-fold greater than that of iopanoic acid.[18] Ipodate and iocetamic acid are also more water soluble than iopanoic acid. Thus, under these limited conditions, one might anticipate that the most widely used agent, iopanoic acid, would be so insoluble in the intestine that absorption might not occur.

Fortunately, the aqueous solubility of these polar lipids is also affected by the presence of bile salts in the intestinal lumen.[41] Bile salts are excreted by the liver, stored in the gallbladder, and emptied into the intestine in response to the hormone cholecystokinin (stimulated by fat and peptides in the intestinal lumen).[48] Bile salts increase the aqueous solubility of compounds such as iopanoic acid by forming micelles,[48] which are molecular aggregates formed by spatial orientation of the bile salt molecules. The bile salt molecules cluster together so that the hydrophobic portions of the molecules form a nonpolar lipid environment in the center of the micelle in which fat-soluble substances such as iopanoic acid can dissolve. The bile salts are reabsorbed largely in the terminal ileum and returned to the liver. The entire pool of bile salts (2 to 4 gm) is recycled two to three times with each meal, and in this manner adequate concentrations of bile salts are maintained in the intestinal lumen for micellar solubilization of lipids. In the fasting state, almost the entire pool of bile salts is stored in the gallbladder. Therefore, in a fasting patient one would anticipate that solubility and absorption of fat-soluble compounds would be impaired.

In vitro, bile salts markedly increase the

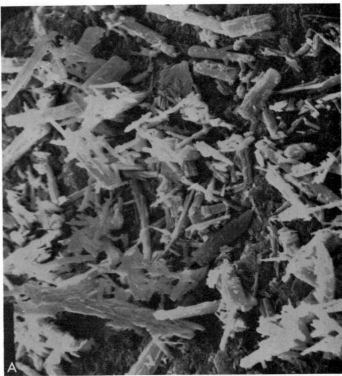

Figure 3–2. Iopanoic acid crystals (electron micrographs). *A*, Commercial Telepaque tablets. *B*, Acid precipitate of sodium salt of iopanoate. These crystals are smaller and have a higher surface area-to-weight ratio than does the commercial form.

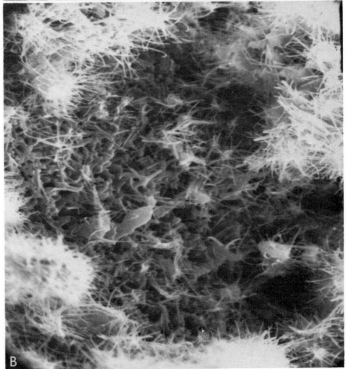

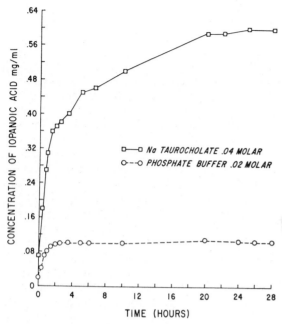

Figure 3–3. Rate of solution and solubility of iopanoic acid in phosphate buffer and in sodium taurocholate at pH 6.5. The rate of solution and solubility is higher in the presence of bile salts. (From Goldberger, L. E., et al.: Invest. Radiol. 9:16, 1974. Courtesy of J. B. Lippincott Co., Publisher.)

in the intestine, the biliary excretion of iopanoic acid is markedly increased (Fig. 3–4).[41] Therefore, it appears likely that if bile salts are sequestered in the gallbladder, the aqueous solubility of a compound such as iopanoic acid would be severely limited, absorption would be incomplete, and ultimate radiographic opacification of the gallbladder might be impaired. This would be expected to occur in a patient who is fasting or on a low-fat and low-protein diet, whereby there are no stimuli to release cholecystokinin and bile salts are not evacuated from the gallbladder into the duodenum. Conversely, if a meal containing fat and/or protein were given with the iopanoic acid, the enterohepatic circulation of bile salts would be enhanced, and the solubility and absorption of iopanoic acid would be facilitated.

The results of clinical studies support the thesis that impaired visualization of the gallbladder in normal patients after the first-dose cholecystogram is due, at least in part, to poor intestinal absorption of iopanoic acid. Evens, Schroer, and Koehler studied the amount of unabsorbed iopanoic acid visible on abdominal radiographs of patients with nonvisualization of the gallbladder after a single dose of iopanoic acid.[51] If large amounts of unabsorbed iopanoic acid were visible, good visualization of the gallbladder was achieved in 85 per cent of these patients with a second-dose cholecystogram. If little or no residual contrast material was observed in the colon after the first study, good gallbladder visualization occurred in only 25 per cent of patients on the second examination. Thus, it appears that impaired visual-

solubility of the oral cholecystographic agents (Fig. 3–3).[41] *In vivo*, this would appear to be more important for the more poorly water-soluble agents like iopanoic acid.[18] In studies in dogs, iopanoic acid is poorly absorbed when bile is diverted away from the intestine, but when bile salts are mixed with iopanoic acid

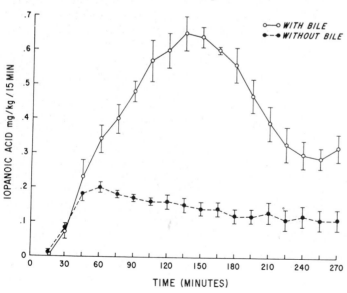

Figure 3–4. Biliary excretion of iopanoate in dogs when iopanoic acid is injected into duodenum with Ringer's lactate or bile. Each point represents the mean and standard error of the mean of data from four dogs in each group. Greater iopanoate excretion is present when iopanoic acid is mixed with bile. (From Goldberger, L. E., et al.: Invest. Radiol. 9:16, 1974. Courtesy of J. B. Lippincott Co., Publisher.)

ization of a normal gallbladder after the first dose of iopanoic acid usually can be related to impaired solubility and poor absorption of the contrast material. Loeb and colleagues showed that only two of ten normal volunteers had satisfactory opacification of the gallbladder when iopanoic acid was administered in the fasting state.[49] All ten had good visualization when the iopanoic acid was given with a meal. Using computerized tomography (CT) to determine the degree of gallbladder opacification, Fon and coworkers showed that feeding similarly affected gallbladder opacification in dogs.[50]

Bile salts also increase the aqueous solubility of each of the other oral cholecystographic agents so that, even in the presence of bile salts, iopanoic acid is the least soluble in the intestinal lumen of all of the oral cholecystographic agents.[18] Thus, if absorption is limited by the rate of solution in the intestine, one would expect that compounds such as tyropanoate and ipodate would be absorbed more rapidly and consistently than iopanoic acid. Indeed, clinical studies suggest that intestinal absorption of ipodate and tyropanoate might be more complete than absorption of iopanoic acid.[21-24, 49] However, the absence of opaque residue in the intestine on abdominal radiographs when the more water-soluble agents are used does not necessarily indicate that they have been completely absorbed. The more water-soluble compounds may be dispersed and in solution in the intestine and therefore are not detectable on the radiographs.

Although rate of solution appears to be the limiting factor in the absorption of iopanoic acid, the rate of permeation across the lipid barrier of the intestinal mucosa also can influence the ultimate rate of disappearance of the oral cholecystographic compounds from the intestinal lumen.[18, 37-39] The permeation of a compound across a lipid membrane depends on the relative solubility of the compound in the lipid membrane and in the aqueous milieu in the intestinal lumen, that is, the degree of partitioning between lipid and aqueous media. Results of studies of the partition coefficients of the oral agents between the lipid solvent benzene and water indicate that the more water-soluble agents, such as tyropanoate, are much less soluble in lipid than the poorly water-soluble compound iopanoic acid.[18] Increasing the pH of the aqueous solution reduces the partitioning into the lipid solvent as it increases ionization of the compounds and aqueous solubility. Studies *in vivo*, whereby isolated loops of a dog jejunum are perfused with solutions of the oral cholecystographic compounds without bile salts, indicate that there is a direct relationship between the lipid solubility of the compound and the rate of absorption from the intestine.[18] Thus, iopanoic acid, once in solution, is absorbed more rapidly than is tyropanoate or ipodate. Ultimate absorption of iopanoic acid, therefore, is limited by its solubility in the intestinal lumen. The more water-soluble agents, such as tyropanoate, dissolve more rapidly in the intestinal lumen but, once in aqueous solution, are not absorbed across the mucosa as rapidly as iopanoic acid. From the data currently available it appears likely that in the absence of bile salts, the more water-soluble compounds, such as ipodate and tyropanoate, would be absorbed more rapidly than iopanoic acid. However, in the presence of bile salts, one cannot predict which agent will be absorbed most rapidly. Although with bile salts the aqueous solubility of all of the compounds would increase, the more water-soluble compounds would still be considerably more soluble than iopanoic acid. The iopanoic acid that is in solution would pass through the lipid membrane more rapidly than the other agents. Therefore, additional studies are needed to define the relative absorption rates of oral cholecystographic agents with or without bile salts.

TRANSPORT IN BLOOD

Once the oral cholecystographic agents diffuse across the intestinal mucosa, it appears that they enter the portal circulation. Studies in animals, in which lymphatic and portal venous concentrations of iopanoic acid were measured after intestinal administration of iopanoic acid, reveal that the vast majority of iopanoate is recovered in the portal blood.[52] Iopanoate probably enters the portal circulation, rather than the lymphatics, because blood has one and one-half times the capacity to bind iopanoate than intestinal lymph and because portal blood flow is about 500 times greater than intestinal lymph flow.

Both oral and intravenous cholecystographic contrast materials are transported in blood bound to albumin by hydrophobic bonds.[15, 53, 54] The degree of binding correlates closely with the octanol-water partition coefficients.[53] Iopanoic acid, which contains only one hydrophilic group and which is the most hydrophobic of the contrast materials, is strongly bound to albumin. Albumin binding, therefore, appears to be important in increasing the solubility in plasma of the poorly water-soluble oral cholecystographic compounds.

However, the degree of binding to albumin is also related to the relative toxicity of the compounds in animals. Lasser and associates studied the binding potential of various contrast materials with serum from a number of animal species and found a linear relation between LD_{50} values and binding to serum proteins.[54] These authors postulated that the greater toxicity of the more highly bound contrast materials was due to binding of the contrast material to critical enzymes. Iodipamide, which is more toxic than the renal contrast agents, is bound more highly to serum proteins.

UPTAKE BY THE LIVER

Once the oral and intravenous contrast agents enter the circulation, they pass through the hepatic sinusoids, enter the space of Disse, and are taken up by the hepatocytes across the sinusoidal hepatic cell membrane.[1, 4] Direct communication between the space of Disse and the bile canaliculi is limited by the tight junction between the intercellular space and the canalicular lumen, and it is unlikely that the contrast agents are excreted directly in bile without passing through the hepatocyte.[55] The factors that determine the rather selective hepatic uptake and biliary excretion of these organic compounds have not been precisely delineated.[2, 54] Binding of the contrast agents to plasma albumin partially limits their distribution to the vascular compartment and probably plays a role in reducing renal excretion by limiting glomerular filtration or tubular secretion. However, the degree of binding to plasma albumin of an organic compound is not necessarily related to the ultimate appearance of that compound in bile.[17] Indeed, studies with the intravenous contrast agent iodipamide[56] and with the organic anion sulfobromophthalein (BSP)[57] indicate that albumin binding impedes the hepatic excretion in bile of these organic compounds. Song, Beranbaum, and Rothschild found that both the initial clearance and the half-time of transfer of iodipamide from plasma into bile were decreased in the isolated perfused rabbit liver when albumin was added to the perfusate.[56] Studies in patients with hypoalbuminemia secondary to

the nephrotic syndrome reveal decreased BSP clearance after albumin is administered intravenously.[57]

Receptors on the sinusoidal liver cell membrane or in the cytoplasm may be the factors that determine the preferential hepatic excretion of the biliary contrast agents. Isolated liver cell membranes have been shown to contain saturable binding sites for a number of other organic anions that are excreted in bile.[58] Unfortunately, with this experimental preparation, it is not possible to separate receptors on the sinusoidal membrane from those on the canalicular membrane. The Y and Z hepatic cytoplasmic proteins discovered by Levi, Gathmaitan, and Arias may be the postulated hepatic receptors.[59] These low molecular weight, soluble, basic proteins have been shown to bind bilirubin and sulfobromophthalein after injection in vivo or after incubation in vitro with the liver-cell supernate. In vitro studies with both the intravenous agent iodipamide and the oral agent iopanoic acid demonstrate that these agents bind to these proteins, whereas iothalamate, a urinary contrast agent, has no affinity for these soluble proteins.[60]

It is also possible that the hepatic uptake or storage of the biliary contrast agents is the same for compounds, such as the renal contrast agents, that are not preferentially excreted in bile. This would be the case if processes involved in the active excretion from the liver cell into bile were responsible for the preferential biliary excretion of the biliary contrast agents.

However, pharmacokinetic data obtained with other organic compounds indicate that hepatic uptake is mediated by a rate-limiting active transport process.[61, 62] Competition for hepatic uptake may explain the transient hyperbilirubinemia and the sulfobromophthalein retention that have been demonstrated in some patients after the administration of iopanoic acid.[63] It may also explain the diminished biliary excretion of iodipamide found in dogs when iopanoic acid and iodipamide are administered together.[64]

BIOTRANSFORMATION IN THE LIVER

Current data indicate that the intravenous contrast agents are not altered chemically during transport through the liver but are excreted in the bile without structural modification.[26] The oral contrast agents, which are less soluble in water, appear to be converted to more water-soluble conjugates prior to excretion in bile.[14, 65, 66] Experimental data indicate that iopanoic acid is conjugated with glucuronic acid in the liver. Initially, McChesney and Hoppe found that iopanoic acid, when fed to cats, was excreted in an altered form in bile.[14] Studies in dogs indicated that the metabolic product of iopanoate found in bile met the analytical requirements of an ester of glucuronide.[65] Studies in human volunteers who were administered iopanoic acid revealed that the urine contained the glucuronide conjugate.[65] Data summarized by Knoefel suggest that tyropanoate, ipodate, and iocetamic acid are also excreted as the glucuronide conjugate.[17]

The hepatic biotransformation of these oral contrast agents is similar to that of the endogenous organic anion bilirubin except that bilirubin is excreted predominantly as a diglucuronide rather than a monoglucuronide, as is iopanoic acid.[67, 68] It is generally accepted that iopanoic acid, like bilirubin, is conjugated by the action of the microsomal enzyme glucuronyl transferase, which catalyzes the transfer of glucuronic acid from the nucleotide uridine diphosphate glucuronic acid.[65] However, the results of preliminary studies with bilirubin suggest that the second glucuronide is added by enzymatic action at the canalicular membrane.[69] In vitro studies with the oral contrast agents to identify the site of glucuronidation have not been performed. In any case, conjugation appears to provide a more water-soluble molecule of increased molecular weight for excretion into bile that cannot diffuse back into the liver across the lipid membrane of the canaliculi as readily as the unconjugated, fat-soluble compound. Furthermore, if the oral cholecystographic compounds are completely conjugated prior to excretion in bile, conjugation may be a structural requirement for active transport from the liver into bile. This is not the case for sulfobromophthalein, which is excreted in bile, in part, without prior conjugation with glutathione.[70] With the oral contrast agents, conjugation may be the rate-limiting step in the hepatic excretion, since the glucuronide of iopanoate, when administered intravenously, produces good radiographic opacification of the gallbladder within one hour, whereas an equivalent dose of unconjugated iopanoic acid administered intravenously produces visualization after an eight-hour delay.[65]

EXCRETION IN BILE

Considerable data have been accumulated to indicate that excretion in bile of both the oral and intravenous contrast agents is mediated by an active transport process involving enzymes in the liver that become saturated, thereby limiting the maximum rate of excretion of the contrast agent.[27, 35, 36, 71-76] The site of this rate-limiting transport process for organic compounds has not been delineated, although it is generally believed to be located at the canalicular membrane.

Among the biliary contrast agents studied, iopanoic acid is unique in that the rate of excretion of bile salts in bile has a profound influence on the rate of biliary excretion of iopanoate.[71, 72, 76-78] The results of several studies reveal a linear relation between the rate of iopanoate excretion in bile and the rate of bile flow produced by the infusion of the bile salt taurocholate (Fig. 3–5A).[77-79] The mechanism by which taurocholate enhances the biliary excretion of iopanoate is poorly understood. When excreted in bile, it results in an increase in bile flow (choleresis) by stimulating water movement across the canaliculi.[55] In addition, bile salts form micelles in bile that are important in the solubilization of cholesterol in bile, preventing the formation of cholesterol gallstones.[80] Choleresis per se, whether produced by secretin,[81] which stimulates water excretion across the bile ducts, or by a substance that stimulates bile salt–independent canalicular bile flow (SC2644),[55, 77] does not affect the excretion rate of iopanoate (Fig. 3–5B). Therefore, it is clear that bile salts per se, independent of their choleretic effect, are the important determinants of iopanoate excretion. Since the bile salt dehydrocholate, a triketo bile salt that forms micelles poorly, also facilitates the biliary excretion of iopanoate, it originally was postulated that bile salts enhance iopanoate excretion independent of their micellar effect (Fig. 3–5C).[77] However, it has been shown subsequently that some of the metabolic products of dehydrocholate that appear in bile form micelles.[82] Therefore, micellar solubilization of iopanoate cannot be excluded as the mechanism whereby bile salts increase the excretion of iopanoate in bile. The biliary excretion of ipodate and tyropanoate is not affected by bile salt excretion.[74] These compounds, as noted previously, are more soluble in aqueous solution than iopanoic

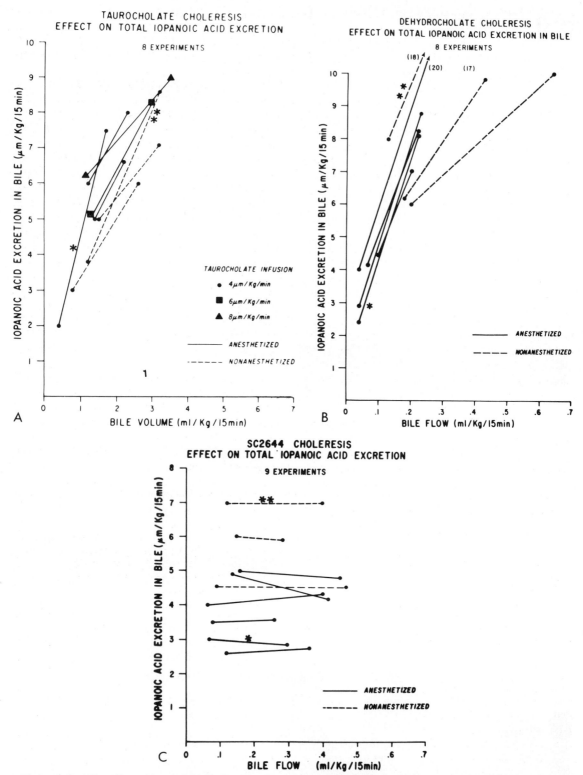

Figure 3–5. The effect of increased bile flow due to taurocholate *(A)*, dehydrocholate *(B)*, and SC2644 *(C)* on the rate of biliary excretion of iopanoate in dogs. The average 15-minute iopanoate excretion and the average 15-minute bile flow are plotted before and after the infusion of the choleretic. The failure of the choleresis produced by SC2644 to increase the rate of iopanoate excretion indicates that the increased excretion of iopanoate is due to the bile salts *per se* rather than the increase in bile flow. (From Berk, R. N., Goldberger, L. E., and Loeb, P. M.: Invest. Radiol. 9:7, 1974. Courtesy of J. B Lippincott Co., Publisher.)

acid, which may explain why the biliary excretion of ipodate and tyropanoate is not affected by biliary bile salt micelles. Likewise, the intravenous biliary contrast agents iodipamide and iotroxamide are highly soluble in aqueous solutions and also are not affected by bile salt excretion.[36] However, the relative solubility of the conjugated form of iopanoate, ipodate, and tyropanoate is not known, and the necessity for bile salt micelles in order to solubilize these compounds in bile also has not been determined.

Another possible mechanism by which bile salts could facilitate the biliary excretion of iopanoate is by means of a direct action on the rate-limiting transport protein. This was postulated originally by Forker and Gibson as the mechanism by which bile salts enhance the biliary excretion of BSP.[83] They suggest that a carrier for BSP on the canalicular membrane would bind taurocholate and by an allosteric interaction produce, in effect, a second carrier with a greater capacity to transport BSP. Allosteric means a physical change in the geometry of protein molecules or enzymes that alters the efficiency of the catalytic function of the enzyme. Since ipodate and tyropanoate are similar in chemical structure to iopanoate, one might expect them to bind the same transport proteins and to be affected by the same factors as iopanoate (Fig. 3–1). Consequently, the failure of bile salts to facilitate the excretion of ipodate and tyropanoate is evidence against an allosteric interaction of bile salts with a carrier protein.[74] Goresky and colleagues found a similar, but quantitatively smaller, effect of bile salts on the maximum rate of biliary excretion of bilirubin.[84] These investigators postulated that, with low rates of taurocholate infusion, the extraction of taurocholate is completed in the periphery of the hepatic lobule, and, with higher bile salt infusion rates, the centrilobular canaliculi are utilized for the excretion of bile salts. Goresky and coworkers suggested that the recruitment of the centrilobular area of the liver increases the capacity of the liver to transport bilirubin.[85]

Studies in dogs indicate that there is a linear relation between the transport maximum of iopanoate and the rate of bile salt excretion, so that, for each additional micromole of bile salt excreted in bile, there is an increase of 0.84 μmol in the transport maximum of iopanoate.[78, 86] Unfortunately, this coupling of bile salts and iopanoate in bile during maximum excretion of iopanoate does not provide information that allows one to determine whether

bile salts act by affecting a transport protein; by concentrating iopanoate in bile by means of micellar solubilization; or by influencing uptake, conjugation, or intracellular transport of iopanoate.

However, it is clear that in the absence of circulating bile salts the biliary excretion rate of iopanoate is markedly reduced. Thus, when a patient is fasting or on a low-fat and low-protein diet, sequestration of the bile salt pool in the gallbladder results in a reduction of the biliary excretion rate of bile salts. This not only impairs the intestinal solubility and absorption of iopanoate, as noted earlier, but limits the rate of biliary excretion of iopanoate. Consequently, the effect of bile salts on the biliary excretion of iopanoate must be taken into consideration when iopanoic acid is compared with other biliary contrast agents (Table 3–3). Studies in dogs show that when the oral agents are infused intravenously, the transport maximum for ipodate (Oragrafin) and tyropanoate (Bilopaque) is greater than that for iopanoate (Telepaque) at a low bile salt infusion rate (0.5 μmol/min/kg) (Fig. 3–6).[74, 76] At a higher bile salt infusion rate (2.0 μmol/min/kg), the transport maximum for iopanoate is not different from that for ipodate or tyropanoate. However, with an even higher infusion rate of bile salt (3.5 μmol/min/kg), the transport maximum of iopanoate becomes greater than that of the other compounds.[86] The excretion rate of bile salts in humans during fasting and during eating is variable, but in the fasting state bile salt excretion is probably 0.5

Table 3–3. MAXIMUM BILIARY EXCRETION RATES OF BILIARY CONTRAST AGENTS*

Taurocholate Infusion	0.5†	2.0†
Oral contrast agents		
Iopanoic acid‡	0.671	1.326
Ipodate‡	1.472	1.419
Tyropanoate	0.956	1.116
Intravenous contrast agents		
Iodipamide§	1.201	1.146
Ioglycamide‖	0.977	††
Iodoxamate§	1.595	††
Iotroxamide**	1.626	1.662

*Derived from the relation of plasma concentration to biliary excretion rate in chronic bile-fistula dogs.
†μmol/min/kg.
‡See reference 74.
§See reference 35.
‖See reference 75.
**See reference 36.
††Not studied.

BILIARY EXCRETION VS. INFUSION RATE

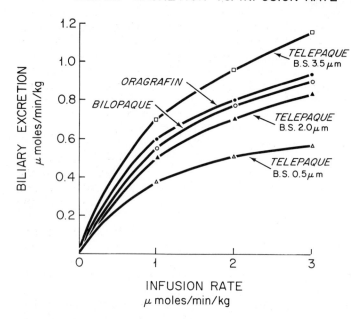

Figure 3–6. Relation between biliary excretion rate and infusion rate of iopanoic acid (Telepaque) at three different bile salt (BS) infusion rates (μmoles/min/kg) and ipodate (Oragrafin) and tyropanoate (Bilopaque). BS infusion rates have no effect on Oragrafin or Bilopaque (see Table 3–3).

μmol/min/kg or less, in which case the biliary excretion of iopanoate would be less than that of the other two agents.[87]

Despite the similarity in structure of the intravenous contrast agents, differences in the transport maximums for these agents can be detected in animals (Table 3–3).[27, 35, 36, 75] Two new agents, iodoxamate and iotroxamide, have maximum biliary excretion rates that exceed those of iodipamide and ioglycamide by significant amounts (Fig. 3–7). It is of interest that the transport maximum per micromole of the intravenous agents is approximately equal to that of the oral agents. However, the rate of excretion of iodine is twice as great with the intravenous agents, since they contain six iodine atoms per molecule rather than three (Fig. 3–1).

DETERMINANTS OF CONCENTRATION IN BILE DUCTS

In the bile ducts, there is little or no reabsorption of water immediately after hepatic excretion. Therefore, the concentration of bil-

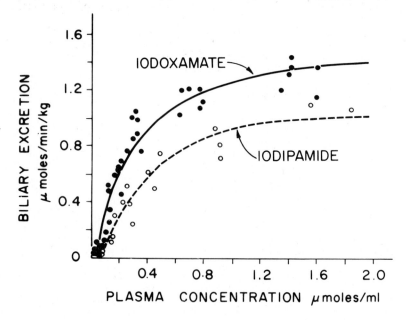

Figure 3–7. Relation between the biliary excretion of iodoxamate (solid circles, solid line) and iodipamide (open circles, dashed line) and the plasma concentration. The biliary excretion rate of iodoxamate (which is similar to iotroxamide) exceeds iodipamide (which is similar to ioglycamide) at any given plasma concentration. (From Berk, R. N., et al.: Radiology *119*:529, 1976. Courtesy of Radiological Society of North America, Publisher.)

iary contrast agents as they are excreted in the bile ducts is determined by the rate of excretion of the contrast agent, the choleresis associated with the excretion of the agent, and the basal bile flow (bile flow independent of that associated with the contrast material).[2, 4]

Bile appears to be formed by diffusion of water secondary to the active excretion of solutes across the liver-cell canalicular membrane (canalicular bile flow) and across the bile ductular epithelium (ductular bile flow).[55] Canalicular bile flow is the sum of choleresis associated with bile salt excretion (bile salt–dependent canalicular bile flow) and choleresis independent of bile salts (bile salt–independent canalicular bile flow). The intravenous cholangiographic contrast agents, unfortunately, are all potent choleretics. They all stimulate water flow across the bile canaliculus, which is independent of bile salt excretion.[35, 36, 75, 88, 88a] This imposes an inherent limitation on the concentration of contrast material that can be achieved in the bile ducts. Each millimole of each of the four intravenous agents is coupled with approximately 22 ml of water as it is excreted in bile (Fig. 3–8). If there were no basal bile flow, the concentration of the contrast materials would, therefore, be constant and equal for any excretion rate, 1 mmol/22 ml or 45 μmol/ml.[35] However, the concentration of the contrast agents in bile is less than this theoretic value because of the dilutional effect of the basal bile flow, as illustrated by the family of curves in Figure 3–9. Here the bile concentration of iodipamide is compared with that of iodoxamate at increasing basal bile flows. The curves for ioglycamide

would be similar to those for iodipamide, and the curves for iotroxamide would be similar to those for iodoxamate. The greater the basal bile flow, the greater the dilution of the contrast material. When smaller amounts of the contrast material are excreted in bile at slower infusion rates, the basal bile flow constitutes a larger proportion of the total bile flow and the dilution of the contrast material is greater. At higher rates of excretion of the contrast agent, the basal bile flow contributes a smaller fraction of the total bile flow, and the dilution of the contrast agent is less. This effect of the basal bile flow results in a hyperbolic relation between the biliary concentration and the plasma concentration.

When studies were performed in bile-fistula dogs infusing sodium taurocholate at a low infusion rate (0.5 μmol/min/kg), little difference in the biliary concentration could be detected among the four intravenous agents at high infusion rates of the contrast agents (Fig. 3–9, curve C).[35, 36, 75] Only at low infusion rates of the contrast agent does the more rapid excretion rate of iodoxamate (or iotroxamide) produce higher concentrations of contrast material in bile than iodipamide (or ioglycamide). When the basal bile flow is reduced by decreasing bile acid excretion rates, the concentration of the contrast agents in bile is increased. However, the differences between the intravenous contrast agents become less apparent, as illustrated by curve B in Figure 3–9.

The oral contrast agents are much less potent choleretics than are the intravenous contrast agents (Fig. 3–10). Iopanoic acid is not a choleretic, and the concentration of iopanoate

Figure 3–8. Relation between bile flow and biliary excretion of iodoxamate (solid circles, solid line) and iodipamide (open circles, dashed line). (From Berk, R. N., et al.: Radiology *119*:529, 1976. Courtesy of Radiological Society of North America, Publisher.)

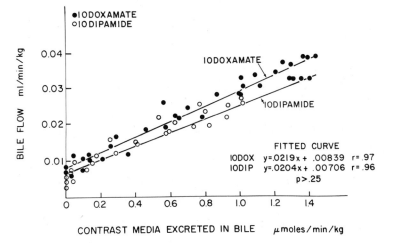

BILE FLOW VS. EXCRETION IN BILE

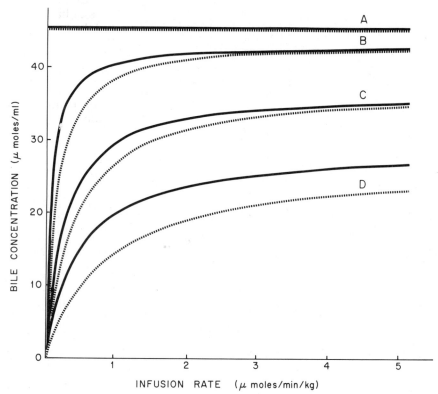

Figure 3–9. The theoretic relation between the bile concentration of iodoxamide (solid line) and iodipamide (dashed line) and the infusion rate derived from experiments in dogs. Line A represents the bile concentration when there is no basal bile flow. Curve B is the calculated bile concentrations when the basal bile flow is low (.002 ml/min/kg). Curve C represents actual experimental data when the basal bile flow is 0.0068 ml/min/kg. Curve D is the calculated bile concentrations when the basal bile flow is high (0.02 ml/min/kg). (From Berk, R. N., et al.: Radiology *119*:529, 1976. Courtesy of Radiological Society of North America, Publisher.)

in bile is determined only by the dilutional effect of the basal bile flow.[71, 76, 89] However, any reduction in the basal bile flow caused by reduction in bile salt excretion rate also decreases the excretion rate of iopanoate, since the excretion rate of iopanoate is influenced by bile salt excretion rate. In experiments in dogs, because bile salts are more efficient in stimulating water flow than in augmenting iopanoate excretion, the concentration of iopa-

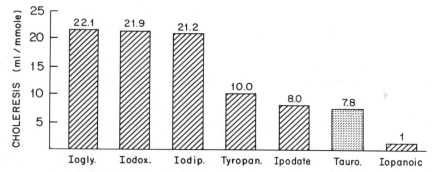

Figure 3–10. Choleresis produced by the excretion of contrast agents and taurocholate in unanesthetized bile-fistula dogs. Iogly. = ioglycamide; iodox. = iodoxamate; iodip. = iodipamide; tyropan. = tyropanoate; tauro. = taurocholate.

noate in bile is decreased when additional bile salts are infused.[76] Ipodate and tyropanoate are associated with approximately 8 ml/mmol of compound excreted in bile.[78] The maximum concentrations achieved in bile of iopanoate, tyropanoate, and ipodate are approximately twice those of the intravenous cholangiographic agents on a molar basis. However, when one takes into consideration that there are only three iodine atoms per molecule for the oral agents, compared with six iodine atoms per molecule for the intravenous agents, it is apparent that the biliary concentration of iodine per milliliter is approximately the same for the two groups of agents (Fig. 3–1). Since the biliary concentration of iodine is the major determinant of the degree of radiographic opacification, the use of the oral agents, administered intravenously, would appear to offer no advantage over the agents currently used for intravenous cholangiography.

CONCENTRATION IN THE GALLBLADDER

When the cystic duct is patent, although a small portion of the biliary contrast materials is lost by flow of bile into the duodenum, most of the contrast material enters the gallbladder. Once in the gallbladder, the contrast material can be concentrated by the reabsorption of water by the gallbladder mucosa. A concentration of 1.2 to 6.5 mg I/ml is required in the gallbladder for radiographic visualization.[90, 91] When the contrast material enters the gallbladder, it is diluted by the bile already present there. After intravenous cholangiography, the contrast material is sufficiently concentrated to visualize the bile ducts, but once it enters the gallbladder it is dispersed and diluted. Visualization of the gallbladder may be present but usually is faint, at least initially. With the oral cholecystographic agents, the contrast material is excreted by the liver in low concentrations owing to the slow rate of intestinal absorption, and the bile ducts usually are not visualized. The gallbladder becomes radiopaque over a period of many hours, as it fills with contrast material that is gradually concentrated.

With iopanoic acid, peak radiographic opacification of the gallbladder occurs 14 to 19 hours after ingestion of the contrast material.[92] Poor radiographic opacification of the gallbladder during cholecystography could be due to the fact that the radiographs are routinely obtained 12 hours after ingestion of the mate-rial. In some cases this interval may not allow enough time for optimal concentration in the gallbladder. With tyropanoate, peak radiographic opacification occurs at ten hours, so the radiographs should be made earlier with this contrast agent.[22, 23] It is likely that if the patient were fasted for 6 to 12 hours after the administration of an intravenous cholangiographic agent, better visualization of the gallbladder could be obtained when sufficient time had elapsed for concentration of the contrast material.

Since the first cholecystogram was reported by Graham and Cole in 1924, failure of the gallbladder to reabsorb water and to concentrate the contrast material has been assumed to be the major cause of nonvisualization of the gallbladder when cystic duct obstruction or extra biliary problems are eliminated. Hence, the term "nonfunctioning gallbladder" is used in this circumstance. In 1972, Berk and Wheeler studied *in vitro* water reabsorption in 43 human gallbladders with cholecystitis and cholelithiasis immediately after cholecystectomy.[94] By utilizing a perfusion apparatus, the rate of water reabsorption *in vitro* was compared with the results of the preoperative cholecystograms. From these studies, it is apparent that some gallbladders that fail to visualize on cholecystography have the ability to transport water normally *in vitro* (cystic duct obstruction excluded). Therefore, in some cases, nonvisualization cannot be attributed to failure of the gallbladder to reabsorb water and to concentrate the contrast material. In his classic review of gallbladder physiology in 1934, Ivy suggested that reabsorption of contrast material by the gallbladder mucosa could also contribute to nonvisualization.[95] Indeed, Berk and Lasser were able to demonstrate that conjugated iopanoate is readily reabsorbed from the inflamed gallbladder.[96] Thus, nonvisualization of the gallbladder may result from inadequate concentration of contrast material in the gallbladder due to failure to reabsorb water and/or the contrast material from the gallbladder.

GASTROINTESTINAL EXCRETION

After administration of an oral biliary contrast agent, most of the contrast material that is not absorbed and the contrast material that has been conjugated in the liver, stored in the biliary tree, and excreted into the duodenum eventually appears in the stool. Although the more polar glucuronide conjugate permeates poorly through the lipid barrier of the intestine, bacteria in the intestinal tract, primarily in the colon, may deconjugate the contrast material and permit the more lipid-soluble unconjugated compound to be reabsorbed. Goldberg and associates placed conjugated iopanoate in the duodenum of a dog and found that approximately 40 per cent of the iopanoate was absorbed and excreted in bile over eight hours.[97] Schroder and Rooney found iopanoate in human stools five days after administration of an oral dose.[98] During this period about 65 per cent of the administered dose was recovered in the stool. These studies do not delineate whether conjugated iopanoate is reabsorbed or whether the iopanoate is deconjugated in the intestine and reabsorbed as unconjugated iopanoate. The fraction of the intravenous contrast materials that enters the biliary tree would most likely be entirely excreted in the stool, since these highly water-soluble compounds essentially are not absorbed from the intestinal tract.

RENAL EXCRETION

Renal excretion is the other major route of elimination of the biliary contrast agents. Data currently available suggest that only the water-soluble conjugated form of the oral contrast agents appears in urine.[65, 66] Thus, iopanoate must first be taken up by the liver, conjugated with glucuronide, and re-entered in the plasma before it can be excreted in the urine. The water-soluble intravenous contrast agents are excreted directly by the kidneys without chemical modification by the liver. Above a minimal plasma concentration, the renal excretion of both the intravenous contrast agents and the oral agents is linearly related to the plasma concentration of the compound.[27, 35, 36, 74-76] With the oral contrast agents, this is more accurately related to the concentration of the conjugated form of the contrast agent in plasma. Therefore, unlike excretion in bile, the urinary excretion of the biliary contrast materials appears to be a passive process across the glomerulus or renal tubule.

When one of the oral contrast materials iopanoic acid, ipodate, or tyropanoate is infused intravenously in unanesthetized bile-fistula dogs in acute experiments, no more than 5 per cent of the infused dose is excreted in the urine.[74, 76] However, in studies in human subjects, 15 to 35 per cent of an orally administered dose of iopanoate is excreted in the urine.[66, 98] The amount excreted in the urine for each 24-hour period is about one-half that for the preceding 24 hours, so that by the fifth day only traces of iopanoate appear in the urine. If these studies are accurate, they suggest that in the several days after administration of iopanoic acid, stored (probably in the liver) conjugated iopanoate diffuses back into the plasma and is excreted in urine or that some conjugated compound excreted in the bile into the duodenum is reabsorbed into the circulation and is subsequently excreted in the urine. It is of clinical interest that iopanoate glucuronide in the urine produces a false-positive protein-precipitation test for albumin; positive reactions should be verified by a colorimetric dipstick method.[99]

With the intravenous biliary contrast agents, the urine excretion rate also is linearly related to the plasma concentration or infusion rate of the compound (Fig. 3–11).[27, 35, 36, 75] Studies in dogs have demonstrated that at high infusion rates, more than 20 per cent of the infused dose is excreted in the urine. With slow infusion rates, less than 5 per cent of the infused dose is excreted in the urine. As the maximum capacity of the liver for excretion of the contrast agents is approached with faster rates of

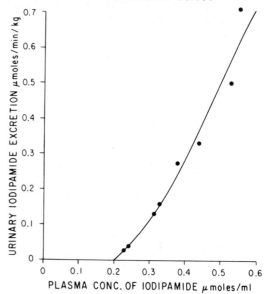

Figure 3–11. Relation between plasma concentration and urinary excretion of iodipamide. (From Loeb, P. M., et al.: Gastroenterology 68:554, 1975. Courtesy of the Williams & Wilkins Co., Publisher.)

infusion of the contrast agent, the biliary excretion rate of the compound is increased by progressively smaller increments, and greater proportions of the infused dose appear in the urine.[27] In human studies, between 15 and 20 per cent of the administered dose of iodipamide is eliminated in the urine.[30, 100, 101] This explains why a pyelogram is sometimes obtained during intravenous cholangiography. Obviously, the percentage of the infused dose that appears in the urine is directly related to the rate of administration of the compound. From experimental data in bile-fistula dogs, it appears that biliary concentrations adequate for radiographic visualization can be obtained with low plasma concentrations and minimal renal excretion.[27] Studies in dogs with experimentally produced liver injury or partial biliary obstruction reveal that biliary excretion of iodipamide is reduced and renal excretion is increased.[102, 103]

Attempts to improve radiographic opacification of the biliary tree during intravenous cholangiography by blocking the renal excretion of iodipamide with probenecid have been unsuccessful.[104]

TOXICITY

Serious toxic reactions are apparently much more common with the intravenous contrast agents than with the oral contrast agents. In a survey by Ansell, iodipamide was associated with a higher incidence of toxicity than the renal contrast materials.[105] In his series, there was 1 death per 5000 examinations with iodipamide, compared with 1 death per 40,000 examinations with intravenous pyelograms. However, in an uncontrolled survey of this sort, it is impossible to validate any conclusion statistically. The primary reactions associated with iodipamide are skin rash, cardiovascular collapse, and renal dysfunction.[105-113] The mechanisms involved in the production of adverse reactions have not been clearly defined but probably involve hypersensitivity reactions, direct cellular toxicity, critical enzyme inhibition, or vasoactive alterations in hemodynamics.[17, 53, 54] It is generally assumed that the incidence of adverse reactions is related to the dose and rate of administration of the contrast material. However, as noted hereafter, this is difficult to confirm in clinical studies. If toxicity is related to allergic phenomena, the incidence of adverse reactions may have no relation to dose or rate of admin-

istration of the compound. Peters, Hodgson, and Donovan, in an uncontrolled study, found that toxic reactions were reduced to 6 per cent in 1,830 patients given the antihistamine chlorpheniramine (6 to 10 mg intramuscularly) five minutes prior to the intravenous injection of iodipamide, whereas 24 per cent of 854 patients who did not receive the premedication had a reaction.[109]

With the oral cholecystographic contrast materials, significant morbidity and mortality are rare. Poor intestinal absorption of iopanoic acid may be a major factor in preventing serious toxic reactions when large and/or multiple doses are given. Minor side effects, including nausea, vomiting, and diarrhea, occur in nearly 50 per cent of patients administered any of the oral cholecystographic agents.[19-23, 114-118] These problems appear to be dose related and may be due to a direct effect on the intestinal mucosa. Transient diarrhea is the most frequent side effect and occurs most commonly with iopanoic acid. The diarrhea may be related to failure to absorb the latter. Although the cathartic action of the oral contrast agents may eliminate fecal material from the colon overlying the gallbladder and improve radiographic visualization, care should be used in patients with inflammatory bowel disease in whom subsequent diarrhea may be severe.

Impairment of renal function can occur after both oral and intravenous contrast studies and is the most serious toxic reaction.[105-110, 119-125] Renal toxicity usually occurs after oral cholecystography in patients given large or multiple doses of the contrast materials, in those administered a combination of an oral and intravenous cholangiographic contrast material, and/or in those with associated liver disease. Three of the five deaths associated with iodipamide reported by Ansell had an oral cholecystogram within 24 hours of an intravenous cholangiogram.[105] Simultaneous administration of two contrast agents, large doses of one agent, or impaired biliary excretion appears to be related to renal injury because, in each of these circumstances, renal excretion of the contrast agent would most likely be increased. It is of interest that nephrotoxicity following oral cholecystography often occurs in patients with previously normal renal function.[122] Careful monitoring of renal function may reveal a higher incidence of minor renal injury.

Current data do not provide information to help distinguish the mechanism by which the contrast agents produce nephrotoxicity.[126] Obstructive crystalluria, direct cellular toxicity, renal vasoconstriction, and an immunologic reaction are all potential mechanisms. The oral cholecystographic materials are potent uricosuric agents that enhance secretion of uric acid by the tubules and are comparable with some drugs routinely used in the treatment of gout.[127, 128] The uricosuric action of iopanoic acid persists for five or six days and results in a transient decrease in serum uric acid.[129] The intravenous cholangiographic agent iodipamide appears to have a less potent uricosuric action that lasts only for one day.[129] Obstructive crystalluria from precipitated uric acid in the kidney has not been directly demonstrated to be a cause of nephrotoxicity. Renal complications do appear to be related to the dose of contrast agent and to oliguria. Precipitation of contrast materials in the renal tubules is also a possible, but unproved, cause of nephrotoxicity. This might be expected to occur in the presence of an acidic and concentrated urine after the administration of the less water-soluble oral contrast agents.

Renal injury may result from systemic hypotension produced by a contrast agent.[130, 131] Hypotension has been reported to be more frequent in patients with impaired hepatic excretion of a contrast agent.[122, 131] Renal ischemia also could result from hypotension, especially if the patient is dehydrated, and adequate hydration is advisable in those undergoing biliary contrast studies. Excessive doses and combinations of oral and intravenous contrast agents should be avoided. Caution must be used in giving cholecystographic agents to patients with liver disease. In hyperuricemic patients, alkalinization of the urine as well as hydration is recommended to prevent formation of urate crystals.

DOSE AND METHOD OF ADMINISTRATION

Oral Cholecystographic Agents

Although oral cholecystography is a valuable technique for the detection of gallbladder disease, there are significant limitations to its use in clinical practice. When iopanoic acid is administered in a single dose of 3.0 gm after a low-fat meal, as many as 47 per cent of patients with apparently normal gallbladders fail to have adequate radiographic opacification of the gallbladder.[24, 132-136] This occurs even if one excludes those patients in whom there is an obvious cause for nonvisualization such as failure to take the contrast material, vomiting, delayed gastric emptying, or impaired hepatic function (see Chapter 4). Therefore, a second dose of iopanoic acid is required in these patients before the presence of gallbladder disease can be established. An equally serious limitation of oral cholecystography is that in up to two-thirds of patients with acute pancreatitis, visualization of the gallbladder is not obtained despite the fact that the biliary tract subsequently is shown to be normal.

On the basis of current studies in experimental animals, it appears likely that the administration of a low-fat meal on the night of the examination or fasting the patient (as might be the treatment in pancreatitis or other acute abdominal problems) results in sequestration of bile salts in the gallbladder and impaired absorption and biliary excretion of iopanoic acid. In addition, it is possible, but not likely, that in this situation the gallbladder is filled with bile so that an adequate amount of contrast material cannot enter the gallbladder. This theory of cholecystostasis was proposed originally by Stewart and Ryan[137] and later discussed by Zboralske and Amberg.[138]

The results of clinical studies provide indirect and direct evidence that bile salts are important in the adequate opacification of the gallbladder with iopanoic acid. Zboralske and Amberg found that a high percentage of normal volunteers did not have adequate radiographic visualization of the gallbladder if placed on low-fat diets.[138] Stanley and colleagues reported that only 47 per cent of patients given iopanoic acid with a nonfat meal had satisfactory first-day examinations compared with 70 per cent when the iopanoic acid was given with a high-fat meal.[24] Mauthe, however, failed to detect any difference in the incidence of first-dose visualization in patients given iopanoic acid with a fatty meal compared with those in whom iopanoic acid was given with a low-fat meal.[135] Since he administered 0.5 gm of iopanoic acid per 20 lb of body weight, it appears that these patients generally were given more than the usual 3-gm dose of iopanoic acid. This larger dose may have overcome the difficulties in intestinal absorption and hepatic excretion that would be expected to occur in the absence of circulating bile salts. Studies by Roller and associates indicate that a high percentage of nonjaundiced patients with acute pancreatitis can be successfully examined if the oral cholecystogram is performed after they have been on a solid diet for two days.[139] Thus, when iopanoic acid is administered, it is rational to feed the patient a high-fat diet before the tablets are administered. Obviously, the patient should then be fasted until the radiographs are obtained to prevent evacuation of the iopanoate from the gallbladder. However, it also is apparent that factors other than lack of bile salts are responsible for some cases of impaired visualization of the gallbladder on first-dose visualization, since, in 30 per cent of the normal patients studied by Stanley and coworkers, gallbladder visualization was not obtained initially when the iopanoic acid was given after a high-fat meal.[24]

Increasing the dose of iopanoic acid is another possible way to improve visualization of the gallbladder. However, this will also increase the likelihood of the patient's having a significant reaction. Although the optimal dose of iopanoic acid has not been sufficiently delineated, a double dose (6 gm) would not appear to be warranted, since most reported cases of renal failure due to oral cholecystographic materials occurred in patients receiving high doses of the compounds.

Burhenne and Obata circumvent the necessity of performing a second cholecystogram in patients with initial nonvisualization or poor visualization of the gallbladder by administering two consecutive doses of contrast material before the radiographs are made (see Chapter 4).[140] Their results suggest that failure of the gallbladder to opacify under these circumstances is reliable evidence of gallbladder disease, if extrabiliary causes of nonvisualization (such as liver disease) are excluded. The reason why two consecutive doses of contrast material may be successful in opacifying the gallbladder, when a single-dose examination fails, is not completely understood. If the patients remain on a low-fat diet throughout the study, the additional dose and time may permit a larger fraction of the iopanoic acid to be absorbed and may allow more time for hepatic excretion and gallbladder concentration. If the patient ingests a fatty meal after the initial dose of iopanoic acid, the second dose may be more efficiently absorbed and excreted in bile, even though the fatty meal would result in emptying from the gallbladder any contrast material that might have accumulated after the first dose. Another method to reduce first-dose nonvisualization is to fractionate the dose over a six-hour period the day before the study, as reported by Koehler and Kyaw (see Chapter 4).[141]

The use of oral contrast agents other than iopanoic acid is probably the most promising mode of improving oral cholecystography. Ipodate and tyropanoate, because of their greater solubility in water and because their biliary excretion is not affected by bile salts, do not appear to depend on the enterohepatic circulation of bile salts for a successful cholecystogram.[74] Although clinical results of studies with these agents are interpreted optimistically, adequately controlled, double-blind studies are not available.[16, 20-25, 142] Stanley and associates did not find that visualization of the gallbladder with iocetamic acid or tyropanoate was affected by the presence or absence of fat in the diet.[24] However, visualization of the gallbladder after a single dose of these agents was not superior to visualization when iopanoic acid was administered with a fatty meal.

Therefore, if iopanoic acid is to be used, it should be administered with a fatty meal and radiographs should be obtained no sooner than 14 hours later to allow adequate time for visualization. If oral cholecystography must be performed in a patient who is on a low-fat diet, who is fasting, or who perhaps has a malabsorptive state owing to bile salt deficiency, it would seem more logical to utilize one of the more water-soluble agents, such as tyropanoate or ipodate, whose biliary excretion does not depend on bile salts.

Intravenous Cholangiographic Agents

The degree of bile duct opacification is determined by a number of interrelated factors.[24] Impaired hepatic clearance of the contrast agent due to liver disease or bile duct obstruction, the diameter of the common duct, the rate of emptying of the biliary tree, and radiographic technical factors are all important. The rate of biliary excretion and the concentration of the contrast agent in bile are related to the pharmacokinetic properties of the contrast agent. The concentration of the contrast agent alone does not determine the degree of radiographic visualization. For example, radiographic opacification of the kidney during intravenous pyelography is more accurately related to the amount of contrast material in the renal pelvis.[143] This would also appear to apply to opacification of the biliary tree. The x-ray beam "measures" the total number of iodine atoms in its path, not the concentration. Therefore, a bile duct distended with a large volume of a contrast agent would be more radiopaque than a duct containing a smaller volume of contrast material at the same concentration. Therefore, if experimental data in animals can be applied to man, iodoxamate and iotroxamide have more desirable pharmacokinetic properties than iodipamide or ioglycamide.[35, 36] The greater biliary excretion rates achieved with iodoxamate and iotroxamide by any given infusion rate, although not necessarily producing significantly higher biliary concentrations, would cause more rapid filling of the biliary tree, perhaps distend it more fully, and wash out pre-existing nonopaque bile more rapidly.

With each of the intravenous contrast agents, the rate of hepatic excretion is limited by a transport maximum, so that infusion rates of the compounds that exceed the transport maximums result in higher plasma concentrations of the compound and increased renal excretion without increasing bile duct opacification. Furthermore, it is likely that toxicity from these agents is related, at least in part, to plasma concentration and renal excretion. The dose of iodipamide (the only agent approved for use in the U.S.) as recommended by the manufacturers is 20 ml of the 52 per cent solution (6.8 mmol) injected over a ten-minute period. This would be approximately 0.3 ml/kg (.097 mmol/kg) in a 70-kg man. This dose is derived from studies by Fischer in dogs in which it was found that a bolus dose of iodipamide larger than 0.6 ml/kg did not result in significantly higher iodine concentrations in bile.[100, 104, 144] Based on these experiments, a dose of iodipamide equivalent to 0.6 ml/kg (40 ml) is often used in man. However, the dose of 0.3 ml/kg given over even 30 minutes would be 0.01 ml/min/kg, or 9.7 μmol/min/kg. This is nine times greater than the dose estimated (1 μmol/min/kg) in dogs that would produce a biliary concentration required for adequate radiographic visualization (13 to 16 μmol/ml).[27] This dose, of course, does not take into consideration the amount of iodipamide needed to achieve equilibrium between vascular and extravascular compartments or reduction in the transport capacity of the liver for contrast material in the presence of liver or biliary tract disorders.

These findings in dogs provide experimental support for the clinical attempt of investigators to administer iodipamide by slow infusions. Slower infusions will produce lower plasma concentrations that do not exceed the maximum excretory capacity of the liver, less urine excretion, and a greater proportion of the administered dose entering the bile. The slower infusions can be stopped before the total dose is administered if opacification of the biliary tree is obtained or if an adverse reaction occurs.[145, 146] However, contrary to what has been suggested by other investigators,[147] slower infusion rates do not allow more biliary excretion and less urine excretion of the contrast agent by means of more complete binding to albumin. Binding to albumin of the contrast agent limits the biliary excretion as well as the renal excretion.[56] The choleretic effect of iodipamide is not reduced by slow infusion techniques, since the choleresis associated with the excretion of the contrast agent is equal over all ranges of excretion in bile. Reducing the rate of excretion of iodipamide decreases the concentration of the contrast material in bile by increasing the dilutional effect of basal bile flow, as discussed previously.[88, 148, 149] Slow infusion rates have no apparent effect on bile salt excretion and do not decrease basal bile flow.[35, 36] The initial suggestion that the intravenous administration of hypertonic glucose with the iodipamide would cause an increase in concentration of contrast material in bile has not been confirmed.[150-152] Moss, Nelson, and Amberg, using bile-fistula dogs, showed that dilution of iodipamide with 5 per cent glucose hypertonic glucose, sorbitol, or saline had no effect on biliary iodine concentrations.[152] Whitney and Bell, using a monkey model, found that when iodipamide was diluted with 20 per cent glucose or normal saline, there was no effect on the concentration of iodipamide in bile.[149]

The finding that basal bile flow dilutes the contrast agent in bile and produces lower concentrations suggests that attempts should be made to reduce basal bile flow in patients having intravenous cholangiography.[35, 75] Therefore, it would be rational to maintain patients on a low-fat, low-protein diet prior to intravenous cholangiography, since these substances cause release of cholecystokinin, which stimulates the gallbladder to contract and releases bile salts into the enterohepatic circulation.[153] If bile salts can be retained in the gallbladder, the bile salt–dependent portion of the basal bile flow will be reduced, the concentration of iodipamide in the biliary tree will be greater, and radiographic opacification of the bile ducts will be improved. Other potential mechanisms to reduce basal bile flow include administration of cholestyramine to bind bile salts in the intestine, preventing their enterohepatic circulation, and the use of anticholinergic drugs to reduce the dilutional effect of ductular bile flow.[35]

Most of the reported clinical studies that

attempt to define the optimal dose and rate of administration of intravenous contrast agents have been performed with iodipamide, and most offer little useful information because they do not provide controls and because they fail to randomize or properly blind variables, especially the duration, stage, or severity of hepatobiliary disease. The patients in most reports are not properly matched for age, the presence of associated disease (especially alcoholism with concomitant liver disease or pancreatitis), and the recent administration of other radiographic contrast materials. Often the studies involve a comparison of one dose of iodipamide given by bolus with a different dose for slow infusion. Radiographic technique and the technical quality of the radiographs may have more influence on the degree of opacification of the biliary tract than the method of administration and the dose of the contrast material.[154] The time at which the radiographs are made, the total length of the examination, and the use of tomography are not discussed in many studies. Finally, the methods of determination of the relative degree of radiographic opacification are subjective. In many cases the radiographs apparently were interpreted with full knowledge of the dose and method of administration of the contrast agent. It is not always clear if the common duct or gallbladder opacification is used for assessment of visualization. Side effects also are difficult to evaluate, since the definition and method of detection of toxicity are not always precise and vary among different authors.

Despite these obstacles, some attempt has been made from the reports in the literature to assess the effect of dose and duration of infusion on the degree of opacification and the incidence of side effects (Tables 3–4 and 3–5).[4] There are no controlled studies to determine whether increasing the dose of a bolus injection of iodipamide (administered in less than ten minutes) more than 20 ml provides better radiographic opacification or an increased incidence of side effects. Only two reports are available that compare a 20-ml bolus injection of iodipamide with 20 ml infused over longer periods, and the results of the two studies are conflicting.[146, 155] Scholz, Johnston, and Wise found a slightly lower incidence of both good visualization and side effects when 20 ml of iodipamide were infused over 30 minutes compared with a bolus injection of 20 ml.[155] Sinclair reported that the side effects were reduced and that the incidence of

good visualization increased when about 20 ml of iodipamide were infused at much slower rates so that the infusion lasted as long as 143 minutes.[146]

When a 20-ml bolus dose is compared with 20 ml or 40 ml infused over 10 to 60 minutes, no consistent difference can be detected in incidence of good visualization or reactions (Table 3–4).[130, 146, 155-157] However, in studies by Payne[158] and Isdale,[159] when the infusion dose was increased to 60 ml and the period of infusion to 60 to 120 minutes, it appeared that the incidence of good visualization was increased without an increase in reactions. However, since the frequency of good visualization with a 20-ml bolus was lower than in most other studies, 48 and 26 per cent, respectively, the results are difficult to assess. In one of the best-designed studies, McNulty found that a 40-ml infusion over 120 minutes, compared with a 40-ml bolus, resulted in improved radiographic visualization and a decrease in toxicity in patients with and without elevated serum bilirubin concentrations.[160] Thus, from available studies, there is no firm evidence that a 20-ml bolus dose results in less frequent radiographic visualization or a higher incidence of side effects than a 20-ml or larger dose of iodipamide infused over long periods. If a 40-ml dose is used, it is safer and more efficacious to infuse it over 120 minutes.

Only two studies are available to compare the effects of different infusions (Table 3–5). Sinclair compared doses of less than 20 ml given by infusion for up to 143 minutes with a 40-ml dose given over 15 to 20 minutes.[146] The larger dose infused more rapidly increased the rate of visualization and the incidence of reactions. Scholz, Johnston, and Wise found that 40 ml infused over 30 minutes increased both incidence of good visualization and toxicity when compared with 20 ml infused over 30 minutes.[155]

Therefore, the data are conflicting concerning the postulate that by increasing the dose or prolonging the infusion, the incidence of good visualization will be increased. However, it does appear that the more rapidly the dose is administered (in ml/min), the higher the incidence of toxicity if a dose larger than 20 ml is used. The reason for failure to improve visualization with all of these doses and infusion rates is probably that in virtually all of them, plasma concentrations are produced that saturate the transport process for hepatic excretion. Even a 20-ml dose infused over 150 minutes would be equivalent to an infusion

Table 3–4. CLINICAL STUDIES COMPARING BOLUS VERSUS INFUSION OF IODIPAMIDE*

Bolus Dose (ml)‡	Infusion Dose (ml)	Infusion Duration (min)	Reference	No. of Pat.	Serum Bilirubin (mg %)	Solution Amount (ml)	Solution Composition	Visualization (%) Good	Poor	None	Reactions (%) Moderate	Severe	Life Threat.	Author's Comments
20	≤20	≤143	Sinclair[146]	18	≤1.0	—	—	50	22	28	50	0	0	Infusion gives better visualization and fewer reactions.
				18	≤1.0	—	—	61	28	11	0	0	0	
20			Scholz[155]	150	V	—	—	52	37	11	6	4	0	Both infusions decrease ductal opacification; reactions unchanged.
	20	30		76	V	20	N saline	43	50	7	1	4	0	
	20	30		71	V	80	N saline	39	46	14	4	8	0	
20			Russell[156]	60	V	—	—	43	38	18	NG	NG	NG	Infusion gives better opacification.
	40	10		88	V	400	20% glucose	64	29	7	22	3	1	
20			Foy[130]	53	<4.0	—	—	58		←42→	NS	0	0	No significant difference between groups; injection favored.
	40	15		53	<4.0	50	N saline	57		←43→	4	0	0	
20			Sinclair[146]	18	≤1.0	—	—	50	22	28	50	0	0	Double-dose infusion too toxic; single-dose infusion favored.
	40	15–20		14	≤1.0	200	20% glucose	79	7	14	21	0	0	
20			Scholz[155]	150	V	—	—	52	37	11	6	4	0	Opacification not significantly higher with double-dose infusion; toxicity considerably higher.
	40	30		145	V	40	N saline	59	36	5	6	14	0	
20				25	<1.0	—	—	84	←(16→)		0	0	0	With all technical factors remaining the same, no difference in opacification; injection favored.
20				8	1.0–3.0	—	—	75	←(25→)		0	0	0	
20				6	>3.0	—	—	0	←(100→)		0	0	0	
		60	Howland[157]	97	<1.0	250	20% glucose	33	←(17→)		NS	0	0	
		60		22	1.0–3.0	250	20% glucose	60	←(40→)		NS	0	0	
		60		8	>3.0	250	20% glucose	0	←(100→)		NS	0	0	
20			Payne[158]	25	V	—	—	48	28	24	8	0	0	Infusion improves bile duct opacification; infusion favored.
	60	60		25	V	250	30% glucose	76	16	8	12	0	0	
20				42	<1.5	—	—	26	71	2	NS	NS	0	Infusion improves bile duct opacification; infusion favored.
20				8	>1.5	—	—	0	13	87	NS	NS	0	
	60	120		96	<1.0	250	5% glucose	78	20	2	NS	NS	0	
	60	120		20	1.0–3.0	250	5% glucose	40	60	0	NS	NS	0	
	60	120	Isdale[159]	6	3.0–5.5	250	5% glucose	33	67	0	NS	NS	0	
	60	120		8	>5.5	250	5% glucose	0	0	100	NS	NS	0	
40				25	≤1.0	—	—	64	24	12	50	0	0	Infusion improves quality of opacification and decreases renal excretion; adverse reactions are drastically reduced.
40			McNulty[160]	21	>1.0	—	—	29	43	28	50	0	0	
	40	120		25	≤1.0	250	5% glucose	92	8	0	0	0	0	
	40	120		21	>1.0	250	5% glucose	57	29	14	0	0	0	

*Adapted from reference 4.
†All data converted to 52 per cent solution of Cholografin (iodipamide).
‡Bolus dose = 10 min or less.
V = varied.
NS = not significant.
NG = not given.

Table 3–5. CLINICAL STUDIES COMPARING INFUSION METHODS OF IODIPAMIDE

Infusion			Serum	Solution		Visualization (%)			Reactions (%)			
Dose (ml)	Duration (min)	Reference	No. of Pat.	Bilirubin (mg %)	Amount (ml)	Composition	Good	Poor	None	Moderate	Severe	Life Threat.	Author's Comments
20	≤143	Sinclair[146]	18	≤1.0	—	—	61	28	11	0	0	0	Low-dose infusion decreases opacification but also decreases reactions; hence it is preferred.
40	15–20		14	≤1.0	200	20% glucose	79	7	14	21	0	0	
20	30	Scholz[155]	76	V	20	N saline	43	50	7	1	4	0	Double-dose infusion improves opacification significantly but also increases incidence of reactions.
20	30		71	V	80	N saline	39	46	14	4	8	0	
40	30		145	V	40	N saline	59	36	5	6	14	0	

V = varied.

rate of approximately 2 µl/min/kg in a 70-kg man (perhaps twice that needed to achieve satisfactory visualization).[27] Pharmacokinetic data derived from animals, using these relatively large doses, indicate no difference in the biliary iodine concentration when the bolus and infusion methods are compared.[149, 152] The clinical studies of Ansell and Faux[145] and Sinclair[146] indeed suggest that doses smaller than 20 ml can be administered successfully.

In jaundiced patients, the use of prolonged infusions with larger doses may be of value. Fuchs and Presig infused 40 ml of ioglycamide diluted in 500 ml of normal saline over 12 hours and achieved successful cholangiograms in about 75 per cent of 45 patients with previously unsuccessful conventional cholangiograms.[161] This occurred despite the fact that almost one-half of the patients had serum bilirubin concentrations greater than 2 mg per cent.

In normal patients, maximum visualization of the bile ducts with iodipamide and iodoxamate occurs at 45 to 60 minutes.[154] Experimental studies in animals indicate that impaired hepatic excretion of iodipamide results from liver injury or bile duct obstruction.[102, 103] In patients with liver disease, the radiographic examination should be continued for at least four hours if bile duct opacification is not obtained earlier. Robbins and coworkers found that radiographic opacification of the bile duct frequently was not obtained until four hours had passed.[33] In his classic monograph, Wise delineated the relation between visualization of the bile ducts and the level of the serum bilirubin.[5] Radiographic visualization was obtained in only 10 per cent of patients with a serum bilirubin concentration greater than 4 mg per cent.

It is possible that the two new agents iodoxamate and iotroxamide, in view of their apparently superior pharmacokinetic properties, will be useful in patients with biliary tract and/or liver disorders.[35, 36] The clinical experience with iodoxamate recently reported by Robbins and colleagues is encouraging.[33] They were able to obtain successful opacification of the bile ducts in 71 per cent of patients with serum bilirubin between 4 and 6 mg per cent and in 25 per cent of those with serum bilirubin between 6 and 8 mg per cent.

Until better data are available for iodipamide or until the effectiveness of iotroxamide and iodoxamate is further evaluated, it would appear that the best available technique for intravenous cholangiography would be to limit the amount of iodipamide to 20 ml in most cases. An infusion over 10 to 15 minutes would be most convenient and would facilitate control of toxicity, if it occurs. If larger doses of iodipamide are to be used, they should be infused over longer periods.

References

1. Berk, R. N., Loeb, P. M., and Goldberger, L. E.: Oral cholecystography with iopanoic acid. N. Engl. J. Med. *290*:204, 1974.
2. Berk, R. N., and Loeb, P. M.: Pharmacology and physiology of the biliary radiographic contrast materials. Sem. Roentgenol. *11*:147, 1976.
3. Berk, R. N., and Loeb, P. M.: Contrast materials for oral cholecystography. *In* Miller, R. E., and Skucas, T. S. (eds.): Radiological Contrast Agents. Baltimore: University Park Press. 1977, pp. 195–215.
4. Berk, R. N., Loeb, P. M., and Ellzey, B. A.: Contrast materials for intravenous cholangiography. *In* Miller, R. E., and Skucas, T. S. (eds.): Radiological Contrast Agents. Baltimore: University Park Press. 1977, pp. 223–236.
5. Wise, R. E.: Intravenous cholangiography. Springfield: Charles C Thomas, 1962.
6. Abel, J. J., and Rowntree, L. G.: On the pharmacological action of some phthaleins and their derivatives with special reference to their behavior as purgatives. J. Pharmacol. Exp. Ther. *1*:231, 1909.
7. Rous, P., and McMaster, P. O.: The concentrating function of the gallbladder. J. Exp. Med. *34*:47, 1921.
8. Graham, E. A., Cole, W. H., and Copher, G. H.: Visualization of gallbladder by the sodium salt of tetrabromophthalein. J.A.M.A. *82*:1777, 1924.
9. Graham, E. A.: The story of the development of cholecystography. Am. J. Surg. *12*:330, 1931.
10. Cole, W. H.: Historical features of cholecystography. Radiology *76*:354, 1961.
11. Archer, S. J., Hoppe, J. O., and Lewis, T. R.: The preparation and cholecystographic properties of some aminotriiodophenylalkanoic acids. J. Am. Pharm. Assoc. *40*:617, 1951.
12. Archer, S., et al.: The preparation of some iodinated phenyl- and pyridylalkanoic acids. J. Am. Pharm. Assoc. *40*:143, 1951.
13. Hoppe, J. O., and Archer, S.: Observations on a series of aryl triiodo alkanoic acid derivatives with particular reference to a new cholecystographic medium, Telepaque. Am. J. Roentgenol. *69*:631, 1953.
14. McChesney, E. W., and Hoppe, J. O.: Observations on the metabolism of iopanoic acid. Arch. Int. Pharmacodyn. Ther. *99*:127, 1954.
15. Lasser, E. C.: Pharmacodynamics of biliary contrast media. Radiol. Clin. North Am. *4*:511, 1966.
16. Hoppe, J. O., et al.: Sodium tyropanoate, a new oral cholecystographic agent. J. Med. Chem. *13*:997, 1970.
17. Knoefel, P. K.: Radiocontrast Agents, Vol. 2. New York: Pergamon Press, 1971.
18. Janes, J. O., Dietschy, J. M., Berk, R. N., and Loeb, P. M.: The physiochemical determinants of the rates of intestinal absorption of the oral cholecystographic contrast agents. Gastroenterology *76*:970, 1979.
19. Benisek, G. J., and Gunn, J. A.: A preliminary clinical evaluation of a new cholecystographic medium, Bilopaque. Am. J. Roentgenol. *88*:792, 1962.

20. Burhenne, H. J.: Bilopaque: a new cholecystographic medium. Radiology *81*:629, 1963.
21. Han, S. Y., and Witten, D. M.: Clinical trial of Bilopaque oral cholecystography. Evaluation of time of optimal and peak opacification of the gallbladder. Radiology *112*:529, 1974.
22. Moskowitz, H., Milikow, E., and Osmun, G. P.: Sodium tyropanoate evaluation of new oral cholecystographic agent. N.Y. State J. Med. *73*:271, 1973.
23. Parks, R. E.: Double blind study of four oral cholecystographic preparations. Radiology *112*:525, 1974.
24. Stanley, R. J., et al.: A comparison of three cholecystographic agents: a double study with and without a prior fatty meal. Radiology *112*:513, 1974.
25. Wishart, D. L., and Dotter, L. T.: Comparison of the opacifying characteristics and pharmacologic responses of iocetamic acid, a new oral cholecystographic agent with sodium tyropanoate. Am. J. Roentgenol. *119*:428, 1972.
26. Sperber, I., and Sperber, G.: Hepatic excretion of radiocontrast agents. In Knoefel, P. E. (ed.): International Encyclopedia of Pharmacology and Therapy, Section 76. New York: Pergamon Press, 1971.
27. Loeb, P. M., et al.: Biliary excretion of iodipamide. Gastroenterology *68*:554, 1975.
28. Corman, L. A., et al.: Human pharmacologic and pharmacokinetic studies of ioglycamate, a cholegraphic radiopaque agent. Curr. Ther. Res. *9*:99, 1967.
29. Brismar, J., Lindgren, P., and Saltzman, G. F.: Ioglycamide (Bilivistan) as a contrast medium for intravenous cholegraphy. Acta Radiol. *2*:129, 1971.
30. Benness, G. T., and Soschko, M.: Cholangiographic excretion studies. Iodipamide and ioglycamic acid comparison. Austr. Radiol. *6*:383, 1972.
31. Parkin, G. Q., and Herlinger, H.: Simplified cholangiography using ioglycamide. Gut *15*:268, 1974.
32. Cantwell, D. F.: Intravenous cholangiography using ioglycamide (Biligram) infusion: a report of 150 cases. Ir. J. Med. Sci. *148*:325, 1974.
33. Robbins, A. H., et al.: Successful intravenous cholecystocholangiography in the jaundiced patient using meglumine iodoxamate (Cholevue). Am. J. Roentgenol. *126*:70, 1976.
34. Rosati, G., and Schiantarell, P.: Biliary excretion of contrast media. Invest. Radiol. *5*:232, 1970.
35. Berk, R. N., et al.: Saturation kinetics and choleretic effects of iodoxamate and iodipamide—an experimental study in dogs. Radiology *119*:529, 1976.
36. Loeb, P. M., et al.: Iotroxamide—a new intravenous cholangiographic agent (comparison with iodipamide and the effect of bile salts). Radiology *125*:323, 1977.
37. Hogben, C. A. M., et al.: On the mechanism of the intestinal absorption of drugs. J. Pharmacol. Exp. Ther. *125*:275, 1959.
38. Jollow, D. J., and Brodie, B. B.: Mechanisms of drug absorption and of drug solution. Pharmacology *8*:21, 1972.
39. Wilson, F. A., and Dietschy, J. M.: Characterization of bile acid absorption across the unstirred water layer and brush border of the rat jejunum. J. Clin. Invest. *51*:3015, 1972.
40. Gibaldi, M.: Introduction to Biopharmaceutics. Philadelphia: Lea & Febiger, 1971.
41. Goldberger, L. E., Berk, R. N., and Loeb, P. M.: Biopharmaceutical factors influencing intestinal absorption of iopanoic acid. Invest. Radiol. *9*:16, 1974.
42. Levy, G.: Effect of particle size on dissolution and gastrointestinal absorption rates of pharmaceuticals. Am. J. Pharmacol. *135*:78, 1963.
43. Holmdahl, K. H., and Lodin, H.: Absorption of iopanoic acid and its sodium salt. Acta Radiol. *51*:247, 1959.
44. Peterhoff, R.: Cholecystography with the sodium salt of iopanoic acid. Acta Radiol. *46*:719, 1956.
45. Taketa, R. M., et al.: The effect of pH on the intestinal absorption of Telepaque. Am. J. Roentgenol. *114*:767, 1972.
46. Nelson, J. A., et al.: Gastrointestinal absorption of iopanoic acid. Invest. Radiol. *8*:1, 1973.
47. Fordtran, J. A., and Locklear, T. W.: Ionic content of small bowel fluid. Am. J. Dig. Dis. *11*:503, 1966.
48. Carey, M. C., and Small, D. M.: Micelle formation by bile salts: physical, chemical and thermodynamic considerations. Arch. Intern. Med. *130*:506, 1972.
49. Loeb, P. M., Berk, R. N., et al.: The effect of fasting on gallbladder opacification during oral cholecystography: a controlled study in normal volunteers. Radiology *126*:395, 1978.
50. Fon, G. R., Hunter, T. B., Berk, R.N., and Capp, M. P.: The effect of diet and fasting on gallbladder opacification in dogs as measured by CT. Radiology *136*:585, 1980.
51. Evens, G., Schroer, C., and Koehler, P. R.: Importance of contrast absorption in evaluation of nonvisualized gallbladder. Radiology *98*:365, 1971.
52. Reinke, R. T., and Berk, R. N.: The mode of Telepaque absorption from the intestine. Am. J. Roentgenol. *113*:578, 1971.
53. Lang, J. H., and Lasser, E. C.: Binding of roentgenographic contrast media to serum albumin. Invest. Radiol. *2*:396, 1967.
54. Lasser, E. C., et al.: The significance of protein binding of contrast media in roentgen diagnosis. Am. J. Roentgenol. *87*:338, 1962.
55. Erlinger, S.: Hepatocyte bile secretion: current views and controversies. Hepatology *1*:352, 1981.
56. Song, C. S., Beranbaum, E. R., and Rothschild, M. A.: The role of serum albumin in the hepatic excretion of iodipamide. Invest. Radiol. *11*:39, 1976.
57. Grauz, H., and Schmid, R.: Reciprocal relation between plasma albumin level and hepatic sulfobromophthalein removal. N. Engl. J. Med. *274*:1403, 1971.
58. Cornelius, C., Ben-Ezzer, J., and Arias, I. M.: Binding of sulfobromophthalein sodium (BSP) and other organic anions by isolated hepatic cell plasma membranes in vitro. Proc. Soc. Exp. Biol. Med. *124*:665, 1967.
59. Levi, A. J., Gathmaitan, Z., and Arias, I. M.: Two hepatic cytoplasmic protein fractions, Y and Z, and their possible role in the hepatic uptake of bilirubin, sulfobromophthalein and other anions. J. Clin. Invest. *48*:2156, 1969.
60. Sokoloff, J., et al.: The role of the Y and Z hepatic proteins in the excretion of radiographic contrast materials. Radiology *106*:519, 1973.
61. Goresky, C. A.: The hepatic uptake and excretion of sulfobromophthalein and bilirubin. Can. Med. Assoc. J., *92*:851, 1965.
62. Scharschmidt, B. F., Waggoner, J. G., and Berk, R. N.: Hepatic organic anion uptake in the rat. J. Clin. Invest. *56*:1280, 1975.
63. Bolt, R. J., Dillon, R., and Pollard, H. M.: Interference with bilirubin excretion by a gallbladder dye: report of a case. N. Engl. J. Med. *265*:1043, 1961.
64. Georgen, T., Goldberger, L. E., and Berk, R. N.: The combined use of oral cholecystopaque media and iodipamide. Radiology *111*:543, 1974.
65. McChesney, E. W., and Hoppe, J. L.: Observations on the absorption and excretion of the glucuronide

of iopanoic acid by the cat. Arch. Int. Pharmacodyn. Ther. *105*:306, 1956.

66. Barnhart, J. L., Parkhill, B. J., Berk, R. N., et al.: Iopanoate glucuronide: Procedure for its isolation and purification and pharmacokinetics of its biliary excretion. Invest. Radiol. *13*:347, 1978.

67. Gartner, L. M., and Arias, I. M.: Formation, transport, metabolism and excretion of bilirubin. N. Engl. J. Med. *280*:1339, 1969.

68. Schmid, R.: Bilirubin metabolism in man. N. Engl. J. Med. *288*:703, 1973.

69. Jansen, P. L. M., et al.: An enzyme in liver plasma cell membrane which converts bilirubin monoglucuronide to bilirubin diglucuronide. Clin. Res. *24*:433A, 1976.

70. Barnhart, J. L., and Combes, B.: Biliary excretion of dye in dogs infused with BSP or its glutathione conjugate. Am. J. Physiol. *231*:399, 1976.

71. Cooke, W. J., and Mudge, G. H.: Biliary and urinary excretion of iopanoic acid in the dog. Invest. Radiol. *10*:25, 1975.

72. Nelson, J. A., Staubus, A. E., and Roegelman, S.: Saturation kinetics of iopanoate in the dog. Invest. Radiol. *10*:371, 1975.

73. Rosati, G., and Schiantaretti, P.: Biliary excretion of contrast media. Invest. Radiol. *5*:232, 1970.

74. Berk, R. N., et al.: The biliary and urinary excretion of sodium tyropanoate and sodium ipodate in dogs. Invest. Radiol. *12*:85, 1977.

75. Loeb, P. M., et al.: The biliary and urinary excretion of ioglycamide in dogs. Invest. Radiol. *11*:449, 1976.

76. Berk, R. N., et al.: Saturation kinetics of iopanoic acid—an experimental study in dogs. Radiology *120*:41, 1976.

77. Berk, R. N., Goldberger, L. E., and Loeb, P. M.: The role of bile salts in the hepatic excretion of iopanoic acid. Invest. Radiol. *9*:7, 1974.

78. Loeb, P. M., Barnhart, J. L., Berk, R. N.: Dependence of the biliary excretion of iopanoic acid on bile salts. Gastroenterology *74*:174, 1978.

79. Dunn, C. R., and Berk, R. N.: The pharmacokinetics of Telepaque metabolism: the relation of blood concentration and bile flow to the rate of hepatic excretion. Am. J. Roentgenol. *114*:758, 1972.

80. Admirand, W. H., and Small, D. M.: The physicochemical basis of cholesterol gallstone formation in man. J. Clin. Invest. *47*:1043, 1968.

81. Berk, R. N., and Dunn, C. R.: The effects of secretion on the hepatic excretion of Telepaque. Radiology *103*:585, 1972.

82. Soloway, R. D., et al.: Triketocholangic (dehydrocholic) acid. Hepatic metabolism and effect on bile flow and biliary lipid secretion in man. J. Clin. Invest. Radiol. *52*:715, 1973.

83. Forker, E. L., and Gibson, G.: Interaction between BSP and taurocholate: The kinetics of transport from liver cells to bile in rats. *In* Baumgartner, G., and Preisig, R. (eds.): Liver: Quantitative Aspects of Structure and Function. Basel: S. Karger, 1973, pp. 326–336.

84. Goresky, C. A., et al.: The enhancement of maximal bilirubin secretion with taurocholate-induced increment in bile flow. Can. J. Physiol. Pharmacol. *52*:389, 1974.

85. Goresky, C. A., Bach, G. G., and Nadeau, B. E.: On the uptake of materials by the intact liver: the transport and net removal of galactose. J. Clin. Invest. *52*:991, 1973.

86. Berk, R. N., Barnhart, J. L., and Goldberger, L.

E.: The enhancement of iopanoate excretion by taurocholate. Invest. Radiol. *15*:S116, 1980.

87. Grundy, S. M., and Metzger, A. L.: A physiological method for estimation of hepatic secretion of biliary lipids in man. Gastroenterology *62*:1200, 1972.

88. Feld, G. K., et al.: The choleretic effect of iodipamide. J. Clin. Invest. *55*:528, 1975.

88a. Hoenig, V., and Presig, R.: Organic-anionic choleresis in the dog: comparative effects of bromsulfalein, ioglycamide and taurocholate. Biomedicine *18*:23, 1973.

89. Mudge, G. H., and Cooke, W. J.: Oral cholecystography: osmotic activity of iopanoic acid glucuronide in bile. Johns Hopkins Med. J. *137*:65, 1975.

90. Edholm, P., and Jacobson, B.: Quantitative determination of iodine *in vivo*. Acta Radiol. *52*:337, 1959.

91. Janower, M. L., and Lundstrom, P.: Biliary tract opacification: effect of iodine concentration and luminal size. Am. J. Roentgenol. *126*:515, 1981.

92. Whalen, J. P., Rizzuti, R. J., and Evans, J. A.: Time of optimal gallbladder opacification with Telepaque (iopanoic acid). Radiology *105*:523, 1972.

93. Oliphant, M., Whalen, J. P., and Evans, J. A.: Times of optimal gallbladder opacification with Bilopaque (tyropanoate sodium). Radiology *112*:531, 1974.

94. Berk, R. N., and Wheeler, H. O.: The role of water reabsorption by the gallbladder in the mechanism of nonvisualization at cholecystography. Radiology *103*:37, 1972.

95. Ivy, A. C.: The physiology of the gallbladder. Physiol. Rev. *14*:1, 1934.

96. Berk, R. N., and Lasser, E. C.: Altered concepts of the mechanism of nonvisualization of the gallbladder. Radiology *82*:296, 1964.

97. Goldberg, H. I., Lin, S. K., Thoeni, R. F., et al.: Recirculation of iopanoic acid after conjugation in the liver. Invest. Radiol. *12*:537, 1977.

98. Schroder, J. S., and Rooney, D.: Excretion of 3-(3-amino-2,4,6-triiodophenyl)-2-ethylpropanoic acid (Telepaque) by man. Proc. Soc. Exp. Biol. Med. *83*:544, 1953.

99. Holonbek, J. E., et al.: Evaluation of pseudoalbuminuria following cholecystography in 76 cases. J.A.M.A. *153*:1018, 1953.

100. Fischer, H. W.: Physiologic and pharmacologic aspects of cholangiography. Radiol. Clin. North Am. *4*:625, 1966.

101. Shames, D. M., and Moss, A. A.: Iodipamide kinetics in the dog. A multicompartmental analysis. Invest. Radiol. *9*:141, 1974.

102. Burgener, F. A., and Fischer, H. W.: Intravenous cholangiography in normal subsequently liver-damaged dogs. Radiology *114*:519, 1975.

103. Burgener, F. A., Fischer, H. W., and Adams, J. T.: Intravenous cholangiography in different degrees of common bile duct obstruction. Invest. Radiol. *10*:342, 1975.

104. Fischer, H. W.: Attempts to improve iodipamide intravenous cholangiography. Am. J. Roentgenol. *96*:477, 1966.

105. Ansell, G.: Adverse reactions to contrast agents. Invest. Radiol. *5*:374, 1970.

106. Finby, N., and Blasberg, G.: A note on the blocking of hepatic excretion during cholangiographic study. Gastroenterology *46*:276, 1964.

107. Berndt, W. O., and Mudge, G. H.: Renal excretion of iodipamide. Invest. Radiol. *3*:414, 1968.

108. Lindgren, P., Nordenstram, H., and Saltzman, G. F.: Effects of iodipamide on the kidneys. Acta Radiol. (Diagn.) 4:129, 1966.

109. Peters, G. A., Hodgson, J. R., and Donovan, R. J.: The effect of premedication with chlorpheniramine on reactions to methylglucamine iodipamide. J. Allergy 38:75, 1966.

110. Craft, I. L., and Swales, J. D.: Renal failure after cholangiography. Br. Med. J. 2:736, 1967.

111. Groth, C. G., Lofstrom, B., and Saltman, G. F.: Effect of dextran solutions on intravenous iodipamide toxicity. Acta Radiol. 10:458, 1970.

112. Stillman, A. E.: Hepatoxic reaction to iodipamide meglumine injection. J.A.M.A. 228:1420, 1974.

113. Lindgren, P., and Saltzman, G. F.: Increase of subcapsular renal pressure after intravenous iodipamide and other parenteral contrast media. Acta Radiol. (Diagn.) 15:273, 1974.

114. White, W. W., and Fischer, H. W.: A double blind study of Oragrafin and Telepaque. Am. J. Roentgenol. 87:745, 1962.

115. Juhl, J. H., Cooperman, L. R., and Crummy, A. B.: Oragrafin, a new cholecystographic medium. Radiology 80:88, 1963.

116. Hekster, R. E. M.: Results of comparative radiographic, clinical and clinical-chemical studies in iocetamic acid and iopanoic acid. Radiol. Clin. Biol. 37:338, 1968.

117. Tishler, J. M., and Gold, R.: A clinical trial of oral cholecystographic agents: Telepaque, sodium Oragrafin and calcium Oragrafin. J. Can. Assoc. Radiol. 20:102, 1969.

118. Russell, J. G., and Frederick, P. R.: Clinical comparison of tyropanoate sodium, ipodate sodium and iopanoic acid. Radiology 112:519, 1974.

119. Rene, R. M., and Mellinkoff, S. M.: Renal insufficiency after oral administration of a double dose of cholecystographic medium; report of 2 cases. N. Engl. J. Med. 261:589, 1959.

120. Fink, H. E., Roenick, W. J., and Wilson, G. P.: An experimental investigation of the nephrotoxic effects of oral cholecystographic agents. Am. J. Med. Sci. 247:201, 1964.

121. Teplick, J. G., Myerson, R. M., and Sanen, F. J.: Acute renal failure following oral cholecystography. Acta Radiol. (Diagn.) 3:353, 1965.

122. Harrow, B. R., and Winslow, O. P.: Renal toxicity following oral cholecystography with Oragrafin. Radiology 87:721, 1966.

123. Canalis, C. O., et al.: Acute renal failure after the administration of iopanoic acid as a cholecystographic agent. N. Engl. J. Med. 281:89, 1969.

124. Meway, J., McGeown, M. G., and Kumar, R.: Renal failure after radiological contrast material. Br. J. Med. 4:717, 1970.

125. Gelfand, D. W., Ott, D. J., and Klein, A. A.: Massive iopanoic acid (Telepaque) overdose without ill effects. Am. J. Roentgenol. 130:1174, 1978.

126. Mudge, G. H.: Some questions of nephrotoxicity. Invest. Radiol. 5:407, 1970.

127. Mudge, G. H.: Uricosuric action of cholecystographic agents: a possible factor in nephrotoxicity. N. Engl. J. Med. 284:929, 1971.

128. Postethwaite, A. E., and Kelley, W. H.: Radiocontrast agents and aspirin. J.A.M.A. 219:1479, 1972.

129. Postethwaite, A. E., and Kelley, W. H.: Uricosuric effect of radio-contrast agents, a study in man of four commonly used preparations. Ann. Intern. Med. 74:845, 1971.

130. Foy, R. E.: Slow-infusion compared with direct injection cholangiography. Radiology 90:576, 1968.

131. Saltzman, G. F., and Sandstrom, K. A.: Influence of different contrast media for cholegraphy on blood pressure and pulse rate. Acta Radiol. 54:353, 1960.

132. Rosenbaum, H. O.: The value of re-examination in patients with inadequate visualization of the gallbladder following a single dose of Telepaque. Am. J. Roentgenol. 82:1011, 1959.

133. Berk, R. N.: Consecutive dose phenomenon in oral cholecystography. Am. J. Roentgenol. 110:230, 1970.

134. Berk, R. N.: The problem of impaired first-dose visualization of the gallbladder. Am. J. Roentgenol. 113:186, 1971.

135. Mauthe, H.: The low-fat meal in gallbladder examinations. Radiology 112:5, 1974.

136. Mujahed, Z., Evans, J. A., and Whalen, J. P.: The nonopacified gallbladder on oral cholecystography. Radiology 112:1, 1974.

137. Stewart, W. H., and Ryan, E. Q.: Further development in the jejunal and oral administration of tetraiiodopyenolphthalein. Am. J. Roentgenol. 14:504, 1924.

138. Zboralske, F. F., and Amberg, J. R.: Cholecystostasis: a cause of cholecystographic error: Am. J. Dig. Dis. 7:339, 1962.

139. Roller, J., et al.: Oral cholecystography in patients with acute alcoholic pancreatitis. Gastroenterology 73:218, 1977.

140. Burhenne, H. J., Morris, D. C., and Graeb, D. A.: Single visit oral cholecystography for inpatients. Radiology 104:505, 1981.

141. Koehler, P. R., and Kyaw, M. M.: Effect of fractionated administration of Telepaque on gallbladder visualization. Radiology 103:517, 1973.

142. Benness, G. T., et al.: Cholangiographic excretion studies. Solu-biloptin and Biligrafin comparison. Invest. Radiol. 10:526, 1975.

143. Dure-Smith, P., et al.: Opacification of the urinary tract during excretory urography: concentration vs. amount of contrast medium. Invest. Radiol. 7:407, 1972.

144. Fischer, H. W.: The excretion of iodipamide. Relation of bile and urine output to dose. Radiology 84:483, 1965.

145. Ansell, G., and Faux, P. A.: Low-dose infusion cholangiography. Clin. Radiol. 24:95, 1973.

146. Sinclair, D. J.: Intravenous cholangiography—a comparative study of techniques. J. Assoc. Can. Radiol. 23:116, 1972.

147. Martinez, L. O., et al.: Present status of intravenous cholangiography. Am. J. Roentgenol. 113:10, 1971.

148. Whitney, B., and Campbell, C. B.: Effect of interruption of the enterohepatic circulation of bile on the secretion of iodipamide in the bile of the Rhesus monkey. Invest. Radiol. 7:83, 1972.

149. Whitney, B., and Bell, G. D.: Single bolus injection or slow infusion for intravenous cholangiography? Measurement of iodipamide (Biligrafin) excretion using a rhesus monkey model. Br. J. Radiol. 45:891, 1972.

150. Watson, A., Russell, H. G. B., and Torrance, H. B.: Hepatic blood flow and Biligrafin excretion during intravenous cholangiography. Br. J. Radiol. 43:248, 1970.

151. Nolan, D. J., and Gibson, M.J.:Improvements in intravenous cholangiography. Br. J. Radiol. 43:652, 1970.

152. Moss, A. A., Nelson, J., and Amberg, J. R.: Intravenous cholangiography: An experimental evaluation of several currently proposed methods. Am. J. Roentgenol. *117*:406, 1973.

153. Small, D. M., Dowling, R. H., and Redinger, R. N.: The enterohepatic circulation of bile salts. Arch. Intern. Med. *130*:552, 1972.

154. Wise, R. E., and Scholz, F. J.: Radiology of the liver and biliary tract. Gastroenterology *65*:967, 1973.

155. Scholz, F. H., Johnston, D. O., and Wise, R. E.: Intravenous cholangiography. Radiology *114*:513, 1975.

156. Russell, J. G. B.: Drip infusion cholangiography. Proc. R. Soc. Med. *61*:262, 1968.

157. Howland, W. J., et al.: Drip-infusion cholangiography: a second look. Radiology *107*:71, 1973.

158. Payne, R. F.: Drip infusion cholangiography. Clin. Radiol. *19*:291, 1968.

159. Isdale, J. M.: Assessment of the slow drip-infusion technique in cholangiography. S. Afr. Med. J. *44*:1328, 1970.

160. McNulty, J. G.: Drip-infusion cholecystocholangiography. Radiology *90*:570, 1968.

161. Fuchs, W. A., and Presig, R.: Prolonged drip-infusion cholangiography. Br. J. Radiol. *48*:539, 1975.

ORAL CHOLECYSTOGRAPHY

by Robert N. Berk, M.D.

4

Most physicians consider oral cholecystography an uncomplicated radiologic procedure that is simple to perform and easy to interpret. However, in reality, few examinations in radiology require more expertise. The proper performance of oral cholecystography demands sound judgment based on knowledge of the pathophysiology of the diseases of the hepatobiliary system, familiarity with the clinical manifestations of these diseases, and an understanding of the pharmacology of biliary contrast materials. Radiographs of excellent technical quality are a prerequisite. Only with this background can oral cholecystography be conducted with sufficient competence to ensure maximum accuracy, efficiency, and safety.

The major use of oral cholecystography is for the diagnosis of cholelithiasis. Considering that nearly 20 million people in the United States have gallstones and that more than one-half million require hospitalization each year for problems related to that disease,[1] it is not surprising that more than 2 million oral cholecystograms are performed each year in this country.[2] At present, the examination is done only when clinical findings suggest the presence of cholelithiasis. It is not customary to perform the study to detect gallstones in asymptomatic individuals, although this may be worthwhile in exceptionally high risk groups such as diabetics, American Indians, and patients with hemolytic anemia, Crohn's disease, and cirrhosis.[3] Oral cholecystography should not be attempted in patients with impaired liver function or biliary obstruction in whom the serum bilirubin is 2.0 mg per cent or higher, because with this degree of cholestasis the possibility of opacification of the gallbladder is negligible.

The introduction of sonography for the evaluation of the gallbladder has had a profound influence on the use of oral cholecystography in clinical practice.[4] Whereas previously oral cholecystography alone occupied center stage as the paradigm of diagnostic procedures, now its shortcomings (dependence on liver function, the use of contrast material and radiation) are becoming ever more glaring to the extent that the future of the technique is in doubt. Moreover, sonography is still evolving and will, no doubt, be refined even further, compared with oral cholecystography, which has not been improved substantially in the last several years and is not likely to command a high priority for research in the future. Utilization data from the Massachusetts General Hospital show a decline of approximately 40 per cent in the annual number of cholecystograms performed between 1976 and 1980, with a commensurate increase in the use of sonography during the same period.[4] Most authorities believe that the move away from oral cholecystography and toward sonography for gallbladder imaging is inexorable, and it is likely that, with a few exceptions, sonography will sooner or later become the primary modality for diagnosing cholelithiasis.[4] It is only a matter of the availability of experienced radiologists and the necessary equipment; the trend will accelerate as newly trained radiologists go into practice and equipment is updated.

In addition to deficiencies compared with sonography, there are several problems related to oral cholecystography.[2] These include: (1) overrated sensitivity in the diagnosis of gallstones; (2) the waste of time, money, and radiation exposure associated with the necessity of performing a second examination when there is poor visualization of the gallbladder after a single dose of contrast material; (3) uncertainty regarding the significance of non-visualization of the gallbladder after two consecutive doses of contrast material because of the difficulty in accurately excluding extrabiliary causes for the nonvisualization; (4) failure of cholecystokinin cholecystography in the diagnosis of acalculous cholecystitis, biliary dyskinesia, and the cystic duct syndrome; and (5) difficulty in distinguishing cholesterol from pigment gallstones to establish the efficacy of medical therapy.

THE ACCURACY OF ORAL CHOLECYSTOGRAPHY

The results of reports indicating an accuracy rate for oral cholecystography in the range of 97 to 99 per cent are misleading in that they concern specificity rather than sensitivity and involve only patients in whom a positive oral cholecystogram was correlated with the pathologic findings at surgery.[5-12] These data indicate that the interpretation of an oral cholecystogram is nearly 100 per cent correct when gallstones are visible in an opacified gallbladder or when there is nonvisualization of the gallbladder following two consecutive doses of contrast material. Hence, the studies show that the specificity of the cholecystogram is high; false-positive results are exceedingly rare. However, they give no indication concerning the sensitivity of the test; i.e., the number of patients who have gallstones in whom the cholecystogram is interpreted as normal (false negatives). Until the availability of sonography, this information was impossible to obtain, because performing a cholecystectomy indiscriminately is not justified in patients who have an apparently normal oral cholecystogram.

The results of numerous studies comparing the sensitivity of oral cholecystography and sonography indicate that the incidence of overlooked gallstones on cholecystography is in the range of 6 to 8 per cent.[13-21] It seems likely that, even with ideal radiographic technique and good opacification of the gallbladder, gallstones that are 2 to 3 mm or less in diameter occasionally may be missed when only one or two are present. The accuracy of oral cholecystography in detecting gallstones is probably closer to 92 to 95 per cent than to 98 per cent. Consequently, when a patient's symptoms are highly suggestive of gallbladder disease or

when there is acute pancreatitis that may be due to cholelithiasis, a normal oral cholecystogram should not be taken as conclusive evidence against the presence of gallstones.

TECHNIQUES OF PERFORMING ORAL CHOLECYSTOGRAPHY

Preparation of the Patient

Experimental data in dogs indicate that the active enterohepatic recirculation of bile salts plays a major role in facilitating both the intestinal absorption and hepatic excretion of Telepaque (see Chapter 3).[22, 23] Therefore, it is important to ensure that fat is given in the diet at the same time Telepaque is administered. Fat stimulates the release of cholecystokinin, which causes the gallbladder to contract and empty bile salts stored in the gallbladder into the intestine. The fat content of the diet given with the other, more water-soluble oral cholecystographic materials appears to be less important.

Data reported by Stanley and coworkers provide clinical evidence that fat in the diet is important in the adequate opacification of the gallbladder with Telepaque.[24] In their study, 47 per cent of patients given Telepaque with a nonfat supper had satisfactory first-day examinations compared with 70 per cent when the Telepaque was given with a high-fat meal. Opacification with Cholebrine and Bilopaque was unaffected by the presence or absence of fat in the diet. Nonvisualization of the gallbladder with Telepaque in volunteers on a low-fat diet, reported by Zboralske and Amberg,[25] may be due to poor absorption and excretion of the Telepaque rather than to stasis of nonopaque bile in the gallbladder, as suggested by the authors.

Loeb and associates studied the effect of fasting on gallbladder opacification during oral cholecystography in ten normal volunteers with Telepaque and Bilopaque.[26] There was good opacification in all ten subjects when Telepaque was administered with a meal and when Bilopaque was given in the fasting state. Only two of the ten subjects had satisfactory visualization when Telepaque was given in the fasting state. Three of the ten had good opacification when Bilopaque was given with a meal. Consequently, food plays an important role in gallbladder visualization. Care should be taken to ensure that Telepaque is administered with a meal, whereas Bilopaque should be given in a fasting state.

The optimal dose of Telepaque and the other oral cholecystographic contrast agents has not been studied sufficiently. Some use 2.0 gm rather than the usual 3.0-gm dose to avoid opacification of the gallbladder so dense that gallstones may be obscured.[27] This is not a problem if compression spot films are made. Administering more than 3.0 gm of Telepaque may be necessary in obese patients, but the routine use of large doses should be avoided because of the likelihood that the degree of toxicity produced by the contrast agent is proportional to the amount of the compound given. The routine use of a double dose (6.0 gm) is not warranted, because most reported cases of renal failure due to oral cholecystographic contrast materials have been in patients who received high doses of the compound.[28] More than two consecutive doses are not indicated, because such examinations are not associated with a higher incidence of improved gallbladder opacification.[9]

Care should be taken not to dehydrate the patient following the administration of the contrast agent because of the potent uricosuric effects of the compounds.[28] Water should be allowed *ad lib*. If the patient is known to have gout, fluid intake should be encouraged, and the urine should be alkalinized to avoid precipitation of urate crystals in the urine. A small dose of aspirin may be given to reduce the uricosuria associated with Telepaque. When 600 mg (2 tablets) of aspirin are given with 3.0 gm of Telepaque, followed by an additional dose of 600 mg of aspirin two hours later, the uricosuric effect of Telepaque is reduced by a factor of ten.[29]

Because Telepaque frequently has a cathartic effect, it is not necessary to routinely administer a laxative to eliminate fecal material in the colon that might interfere with optimal visualization of the gallbladder. Conversely, it has been shown that castor oil does not interfere with opacification of the gallbladder when it is given with Telepaque.[30, 31] Since castor oil stimulates the gallbladder to contract, there is experimental evidence to suggest, at least, that it could improve the absorption and excretion of Telepaque.[28]

Patients should be evaluated for a history of previous allergic reaction to any of the radiographic contrast materials before proceeding with oral cholecystography. Cross-over reactions with the urographic and angiographic contrast materials may occur. Adverse reactions in a patient with a known allergy to contrast material can be avoided by treatment with corticosteroids and antihistaminics before administering the cholecystographic contrast agent.

Radiographic Technique

Ideally, a preliminary plain abdominal radiograph should be made prior to the administration of contrast material to detect radiopaque gallstones that might be obscured by contrast material in the gallbladder and to recognize milk of calcium bile, which could be confused with a normally opacified gallbladder. This is in keeping with the basic radiologic tenet that a preliminary radiograph should be made before any contrast agent is used. However, it is impractical in most cases to require patients to make an additional trip to the radiology department for the preliminary examination. Consequently, one must weigh the inconvenience and expense of the preliminary radiograph against the number of times gallbladder disease will be overlooked without it. In a series of 467 cases of cholecystography reported by Harned and LaVeen, the plain abdominal radiograph would have prevented a false-negative diagnosis in less than 1 per cent.[32] These and other investigators[33] concluded that this small yield is not worth the cost and effort involved. If upright spot films of the gallbladder are made with graded compression, it is particularly unlikely that radiopaque gallstones will not be identified in the fundus of the opacified gallbladder. However, two such cases were reported by Moadel and Bryk,[34] and undoubtedly others occur. One must keep in mind that such false-negative cholecystograms may happen if the preliminary radiograph is omitted. In special cases, e.g., patients with apparently normal cholecystograms who have characteristic symptoms of biliary colic and/or those in whom significant symptoms persist, a plain abdominal radiograph should be made at some point in the radiologic work-up.

Care must be taken to make the radiographs of the gallbladder at the appropriate time following the administration of the contrast material. Poor gallbladder opacification will occur if the radiographs are taken prematurely or if they are delayed. Whalen, Rizzuti, and Evans studied 50 patients having cholecystog-

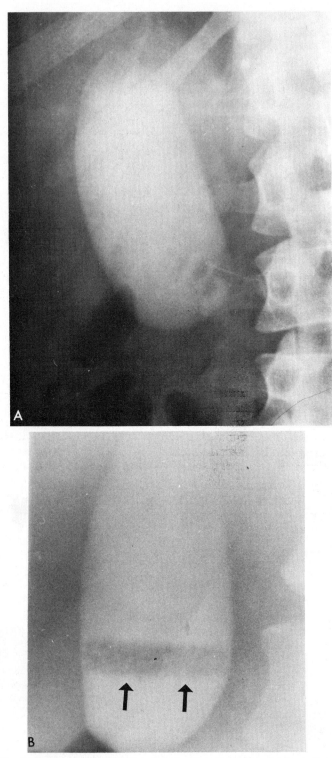

Figure 4–1. *A*, Supine radiograph made during oral cholecystography, showing no gallstones in the gallbladder. *B*, Upright spot film of the gallbladder in the same patient using fluoroscopy. A layer of small gallstones is visible, which was not evident on supine or prone radiographs (arrows). *C*, Upright spot film made in another patient, showing a layer of radiolucent gallstones (arrows). The supine radiographs were normal.

Illustration continued on opposite page

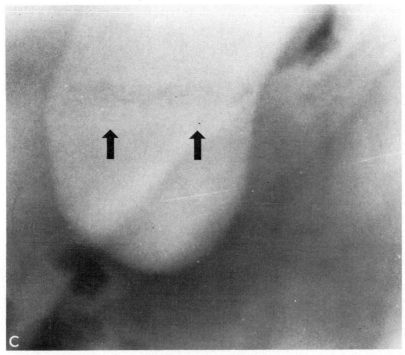

Figure 4–1. *Continued*

raphy with Telepaque and showed that peak opacification of the gallbladder occurred between 14 and 19 hours after ingestion of the contrast material.[35] Using Bilopaque in 50 patients, Oliphant, Whalen, and Evans determined that optimal gallbladder opacification occurred at ten hours.[36] Consequently, timing of the radiograph depends upon which contrast material is used.

The actual number and type of radiographs that are made as part of a cholecystogram vary depending upon the individual preference of the radiologist, but in all cases the following principles must be observed. (1) Upright spot films made with fluoroscopy or right lateral decubitus radiographs should be included if gallstones are not evident on prone or supine radiographs (Figs. 4–1 and 4–2).[37-39] (2) At least one radiograph should include the entire abdomen. (3) The radiographs should be of excellent technical quality and should be made using a low kilovoltage technique. (4) The radiographs should be viewed before the patient leaves the department so that additional films can be obtained if necessary.

Small gallstones are often visible on supine and prone abdominal radiographs, even when they are numerous. The accuracy of the cholecystogram is significantly impaired unless up-right or decubitus projections of the gallbladder are obtained to allow the calculi to collect by gravity in the dependent portion of the gallbladder or to form a layer in the bile (Figs. 4–1 and 4–2).[37-39] Upright spot films made at fluoroscopy with graded compression of the gallbladder are indispensable unless gallstones are obvious on the supine or prone radiographs. Fluoroscopy allows graded compression of the gallbladder under direct vision, so that an optimum radiograph can be composed. The obliquity of the patient can be varied as necessary to free the fundus of overlying fecal material, gas, and bone. The appropriate degree of compression applied under direct visual control improves radiographic detail and reduces the density of the gallbladder. The latter may be important when small or radiopaque gallstones are present. Jensen and Kaude showed that fluorography with 70-mm film from the output screen of the image intensifier is an acceptable substitute for full-scale spot film radiography.[40]

A right lateral decubitus projection of the abdomen is helpful when spot films are unsuccessful and is recommended by some to replace fluoroscopy (Fig. 4–2).[41] However, decubitus views usually are not as good technically unless the radiographic table is equipped with a spe-

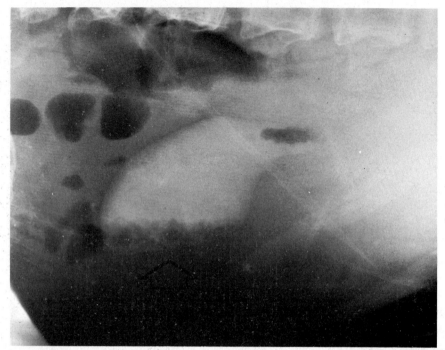

Figure 4–2. Decubitus abdominal radiograph made during cholecystography with the right side down. Numerous gallstones are evident in the dependent portion of the gallbladder (arrow). The diagnosis of cholelithiasis was inconclusive on supine and prone radiographs because of overlying gas and fecal material in the colon.

cial attachment. A simple device for this purpose is recommended by Miller.[42] With the decubitus projections, visualization of the dependent portion of the gallbladder is left to chance and compression under direct visual control is impossible. Amberg, Zboralske, and Johnson recommend elevating the patient's hips in the lateral decubitus position to improve visualization of the dependent portion of the gallbladder when it is obscured on the conventional decubitus projection.[43] Others recommend an oblique bending position for this purpose.[44]

One radiograph should include the entire abdomen so that a gallbladder in an unusual position will not be overlooked and a mistaken diagnosis of nonvisualization will be avoided.[45] It is helpful to make this radiograph in a slightly oblique position so that the gallbladder is not obscured by the spine. This projection serves as a guide for the fluoroscopist and is also useful in searching for other abdominal abnormalities that may be present incidentally (Fig. 4–3).

Both spot films and conventional radiographs must be of excellent technical quality so that subtle, small stones lying in the fundus of the gallbladder or layered in the bile will be visible. A low kilovoltage technique (70 kVp)

should be used to optimize the density of the contrast material in the gallbladder. This is particularly important when there is poor opacification of the gallbladder and also in obese patients. Failure to observe the basic principles of good radiographic technique is a leading cause of false-negative cholecystograms.[46]

There has been considerable debate as to whether the radiographs should be made with a high- or low-ratio grid or even without a grid. Miller and Besozzi studied 50 patients without a grid, with one 6:1 grid, and with two crossed 6:1 grids.[47] A 12:1 linear grid was not evaluated because of mechanical and electrical limitations. The results showed that a crossed 6:1 grid was superior in 80 per cent of the cases. In those cases in which no grid or one grid was superior, there was a shorter exposure time or no movement by the patient. The investigators concluded that for routine cholecystography, high-ratio grids should be used in combination with short exposure times.

The radiographs of every patient having cholecystography must be reviewed by a radiologist or a knowledgeable surrogate before the patient leaves the x-ray department so that additional projections can be made if the first films are inadequate. Hence, the examination

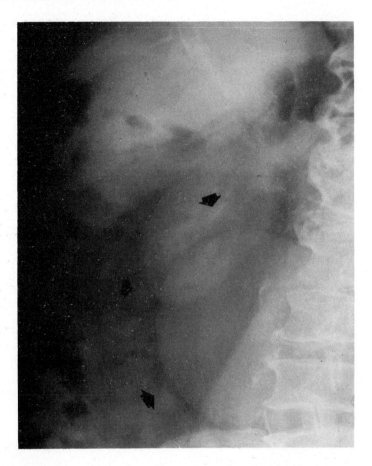

Figure 4–3. Supine radiograph of the abdomen made during an oral cholecystogram after two doses of Telepaque. Failure of the gallbladder to opacify was shown subsequently to be due to cholelithiasis with obstruction of the cystic duct. The abdominal mass noted incidentally was a large renal cyst (arrows).

must be tailored to the special needs of each patient. If the spot films or decubitus projections fail to demonstrate the fundus of the gallbladder satisfactorily, these examinations should be repeated. If the fundus of the gallbladder still cannot be freed of overlying fecal material, an enema may eliminate the problem. In some cases, a fatty meal is useful to contract the gallbladder so that the fundus can be demonstrated adequately. When these maneuvers fail, tomography, stereoscopic radiographs, or ultrasound studies of the gallbladder may be necessary. Occasionally, there is no alternative but to repeat the examination at a later date before attempting to make a definite diagnosis.

The Fatty Meal

The routine use of a fatty meal in oral cholecystography has been recommended by various authors[41, 48, 49] to (1) free the gallbladder from overlying gas and fecal material in the colon; (2) evaluate gallbladder function as a determinant of acalculous cholecystitis and the cystic duct syndrome; (3) detect small gallstones, especially those that lie in the neck of the gallbladder; (4) visualize the cystic and common ducts; (5) diagnose cholesterolosis and adenomyomatosis; and (6) differentiate a gallstone from a fixed filling defect in the gallbladder wall.

The use of a fatty meal to demonstrate the fundus of the gallbladder on upright spot films or decubitus radiographs when visualization free of feces and gas cannot be accomplished has already been mentioned. It is generally agreed that the response of the gallbladder to a fatty meal is too variable to permit valid conclusions regarding its ability to empty normally.[4, 50-52] Cholecystokinin has replaced a fatty meal for this purpose, and the subject of cholecystokinin cholecystography in the diagnosis of acalculous cholecystitis, the cystic duct syndrome, and biliary dyskinesia on the basis of abnormal contractions and emptying will be discussed later in this chapter.

Miller, Chernish, and Rodda emphasized

importance of giving a fatty meal routinely to visualize the neck of the gallbladder, where they believe stones are often missed.[41] However, Laufer and Gledhill compared the diagnoses before and after a fatty meal in 231 patients undergoing cholecystography and found only one patient in whom a stone was detected only on the postfat radiograph.[53] In this case, the stone was missed on the original film because of overlying gas and not because it was hidden in the neck of the gallbladder. Similar results were reported by Harvey, Thwe, and Low-Beer.[48]

Visualization of the cystic and common ducts is not justification for the routine use of a fatty meal. If the gallbladder is opacified on the oral cholecystogram, it is reasonable to assume that there are no calculi in the cystic duct. Furthermore, it also can be assumed that there are no gallstones in the common duct if there are none in the gallbladder, except in the most unusual circumstances. Choledocholithiasis is exceedingly rare in the absence of gallstones in the gallbladder in patients without cholecystectomy. If a patient has cholelithiasis, the common duct should be opacified by operative cholangiography performed routinely during cholecystectomy.[2] Consequently, there is no need to attempt to visualize the common duct preoperatively.

Another putative indication for giving a fatty meal is the detection of cholesterolosis and adenomyomatosis on the postfat meal radiography when these abnormalities are not evident on the initial films. In Laufer and Gledhill's series of 231 patients, this occurred only three times.[53] In addition, since the clinical significance of cholesterolosis and adenomyomatosis is uncertain, one might question the importance of establishing the diagnosis of these diseases, especially in patients in whom the changes are so mild that they are not apparent on prefatty meal radiographs of the gallbladder. However, a fatty meal is useful to evaluate a compartmentalized gallbladder for circumscribed adenomyomatosis.

In view of the considerable inconvenience, expense, and additional radiation exposure involved in obtaining a radiograph after a fatty meal, there are few objective data to justify the routine use of a fatty meal in cholecystography. A fatty meal may be useful in specific circumstances, such as when the fundus of the gallbladder cannot otherwise be separated from fecal material in the colon and when the initial radiograph suggests the presence of adenomyomatosis or cholesterolosis.

THE PROBLEM OF IMPAIRED FIRST-DOSE VISUALIZATION OF THE GALLBLADDER

Repeat examination in cases of impaired visualization of the gallbladder on a single-dose oral cholecystogram is required with disturbing regularity and represents an important practical problem.[54] The incidence varies, depending on the degree of gallbladder opacification that individual radiologists are willing to accept as adequate for diagnosis on the first-dose examination. In both Rosenbaum's[55] and Berk's[56] series of patients having cholecystography, 15 per cent required a second examination because of impaired first-dose visualization. Mujahed, Evans, and Whalen[9] found a second-dose examination necessary in 25 per cent of their cases, whereas approximately 50 per cent of Stanley's patients required a second study.[24]

The difficulty arises from the fact that gallbladder opacification is not always maximum on the first study and sometimes can be improved by a second dose of contrast material.[54] As a result, initial nonvisualization of the gallbladder is not a definite indication of the presence of gallbladder disease, and a second study is required before a diagnosis can be made. Between 10 and 20 per cent of patients with *no* visualization of the gallbladder after a single dose of contrast material have a normal cholecystogram on the second-dose examination.[54] Equally troublesome is *faint* opacification at the first study. The initial visualization may be so poor, even in the absence of disease, that a second examination is necessary to obtain maximum opacification in an attempt to identify or exclude gallstones accurately. In this group, 65 to 75 per cent of the cases are normal on the second examination.[54] In either case, failure to repeat the cholecystogram significantly vitiates the diagnostic accuracy of the procedure and invites unacceptable diagnostic error.

Poor visualization of the gallbladder after a single dose of contrast material occurs not only in a significant percentage of apparently normal patients but also regularly in those with acute pancreatitis[57-60] or acute peritonitis[61]; after trauma,[62, 63] surgery,[61] and fasting[25, 26]; and in patients with pernicious anemia,[64] infants under six months of age,[65] and women in the late months of pregnancy.[66] Kaden, Howard, and Doubleday showed that two-thirds of 25 patients with acute pancreatitis had nonvisualization or poor visualization of the gallbladder when the examination was performed during the first week of an acute exacerbation of the disease.[57] Subsequent cholecystograms performed after recovery showed that the gallbladders in these patients were normal (Fig. 4–4). Similar results were obtained by Silvani and McCorkle in their series of 28 patients with acute pancreatitis.[60] The nonvisualization of the gallbladder in patients with acute pancreatitis cannot be attributed to common bile

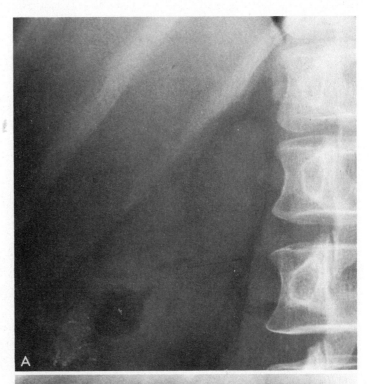

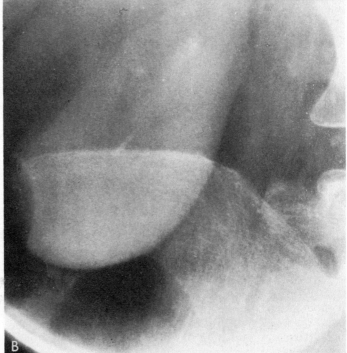

Figure 4–4. *A*, Oral cholecystogram in a patient with acute pancreatitis, performed with Telepaque during an acute exacerbation of the disease, shows nonvisualization of the gallbladder. The serum bilirubin and serum alkaline phosphatase were normal. *B*, Oral cholecystogram performed with Telepaque one month later during a remission. There is excellent opacification of the gallbladder and no evidence of cholelithiasis.

Illustration continued on following page

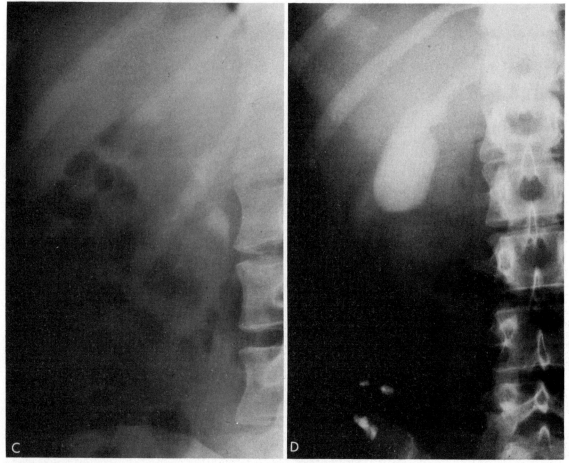

Figure 4–4. *Continued C,* Intravenous cholangiogram in another patient with acute pancreatitis shows nonvisualization of the biliary tree. Renal excretion is evident. *D,* Excellent opacification of a normal gallbladder on an oral cholecystogram performed after recovery from the acute illness.

duct obstruction secondary to inflammation of the pancreas, since there is no correlation between failure of the gallbladder to visualize and serum bilirubin concentration. If obstruction were a factor, one would expect failure to excrete Telepaque to occur only in those patients who were also unable to excrete bilirubin and who had increased serum bilirubin concentrations.

Sanchez-Ubeda, Ruzicka, and Rousselot showed that gallbladder opacification is impaired not only in most patients with acute pancreatitis but in most cases of peritonitis owing to a variety of causes such as a perforated ulcer and appendicitis; in patients with an active duodenal ulcer; and in the postoperative period following abdominal surgery.[61] In their series, the impaired visualization persisted up to 12 weeks after recovery in many cases, despite the resumption of a normal diet.

The cause of inadequate radiographic visu-

alization of the gallbladder in the absence of gallbladder disease has not been clearly defined. Impaired first-dose opacification in apparently normal patients may be due to impaired intestinal absorption and/or deficient hepatic excretion of Telepaque in the absence of circulating bile salts (see Chapter 3). This occurs in patients who are fasting or on a low-fat diet in whom bile salts are sequestered in the gallbladder (Fig. 4–5). Poor absorption of the contrast material also may be related to diminished secretion of pancreatic juice with an associated decrease in intestinal pH.[28] Stagnation of nonopaque bile in the gallbladder in fasting patients may prevent filling of the gallbladder with contrast material and may prevent opacification.[25] Poor visualization in patients with acute pancreatitis may be related to the fact that they usually are fasting because of abdominal pain and as part of their therapy. This would not explain the persistent failure

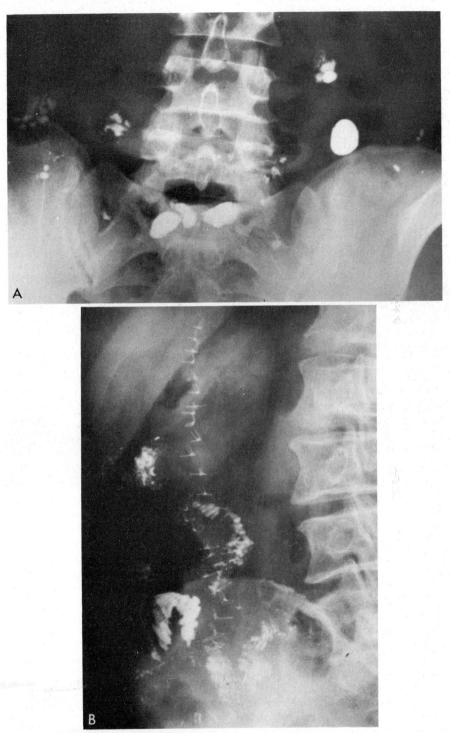

Figure 4–5. *A*, Abdominal radiograph made 14 hours after ingestion of 3.0 gm of Telepaque in a patient who had been fasting for three days. The Telepaque tablets have only begun to disintegrate. The gallbladder failed to opacify. Bile salts in fasting patients are sequestered in the gallbladder and therefore are not available to make the Telepaque in the intestine soluble. A cholecystogram performed when the patient had resumed a normal diet was normal. *B*, Excessive unabsorbed Telepaque in the intestine in another patient whose gallbladder was not visible because of poor absorption of the Telepaque.

of the gallbladder to visualize after a patient has resumed a normal diet, as described by Sanchez-Ubeda, Ruzicka, and Rousselot.[61] However, these data may be in error in light of the more current report of Roller and associates,[67] who were able to obtain satisfactory gallbladder opacification in 89 per cent of patients with acute pancreatitis before discharge from the hospital when the examination was performed after solid food was resumed. Others performed successful oral cholecystography with Bilopaque early in the course of acute pancreatitis.[68]

Cholecystography in patients who are fasting and/or have acute pancreatitis should be delayed until a normal diet can be resumed; alternatively, the examination should be performed with other contrast agents such as Bilopaque and Oragrafin. These compounds, because of their greater water solubility, are not dependent on circulating bile salts for their absorption. Fortunately, the problem of uncertain visualization of the gallbladder in patients with acute pancreatitis is moot when sonography is available.

TECHNIQUES TO ELIMINATE THE NEED FOR A SECOND-DOSE CHOLECYSTOGRAM

Burhenne and Obata recommend administering two consecutive 3.0-gm doses of Telepaque each evening prior to the day the radiographs are made to avoid having to perform a second cholecystogram in patients with initial nonvisualization or poor visualization of the gallbladder.[69] Their data from over 600 single-visit oral cholecystograms indicate that failure of the gallbladder to opacify under these circumstances is reliable evidence of gallbladder disease when extrabiliary causes of nonvisualization, such as liver disease, are excluded. Their technique requires that the patient be relied upon to take the contrast material consecutively as directed. If the method is used in hospitalized patients, an additional day in the hospital may be necessary. To avoid this difficulty, Burhenne, Morris, and Graeb recommend a one-day medication schedule using both Telepaque and Oragrafin sodium on the day prior to making the radiographs.[70] Their results in 45 patients demonstrate the accuracy of the procedure and its usefulness in hospitalized patients. Both regimens are clever solutions to the problem of having to perform second-dose cholecystograms.

In most centers in the United States, patients with initial poor opacification or nonvisualization of the gallbladder are now routinely referred for sonography. Numerous reports prove the accuracy of sonography for the detection of cholelithiasis.[13-21] The direct identification of gallstones provided by sonography is preferable to the presumptive evidence available when there is consecutive-dose nonvisualization of the gallbladder on oral cholecystography.

Koehler and Kyaw[71] were able to reduce the incidence of poor first-dose opacification of the gallbladder from 54 to 15 per cent by giving the Telepaque tablets over a six-hour period the day before the study rather than using the conventional method (i.e., giving the total dose with supper the evening before the examination). It may be that the more prolonged administration of the Telepaque increases the probability that bile salts are available to mix with the contrast material and that this therefore improves the rate of intestinal absorption and hepatic excretion of the Telepaque. Similar results were reported by Nelson.[72] Fischer and Burgener[73] showed in nine volunteers that a 3.0-gm dose of Bilopaque given in four divided doses over six hours produced at least the same radiographic density of the gallbladder as a single 3.0-gm dose. They recommend the fractionated dose because the lower peak blood concentrations of the Bilopaque achieved with the divided dose should predispose to fewer toxic reactions than the single-dose method. In distinction to the value of fractionating the dosage with Telepaque, Michal, Nelson, and Koehler[74] demonstrated that fractionating the dosage of Cholebrine was counterproductive, in that gallbladder visualization was significantly better when Cholebrine was given in a single dose. The reason for this difference between Cholebrine and Telepaque is not known.

Administering Oragrafin calcium to patients with first-dose nonvisualization or poor visualization of the gallbladder is a useful alternative to performing a second-day cholecystogram (reinforcement cholecystography) (Fig. 4-6),[75-77] and this technique may thus save the patient a day of hospitalization. Radiographs made four hours after administering 6.0 gm of Oragrafin calcium showed sufficient improvement in opacification to allow a diagnosis in 80 per cent of Beseman's patients with initial poor visualization.[75] When the original cholecystogram showed nonvisualization of the gallbladder, the chance of increased opacification

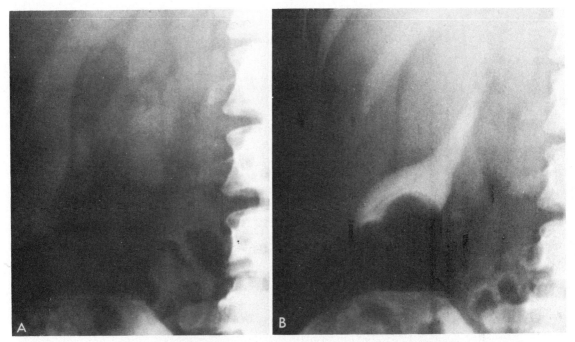

Figure 4–6. *A*, Oral cholecystogram performed 14 hours after the ingestion of 3.0 gm of Telepaque shows poor opacification of the gallbladder. *B*, Five hours later, after the administration of a reinforcing dose of 3.0 gm of calcium ipodate, opacification of the gallbladder has improved sufficiently to show that the gallbladder was normal.

with Oragrafin was only 13 per cent. In a series of 115 patients with initial nonvisualization, Crummy showed that persistent failure of the gallbladder to visualize on radiographs made five hours after a second 3.0-gm dose of Oragrafin calcium is conclusive evidence of gallbladder disease when extrabiliary causes of nonvisualization are excluded.[76]

Visualization of the common duct is accurate evidence that there has been adequate intestinal absorption and hepatic excretion of the contrast material to opacify the gallbladder (Fig. 4–7). Nonvisualization of the gallbladder in this circumstance indicates the presence of cystic duct obstruction. Tomography of the right upper quadrant of the abdomen can reduce the need for a second cholecystogram by demonstrating opacification of the common bile duct in the absence of gallbladder visualization in 70 to 80 per cent of patients with nonvisualization of the gallbladder on cholecystography.[78-82] Tomography may reveal calcification in the obstructing cystic duct calculus that is not visible on the conventional cholecystogram or may identify the stone as a crescentic filling defect in the cystic duct.[82] Frequently, tomography of the nonopacified gallbladder will permit identification of stones that are not obvious or definite on the initial films. Calcified gallstones that are obscured by over-

lying ribs and costal cartilage and stones that are too faintly calcified to be identified on plain films may be shown clearly on tomography.[82] Tomography sometimes reveals nonopaque stones in a faintly opacified gallbladder that was believed to be nonopacified on the initial films. Often the gallbladder can be visualized on retrospective review of the conventional films. When tomography does not reveal a stone or opacification of the gallbladder or bile ducts, an extrinsic cause for the lack of gallbladder opacification should be considered. Tomography also may be rewarding in the presence of a faintly opacified gallbladder in which gallstones cannot be recognized or excluded with certainty.[82] The use of tomography is unnecessary in patients who have nonvisualization of the gallbladder after two doses of contrast material, because this in itself is usually considered to be accurate evidence of gallbladder disease when other causes of nonvisualization are excluded.[9] However, tomography is valuable in patients with failure to opacify the gallbladder on a second-dose cholecystogram if extrabiliary causes cannot be excluded with certainty and in patients with first-dose impaired gallbladder opacification when it is important to establish a diagnosis without further delay. Sonography is more efficacious in these circumstances. Routine to-

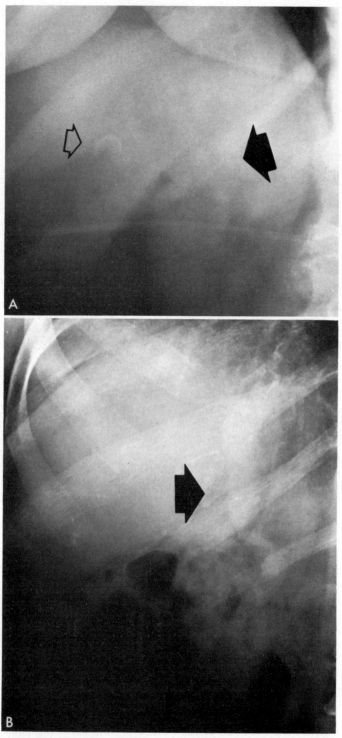

Figure 4–7. *A,B,* Visualization of the common duct (closed arrows) with nonvisualization of the gallbladder on oral cholecystography in different patients. A partly calcified gallstone in the gallbladder is visible in *A* (open arrow). Opacification of the common duct with failure to visualize the gallbladder is accurate evidence of gallbladder disease.

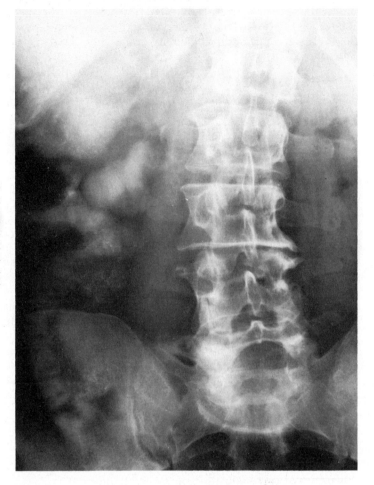

Figure 4–8. Radiograph made 12 hours after the ingestion of 3 gm of Telepaque shows the homogeneous appearance of conjugated Telepaque in the small intestine. Identification of conjugated Telepaque indicates that the contrast material has been absorbed from the intestine and excreted by the liver. Compare this with the particulate appearance of unabsorbed Telepaque shown in Figure 4–5B.

mography is not recommended because of the additional time, expense, and radiation exposure required.

Another possible alternative to performing a second-day cholecystogram in patients with initial nonvisualization of the gallbladder is to perform an intravenous cholangiogram with Cholografin on the same day as the first examination. This is not recommended because the cholangiogram is more hazardous for the patient than the oral study, since Cholografin is more toxic than Telepaque[28] and since the examination is more time consuming for the radiology department. However, if the common duct opacifies without visualization of the gallbladder after four hours, the intravenous cholangiogram provides accurate direct evidence of gallbladder disease (see Chapter 5).[83] Opacification of the gallbladder without evidence of gallstones during an intravenous cholangiogram does not exclude their presence. In one series of patients with consecutive nonvisualization of the gallbladder following Tel-

epaque and in whom gallbladder disease was ultimately proved at surgery, 17 per cent had a normal intravenous cholangiogram.[9] Consequently, a normal intravenous cholangiogram in a patient with nonvisualization of the gallbladder on oral studies does not exclude gallbladder disease. In these patients, the oral cholecystogram should be repeated at a later date, or a sonogram should be performed.

Nathan and Newman point out that detection of conjugated Telepaque in the intestine on the radiographs of patients with nonvisualization of the gallbladder after a single dose of Telepaque has the same significance as visualization of the common bile duct and indicates cystic duct obstruction.[84] Conjugated Telepaque may be identified on the radiograph as a homogeneous uniform density easily distinguishable from the granular particulate appearance of unabsorbed, unconjugated contrast material (Fig. 4–8). Its presence in the small bowel or colon indicates that the Telepaque has been adequately absorbed from the intestine and properly excreted by the liver. Therefore, failure of the gallbladder to opacify in these circumstances is due to cystic duct obstruction.

SIGNIFICANCE OF NONVISUALIZATION OF THE GALLBLADDER AFTER A SECOND-DOSE CHOLECYSTOGRAM

Failure of the gallbladder to visualize after administration of two consecutive doses of cholecystographic contrast material is considered by many authorities to be reliable evidence of gallbladder disease if other causes of nonvisualization, such as impaired liver function, can be excluded.[7, 9, 27, 51, 55] However, in many patients extrabiliary reasons for poor opacification are difficult to exclude with certainty. Consequently, the accuracy of the cholecystogram in these circumstances is flawed by this difficulty, and conclusions often depend too heavily on clinical impressions rather than anatomic evidence.[4] Now that direct morphologic data are readily obtainable by ultrasonography, it is no longer necessary to rely on the indirect evidence that the second-dose cholecystogram provides.

In a series of 5000 patients having oral cholecystography reported by Mujahed, Evans, and Whalen,[9] all of the patients who had consecutive nonvisualization of the gallbladder with no apparent extrabiliary reason and who were operated on had gallbladder disease at surgery. The pathologic diagnosis in nearly all cases was chronic cholecystitis and cholelithiasis. However, these results may be biased by the fact that many patients with nonvisualization were not operated on, and the accuracy of the pathologic diagnosis in some of those who were operated on can be questioned. In fact, the histologic criteria for the diagnosis of cholecystitis, especially chronic acalculous cholecystitis, are ambiguous.[4] Inflammatory cellular infiltrates can be identified histologically in the gallbladder wall of many asymptomatic patients after middle age. Certainly, pathologists are reluctant to embarrass the surgeon by suggesting that a normal gallbladder has been removed. Therefore, since only the presence of gallstones serves to objectively identify patients with *bona fide* gallbladder disease, ultrasonography is indicated after nonvisualization of the gallbladder with a two-dose cholecystogram.[4]

In centers where sonography is used to con-firm the diagnosis of gallbladder disease in patients with consecutive-dose nonvisualization of the gallbladder on oral cholecystography when there are no extrabiliary causes, data show that nonvisualization on the oral cholecystogram is not a reliable indication of the presence of gallbladder disease. Lee and coworkers noted that only 82 per cent of their 48 patients with no gallbladder visualization after second-dose cholecystography proved to have gallstones at surgery.[85] Bartrum, Crow, and Foote reported that only 23 such gallbladders were abnormal in their series of 29 patients (79 per cent).[21]

There are a large number of extrabiliary causes for nonvisualization of the gallbladder (Table 4–1). Low-Beer, Heaton, and Roylance presented evidence that small bowel disease is rarely a cause of nonvisualization of the gallbladder on oral cholecystography with Oragrafin. They reported 84 patients with diseases that produce malabsorption (celiac disease, Crohn's disease, ileal resection, small intestine diverticulosis), in whom 95 per cent had satisfactory gallbladder opacification.[86] Goldberg noted that, in his experience, patients with Crohn's disease or ileal resection may have nonvisualization of the gallbladder on oral cholecystography with Telepaque owing to impaired intestinal absorption of the contrast materials, perhaps related to a deficiency of bile salts.[87]

Table 4–1. EXTRABILIARY CAUSES OF NONVISUALIZATION OF THE GALLBLADDER

Fasting
Failure to ingest the contrast material
Vomiting
Nasogastric suction
Esophageal disease
   Zenker's diverticulum
   Epiphrenic diverticulum
   Esophageal obstruction
   Hiatus hernia
Gastric retention
Gastrocolic fistula
Acute pancreatitis
Acute peritonitis
Severe trauma
Postoperative ileus
Liver disease
Dubin-Johnson syndrome
Previous cholecystectomy
Cholestyramine
Infancy
Crohn's disease
Pregnancy
Pernicious anemia

Unabsorbed Telepaque occasionally serves as a useful contrast material for the detection of a number of abnormalities during cholecystography. Telepaque may coat the surface of a tumor or fill an ulcer crater (Fig. 4–9). The contrast material may be retained in diverticula of any type including Zenker's, epiphrenic, duodenal, Meckel's, and colonic (Fig. 4–10). Obstruction of the gastroesophageal junction due to achalasia or tumor may be demonstrated by retention of Telepaque in the esophagus. Telepaque may coat a gastric bezoar, or gastric retention of the contrast material may indicate the presence of pyloric obstruction (Fig. 4–11).[88] Telepaque may accumulate proximal to an intestinal obstruction. Clements demonstrated *in vitro* that Oragrafin coats the surface of tomato seeds, making them radiopaque (personal communication). He was able to make a diagnosis of colonic obstruction on a cholecystogram by identifying the seeds proximal to the obstruction. Finally, the retention of Telepaque in a hiatus, umbilical, or inguinal hernia occasionally allows these abnormalities to be diagnosed on the cholecystogram.[89]

Cholecystokinin Cholecystography

Fatty-food intolerance, heartburn, flatulence, epigastric fullness, and upper abdominal discomfort often are considered to be classic symptoms of cholelithiasis. However, patients with a normal cholecystogram have these dyspeptic complaints as frequently as those with gallstones.[88] Consequently, although it is possible that these symptoms originate in the gallbladder, they are not due to cholelithiasis.

Text continued on page 105

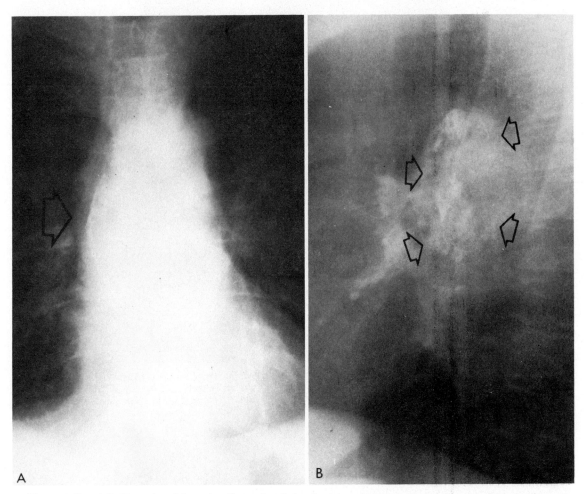

Figure 4–9. *A,B*, Frontal and lateral radiographs of the chest in a patient having cholecystography in whom the Telepaque adhered to the surface of an esophageal tumor and is faintly visible (arrows).

Illustration continued on following page

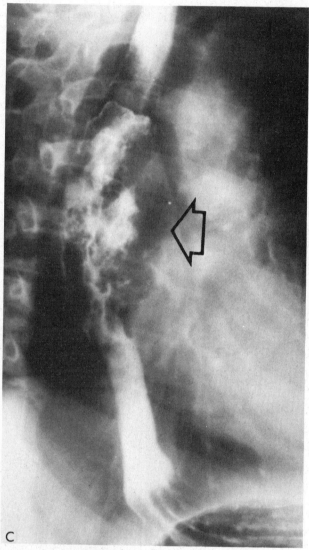

C

Figure 4–9. *Continued   C*, Barium esophagram demonstrates the carcinoma of the esophagus. *D*, An oral cholecystogram shows poor visualization of the gallbladder after a single dose of Telepaque. There is excessive unabsorbed
contrast material in the intestine and an unusual collection of Telepaque to the right of the spine (arrow). Calcification
is visible in the splenic artery. *E*, Barium examination of the stomach confirms the presence of an ulcer crater in the
pylorus.

Illustration continued on opposite page

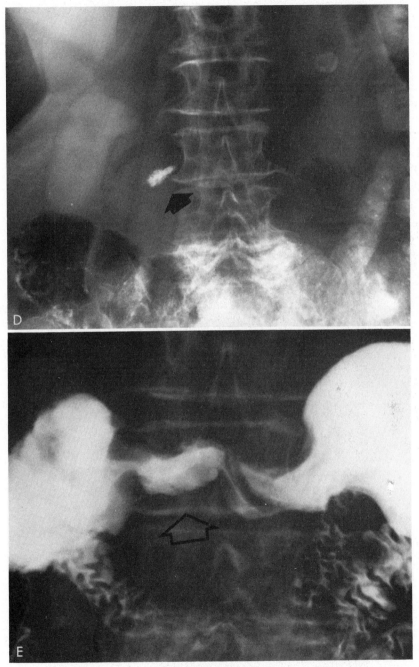

Figure 4–9. *Continued*

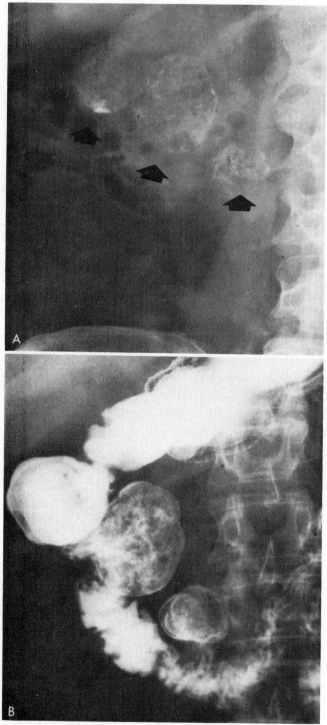

Figure 4–10. *A*, Radiograph from an oral cholecystogram showing three unusual collections of Telepaque on the upper abdomen (arrows). *B*, Radiograph from an upper gastrointestinal examination in the same patient, showing that the Telepaque was retained in duodenal diverticula.

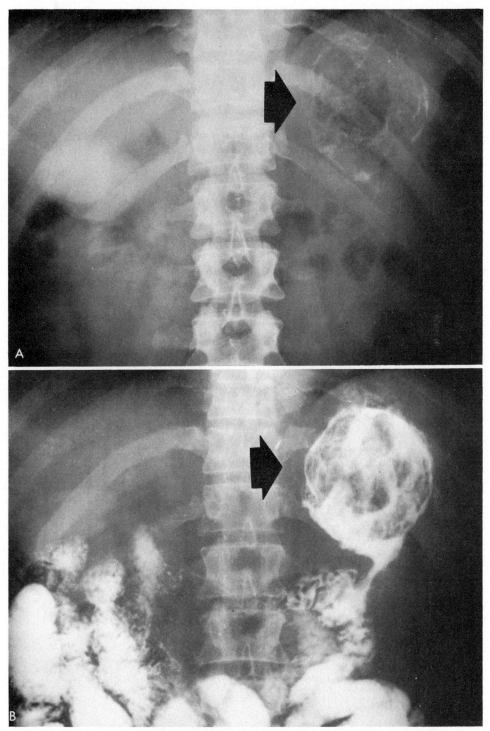

Figure 4–11. *A,* Radiograph from an oral cholecystogram showing opacification of the gallbladder. There is an unusual collection of Telepaque in the left upper quadrant. *B,C,* Radiographs from the upper gastrointestinal examination in the same patient, showing that the Telepaque was on the surface of a bezoar in the stomach (arrow). The patient has had a Billroth II anastomosis. *D,* Radiograph from an oral cholecystogram in another patient. The gallbladder is faintly opacified. There is retention of the Telepaque in the stomach (arrow), suggesting gastric obstruction. Subsequent upper gastrointestinal examination confirmed the presence of gastric obstruction and showed that it was due to antral carcinoma.

Illustration continued on following page

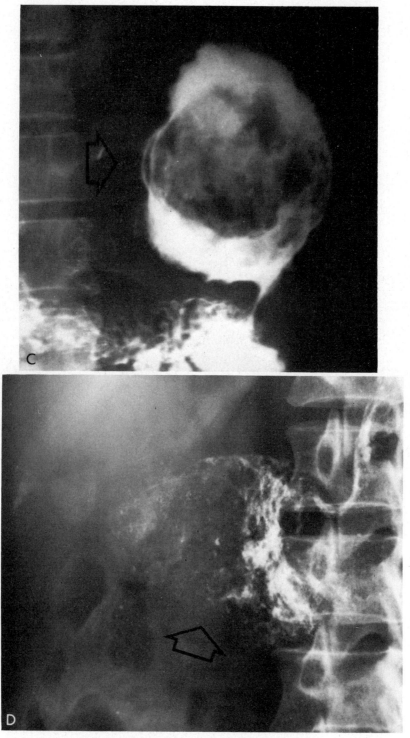

Figure 4–11. *Continued*

In the U.S., the only universally accepted cause for recurrent biliary-type pain is gallstones. Patients with undiagnosed abdominal pain related to the ingestion of fatty foods but who have a normal cholecystogram generally are considered to have psychosomatic disease no matter how much the pain resembles biliary colic. Some of these patients have gallstones that have been missed on cholecystography or diseases such as peptic ulcer or pancreatitis that have been overlooked. However, most suffer from one of a number of marginal organic diseases and questionable physiologic disorders of the biliary tract that present an enigma in terms of their actual existence, diagnosis, and treatment. These syndromes have been variously termed biliary dyskinesia, acalculous chronic cholecystitis, and the cystic duct syndrome. The clinical manifestations, pathologic changes, and results of surgery are so variable in these putative disorders that most surgeons are reluctant to perform a cholecystectomy in these patients. However, this inflexible approach to cholecystectomy for patients complaining of biliary tract pain has probably led to the underdiagnosis of biliary tract disease.[90] A reliable radiographic procedure for the diagnosis of these abnormalities and a technique to determine which patient would benefit from surgery would be exceedingly valuable.

DIAGNOSIS OF BILIARY DYSKINESIA ON ORAL CHOLECYSTOGRAPHY

The fatty meal has been used since the inception of oral cholecystography in an effort to recognize abnormalities in gallbladder evacuation in patients who have symptoms of biliary tract disease but a normal cholecystogram. Unfortunately, the degree of emptying of the normal gallbladder following a fatty meal varies widely and thus has little diagnostic significance. The difficulty arises from the fact that a fatty meal leaves the stomach at different rates, and when it reaches the duodenum it has a variable effect on stimulating the production of cholecystokinin by the duodenal mucosa.

It has recently been suggested that persistent visualization of the gallbladder 36 hours after administration of Telepaque is diagnostic of biliary dyskinesia.[91] The idea was introduced in two reports of prolonged gallbladder opacification in a combined total of 50 patients who had long-standing symptoms of gallbladder disease and who repeatedly had normal cholecystograms.[91, 92] These patients underwent cholecystectomy and were relieved of their symptoms in almost every instance. Two subsequent studies led to the opposite conclusion; that prolonged opacification of the gallbladder is devoid of clinical significance because its frequency was not significantly lower in asymptomatic controls.[93, 94] Prolonged opacification can be related to the enterohepatic recirculation of contrast material, which is known to occur,[95] the degree of initial opacification, and diet. Patients would be expected not to empty their gallbladders if they had little or no fat in their diet following the cholecystogram.

Despite these logical explanations postulated to explain persistent opacification as a normal phenomenon, a recent report from Israel noted that only one of 17 normal volunteers whose diet included a fat supplement had persistent opacification compared with two-thirds of patients with gallstones, two-thirds of patients with biliary-type abdominal pain in whom cholecystography was normal, and two-thirds of healthy subjects deprived of fat.[96] This highly significant difference leaves open the possibility that persistent opacification of the gallbladder in patients taking fat in the diet may be a sign of gallbladder disease. Confirmation of these results by other workers is necessary before the significance of this finding can be determined.

Cholecystokinin

In 1928, Ivy and Oldberg[97] showed that fat in the small intestine stimulates the release of a substance that activates gallbladder contraction. This hormone, which they termed cholecystokinin (CCK), is a polypeptide with the active portion of the molecule residing in the C-terminal octapeptide fragment.[98] The octapeptide, synthesized by Ondetti in 1978,[99] is more easily produced and promises to be an inexpensive alternative to the extracted preparation for use in place of a fatty meal during cholecystography. The octapeptide is available for general use during cholecystography without special government approval.

Technique of CCK Cholecystography

CCK cholecystography is performed by giving 1.0 Ivy dog unit of CCK or the octapeptide intravenously, after first opacifying the gallbladder by oral cholecystography in the usual manner.[100-107] Four or five serial radiographs of the gallbladder are then made in the prone oblique projection during the 15- to 20-minute interval after the injection. The optimal rate of injection has not been defined, but the CCK usually is given over one to three minutes. No change in the patient's position is allowed during the study, since this might affect the gallbladder's size or configuration. A positive examination is defined differently by various investigators, but is generally one in which (1) the CCK induces the patient's symptoms (usually upper abdominal pain);[104, 105] and/or (2) the radiographs show incomplete emptying and/or spasm of the gallbladder.[101, 103, 108] Incomplete emptying implies a reduction in volume of less than 20 to 50 per cent in the 15- to 20-minute interval.[101-103, 106-109]

Accuracy of CCK Cholecystography

Goldstein and colleagues were enthusiastic about their experience with CCK cholecystography performed between 1959 and 1972 in which the diagnosis of the cystic duct syndrome was apparently made correctly on the basis of a positive test in 28 patients.[101-103, 106, 107] The response to CCK was considered abnormal when the gallbladder emptied less than 50 per cent. In many of these cases, the gallbladder assumed a globular configuration (fighting gallbladder), as if it were attempting to empty against increased resistance. All the patients with deficient gallbladder contraction developed upper abdominal pain after the CCK injection. Cholecystectomy was performed in 25 of the 28 patients. All but three were relieved of their symptoms during follow-up periods ranging from six months to 11 years. Histologic examination of the gallbladder showed varying degrees of chronic cholecystitis, with kinks or narrowing of the cystic duct in 18 of the 25 patients. The gallbladder was normal in five, and histologic data were not available in two. CCK cholecystography was performed in 17 control subjects. In every instance the gallbladder contracted 50 per cent or more, and no patients had upper abdominal pain (Table 4–2).

Valberg and co-workers[105] had an equally good experience with CCK in 13 patients with typical attacks of biliary-like pain who had normal conventional cholecystograms. CCK, injected in one minute, produced typical attacks of pain in each patient. Changes in size or shape of the gallbladder were not taken into consideration. Twelve of the 13 patients underwent cholecystectomy and had complete relief of their symptoms. None of the 30 control subjects developed pain after the CCK (Table 4–2).

In a third optimistic report, Nathan and associates[104] compared the results of CCK cholecystography in 141 patients with the results in 142 controls (35 doctors, 107 nondoctors). The radiographic and symptomatic responses after CCK injected in 15 to 30 seconds are given in Tables 4–3 and 4–4. The study of

Table 4–2. CHOLECYSTOKININ CHOLECYSTOGRAPHY

	Goldstein et al.[107]	Valberg[107]	Nathan et al.[104]	Goldberg[150]	Dunn et al.[108]
Rate of injection (min)	3	1	.50	1 to 3	0.75
Definition of positive test	Failure to empty gallbladder more than 50%	Pain	Spasm of gallbladder and/or pain	Failure to empty gallbladder more than 80% and pain	Spasm of gallbladder and/or pain
Cure after cholecystectomy in patients with positive test	22 out of 25 (88%)	12 out of 13 (92%)	77 out of 79 (97%)	14 out of 15 (93%)	17 out of 20 (85%)
Control studies Number	17	30	142	0	44
Results	0 failed to empty gallbladder more than 50%	0 had pain	3% or less had spasm of gallbladder; 9% or less had pain	—	28% had spasm of gallbladder; 27% had pain

Table 4–3. RADIOGRAPHIC FINDINGS AFTER INTRAVENOUS CCK*[†]

	Doctor Controls (35)	Nondoctor Controls (107)	Patients (141)
Fundus	3	0	11
Body	0	0	3
Neck	3	2	55
Cystic duct‡	0	1	23
Cystic duct§	80	88	84

*Data from reference 104.
†Numbers indicate percentage of visualization of spasm.
‡Persists on five-minute radiograph or beyond.
§Lasts less than three to four minutes.

Nathan and colleagues differed from that of Goldstein, Grunt, and Margulies[107] in that it did not consider the degree of gallbladder emptying but only spasm of the gallbladder. Transient spasm of the cystic duct was evident in both the patient and control groups. However, prolonged spasm of the cystic duct or spasm of the fundus, body, or neck of the gallbladder occurred more frequently in the patients than in the control group (Table 4–3) (Fig. 4–12). Nausea and upper abdominal cramps (not defined) occurred with approximately equal frequency in the control and patient groups (Table 4–4). The disproportionate number of doctors who developed symptoms suggests that their response to CCK may have been affected by their medical knowledge and is an indication of the importance of extraneous influences on patients' subjective responses.

Nathan and co-workers defined a positive response to CCK as spasm of the neck, body, or fundus of the gallbladder on the radiograph and/or the production of upper abdominal pain.[104] Subsequently, there were 79 patients in their series with a positive examination who had a cholecystectomy (Table 4–2). The gallbladders in 77 of these had histologic evidence of mild or minimal chronic cholecystitis, and

in two the gallbladders were normal. Marked relief of the patients' symptoms occurred in 94 per cent of those having surgery in follow-up periods ranging from three months to four years.

Goldberg was equally sanguine about the value of CCK cholecystography in detecting patients with disease of the biliary tract in the presence of a normal conventional cholecystogram.[100] He defined a positive test more stringently than did Goldstein and associates[106] or Nathan and coworkers[104] and required that, for the gallbladder to be considered abnormal, it must contract less than 20 per cent on the radiograph and the patient must have reproduction of pain. Goldberg reported that 14 of 15 patients with a positive response to CCK who had a cholecystectomy were completely cured or had marked improvement during the follow-up period of six months to four years.

Consequently, despite the facts that (1) different criteria were used to define a positive response to CCK, (2) the CCK was injected at different rates, (3) the control subjects were evaluated by varying standards according to the investigator, and (4) the patients were followed for different lengths of time postoperatively, all the authors reached the same conclusion (Table 4–2). This was that nearly

Table 4–4. SYMPTOMATIC RESPONSE TO INTRAVENOUS CCK*

	Doctor Controls (35)	Nondoctor Controls (107)	Patients (141)
Nausea	23	6	9
Right upper quadrant and epigastric cramps†	17	5	11
Right upper quadrant and epigastric pain	9	0	46
Reproduction of symptoms	—	—	66

*Data from reference 104; numbers indicate percentage of patients in group.
†Not further defined.

all patients with biliary-type pain who have a cholecystectomy based on a "positive" response to CCK are cured despite having a normal conventional cholecystogram. This indicates that, no matter which of the various criteria are used to define a positive examination or how the CCK is injected, there are exceedingly few false-positive CCK cholecystograms. The incidence of false-negative tests has not been determined by these studies,

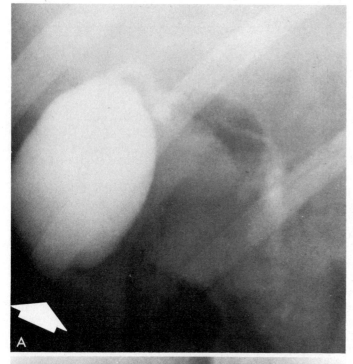

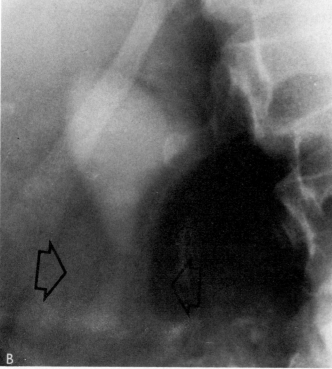

Figure 4–12. Cholecystokinin cholecystograms in three different patients, showing spasm of the fundus (*A,B*) and the body (*C*) of the gallbladder. There is poor emptying (fighting gallbladder) in *A*. The cholecystokinin produced right upper quadrant pain in all three patients. Patients in *A* and *C* underwent cholecystectomies and were relieved of their symptoms. The pathologic diagnosis was mild chronic cholecystitis in both cases. The patient in *B* became asymptomatic without surgery.

Illustration continued on opposite page

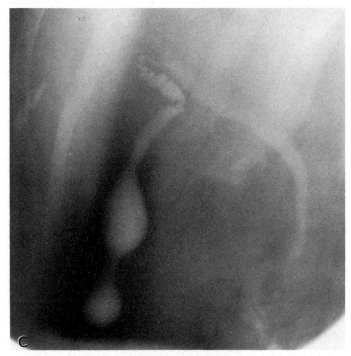

Figure 4–12. *Continued*

because none of the patients with a negative response to CCK had a cholecystectomy.

Despite these favorable reports,[101-107] CCK cholecystography has not been accepted enthusiastically as an accurate diagnostic modality in this enigmatic group of patients. Obviously, one reason is that it is only recently that the octapeptide has become available for use without special government approval in clinical practice, so that experience with the procedure is limited to a few investigators. Some radiologists are skeptical because of their own unsatisfactory experience with a fatty meal during cholecystography in which the response of the gallbladder is variable and the production of symptoms is difficult to evaluate. In addition, there is lack of confidence in CCK cholecystography because investigators do not agree on what constitutes a positive response to CCK. Is it the degree of emptying of the gallbladder that is significant, or is it the presence of spasm in various portions of the gallbladder? If the former, what degree of contraction should be considered abnormal? Less than 50 per cent? Thirty per cent? Twenty per cent? Many clinicians are doubtful about the reliability of putative successful results in patients who have had a cholecystectomy after positive CCK cholecystography. They recognize that clinical symptoms in a group of pa-tients are difficult to evaluate because the symptoms vacillate, are often poorly defined, and sometimes are associated with a potpourri of complaints in other organ systems. In most cases surgeons are still reluctant to operate when the conventional cholecystogram is normal, despite a positive response to CCK, because the pathologic findings in the gallbladder often are marginal and subject to differing interpretations. The importance of the potential placebo effect of surgery *per se* in relieving or altering the complaints in these patients cannot be underestimated. Finally, some skeptics are fearful that the duration of follow-up of the patients in many of the reports is too short and believe that those with initial successful results after cholecystectomy may have an exacerbation of their symptoms as they are observed for longer periods.

The Exegesis

Dunn and colleagues[108] emphasized that none of the previous reports on CCK cholecystography intrepreted the results without knowledge of the patient's clinical condition. Thus, the radiologist who interpreted the radiographs knew which subjects were asymptomatic controls and which had biliary symptoms, so that his analysis of the radiographs could easily have been biased. None of the patients with a negative response to CCK were operated on, so it is impossible to determine whether the CCK cholecystogram could differentiate patients who would benefit from cholecystectomy from those who would not, or whether, indeed, all the patients might not have been cured by surgery if it had been performed.

To overcome these objections, Dunn and coworkers performed CCK cholecystography in 44 control subjects and 74 patients with a history suggestive of gallbladder disease but in whom routine cholecystography was normal. The patients were assigned to one of two categories, possible biliary colic or dyspepsia, depending on their symptoms. To be placed in the possible biliary colic group, the patients must have had distinct attacks of abdominal pain. Patients assigned to the dyspepsia group had pain day after day and generally had epigastric or right upper quadrant discomfort or pain after meals and a feeling of fullness in the epigastrium, with or without food intolerance, belching, and flatulence. These patients had more persistent abdominal discomfort or pain than those in the possible biliary colic group. Some pain was required in order to be included in either category. Those with heartburn, food intolerance, belching, and flatulence were not included in the study unless they also had pain.

The radiographs were evaluated by three radiologists without knowledge of the patient's history. They were interpreted as normal,

probably normal, probably abnormal, or definitely abnormal. The decision was based on changes in gallbladder shape; spasm of the gallbladder fundus, body, or neck; cystic duct spasm; or abnormal patterns of emptying.

The clinical and radiographic responses are shown in Table 4–5. If the interpretations of the three radiologists are averaged, 28 per cent of the controls, 31 per cent of those with possible biliary colic, and 43 per cent of those with dyspepsia had an abnormal or probably abnormal response to CCK. The differences are not significant. In approximately 28 per cent of the cases, the radiologists differed in major ways in their interpretation of the radiographs (i.e., one radiologist read the films as "normal or probably normal," whereas the others interpreted them as "abnormal or probably abnormal"). Not only was there poor correlation when the three interpretations were compared but also when a second interpretation by an individual radiologist was compared with his initial reading.

Biliary-like pain or discomfort was produced in 27 per cent of the controls, 65 per cent of the patients with possible biliary colic, and 44 per cent of the patients with dyspepsia. This was gallbladder-like pain and was carefully differentiated from the abdominal symptoms that can be produced by CCK such as lower abdominal cramping, abdominal fullness, or nausea.

Twenty-nine of the patients were subjected to cholecystectomy because of severe and recurrent abdominal distress (Table 4–6). The decision to operate was made without knowl-

Table 4–5. INTERPRETATION OF RADIOGRAPHS BY THREE RADIOLOGISTS*

	Averge Age (Range)	Radiologist	Normal	Probably Normal	Probably Abnormal	Abnormal	Gallbladder-like Pain After CCK† (% of Patients)
Controls n = 44	33.8 (20–58)	1	48	16	16	20	27
		2	68	18	5	9	
		3	52	14	16	18	
Biliary colic n = 49	37.6 (22–61)	1	47	21	10	22	65
		2	62	12	12	14	
		3	33	31	12	24	
Dyspepsia n = 25	40.5 (17–64)	1	36	16	0	48	44
		2	52	8	12	28	
		3	32	28	12	28	

*Data from reference 108.
†Values given are percentages.

Table 4–6. RESPONSE TO CHOLECYSTECTOMY RELATED TO CLINICAL RESPONSE TO CHOLECYSTOKININ*†

	No. of Patients	No. Cured	No. Improved	No. Same	No. Follow-up
Pain or discomfort reproduced	20	14	3	2	1
Abnormal‡	9	7	2	—	—
Normal§	11	7	1	2	1
Pain or discomfort not reproduced	9	4	2	3	—
Abnormal	3	0	1	2	—
Normal	6	4	1	1	—

*No patient's condition deteriorated as a result of therapy.
†Data from reference 108.
‡Abnormal indicates roentgenogram read as abnormal or probably abnormal by at least two of the three radiologists.
§Normal indicates roentgenogram read as normal or probably normal by at least two of the three radiologists.

edge of the results of the CCK cholecystogram. Forty-one per cent of this group were in the possible biliary colic group and 35 per cent were in the dyspepsia category. Eighty per cent considered themselves cured or definitely improved by cholecystectomy regardless of the results of the CCK cholecystogram (Table 4–7).

Table 4–6 shows the results of cholecystectomy related to the clinical response to CCK. Eighty-five per cent of the patients with pain reproduced by CCK who had a cholecystectomy were cured or improved, whereas 66 per cent of those with a negative symptomatic response to CCK were improved. Follow-up data in patients who did not have a cholecystectomy are given in Table 4–7. Sixty-five per cent of the patients contacted in the biliary colic group were cured or improved, whereas 50 per cent in the dyspepsia group who were contacted were cured or improved.

Goldstein, Grunt, and Margulies[107] criticized Dunn's study on the basis that the rapid injection rate of CCK (45 seconds) used can produce spasm of the cystic duct in most normal individuals. However, the data reported by Nathan and colleagues show that such spasm is transient, rarely lasting longer than three or four minutes.[104] It seems unlikely, therefore, that the rate of injection interfered with the study or influenced the results.

Dunn and associates concluded that CCK cholecystography, as currently performed and interpreted, is of little or no value in the diagnosis and management of patients with possible acalculous biliary tract disease. They give four reasons for their assertion:

(1) The incidence of "abnormal" gallbladder contraction in normal subjects is high (14 to 36 per cent).

(2) CCK cholecystography does not help to predict which patients will be cured by chole-

Table 4–7. FOLLOW-UP IN PATIENTS WHO DID NOT HAVE GALLBLADDER SURGERY*

	No. Cured	No. Improved	No. Same	No. Worse	Average Length of Follow-up (mo)	Range of Follow-up (mo)
Biliary colic (26 of 29 contacted)	6	11	6	3	20.1	6–32
Abnormal†	0	3	1	1	19.6	6–28
Normal‡	6	8	5	2	20.2	7–32
Dyspepsia (14 of 16 contacted)	2	5	4	3	21.7	6–34
Abnormal	1	1	1	1	19.8	11–32
Normal	1	4	3	2	22.7	6–34

*Data from reference 108.
†Abnormal indicates roentgenogram read as abnormal or probably abnormal by at least two of the three radiologists.
‡Normal indicates roentgenogram read as normal or probably normal by at least two of the three radiologists.

cystectomy. Their results show that patients with both normal and abnormal responses to CCK usually are cured or improved by cholecystectomy.

(3) CCK cholecystography does not help to predict histologic findings in the gallbladder. Patients with normal and abnormal CCK responses who had a cholecystectomy had similar histologic findings in their gallbladders.

(4) There is a high degree of observer disagreement (approximately 28 per cent) in the interpretation of the radiographs.

DIFFERENTIATION BETWEEN CHOLESTEROL AND PIGMENT GALLSTONES

Current criteria for the selection of patients for medical treatment of cholelithiasis with chenodeoxycholic acid or similar compounds include the presence of gallbladder visualization on oral cholecystography and radiographic evidence that the stones are either entirely radiolucent or have a calcified center less than 3 mm in diameter.[109, 110] Accuracy in predicting stone composition is a key factor in the success of chemotherapy, since dissolution occurs only with cholesterol stones. If the distinction can be made on oral cholecystography, the role of this procedure in the selection of patients for medical therapy would be considerably expanded.

In an attempt to achieve this goal, Dolgin and coworkers evaluated 56 patients with surgically confirmed cholelithiasis.[111] Only buoyancy as detected on upright radiographs made during cholecystography was highly predictive of gallstone composition; all 14 patients with floating stones had cholesterol stones (Fig. 4–1). However, only one-third of the patients with cholesterol stones had stone buoyancy. Using stepwise discriminant analysis involving multiple variables, ability to identify cholesterol gallstones improved significantly. The sensitivity was 95 per cent (37 of 39 patients with cholesterol stones), specificity was 82 per cent (14 of 17 patients with pigment stones), and efficiency was 91 per cent (51 of 56 patients). The variables employed, in addition to buoyancy, included the number and size of the stones, the type of calcification, and the surface characteristics.

Of interest is the fact that, with few exceptions, gallstones appear to float only during oral cholecystography. Among more than 400 patients with gallstones undergoing sonogra-

phy with upright projections at the Vancouver General Hospital, stones were seen to float in only three patients.[112] In each of these the ultrasound examination was done in combination with an oral cholecystogram. This suggests that contrast material raises the specific gravity of the bile and causes the floating phenomenon. No cases of floating stones were found in the absence of contrast material.

HYPERPLASTIC CHOLECYSTOSES

Hyperplastic cholecystosis is a generic term introduced by Jutras in 1960 for a group of abnormalities of the gallbladder that appear to be separate from inflammatory disease.[113] Hyperplasia implies a benign proliferation of normal tissue elements, whereas cholecystosis indicates a pathologic process that is distinct from inflammation. The two main categories of hyperplastic cholecystoses are cholesterolosis and adenomyomatosis. According to Jutras,[113] both types cause functional abnormalities of the gallbladder consisting of hyperconcentration, hypercontraction, and hyperexcretion. These can be detected on radiographs made during cholecystography and are clues to the diagnosis.

Cholesterolosis

Cholesterolosis, or strawberry gallbladder, is characterized by abnormal deposits of cholesterol esters in fat-laden macrophages in the lamina propria of the gallbladder. The lipid creates coarse, yellow, speckled excrescences on the surface of the reddened hyperemic gallbladder mucosa and gives the latter a "strawberry" appearance. The cause of the cholesterol deposition is unknown, although it has been attributed to excess cholesterol absorption across the gallbladder mucosa. Cholesterolosis is not related to the serum cholesterol concentration, but cholesterol stones develop in 50 to 70 per cent of patients with the abnormality.[114]

When the cholesterol deposits are of sufficient size, the cholecystogram shows fixed radiolucencies, either localized or generalized, in the opacified gallbladder (Fig. 4–13).[113] The lipid protrusions into the gallbladder lumen may be single or multiple, usually vary in size, are unevenly distributed, and may involve any portion of the gallbladder. The lesions often are best seen on radiographs made after partial evacuation of the gallbladder and on radiographs made with compression. Indirect radiographic findings include hyperconcentration and hyperexcretion, which are general features of all the hyperplastic cholecystoses.[113] Cholesterolosis can be differentiated from cholelithiasis by determining that the radiolucent defects are fixed in position within the gallbladder on radiographs made in different positions; gallstones usually are free to move

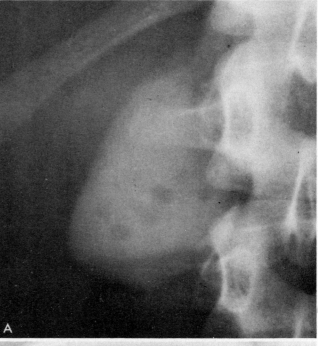

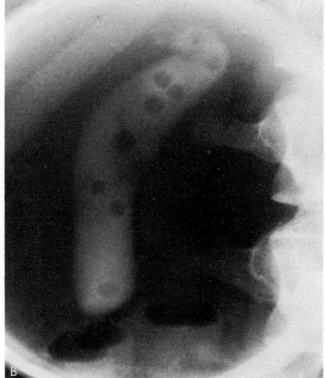

Figure 4–13. *A,B,* Oral cholecystograms in two patients show cholesterolosis of the gallbladder. Numerous round or oval filling defects are visible in the gallbladder. The defects maintained the same location in the gallbladder despite changes in the patient's position during examination, indicating that they are fixed to the wall.

Illustration continued on following page

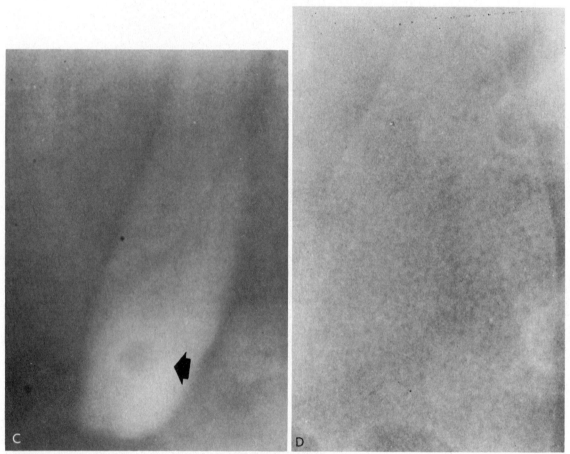

Figure 4–13. *Continued* *C*, Oral cholecystogram shows a single, small, fixed filling defect in the gallbladder due to a single cholesterol polyp (arrow). *D*, Close-up view of the gallbladder from an oral cholecystogram in another patient shows diffuse cholesterolosis of the gallbladder. There is faint opacification of the gallbladder. Innumerable 1- to 3-mm radiolucencies that did not change in position are visible. *E*, Photograph of mucosal surface of gallbladder, showing multiple cholesterol polyps. (Courtesy Loitman, B.S., M.D.)

Illustration continued on opposite page

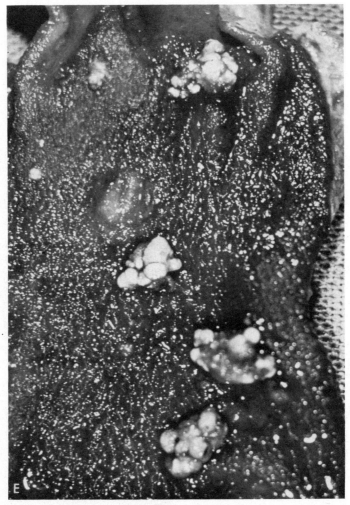

Figure 4–13. *Continued*

about and collect by gravity in the dependent portion of the gallbladder or to form a layer in the bile.

The management of patients with cholesterolosis is uncertain. Some surgeons reserve cholecystectomy in such patients for those who also have cholelithiasis and are symptomatic. However, in 269 cases of cholesterolosis without gallstones reported by Salmenkivi, about 90 per cent had complete or partial relief of symptoms following surgery.[115]

Adenomyomatosis

Adenomyomatosis consists of proliferation of mucosa, increased thickness of the muscle coat, and formation of outpouching of mucosa into or through the muscularis.[113] These diverticula, which are termed Rokitansky-Aschoff sinuses, may be either segmental or diffuse throughout the gallbladder (Fig. 4–14).

Radiographically, the sinuses are seen as multiple or single oval collections of contrast material of varying size adjacent to the lumen of the gallbladder (Fig. 4–15). Any portion of the gallbladder may be involved. At times calcified concretions are present within the diverticula (Fig. 4–16). Adenomyomatosis often is associated with compartmentalization of the gallbladder due to septal folds or annular thickening in the gallbladder wall (Fig. 4–17). Whether compartmentalization is the cause or the effect of adenomyomatosis is not certain. Compartmentalization may be due to circumferential adenomyomatosis, a congenital septum, or adenomyomatosis superimposed on a congenital septum. Aguirre, Boher, and Gur-

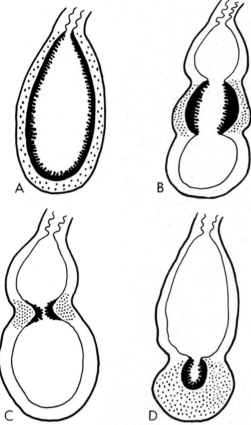

Figure 4–14. Diagram of various types of adenomyomatosis. *A*, Generalized. *B*, Localized. *C*, Circumferential. *D*, Fundal. (From Aguirre, J. R.: Am. J. Roentgenol. *107*:1, 1969.)

aieb believe that the circumferential form of adenomyomatosis producing compartmentalization originates in a congenital septum.[116] It is often difficult to determine by cholecystography whether the stenosis is a simple septum or whether the adenomyomatosis is already present.

The combination of adenomyomatosis and cholesterolosis is not unusual, and gallstones often are present. Like cholesterolosis, adenomyomatosis is often more easily identified and appears more marked on radiographs made after partial emptying of the gallbladder. Fundal adenomyomatosis has various radiologic patterns, ranging from a filling defect or mass in the fundus due to focal hyperplasia of the gallbladder wall to multiple diverticular outpouchings filled with contrast material or small calculi localized to the fundus (Fig. 4–18).

Adenomyomatosis is observed much more commonly pathologically than radiographically. In one series, 50 per cent of patients

Text continued on page 121

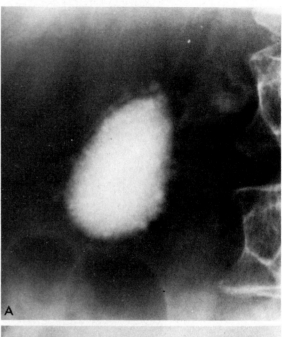

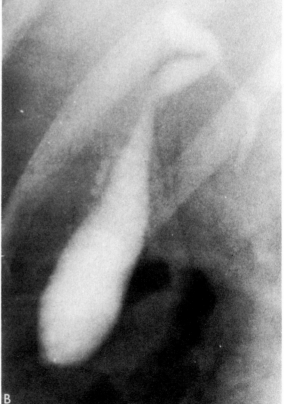

Figure 4–15. *A–C*, Oral cholecystograms in three patients show diffuse adenomyomatosis of the gallbladder. Small outpouches of the gallbladder wall filled with contrast material are visible.

Illustration continued on opposite page

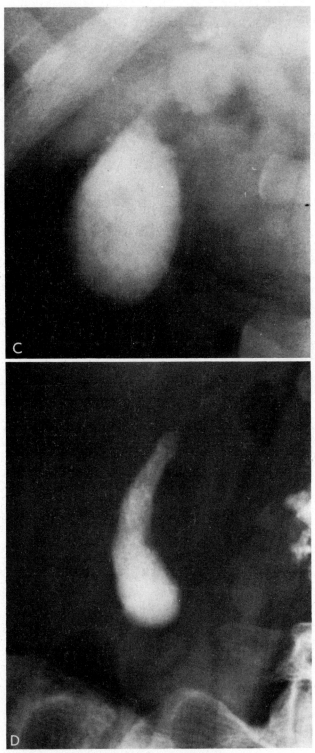

Figure 4–15. *Continued D*, Oral cholecystogram showing an unusual smudged appearance of the gallbladder with good opacification and no evidence of cholelithiasis. The pathologic diagnosis was chronic cholecystitis and cholelithiasis with focal adenomyomatosis. The gallbladder wall was 4 mm thick, the mucosa was edematous, and there were numerous gallstones measuring up to 2 mm in size. Histologically, there was marked thickening of the serosa due to dense fibrous tissue and adenomyomatosis, with only slight chronic inflammatory infiltrate in the submucosa.

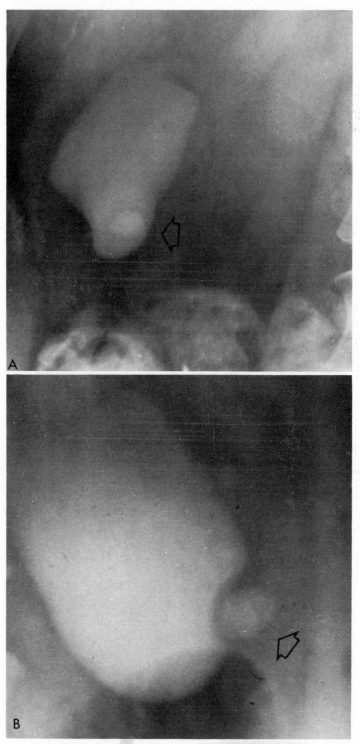

Figure 4–16. Oral cholecystogram shows a gallstone in fundal adenomyomatosis. *A*, The calcification is superimposed on the fundus of the gallbladder. *B*, Spot film made at fluoroscopy shows the gallstone in the wall of the gallbladder.

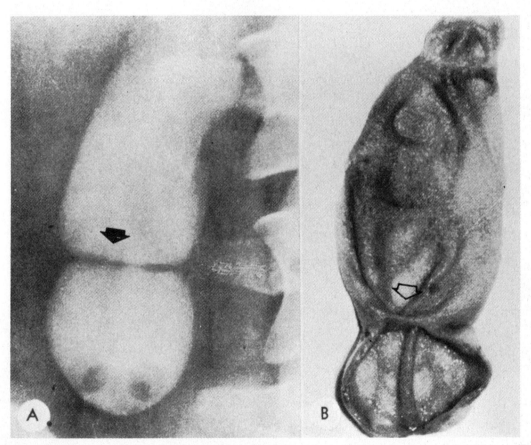

Figure 4–17. *A,B,* Circumferential type of adenomyomatosis with compartmentalization and cholelithiasis. (From Aguirre, J. R.: Am J. Roentgenol. *107*:1, 1969.)

Illustration continued on following page

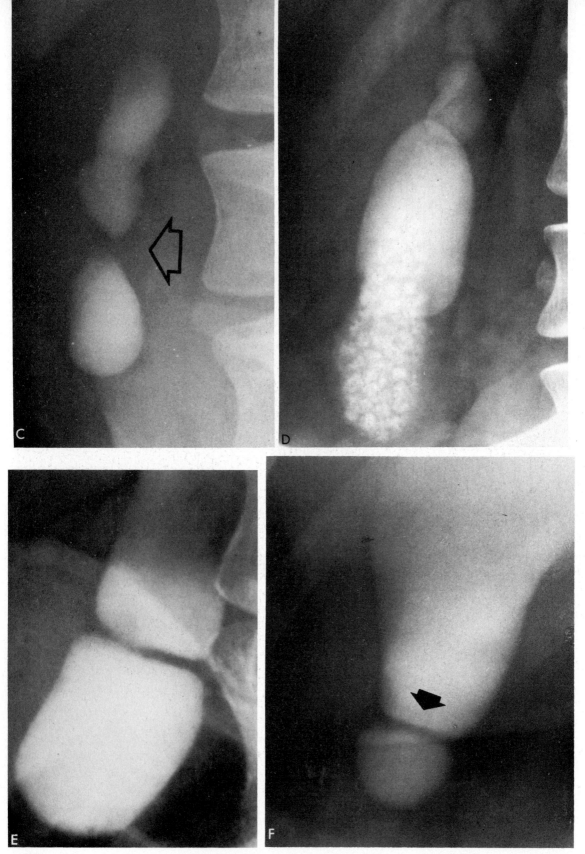

Figure 4–17. *Continued   C–F*, Oral cholecystograms in four patients show compartmentalization of the gallbladder. Note the gallstones in the distal compartment in *D*. Pathologic examination of the gallbladder after surgery in *C* and *D* showed focal adenomyomatosis of the gallbladder in the area of narrowing.

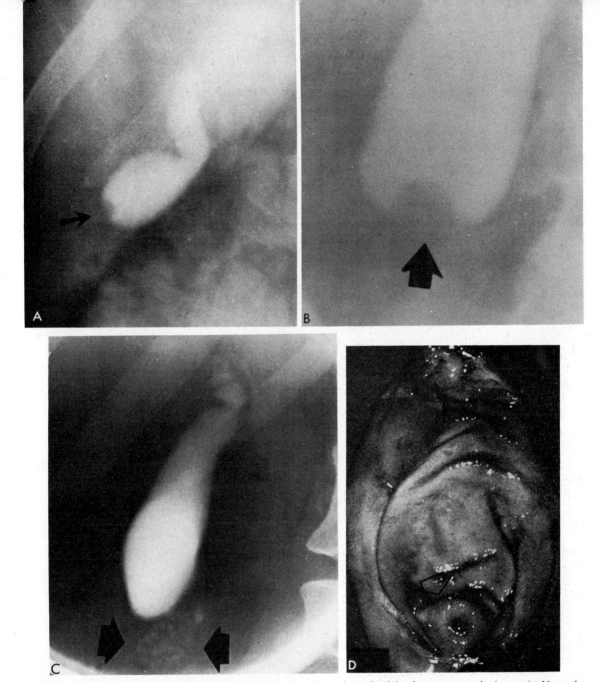

Figure 4–18. *A–C,* Oral cholecystograms in three patients show fundal adenomyomatosis (arrows). Note the multiple small calcifications present in the adenomyomatosis in *C* (arrows). *D,* Photograph showing the fundal adenomyomatosis.

having cholecystectomy for gallstones had associated adenomyomatosis that was not apparent on cholecystography.[117] Whether a cholecystectomy should be performed in a patient with adenomyomatosis depends on the severity and duration of the symptoms and the presence of cholelithiasis.

NORMAL VARIATIONS OF THE GALLBLADDER

The size, shape, and position of the gallbladder as seen on cholecystography vary con-

siderably in normal patients, depending on the body habitus of the patient, the degree of filling of the gallbladder, the amount of distention of the adjacent transverse colon, the position in which the radiograph is made, and the type of contrast material used (Fig. 4–19). Tall, slender individuals tend to have vertically oriented, long gallbladders that may lie in the right iliac fossa; in mesomorphic patients the gallbladder usually is horizontal, tortuous, orientated in a lateral plane, and high in the right upper quadrant of the abdomen. When the gallbladder has no mesentery and is closely applied to the undersurface of the liver, little

Text continued on page 126

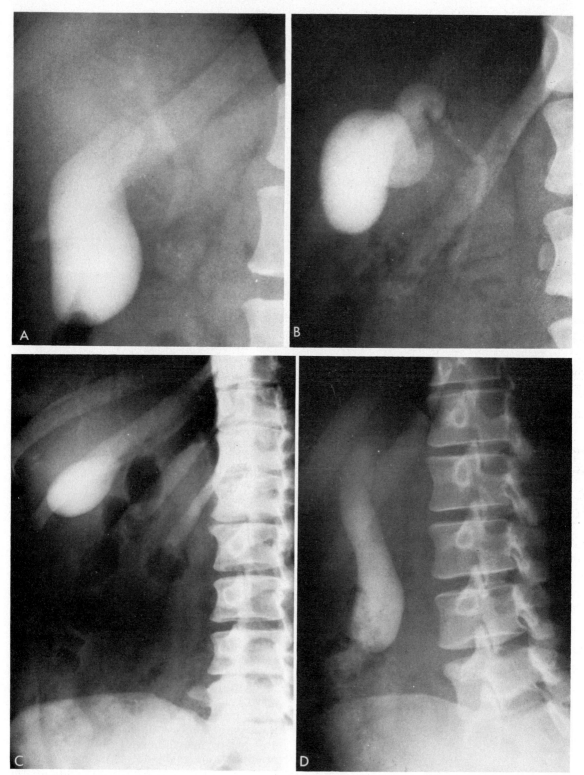

Figure 4–19. *A–G*, Oral cholecystograms in seven different patients, showing normal variations in size, shape, and position of the gallbladder.

Illustration continued on opposite page

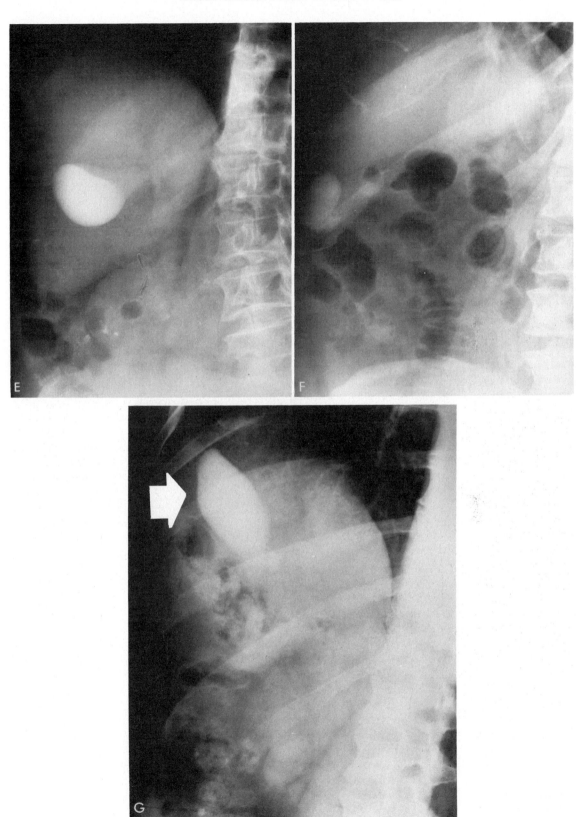

Figure 4–19. *Continued*

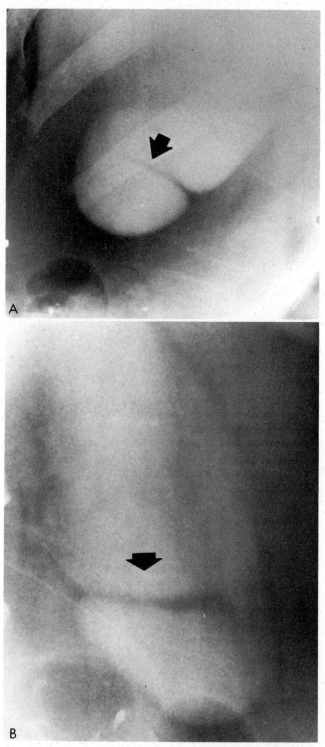

Figure 4–20. *A–E*, Oral cholecystograms in five patients show a phrygian cap of the gallbladder (arrows). The thickness of the septum in the fundus varies. The example in *A* is most characteristic.

Illustration continued on opposite page

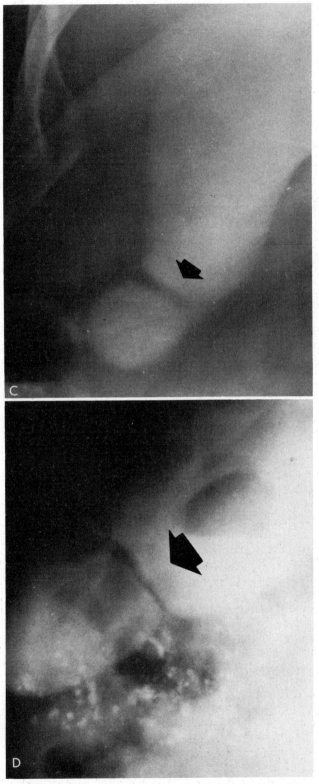

Figure 4–20. *Continued*

Illustration continued on following page

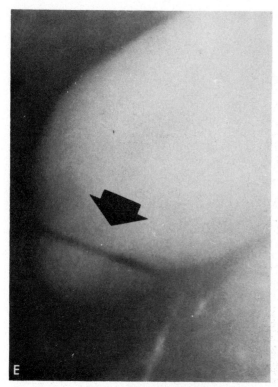

Figure 4–20. *Continued*

change in shape and position occurs with differences in position of the patient, except for the fundus. The liver edge serves as a fulcrum for changes in the position and shape to a considerable extent, depending on gravity. Superimposition of the fundus on the body may simulate duplication of the gallbladder, unless the gallbladder is visualized in profile using fluoroscopy to determine the optimal position.

When the gallbladder is opacified in the course of oral cholecystography, it usually is smaller than when it is visualized during intravenous cholangiography.[118] It may be that the oral contrast agents act as a cholecystogogue that partially empties the gallbladder. More probably, the increase in bile flow associated with the intravenous agent produces greater distention of the gallbladder than do the oral contrast materials, which are not choleretic (see Chapter 3).

Phrygian Cap

A phrygian cap is a normal variation in the shape of the gallbladder in which the fundus appears to be folded on the body (Figs. 4–20 and 4–21). The name is taken from the similarly shaped headdress worn as a sign of lib-

eration by slaves in ancient Greece.[119] In 1935, Boyden studied the morphology and pathogenesis of the phrygian cap and, contrary to the accepted view at that time, recognized that it has no clinical importance.[119] He described two types, depending on whether the serosa of the gallbladder was included in the septum between the fundus and body. Similar folding located more proximally in the body of the gallbladder is not unusual and also has no significance, except that it must be differentiated from compartmentalization of the gallbladder associated with adenomyomatosis. Indeed, such folds may predispose to circumferential adenomyomatosis. When adenomyomatosis involves the septum, the fold or narrowing usually is thicker, and evacuation radiographs of the gallbladder show focal spasm and diverticular outpouchings in the region of the infolding.

Layering of Contrast Material

In the erect position, layers of bile are present in the gallbladder that increase in specific gravity from the neck of the fundus. Visual demonstration of this layering phenomenon occurs during cholecystography in the erect position whenever rapid filling of the gallbladder causes incomplete mixing of nonopaque and contrast-laden bile (Fig. 4–22). When there is incomplete mixing, discrete bands of radiolucent bile can be identified separately from layers of bile containing contrast material on upright radiographs. The layer that has been in the gallbladder the longest has the highest specific gravity and therefore is dependent. Incomplete mixing detected on prone or supine radiographs may simulate cholelithiasis (Fig. 4–23).

Layering of contrast material in the gallbladder is much more common during intravenous cholangiography than during oral cholecystography, because rapid filling of the gallbladder with contrast material during intravenous studies does not allow adequate time for uniform mixing (see Chapter 5). Bryk and Moadel showed that layering of contrast material occurred in only 6 per cent of patients on upright radiographs made during oral cholecystography.[120] However, when a fatty meal was given to these patients, layering was noted in most cases on upright radiographs made two hours later. In these cases, the layering phenomenon appears to be the result of rapid refilling of the gallbladder with nonopaque bile following partial emptying of the gallbladder.

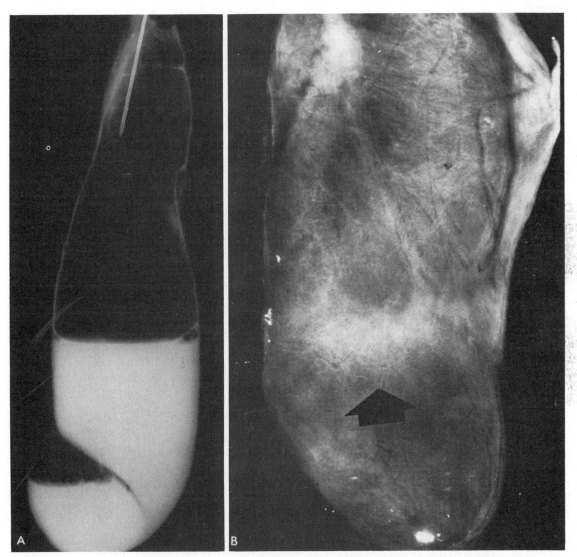

Figure 4–21. *A*, Upright radiograph of a gallbladder *in vitro* shows a phrygian cap. *B*, Photograph of the gallbladder shows the serosal surface. The phrygian cap is not evident from the external surface except for the change in color of the gallbladder wall (arrow).

Illustration continued on following page

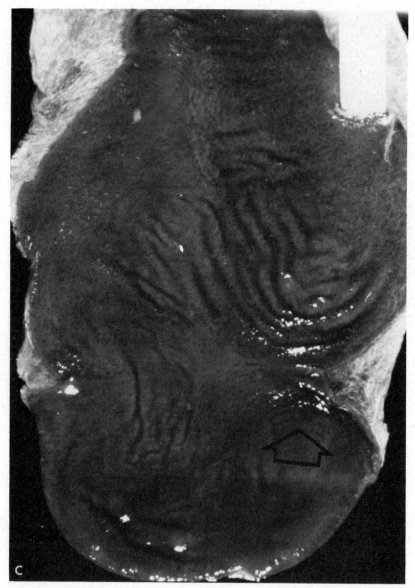

Figure 4–21. *Continued C,* Photograph of the gross specimen showing the mucosal surface of the gallbladder indicates the irregularity of the fundus due to the phrygian cap (arrow). In this variety, the serosa is not included in the infolding.

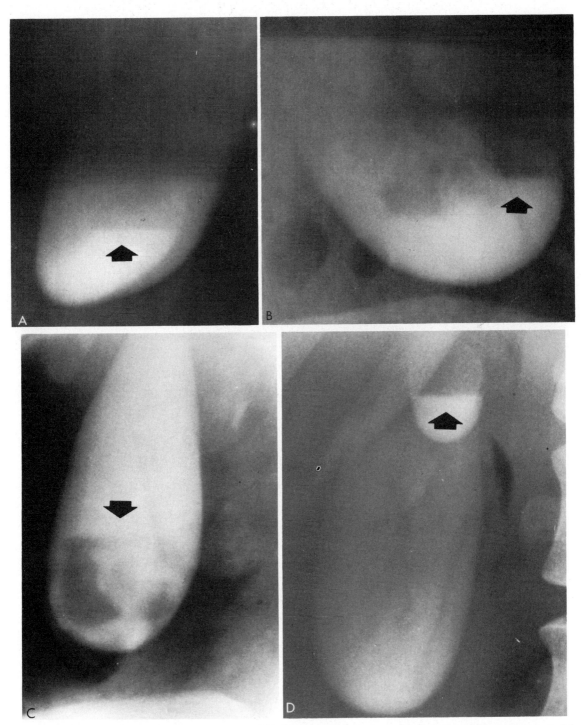

Figure 4–22. Upright radiographs from the oral cholecystograms in patients show layering of the contrast material in the gallbladder. *A,B,* Two projections of the gallbladder in the same patient show a sharp boundary between nonopaque and opaque bile in the fundus (arrow). *C,* Incomplete mixing of Telepaque in the gallbladder (arrow) in this case must be distinguished from a large gallstone. *D,* Note the poorly defined layering in the body of the gallbladder and the sharp stratification of opaque and nonopaque bile in Hartman's pouch (arrow).

Illustration continued on following page

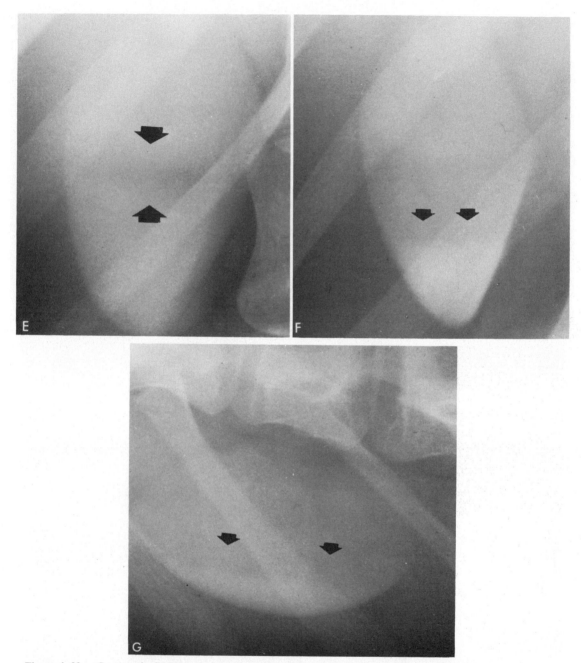

Figure 4–22. *Continued* *E*, There is a poorly defined layer of nonopaque bile (arrows). Opaque bile is dependent in this upright *(F)* and right decubitus projection *(G)* (arrows).

Precipitation of Contrast Material

Since the glucuronide conjugate of Telepaque excreted by the liver is relatively water soluble, the contrast material is neither reabsorbed from the normal gallbladder nor precipitated in the gallbladder lumen (see Chapter 3). Rarely, however, presumably because of the presence in the gallbladder of bacteria capable of producing glucuronidase, Telepaque glucuronide is deconjugated and Telepaque precipitates in the bile.[121] This action produces amorphous radiopaque densities in the gallbladder that collect in the fundus on radiographs made in the upright position (Fig. 4–24).

Differentiation from small radiopaque calculi depends on the fact that the precipitate does not persist on subsequent plain abdominal radiographs, whereas radiopaque calculi remain unchanged (Fig. 4–25). In addition, for reasons that are obscure, Telepaque rarely precipitates a second time on a later cholecystogram.

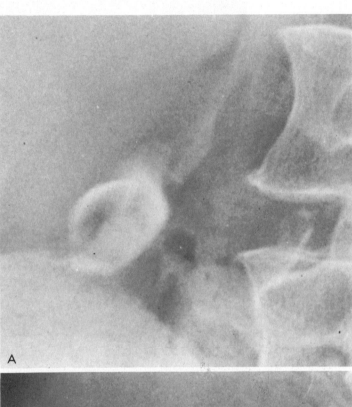

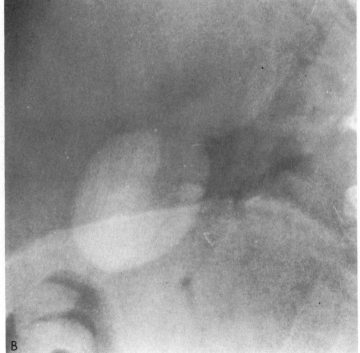

Figure 4–23. *A*, Supine radiograph from the oral cholecystogram shows a poorly defined radiolucency in the gallbladder due to incomplete mixing of opaque and nonopaque bile. *B*, A repeat examination with a second dose of contrast material shows that the gallbladder is normal.

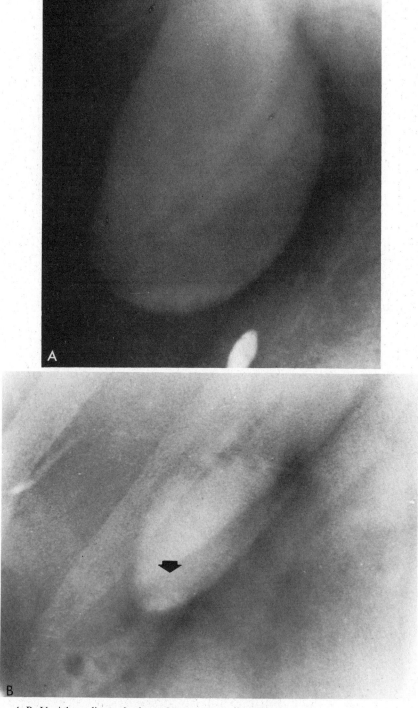

Figure 4–24. *A,B,* Upright radiographs from the oral cholecystograms in two patients show Telepaque precipitate in the fundus of the gallbladder (arrow).

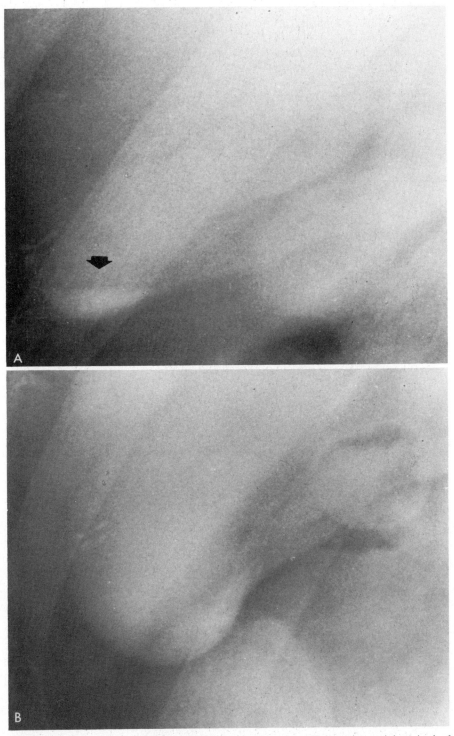

Figure 4–25. *A*, Upright radiograph from an oral cholecystogram shows Telepaque precipitate in the fundus of the gallbladder (arrow). *B*, A repeat examination in the same patient performed one week later demonstrates a normal gallbladder. The precipitation of the Telepaque did not recur on the second examination.

False Filling Defect in the Neck of the Gallbladder

Kriss called attention to a small, false filling defect in the neck of the gallbladder that simulates a tiny gallstone or wall lesion.[122] The radiolucency is 2 to 3 mm in size and occurred in 5 per cent of Kriss's patients. The artifact generally is sharply outlined and lies in the neck of the gallbladder, sometimes assuming a marginal position (Fig. 4–26).

The defect is a projectional artifact due to folding or coiling of the junction between the neck of the gallbladder and the cystic duct on one another. In some cases the defect is caused by viewing the cystic duct opening *en face*, superimposed on the neck of the gallbladder. According to Kriss, the orifice of the cystic

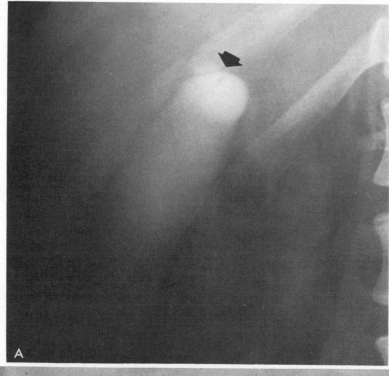

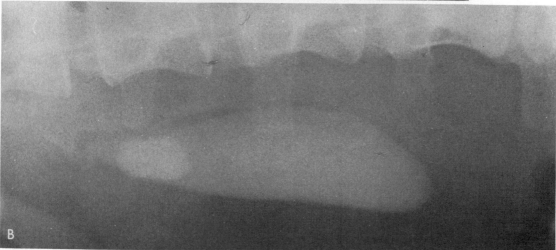

Figure 4–26. *A*, Supine radiograph from an oral cholecystogram shows a false filling defect in the neck of the gallbladder (arrow). *B*, Decubitus projection of the gallbladder in the same patient shows faint opacification of the cystic and common ducts. The filling defect seen in *A* is spurious and is due to superimposition of the cystic duct on the neck of the gallbladder.

duct appears radiolucent because it is not distended when the radiograph is made, creating a summation artifact.

The false filling defect disappears with change in position. This dependence on position and the variability and inconsistency of the finding serve to differentiate these features from true lesions.

CONGENITAL ANOMALIES OF THE GALLBLADDER

Anomalies of Position

Abnormal position of the gallbladder occurs in association with situs inversus.[123] In other cases the gallbladder may be left-sided in relation to the inferior aspect of the left lobe of the liver, in which case the cystic duct may terminate in the right hepatic duct.[124, 125] Rarely, the gallbladder may be on the left, associated with isolated transposition of the liver. In this case the liver and gallbladder usually are located directly anterior to the stomach.

When the gallbladder lies completely within the parenchyma of the liver, major diagnostic and therapeutic difficulties arise if acute cholecystitis occurs (Fig. 4–27). Liver scan, ultrasound studies, and hepatic angiography suggest the presence of an hepatic abscess. Rarely, gallstones can be identified in the gallbladder within the liver on plain abdominal radiographs. The gallbladder may be located behind the liver (retrohepatic) and even may be retroperitoneal or interposed between the liver and the diaphragm (suprahepatic).[123] Isolated cases of an ectopic gallbladder located in the falciform ligament and in the abdominal wall have been reported.[124]

The gallbladder may be unusually mobile when it is on a long mesentery. In such cases, herniation into the foramen of Winslow is possible[126, 127] (Fig. 4–28). Vint reported four surgically proved cases.[126] The key radiologic finding is displacement of the gallbladder medial to the duodenal bulb, which is best seen on frontal projection with the gallbladder and stomach opacified with barium. The gallbladder appears to drape over the apex of the bulb, and the adjacent walls of these structures conform closely to each other. The clinical significance of herniation of the gallbladder is unknown. It may be intermittent and asymptomatic in some patients but in others is believed to be the cause of vague abdominal discomfort.

Duplication of the Gallbladder

The appearance of a double gallbladder on cholecystography most often is proved to be a tortuous gallbladder with overlap of the fundus, body, and neck on one projection or a gallbladder with compartmentalization. To establish the diagnosis, two separate gallbladder lumina and two distinct cystic ducts must be demonstrated. Shehadi and Jacox reported an incidence of 1 in 12,000 cholecystograms[128] (Figs. 4–29 and 4–30).

Roeder, Mersheimer, and Kazarian reported a patient with triplication of the gallbladder in whom one gallbladder had acute cholecystitis and cholelithiasis and another had adenocarcinoma.[129]

Revacuolization of the primitive gallbladder is incomplete in these cases, resulting in a persistent longitudinal septum that divides the gallbladder lengthwise, creating a bifid gallbladder, or a true duplication.[130]

Agenesis of the Gallbladder

Agenesis of the gallbladder is virtually impossible to distinguish radiographically from acute cholecystitis with obstruction of the cystic duct (Fig. 4–31). However, two-thirds of patients with this anomaly have other malformations such as congenital heart lesions, imperforate anus, and rectovaginal fistula.[131] Consequently, the diagnosis should be suspected in patients with multiple congenital anomalies who have opacification of the common bile duct without gallbladder visualization on oral cholecystography or intravenous cholangiography.

Surgical exploration with operative cholangiography may be misleading.[124] A left-sided or intrahepatic gallbladder, an atrophic gallbladder, or one surrounded by adhesions may be mistaken for agenesis of the gallbladder.

Choledochal Cyst

A choledochal cyst is a congenital cystic dilatation of any segment of the extrahepatic biliary ducts, usually involving the main portion of the common bile duct. Babbitt, Star-

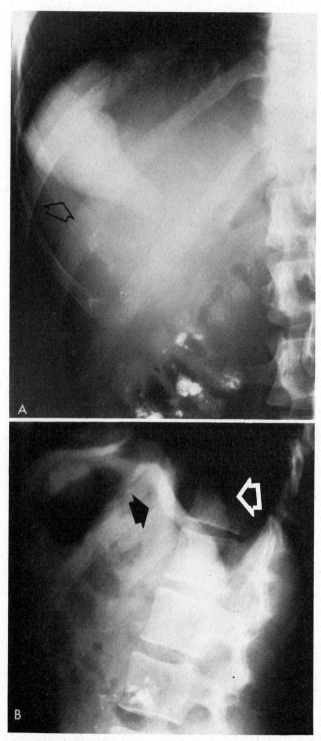

Figure 4–27.   Supine *(A)* and lateral *(B)* projections of an oral cholecystogram demonstrate a gallbladder that is completely in an intrahepatic position (arrows). At surgery for an unrelated condition, the gallbladder was entirely within the hepatic parenchyma.

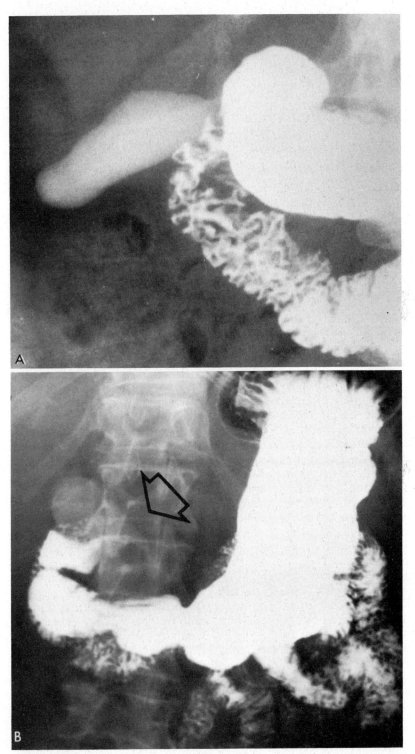

Figure 4–28. Oral cholecystogram and upper gastrointestinal examination in the same patient show herniation of the gallbladder through the foramen of Winslow *(A,B)*. Note the marked change in orientation of the gallbladder between the two projections and draping of the gallbladder to the left of the duodenum in *B* (arrow).

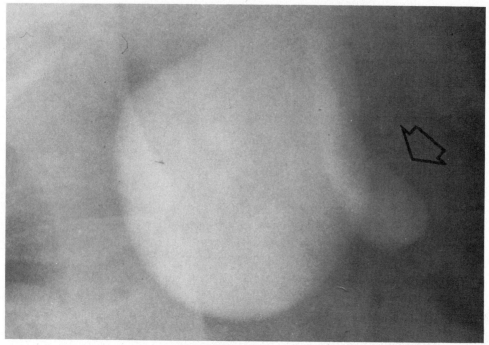

Figure 4–29. An oral cholecystogram shows a double gallbladder (arrow). Two separate lumina and cystic ducts were identified at surgery. (Courtesy Gary Roghair, M.D., Pocatello, Idaho.)

shak, and Clemett postulate that anomalous insertion of the common bile duct into the proximal part of the pancreatic duct several centimeters or more from the papilla of Vater allows reflux of pancreatic enzymes into the biliary tree and leads to inflammation and fibrosis.[132] Subsequent obstruction causes dilatation of the common bile duct. Newborns and infants present with obstructive jaundice. Older children may have a triad of jaundice, abdominal pain, and a mass.

The plain abdominal radiograph may show a right upper quadrant mass (Fig. 4–32). There often is anterior and medial displacement of the duodenal cap and gastric antrum on the upper gastrointestinal study.[133] Total body opacification during intravenous pyelography may demonstrate the fluid-filled cyst as a relatively radiolucent mass in the right upper quadrant.[134] Direct visualization of the choledochal cyst may be accomplished by sonography, scintigraphy, computed tomography, intravenous cholangiography, operative cholangiography, and, rarely, oral cholecystography (Fig. 4–33).[135, 136] Rosenfield and Griscom reviewed 24 cases of choledochal cyst, studied before the new diagnostic modalities were available.[134] Only seven were definitely diagnosed preoperatively; three by rose bengal scanning, two by intravenous cholangiography,

one by oral cholecystography, and one by sulfur colloid scanning followed by angiography. Considerable improvement in diagnostic precision can be expected with the greater availability of sonography and scintigraphy, both of which are highly sensitive techniques for the detection of this lesion.

Multiseptate Gallbladder

Croce defined the multiseptate gallbladder as a solitary gallbladder, usually normal in position and size, characterized externally by a faintly bosselated surface and internally by the presence of multiple septa of variable size and number.[137] The chambers thus formed communicate with each other by one or more orifices from fundus to cystic duct. Histologically, the walls of the septa are characterized by a layer of muscle between the two epithelial surfaces, a finding that appears to exclude the hypothesis that the anomaly is the result of arrested vacuolization of the epithelial bud of the gallbladder or an extension of the valves of Heister from the cystic duct.[138]

Stasis of bile in the gallbladder predisposes to infection and gallstone formation. The diagnosis can be made radiographically as long as complicating gallstones do not occlude the

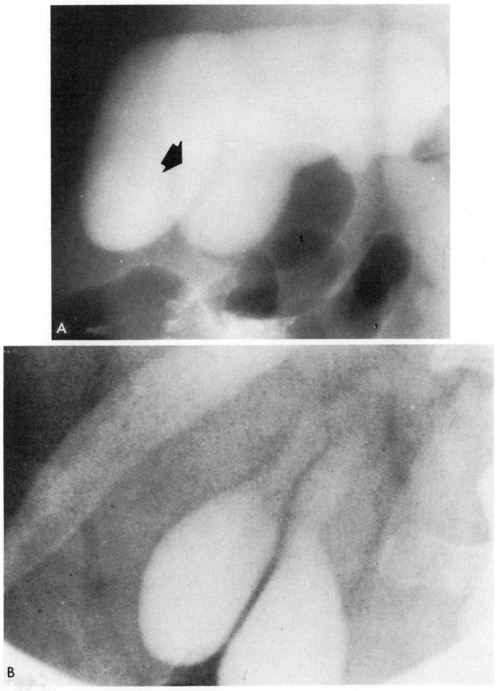

Figure 4–30. *A*, An oral cholecystogram shows a bifid gallbladder. At surgery, the fundus of the gallbladder was divided (arrow), but joined to form a normal body and neck. *B*, An oral cholecystogram showing complete duplication of the gallbladder.

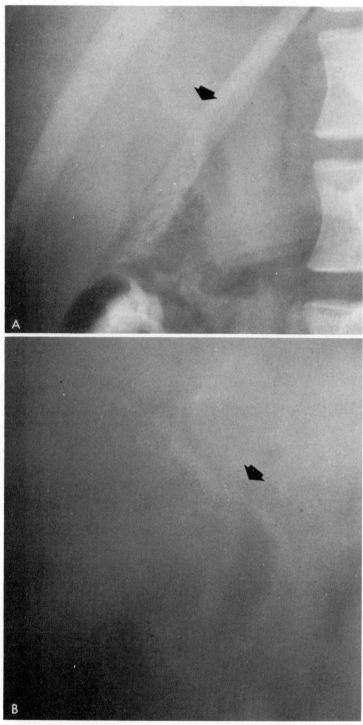

Figure 4–31. *A*, An oral cholecystogram in a patient with agenesis of the gallbladder. The common duct is opacified without visualization of the gallbladder, which ordinarily would suggest obstruction of the cystic duct owing to cholelithiasis (arrow). *B*, Tomogram made during an intravenous cholangiogram in the same patient, again demonstrating opacification of the common duct, but no filling of the gallbladder (arrow). At surgery, the gallbladder and cystic duct were absent.

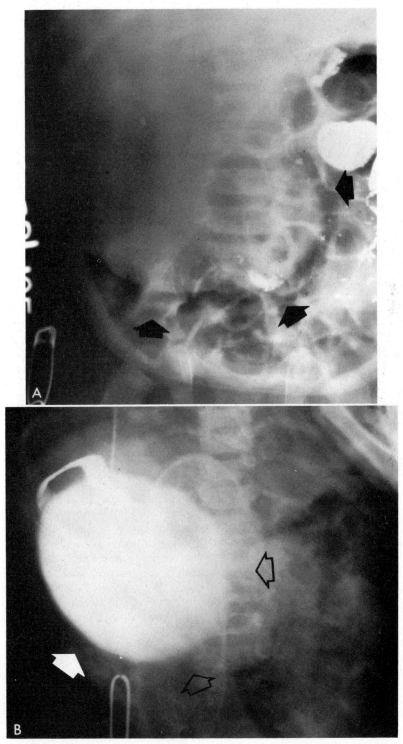

Figure 4–32. *A*, Plain abdominal radiograph of a 1-year-old child with jaundice shows a right upper quadrant mass due to a large choledochal cyst (arrows). Barium is present in the intestine from a previous examination. *B*, Radiograph made at surgery shows the choledochal cyst after the direct injection of contrast material (arrows).

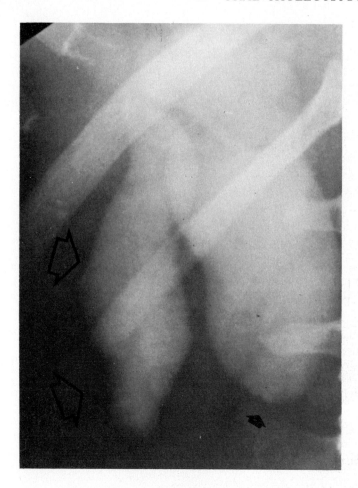

Figure 4–33. An oral cholecystogram in a 35-year-old man demonstrates a choledochal cyst with several small gallstones at the distal end (solid arrow). The gallbladder is opacified (open arrows). The choledochal cyst is unusually well opacified on the oral cholecystogram.

cystic duct and prevent opacification of the gallbladder (Fig. 4–34). The multicystic honeycomb character of the gallbladder is apparent on oral cholecystography.

The multiseptate gallbladder must be differentiated from the hypoplastic changes that occur in the gallbladder in patients with cystic fibrosis of the pancreas.

Heterotopic Pancreatic and Gastric Tissue

Aberrant pancreatic tissue and gastric mucosa occur in a variety of locations throughout the gastrointestinal tract. Rarely, implants of these tissues have been reported in the gallbladder.[139-141] In such cases, the cholecystogram may show a mural nodule in the gallbladder similar to cholesterolosis and various benign tumors. When the lesion is located at the neck of the gallbladder or cystic duct, partial or intermittent obstruction may cause nonvisualization on cholecystography and may result in cholecystitis.

CHOLELITHIASIS

An estimated 15 million Americans have gallstones, 85 per cent of which are composed predominantly of cholesterol.[142] A prerequisite for the formation of cholesterol gallstones is bile containing insufficient bile salts and lecithin in proportion to cholesterol to maintain the cholesterol in solution by the detergent-like property of the bile salts.[143] Such lithogenic bile may result from a decrease in the size of the bile salt pool due to disease or resection of the terminal ileum or to an increased hepatic cholesterol synthesis. Stones composed of bilirubin are less common and occur when there is excessive red blood cell destruction, such as in patients with sickle cell anemia and in patients with cirrhosis and those on parenteral hyperalimentation.

Oral cholecystography is not only a major diagnostic modality for the diagnosis of cholelithiasis, but it also is the main method of observing the results of medical treatment of gallstones. The results of the National Coop-

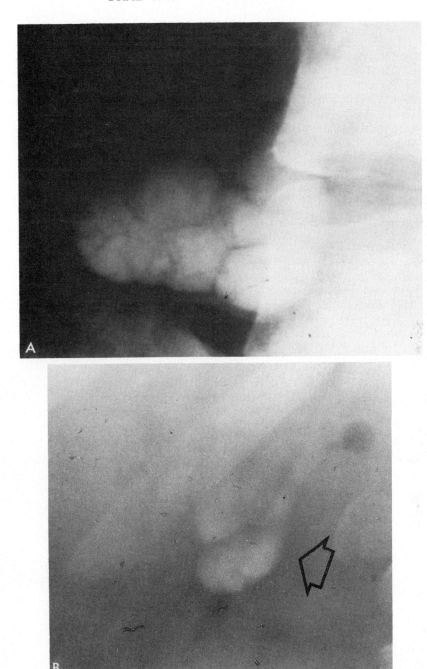

Figure 4–34. *A,B,* Oral cholecystograms in two patients showing congenital multiseptate gallbladders (arrow). At surgery in both cases the gallbladder was hypoplastic with multiple, intercommunicating septa dividing the lumen of the gallbladder.

erative Gallstone study published in 1981 prove that the oral administration of chenodeoxycholic acid, one of the bile salts, results in dissolution of gallstones and is appropriate therapy for gallstones in selected patients. In that study, 916 patients were given either chenodeoxycholic acid (750 or 375 mg) or placebo daily for two years. Serial oral cholecystograms demonstrated complete dissolution of the stones in 14 per cent of the patients on the high dose, 5 per cent on the low dose, and 0.8 per cent on placebo. Partial dissolution of the stones occurred in 41 per cent, 24 per cent, and 11.0 per cent, respectively. Dissolution occurred more frequently in women, in slender patients, and in cases of small or floating stones. Biochemical hepatic abnormalities occurred in 3 per cent and 0.4 per cent of patients on the high and low dose of the drug, respectively, but subsided spontaneously in all patients.

Gallstones vary markedly in number, size, and shape, so that cholecystography may demonstrate gallstones as large as 4 or 5 cm or some that are no more than 1 or 2 mm (Fig. 4–35). A single stone may be present, or there may be as many as 100 or more. When tiny stones are numerous, they often have a sand- or gravel-like consistency and are visible only on upright or lateral decubitus projections of the gallbladder. Gallstones are nearly always freely movable in the gallbladder and readily change position on radiographs made in different positions. The stones usually fall by gravity

to the dependent portion of the gallbladder. Not infrequently they form a layer in the bile, depending on their specific gravity in relation to that of the bile. Occasionally, a stone becomes adherent to the gallbladder wall and simulates a mural lesion such as a cholesterol polyp.

Reports of spontaneous disappearance of gallstones are not rare, so that when there is a significant interval between demonstration of the calculi and surgery, a repeat cholecystogram should be performed (Fig. 4–36).[145, 146] This is especially important if the gallstones are small. In some cases, particularly after pregnancy, it may be that bile that was lithogenic returns to normal and dissolution of the gallstones occurs. In other cases, the gallstones are passed into the duodenum via the cystic and common bile ducts with or without symptoms of biliary colic. As discussed in detail in

Text continued on page 149

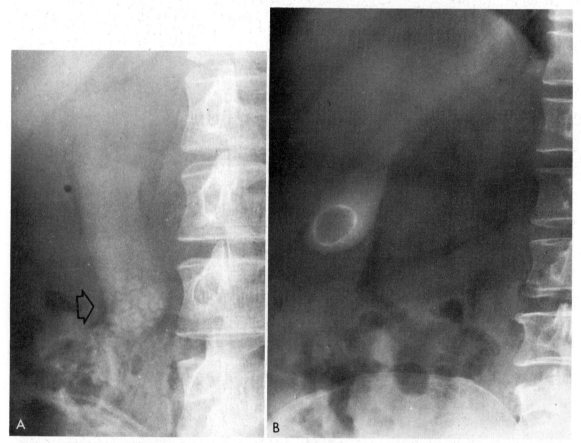

Figure 4–35. *A–N*, Oral cholecystograms from 14 different patients show the wide assortment of sizes and numbers of gallstones that occur. *G,H*, Upright spot films made at fluoroscopy demonstrate gallstones that were not visible on prone and supine projections. The small gallstones are visible, layered at their own specific gravity in the bile, *J*, Innumerable small calculi that have the consistency of sand and that settle in the dependent portion of the gallbladder are visible on upright projections (arrows). *M,N*, Unusually large, partly calcified gallstones.

Illustration continued on opposite page

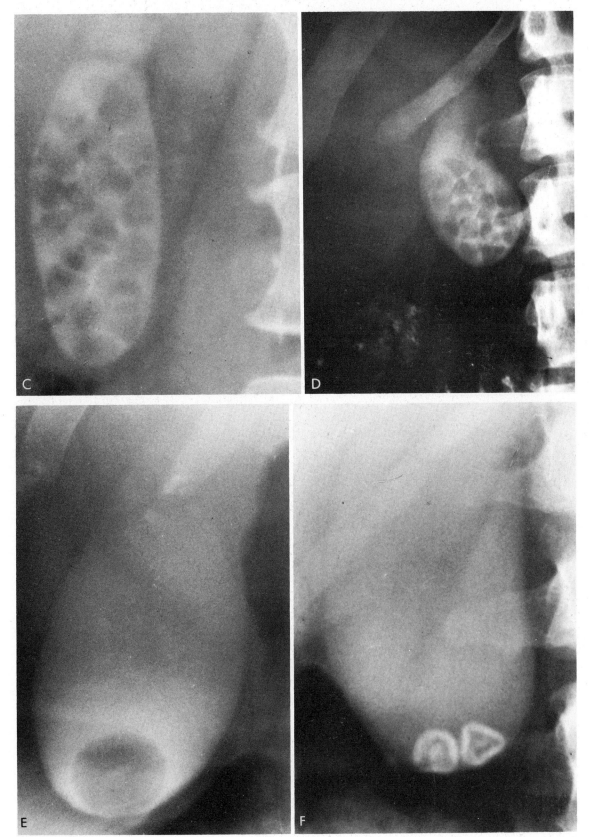

Figure 4–35. *Continued*

Illustration continued on following pages

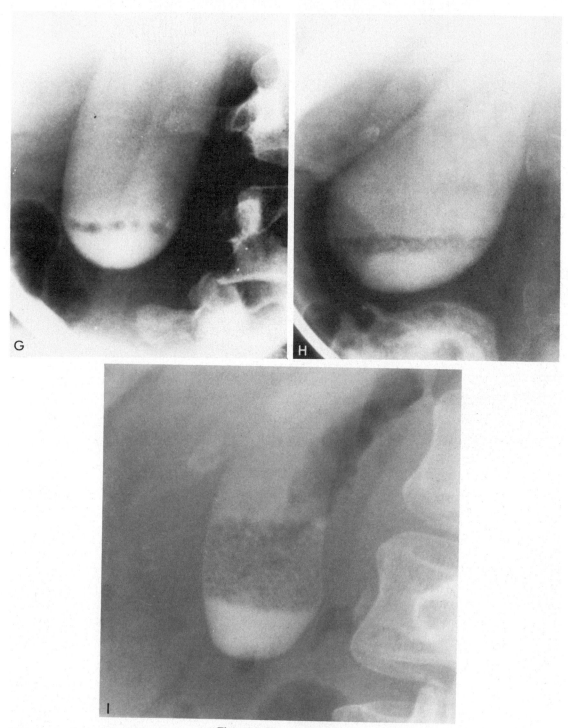

Figure 4–35. *Continued*

Illustration continued on opposite page

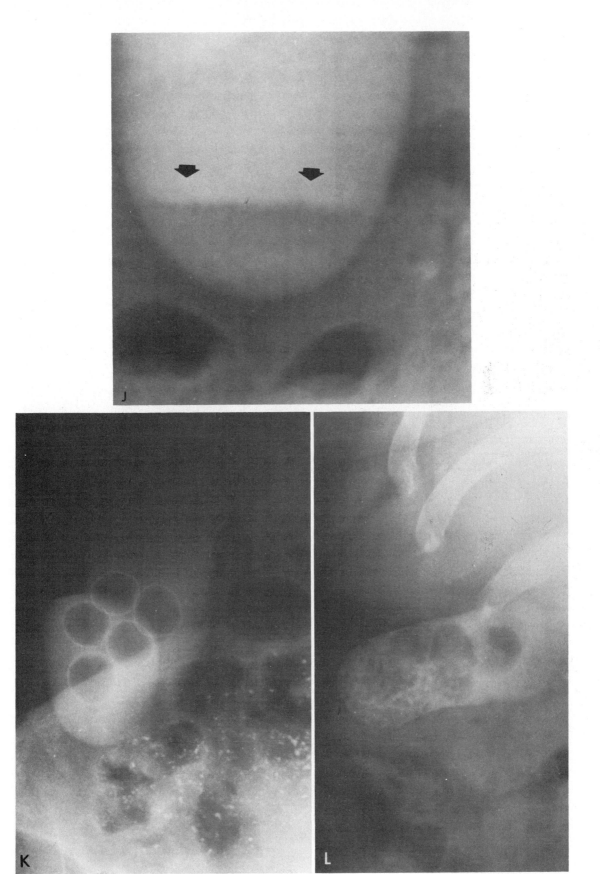

Figure 4–35. *Continued*

Illustration continued on following page

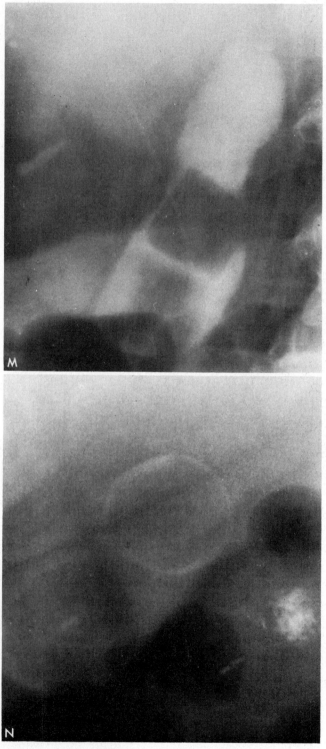

Figure 4–35. *Continued*

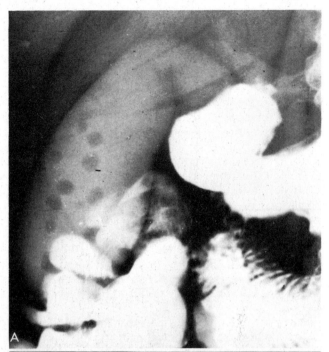

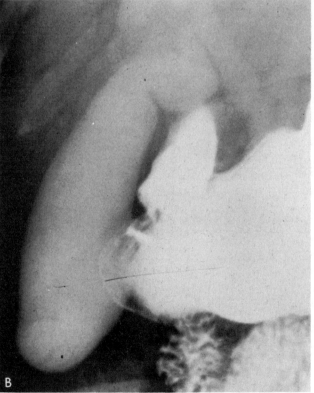

Figure 4–36. *A*, An oral cholecystogram demonstrates cholelithiasis. Barium is in the intestine from an upper gastrointestinal examination. *B*, A repeat examination performed three months later fails to show calculi. The stone must have dissolved or passed spontaneously.

Chapter 1, gas fissuring of gallstones may reduce the specific gravity of the stones so that they float in bile and are more likely to enter the cystic duct and be passed spontaneously.

Splitting of gallstones along the gas-filled faults causes spontaneous fragmentation of the stones, which also predisposes them to spontaneous passage.[147]

NEOPLASMS OF THE GALLBLADDER

Benign Tumors

True benign tumors of the gallbladder are exceedingly rare. Adenomas, the most common type, usually occur as flat elevations located in the body of the gallbladder.[148] Acinar tubular structures are seen beneath the surface epithelium. Adenomas almost invariably occur in or near the fundus and must be distinguished pathologically from adenomyomatosis, which is a hyperplastic change in the gallbladder wall. Papillomas may occur singly or in groups and may be scattered over a large part of the mucosal surface of the gallbladder.[149] Delicate or coarse connective stalks are covered by columns of epithelium not unlike that of the gallbladder mucosa. The papillomas are not precursors of, nor do they predispose to, carcinoma.

When a benign tumor is present, the cholecystogram discloses one or more small, round, or oval radiolucent defects fixed to the wall of an opacified gallbladder (Table 4–8) (Fig. 4–37).[150-152] The lesion often is better delineated after partial contraction of the gallbladder. Radiographs made in various positions and with different degrees of compression confirm that the defect is not freely movable within the gallbladder.

In most patients with a fixed filling defect on cholecystography, surgery proves that the defect is a pseudotumor rather than a true benign neoplasm. Of the many varieties of pseudotumors of the gallbladder that can be

Table 4–8. CAUSES OF FIXED FILLING DEFECTS IN AN OPACIFIED GALLBLADDER

Cholesterolosis
Adenomyomatosis
Adherent gallstone
Adenoma
Papilloma
Carcinoid
Carcinoma
Metastases
Mucosal hyperplasia
Inflammatory polyp
Epithelial cyst
Mucous retention cyst
Spurious defect of infundibulum
Heterotopic pancreatic or gastric tissue
Parasitic granuloma
Metachromatic sulfatides
Varices
Arterial tortuosity and aneurysm

identified during cholecystography, a solitary cholesterol polyp is the most common (Fig. 4–38). However, mucosal hyperplasia, inflammatory polyps, mucous cysts, and granulomata due to parasitic infections also occur (Table 4–8). Polypoid masses containing metachromatic sulfatides produce fixed defects in the wall of the gallbladder and occur in patients with metachromatic leukodystrophy.[153] This disease is one of the sphingolipidoses in which metachromatic sulfatides accumulate in various organs owing to a deficiency of the enzyme arylsulfatase-A. Occasionally, when gallstones are coated with tenacious mucus they adhere to the gallbladder wall and present as a fixed filling defect on oral cholecystography.

Carcinoma of the gallbladder is almost never detected at a resectable stage. Obstruction of the cystic duct by the tumor or lymph nodes occurs early in the course of the disease and causes nonvisualization of the gallbladder at cholecystography. Consequently, sonography is better suited for the detection of this lesion. However, Cimmino reported a case of noninvasive papillary adenocarcinoma in which the tumor was evident as a solitary fixed defect in a well-opacified gallbladder (Fig. 4–39).[154] Others have been reported,[151] but such cases are so unusual that cholecystectomy is not indicated to exclude carcinoma in patients in whom a solitary fixed defect is detected in the gallbladder at cholecystography.

Malignant Tumors

Primary carcinoma of the gallbladder is nearly always a rapidly progressive disease, with a mortality approaching 100 per cent.[155-159] Although it is associated with cholelithiasis in about 80 to 90 per cent of cases, direct proof is lacking to implicate the gallstones as the carcinogenic agent.[160] Patients with porcelain gallbladder also have an increased incidence of carcinoma of the gallbladder (see Chapter 1).[161] The latter condition is twice as common as carcinoma of the bile ducts and occurs most frequently in women 60 years of age and older.

This disease usually arises in the body of the gallbladder and, rarely, in the cystic duct. The tumor infiltrates the gallbladder locally or diffusely, causing thickening and rigidity of the wall. The adjacent liver often is invaded by direct continuity extending through tissue spaces, the ducts of Luschka, and/or the lymph channels. Obstruction of the cystic duct due to direct extension of the tumor or extrinsic

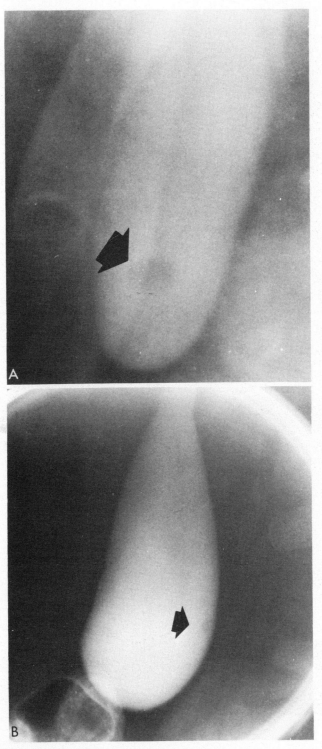

Figure 4–37. *A,B,* Upright radiographs from oral cholecystograms in two patients show solitary adenomyomas of the gallbladder (arrows). In both cases the radiolucency was fixed in position on various projections made during the examination. Adenomyomas are not the same as adenomyomatosis.

Illustration continued on following page

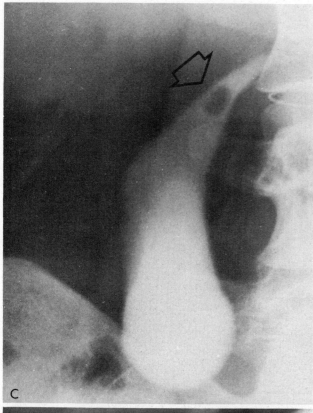

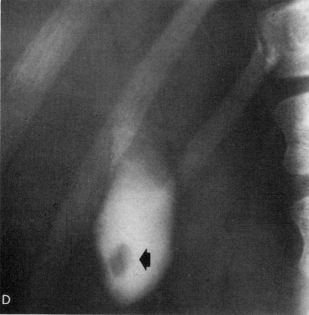

Figure 4–37. *Continued C*, Upright radiograph from an oral cholecystogram in a patient with a single gallstone adherent to the surface of the gallbladder (arrow). The radiolucency was fixed in position on radiographs made in various projections during the course of the examination. *D*, Upright radiograph from an oral cholecystogram, showing a fixed radiolucency due to metachromatic sulfatide in a patient with metachromatic leukodystrophy. (*D* from Kleinman, P., et al.: Gastroenterol. Radiol. *1*:99, 1976.)

compression of involved lymph nodes occurs early in the course of the disease. The tumor is a columnar cell adenocarcinoma, sometimes mucinous in type. Squamous cell carcinoma of the gallbladder occurs but is unusual. Carci-

noma is rarely diagnosed in an early stage preoperatively, which accounts for the extremely poor diagnosis. The availability of sonography may permit earlier diagnosis and possibly improve the grim outlook.

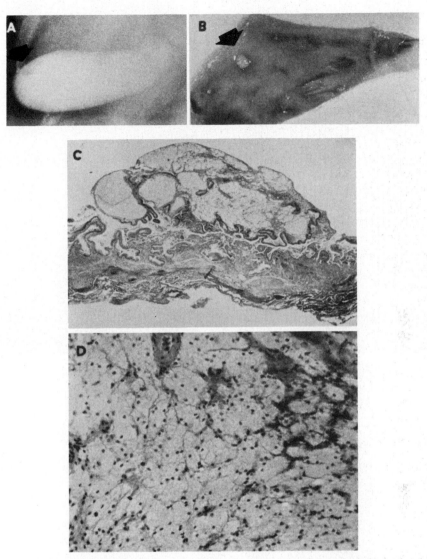

Figure 4–38. *A*, Oral cholecystogram shows a small fixed radiolucency due to a cholesterol polyp (arrow). *B*, Photograph of the gross specimen shows the polyp (arrow). *C*, Low-power histologic section shows the 5-mm cholesterol polyp. *D*, High-power histologic section shows the lipid-filled macrophages. (From Ten Eyck, E. A.: Radiology *71*:840, 1958.)

Keill and DeWeese reviewed the radiologic findings in a series of 33 patients with carcinoma of the gallbladder.[157] Gallstones were evident on plain abdominal radiographs in 15 per cent of patients. The gallbladder failed to opacify on cholecystography in two-thirds of patients. Twelve per cent had abnormalities of the duodenum on upper gastrointestinal studies, 15 per cent had an abnormal barium enema, and 20 per cent had an abnormal liver scan.

Parker and Joffe[162] and Rogers and colleagues[163] reported patients who had mucinous adenocarcinoma of the gallbladder in which fine punctate calcifications were identified in the region of the gallbladder on plain abdominal radiographs. This type of calcification is distinct from that associated with porcelain gallbladder and also has been described in primary and metastatic lesions in cases of mucinous adenocarcinoma of the colon.

When blood-borne metastases to the gallbladder occur, they are often due to melanoma.[164, 165] In Willis' review of 21 reported cases of metastases to the gallbladder, two-thirds were caused by melanoma.[166] Indeed, 15 per cent of patients with metastatic melanoma have gallbladder involvement, indicating

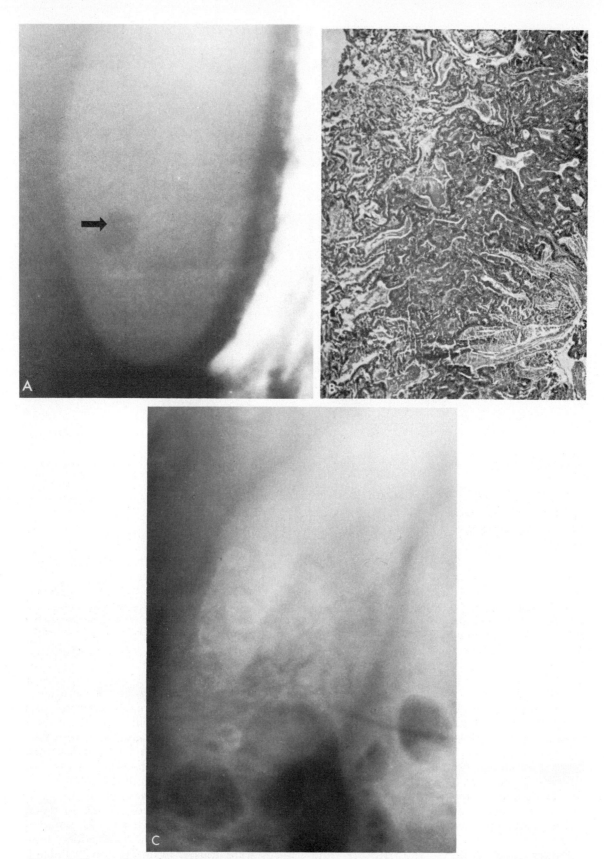

Figure 4-39. *A*, Carcinoma of the gallbladder presenting as a fixed defect in the gallbladder wall (arrow). *B*, Histologic section showing the malignant cells. *C*, An oral cholecystogram in another patient shows faint opacification of the gallbladder and cholelithiasis. At surgery, there was diffuse carcinoma in the gallbladder wall. (*B* from Cimmino, C. V.: Radiology *71*:563, 1958.)

154

that the propensity for melanoma to metastasize to the gastrointestinal tract includes the gallbladder.[165] The metastases usually involve the mucosa of the gallbladder and are accompanied by liver metastases in most instances. According to Shimkin, Soloway, and Jaffe, the metastases first appear as small, flat, subepithelial nodules that become polypoid and even pedunculated as they grow into the gallbladder lumen.[165] A large central ulceration, which is characteristic of intestinal metastases from melanoma, is rare in association with metastatic melanoma of the gallbladder. Most patients have no symptoms referable to the gallbladder unless there is complicating acute cholecystitis.

Oral cholecystography in patients with metastatic melanoma involving the gallbladder may show single or multiple fixed filling defects in an opacified gallbladder. The defects usually are irregular in shape and vary in size from 2 to 15 mm. Angiography may demonstrate the coexisting hepatic metastases and reveal faint contrast staining of the gallbladder nodules.[165]

ABNORMALITIES IN SIZE OF THE GALLBLADDER

Cholecystomegaly

Enlargement of the gallbladder in the absence of obstruction of the biliary tract has been reported by various investigators as a sequela of both truncal and selective vagotomy.[167] In one of the earliest studies on the subject, Johnson and Boyden reported that the fasting gallbladder volume doubles in patients following secretin-induced choleresis. Gallbladder emptying probably remains normal, although this has been the subject of considerable debate.[168-170] Amberg and coworkers showed that the response of the dog gallbladder to cholecystokinin is unchanged after truncal vagotomy.[167] Despite theoretic reasons to expect an increased tendency to form gallstones in patients with an enlarged gallbladder after vagotomy, there is no clinical evidence that this is the case.[170, 171]

Bloom and Stachenfeld reported three pa-

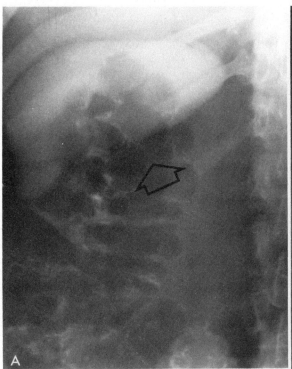

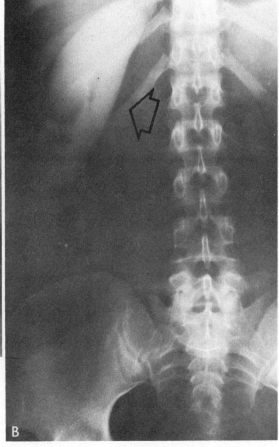

Figure 4–40. *A,B,* The cholecystograms in two patients with diabetes mellitus. In both cases the gallbladder is larger than normal (arrows).

tients with diabetes mellitus in whom the gallbladder was enlarged three to nine times normal size on cholecystography (Fig. 4–40).[172] In their series of 25 patients with diabetes, 16 per cent had an enlarged gallbladder, whereas none were detected in 50 control patients. There was no correlation between cholecystomegaly and the clinical manifestations of diabetes, the severity of the disease, or the mode of therapy. The gallbladder enlargement in these cases probably is related to an autonomic neuropathy. An analogy between postvagotomy and diabetic cholecystomegaly appears likely. However, enlargement of the gallbladder in diabetics may be due to an abnormality of the gallbladder musculature, an alteration of the amount and character of bile, or a change in gallbladder function. Regardless of the pathogenesis, it appears appropriate to evaluate patients with a large gallbladder for diabetes.[173]

Microgallbladder in Mucoviscidosis

A small, contracted, poorly functioning gallbladder with marginal irregularities and mul-tiple web-like trabeculations may be present in patients with cystic fibrosis of the pancreas (Fig. 4–41).[174, 175] The pathologic changes in the gallbladder are presumed to be produced by the thick tenacious bile and mucus that are part of the disease. The findings are similar to those of a congenital multiseptate or hypoplastic gallbladder.

Esterly and Oppenheimer detected gallbladder abnormalities in 30 per cent of their cases with cystic fibrosis studied post mortem.[176] Thick, colorless bile was found characteristically in the gallbladder lumen, and mucous cysts in the wall were frequent. Histologically, mucus was present in normally nonsecreting epithelial lining cells.

Rovsing and Sloth reviewed the radiologic examinations of the biliary tract in 41 patients with cystic fibrosis, noting abnormalities in nearly one-half of the cases.[177] The patients ranged in age from six months to 23 years. There was nonvisualization or poor visualization of the gallbladder in one-fourth of the cases, and the gallbladder was small (microgallbladder) in 15 per cent. Gallstones were present in two cases.

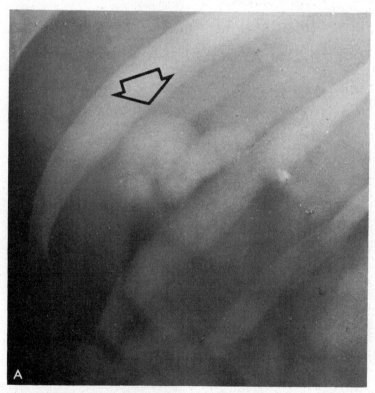

Figure 4–41. *A*, The cholecystogram in a 13-year-old boy with cystic fibrosis of the pancreas. The gallbladder is small and trabeculated and concentrates the contrast material poorly (arrow). *B*, The cholecystogram in a 12-year-old boy with cystic fibrosis. There is good visualization with no marginal irregularities. Cholelithiasis is apparent. *C*, The cholecystogram in a 16-year-old girl with cystic fibrosis, showing a small, trabeculated gallbladder.

Illustration continued on opposite page

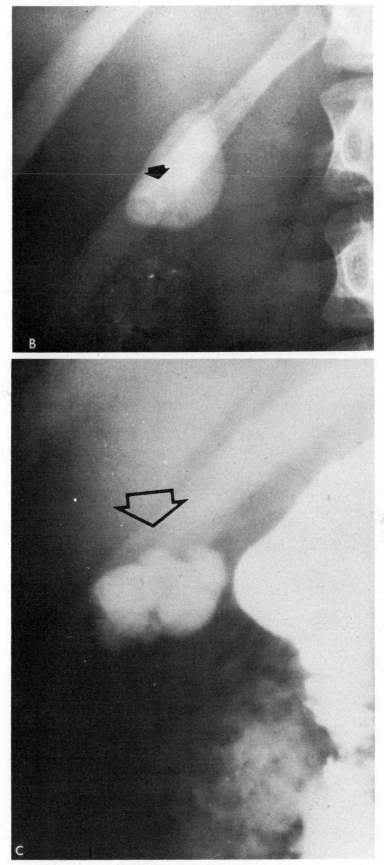

Figure 4–41. *Continued*

The detection of a small, poorly functioning, trabeculated gallbladder in children and young adults allows the radiologist to suggest the diagnosis of cystic fibrosis. This may be particularly important in patients with a mild form of the disease in whom the typical pulmonary findings are minimal or absent and in whom the diagnosis may not have been considered previously.

The clinical significance of microgallbladder or nonvisualization of the gallbladder in patients with cystic fibrosis remains uncertain.

DISPLACEMENT OF THE GALLBLADDER

Displacement and/or deformity of the gallbladder may result from dilatation of adjacent structures, such as the duodenum and colon, or may be produced by mass lesions in the right upper quadrant, particularly those arising in the liver or porta hepatis region.[178] Consequently, deformity of the gallbladder may be the first or only clue to the diagnosis of diseases in a number of organs that are in proximity to the gallbladder.

It can be assumed that any mass adjacent to the gallbladder is capable of deforming its outline. Fisher classified the origin of such masses as either hepatic or extrahepatic and described her own cases of multicentric hepatoma, hepar lobatum due to tertiary syphilis, and lymphadenopathy due to reticulum cell sarcoma in which there were extrinsic pressure defects in the gallbladder.[179]

Other masses in the liver that can displace or deform the contour of the gallbladder include solitary hepatoma, hemangioma, metastases, regenerating nodules, hydatid cysts, polycystic disease and abscesses, or granulomata.[162, 180] Joffe and Babenco emphasized that mass lesions in the liver produce discrete localized defects in the gallbladder that are persistent and reproducible (Fig. 4–42).[178] The deformity tends not to vary in relation to the patient's position. In cases of gallbladder displacement caused by distention of the colon or duodenum, the defect in the contour of the gallbladder is changeable and inconsistent. In these situations, the cause of the abnormality usually is readily apparent.

Extrahepatic masses that may be evident by virtue of their effect on the gallbladder include retroperitoneal tumors; pancreatic pseudocysts; and lymphadenopathy, usually due to one of the lymphomas.

Recognition of defects in the contour of the

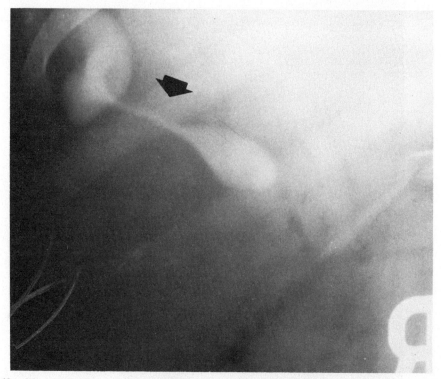

Figure 4–42. The cholecystogram in a man with a large angiosarcoma of the liver. There is striking stretching, displacement, and distortion of the gallbladder due to the adjacent hepatic tumor (arrow).

gallbladder may provide the first evidence that an abnormality is present and that additional studies with ultrasonography, angiography, or computed tomography are indicated to establish a definite diagnosis.

References

1. Ingelfinger, F. J.: Digestive disease as a national problem. Gastroenterology 55:102, 1968.
2. Burhenne, H. J.: Problem areas in the biliary tract. Curr. Probl. Radiol. 5:1, 1975.
3. Amberg, J. R.: Radiography of the biliary tract. In Sleisenger, M. H., and Fordtran, J. S. (eds.): Gastrointestinal Disease. Philadelphia: W. B. Saunders Co., 1973, p. 1101.
4. Berk, R. N., Ferrucci, J. T., Fordtran, J. S., Cooperberg, P. L., and Weissman, H. S.: The radiological diagnosis of gallbladder disease, an imaging symposium. Radiology 141:49, 1981.
5. Alderson, D. A.: The reliability of Telepaque cholecystography. Br. J. Surg. 47:655, 1960.
6. Baker, H. I., and Hodgson, J. R.: Oral cholecystography: an evaluation of its accuracy. Gastroenterology 34:1137, 1958.
7. Baker, H. L., and Hodgson, J. R.: Further studies on the accuracy of oral cholecystography. Radiology 74:239, 1960.
8. Ferguson, A. N., and Palmer, V. L.: Cholecystography: its clinical evaluation. J.A.M.A. 100:809, 1933.
9. Mujahed, Z., Evans, J. A., and Whalen, J. P.: The nonopacified gallbladder on oral cholecystography. Radiology 112:1, 1974.
10. Ochsner, S. F.: Performance and reliability of cholecystography. South. Med. J. 63:1268, 1970.
11. Whitehouse, W. M.: Correlation of surgical pathology with Telepaque cholecystography in doses of two grams. Surg. Gynecol. Obstet. 100:211, 1955.
12. Wickbom, I. G., and Rentzhog, U.: The reliability of cholecystography. Acta Radiol. 44:185, 1955.
13. Crade, M., Taylor, J. W., Rosenfield, A. T., de-Graaff, C. S., and Minihan, P.: Surgical and pathologic correlation of cholecystosonography and cholecystography. A.J.R. 131:227, 1978.
14. Wolson, A. H., and Goldberg, B. B.: Gray scale ultrasonography, a primary screening procedure. J.A.M.A. 240:2073, 1978.
15. McIntosh, D. M., and Penney, H. F.: Gray scale ultrasonography as a screening procedure in the detection of gallbladder disease. Radiology 136:725, 1980.
16. Cooperberg, P. L., and Burhenne, H. J.: Real-time ultrasonography: diagnostic technique of choice in calculous gallbladder disease. N. Engl. J. Med. 302:1277, 1980.
17. deGraaff, C. S., Dembner, A. G., and Taylor, K. J. W.: Ultrasound and false-normal cholecystogram. Arch. Surg. 113:877, 1978.
18. Vas, W., and Salem, S.: Cholecystosonography in diagnosis of cholelithiasis—pathologic radiographic correlation. J. Can. Assoc. Radiol. 31:115, 1980.
19. Krook, P. M., Allen, F. H., Bush, W. J., Jr., Malmer, G., and MacLean, M. D.: Comparison of real-time cholecystosonography and oral cholecystography. Radiology 135:145, 1980.
20. Detwiler, R. P., Kim, D. S., and Longerbeam, J. K.: Ultrasonography and oral cholecystography. A comparison of their use in the diagnosis of gallbladder disease. Arch. Surg. 115:1096, 1980.
21. Bartrum, R. J., Jr., Crow, H. C., and Foote, S. R.: Ultrasound examination of the gallbladder: an alternative to double dose oral cholecystography. J.A.M.A. 236:1147, 1976.
22. Berk, R. N., Goldberger, L. E., and Loeb, P. M.: The role of bile salts in the hepatic excretion of iopanoic acid. Invest. Radiol. 9:7, 1974.
23. Goldberger, L. E., Berk, R. N., and Loeb, P. M.: Biopharmaceutical factors influencing intestinal absorption of iopanoic acid. Invest. Radiol. 9:16, 1974.
24. Stanley, R. J., et al.: A comparison of three cholecystographic agents: a double blind study with and without a fatty meal. Radiology 112:513, 1974.
25. Zboralske, F. F., and Amberg, J. R.: Cholecystocholestasis: a cause of cholecystographic error. Am. J. Dig. Dis. 7:339, 1962.
26. Loeb, P. M., Berk, R. N., Janes, J. O., Perkin, L., and Moore, J.: The effect of fasting on gallbladder opacification during oral cholecystography: a controlled study in normal volunteers. Radiology 126:395, 1978.
27. Hodgson, J. R., and Baker, H. L.: Newer concepts in cholecystography and cholangiography. Postgrad. Med. 26:283, 1959.
28. Berk, R. N., and Loeb, P. M.: Pharmacology and physiology of the biliary radiographic contrast materials. Semin. Roentgenol. 11:147, 1976.
29. Postlethwaite, A. E., and Kelley, W. N.: Radiocontrast agents and aspirin. J.A.M.A. 219:1479, 1972.
30. Sengpiel, G. W.: The compatibility of castor oil and Priodax in concurrent examination of the colon and gallbladder. Radiology 53:75, 1947.
31. McConnell, R. W., and Rice, R. P.: Effect of Neoloid on Telepaque cholecystography. A.J.R. 101:617, 1967.
32. Harned, R. K., and LaVeen, R. F.: Preliminary abdominal films on oral cholecystography: Are they necessary? A.J.R. 130:477, 1978.
33. Anderson, J. F., and Madsen, P. E.: Value of the plain abdominal radiograph prior to oral cholecystography. Radiology 133:309, 1979.
34. Moadel, E., and Bryk, D.: Obscuration of opaque gallstones in oral cholecystography. J. Can. Assoc. Radiol. 25:55, 1974.
35. Whalen, J. P., Rizzuti, R. J., and Evans, J. A.: Time of optimal gallbladder opacification with Telepaque (iopanoic acid). Radiology 105:523, 1972.
36. Oliphant, M., Whalen, J. P., and Evans, J. A.: Times of optimal gallbladder opacification with Bilopaque (tyropanoate sodium). Radiology 112:531, 1974.
37. Ettinger, A.: The value of upright position in gallbladder examinations. Radiology 34:481, 1940.
38. Greenwood, F., and Samuel, E.: The pathological gallbladder. Br. J. Radiol. 21:438, 1948.
39. Lubert, M., and Krause, G. R.: Upright cholecystography using the fluoroscopic spotfilmer with graded compression. Radiology 61:879, 1953.
40. Jensen, R., and Kaude, J.: Oral cholecystography. Acta Radiol. 10:499, 1970.
41. Miller, R. E., Chernish, S. M., and Rodda, B. E.: Cholecystography: a cost reduction study. Radiology 110:61, 1974.
42. Miller, R. E.: Simple apparatus for decubitus films with horizontal beam. Radiology 97:682, 1970.
43. Amberg, J. R., Zboralske, F. F., and Johnson, E. R.: The inclined lateral decubitus position for cholecystography. A.J.R. 92:1128, 1964.

44. Brenner, R. J., Marks, W. M., Sollenberger, R. D., and Laing, F. C.: The oblique bending view in oral cholecystography. Radiology 138:733, 1981.
45. Etter, L. E.: Left-sided gallbladder. A.J.R. 70:987, 1953.
46. Hodgson, J. R.: The technical aspects of cholecystography. Radiol. Clin. North Am. 8:85, 1970.
47. Miller, R. E., and Besozzi, M. J.: Grid selection for oral cholecystography. Radiology 139:234, 1981.
48. Harvey, I. C., Thwe, M., and Low-Beer, T. S.: The value of a fatty meal in oral cholecystography. Clin. Radiol. 27:117, 1976.
49. Sachs, M. D., and Partington, P. F.: The distended gallbladder. A. J. R. 83:835, 1960.
50. Heaton, K. W., and Gibson, M. J.: The use of "fatty meals" in oral cholecystography: report of a postal survey in England and Wales. Clin. Radiol. 24:90, 1973.
51. Lorman, H. G., and Rosenbaum, H. D.: How to do an oral cholecystogram. Semin. Roentgenol. 11:165, 1976.
52. Wise, R. E.: Pitfalls in roentgenographic diagnosis of gallbladder disease. Lakey Clin. Found. Bull. 15:109, 1966.
53. Laufer, I., and Gledhill, L.: The value of the fatty meal in oral cholecystography. Radiology 114:525, 1975.
54. Berk, R. N.: The problem of impaired first-dose visualization of the gallbladder. A.J.R. 113:186, 1971.
55. Rosenbaum, H. D.: The value of re-examination in patients with inadequate visualization of the gallbladder following a single dose of Telepaque. A.J.R. 82:1011, 1959.
56. Berk, R. N.: The consecutive dose phenomenon in oral cholecystography. A.J.R. 110:230, 1970.
57. Kaden, V. G., Howard, J. M., and Doubleday, L. C.: Cholecystographic studies during and immediately following acute pancreatitis. Surgery 38:1082, 1955.
58. Radakovich, M., Greenlaw, R. H., and Strain, W. H.: Iodinated organic compounds as contrast media for radiographic diagnoses. X. Interrelationship of gallbladder pancreas. Soc. Exp. Biol. Med. 77:156, 1951.
59. Radakovich, M., et al.: Iodinated organic compounds as contrast media for radiographic diagnoses. XIV. The influence of pancreatic function on cholecystography. N.Y. State J. Med. 51:2880, 1951.
60. Silvani, H. L., and McCorkle, H. J.: Temporary failure of gallbladder visualization by cholecystography in acute pancreatitis. Ann. Surg. 127:1207, 1948.
61. Sanchez-Ubeda, R., Ruzicka, F. F., and Rousselot, L. M.: Effect of peritonitis of nonbiliary origin on the function of the gallbladder as measured by cholecystography, its frequency and its duration. N. Engl. J. Med. 257:389, 1957.
62. Howard, J. M.: Gallbladder function (cholecystographic studies) following non-specific trauma. Surgery 36:1051, 1954.
63. Sparkman, R. S., and Jernigan, R.: Visualization of gallbladder and bile ducts following trauma. Surgery 41:595, 1957.
64. Lindqvist, T., and Sohrne, G.: X-ray investigation of the gallbladder in pernicious anemia. Acta Med. Scand. 116:117, 1944.
65. Harris, R. C., and Caffey, J.: Cholecystography in infants. J.A.M.A. 153:1333, 1953.
66. Levyn, L., Beck, E. C., and Aaron, A. H.: Further cholecystographic studies in the late months of pregnancy. A.J.R. 30:774, 1933.
67. Roller, J., et al.: Oral cholecystography (OCG) in patients after alcoholic pancreatitis. Gastroenterology 77:218, 1977.
68. Longstreth, G. F., and Slivka, J.: Tyropanoate cholecystography early in the course of acute pancreatitis. J. Clin. Gastroenterol. 3:47, 1981.
69. Burhenne, H. J., and Obata, W. G.: Single-visit oral cholecystography. N. Engl. J. Med. 292:627, 1975.
70. Burhenne, H. J., Morris, D. C., and Graeb, D. A.: Single visit oral cholecystography for inpatients. Radiology 140:505, 1981.
71. Koehler, P. R., and Kyaw, M. M.: Effect of fractionated administration of Telepaque on gallbladder visualization. Radiology 108:517, 1973.
72. Nelson, H. L.: Fractional cholecystography: surgical significance. J. Am. Osteopath. Assoc. 73:440, 1974.
73. Fischer, H. W., and Burgener, F. A.: Fractionated dose administration schedule for cholecystography. Invest. Radiol. 9:24, 1974.
74. Michal, J. A., Nelson, J. A., and Koehler, P. R: The effect of fractionated administration of iocetamic acid (Cholebrine) on gallbladder visualization. Radiology 119:537, 1976.
75. Beseman, E. F.: Can ipodate calcium save the patient one day in hospitalization? A.J.R. 110:226, 1970.
76. Crummy, A. B.: Five-hour reinforcement cholecystography. Gastrointest. Radiol. 1:91, 1976.
77. Pogonowska, M. J., and Collins, L. C.: Immediate repeat cholecystography with Oragrafin-calcium after initial nonvisualization of the gallbladder. Radiology 93:179, 1969.
78. Kalisher, L., Sternhill, V., and Ferrucci, J. T.: Tomographic demonstration of the common bile duct following nonvisualization at oral cholecystography. Am. J. Gastroenterol. 60:623, 1973.
79. Margulies, M., and Wohl, G. T.: Routine tomography in gallbladder nonvisualization: a method for extended positive diagnosis. A.J.R. 117:400, 1973.
80. Filbrow, W. J.: Tomography of the biliary tract during oral cholecystography: a review of 200 cases. Clin. Radiol. 31:189, 1980.
81. Stephens, D. H., Carlson, H. C., and Gisvold, J. J.: Tomography in problem cholecystograms. Radiol. Clin. North Am. 14:15, 1976.
82. Stephens, D. H., Gisvold, J. J., and Carlson, H. C.: Tomography of the gallbladder in oral cholecystography. Gastrointest. Radiol. 1:93, 1976.
83. Berk, R. N.: Radiology of the gallbladder and bile ducts. Surg. Clin. North Am. 53:973, 1973.
84. Nathan, M. H., and Newman, A.: Conjugated iopanoic acid (Telepaque) in the small bowel. Radiology 109:545, 1973.
85. Lee, J. K. T., Melson, G. L., Koehler, R. E., and Stanley, R. J.: Cholecystosonography. Am. J. Surg. 139:223, 1980.
86. Low-Beer, T. S., Heaton, K. W., and Roylance, J.: Oral cholecystography in patients with small bowel disease. Br. J. Radiol. 45:427, 1972.
87. Goldberg, H. I.: Small bowel disease and oral cholecystography. Gastroenterology 71:529, 1976.
88. Price, W. H.: Gallbladder dyspepsia. Br. Med. J. 2:138, 1963.
89. Ochsner, S. F., and Buchtel, B. C.: Nonvisualization of the gallbladder caused by hiatus hernia. A.J.R. 101:589, 1967.
90. Farrar, Z. T.: Underdiagnosis of biliary tract disorders. Gastroenterology 51:1074, 1966.

91. Adams, T. W., and Foxley, E. G.: A diagnostic technique for acalculous cholecystitis. Surg. Gynecol. Obstet. *142*:168, 1976.

92. Hoffmann, T. H., and Glanges, E.: Cholecystitis and delayed emptying of the gallbladder. Surg. Gynecol. Obstet. *151*:170, 1980.

93. Banner, M. P., Bleshman, M. H., and Speckman, J. M.: Persistent gallbladder opacification after iopanoic acid cholecystography: diagnostic implications for acalculous cholecystitis. A.J.R. *132*:51, 1979.

94. Koehler, R. E., Stanley, R. J., and DiCroce, J.: Prolonged gallbladder opacification after oral cholecystography. Radiology *128*:601, 1978.

95. Goldberg, H. I., Lin, S. K., Thoeni, R., Moss, A. A., and Brito, A.: Recirculation of iopanoic acid after conjugation in the liver. Invest. Radiol. *12*:537, 1977.

96. Jacob, C. O., Modan, M., Itschak, Y., Scapa, E., and Neumann, G.: Prolonged opacification of the gallbladder after oral cholecystography: a re-evaluation of its clinical significance. Gastroenterology *81*:938, 1981.

97. Ivy, A. C., and Oldberg, E.: A hormone mechanism for gallbladder contraction and evacuation. Am. J. Physiol. *86*:599, 1928.

98. Rayford, P. L., Miller, T. A., and Thompson, J. C.: Secretin, cholecystokinin and newer gastrointestinal hormones. N. Engl. J. Med. *294*:1093, 1976.

99. Ondetti, M. A., et al.: Cholecystokinin-pancreozymin, recent developments. Am. J. Dig. Dis. *15*:149, 1970.

100. Goldberg, H. I.: Cholecystokinin cholecystography. Semin. Roentgenol. *11*:175, 1976.

101. Goldberg, H. I., et al.: Contractility of the inflamed gallbladder: an experimental study using the technique of cholecystokinin cholecystography. Invest. Radiol. *7*:447, 1972.

102. Cozzolino, H. G., et al.: The cystic duct syndrome. J.A.M.A. *185*:920, 1963.

103. Camishion, R. C., and Goldstein, F.: Partial, noncalculus cystic duct obstruction (cystic duct syndrome). Surg. Clin. North Am. *47*:1107, 1967.

104. Nathan, M. H., et al.: Cholecystokinin cholecystography. A.J.R. *110*:240, 1970.

105. Valberg, L. S., et al.: Biliary pain in young women in the absence of gallstones. Gastroenterology *60*:1020, 1971.

106. Goldstein, F., Grunt, R., and Margulies, M.: Cholecystokinin cholecystography in differential diagnosis of acalculous gallbladder disease. Gastroenterology *62*:756, 1972.

107. Goldstein, F., Grunt, R., and Margulies, M.: Cholecystokinin cholecystography in the differential diagnosis of acalculous gallbladder disease. Am. J. Dig. Dis. *19*:835, 1974.

108. Dunn, F. H., Christensen, E. C., Reynolds, J., Jones, V., and Fordtran, J. S.: Cholecystokinin cholecystography. J.A.M.A. *228*:997, 1974.

109. Iser, J. H., Dowling, R. H., Mok, H. I., and Bell, G. D.: Chenodeoxycholic acid treatment of gallstones: a followup report and analysis of factors influencing response to therapy. N. Engl. J. Med. *293*:378, 1975.

110. Thistle, J. L., Hofmann, A. F., Ott, B. J., and Stephens, D. H.: Chenotherapy for gallstone dissolution. I. Efficacy and safety. J.A.M.A. *239*:1041, 1978.

111. Dolgin, S. M., Schwartz, S., Kressel, H. Y., Soloway, R. D., Miller, W. T., Trotman, B. W., Sollway,

A. S., and Good, L. I.: Identification of patients with cholesterol or pigment gallstones by discriminant analysis of radiographic features. N. Engl. J. Med. *304*:808, 1981.

112. Scheske, G. A., Cooperberg, P. L., Cohen, M. M., and Burhenne, H. J.: Floating gallstones: The role of contrast material. J. Clin. Ultrasound *8*:227, 1980.

113. Jutras, J. A.: Hyperplastic cholecystoses. A.J.R. *83*:795, 1960.

114. Jacobs, L. A., et al.: Hyperplastic cholecystoses. Arch. Surg. *104*:193, 1972.

115. Salmenkivi, K.: Cholesterolosis of the gallbladder, a clinical study based in 269 cholecystectomies. Acta Chir. Scand. (Suppl.) *325*:1, 1964.

116. Aguirre, J. R., Boher, R. O., and Guraieb, S.: Hyperplastic cholecystoses: a new contribution to the unitarian theory. A.J.R. *107*:1, 1969.

117. Lubera, R. J., Clinie, A. R. W., and Kling, G. E.: Cholecystitis and the hyperplastic cholecystoses. A clinical, radiologic and pathologic study. Am. J. Dig. Dis. *12*:696, 1967.

118. Andren, L.., and Theander, G.: Influence of some cholecystographic media on the size of the gallbladder. Acta Radiol. *55*:217, 1961.

119. Boyden, E. A.: The "phrygian cap" in cholecystography. A.J.R. *33*:589, 1935.

120. Bryk, D., and Moadel, E.: Layering of contrast material in oral cholecystography. Am. J. Dig. Dis. *20*:727, 1975.

121. Theander, G.: Pseudoconcretions in precipitate of contrast medium in the gallbladder. A.J.R. *86*:828, 1969.

122. Kriss, N.: False filling defects in neck of gallbladder. N.Y. State J. Med. *71*:1079, 1971.

123. Blanton, D. E., Bream, C. A., and Mandel, S. R.: Gallbladder ectopia. A.J.R. *121*:396, 1974.

124. Taybi, H.: Roentgenology of the biliary tract in children. *In* Alimentary Tract Roentgenology. St. Louis: C. V. Mosby Co., 1967, pp. 1104–1105.

125. Hatfield, P. M., and Wise, R. E.: Anatomic variation in the gallbladder and bile ducts. Semin. Roentgenol. *11*:157, 1976.

126. Vint, W. A.: Herniation of the gallbladder through the epiploic foramen into the lesser sac: radiologic diagnosis. Radiology *86*:1035, 1966.

127. Borkar, B. B., Whelan, J. G., and Creech, J. L.: Herniation of the gallbladder through the foramen of Winslow. Dig. Dis. Sci. *25*:228, 1980.

128. Shehadi, W. H., and Jacox, H. W.: Clinical Radiology of the Biliary Tract. New York: McGraw-Hill, 1963.

129. Roeder, W. J., Mersheimer, W. L., and Kazarian, K. K.: Triplication of the gallbladder with cholecystitis, cholelithiasis, and papillary adenocarcinoma. Am. J. Surg. *121*:746, 1971.

130. Boyden, E. A.: The accessory gallbladder; an embryological and comparative study of aberrant biliary vesicles occurring in man and domestic animals. Am. J. Anat. *38*:177, 1926.

131. Haughton, V., and Lewicki, A. W.: Agenesis of the gallbladder. Is preoperative diagnosis possible? Radiology *106*:305, 1973.

132. Babbitt, D. P., Starshak, R. J., and Clemett, A. R.: Choledochal cyst: a concept of etiology. A.J.R. *119*:57, 1973.

133. Han, S. Y., Collings, L. C., and Wright, R. M.: Choledochal cyst: report of five cases. Clin. Radiol. *20*:332, 1969.

134. Rosenfeld, N., and Griscom, N. T.: Choledochal

cysts: roentgenographic techniques. Radiology *114*:113, 1975.

135. Moseley, J. E.: Radiographic demonstration of choledochal cyst by oral cholecystography. Radiology 68:849, 1957.

136. Yue, P. C. K.: Choledochal cyst: a review of 18 cases. Br. J. Surg. *61*:896, 1974.

137. Croce, E. J.: The multiseptate gallbladder. Arch. Surg. *107*:104, 1973.

138. Simon, M., and Tandon, B. N.: Multiseptate gallbladder. A case report. Radiology *80*:84, 1963.

139. Bentivegna, S., and Hirschel, S.: Heterotopic gastric mucosa in the gallbladder presenting as a symptom-producing tumor. Am. J. Gastroenterol. *57*:423, 1972.

140. Nickerson, W. R., and Boschetti, A. E.: Heterotopic gastric mucosa of gallbladder. Am. J. Surg. *125*:345, 1973.

141. Martinez, L. O., and Gregg, M.: Aberrant pancreas in the gallbladder. J. Can. Assoc. Radiol. *24*:234, 1973.

142. Coyne, M. J., et al.: Treatment of gallstones with chenodeoxycholic acid and phenobarbital. N. Engl. J. Med. *292*:604, 1975.

143. Redinger, R. N., and Small, D. M.: Bile composition, bile acid metabolism and gallstones. Arch. Intern. Med. *130*:618, 1972.

144. Schonfield, L. J., Cachin, J. M., et al.: Chenodiol (chenodeoxycholic acid) for dissolution of gallstones: the national cooperative gallstone study. Ann. Inter. Med. *95*:257, 1981.

145. Arcomano, J. P., Schwinger, H. N., and DeAngelis, J.: The spontaneous disappearance of gallstones. A.J.R. *99*:637, 1967.

146. Lieberman, T. R.: Spontaneous disappearance of gallstones. Gastrointest. Radiol. *4*:265, 1979.

147. Meyers, M. A., and O'Donohue, N.: The Mercedes-Benz sign: an insight into the dynamics of formation and disappearance of gallstones. A.J.R. *119*:63, 1973.

148. Christensen, A. H., and Ishak, K. G.: Benign tumors and pseudotumors of the gallbladder. Arch. Pathol. *90*:423, 1970.

149. McGregor, J. C., and Cordiner, J. W.: Papilloma of the gallbladder. Br. J. Surg. *61*:356, 1974.

150. Grieco, R. V., Bartone, N. F., and Vasiles, A.: A study of fixed filling defects in the well opacified gallbladder and their evaluation. A.J.R. *90*:844, 1963.

151. Ochsner, S. F.: Solitary polypoid lesions of the gallbladder. Radiol. Clin. North Am. *14*:501, 1966.

152. Ten Eyck, E. A.: Fixed defects in the gallbladder wall. Radiology *71*:840, 1958.

153. Kleinman, P., Winchester, P., and Volberg, F.: Sulfatide cholecystosis. Gastrointest. Radiol. *1*:99, 1976.

154. Cimmino, C. V.: Carcinoma in a well-functioning gallbladder. Radiology *71*:563, 1958.

155. Beltz, W. R., and Condon, R. E.: Primary carcinoma of the gallbladder. Ann. Surg. *180*:180, 1974.

156. Holmes, S. L., and Mark, J. B. D.: Carcinoma of the gallbladder. Surg. Gynecol. Obstet. *135*:561, 1971.

157. Keill, R. H., and DeWeese, M. S.: Primary carcinoma of the gallbladder. Am. J. Surg. *125*:726, 1973.

158. Klein, J. B., and Finck, F. M.: Primary carcinoma of the gallbladder. Arch. Surg. *104*:769, 1972.

159. Richard, P. F., and Cantin, J.: Primary carcinoma of the gallbladder. Study of 108 cases. Can. J. Surg. *19*:27, 1976.

160. Milner, L. R.: Cancer of the gallbladder, its relationship to gallstones. Am. J. Gastroenterol. *39*:480, 1963.

161. Berk, R. N., Armbuster, T. G., and Saltzstein, S. L.: Carcinoma of the porcelain gallbladder. Radiology *106*:29, 1973.

162. Parker, G. W., and Joffe, N.: Calcifying primary mucus-producing adenocarcinoma of the gallbladder. Br. J. Radiol. *45*:468, 1972.

163. Rogers, L. F., et al.: Calcifying mucinous adenocarcinoma of the gallbladder. Am. J. Gastroenterol. *59*:441, 1973.

164. Balthazar, E. J., and Javors, B.: Malignant melanoma of the gallbladder. Am. J. Gastroenterol. *64*:332, 1975.

165. Shimkin, P. M., Soloway, M. S., and Jaffe, E.: Metastatic melanoma of the gallbladder. A.J.R. *116*:393, 1972.

166. Willis, R. A.: The Spread of Tumors in the Human Body, 2nd ed. London: Butterworth Ltd., 1952, p. 447.

167. Amberg, J. R., et al.: Effect of vagotomy on gallbladder size and contractility in the dog. Invest. Radiol. *8*:371, 1973.

168. Bouchier, I. A. D.: The vagus, the bile, and gallstones. Gut *11*:799, 1970.

169. Fagerberg, S., et al.: Vagotomy and gallbladder function. Gut *11*:789, 1970.

170. Hopton, D. S.: The influence of the vagus nerves on the biliary system. Br. J. Surg. *60*:216, 1973.

171. Mujahed, A., and Evans, J. A.: The relationship of cholelithiasis to vagotomy. Surg. Gynecol. Obstet. *133*:656, 1971

172. Bloom, A. A., and Stachenfeld, R.: Diabetic cholecystomegaly. J.A.M.A. *208*:357, 1969.

173. Gitelson, S., Oppenheim, D., and Schwartz, A.: Size of the gallbladder in patients with diabetes mellitus. Diabetes *18*:493, 1969.

174. Isenberg, J. N., et al.: Clinical observations on the biliary system in cystic fibrosis. Gastroenterology *65*:134, 1976.

175. Sauvegrain, J., and Feigelson, J.: Cholecystography in mucoviscidosis. Ann. Radiol. *13*:311, 1970.

176. Esterly, J. R., and Oppenheimer, E. H.: Observations in cystic fibrosis of the pancreas. I. The gallbladder. Bull. Johns Hopkins Hosp. *110*:247, 1962.

177. Rovsing, H., and Sloth, K.: Micro-gallbladder and biliary calculi in mucoviscidosis. Acta Radiol. *14*:588, 1973.

178. Joffe, N., and Babenco, G. O.: Localized deformity of the gallbladder secondary to hepatic mass lesions. A.J.R. *121*:412, 1974.

179. Fisher, M. S.: Hepar lobatum and other less exotic causes of gallbladder deformity. Radiology *91*:308, 1968.

180. Brust, R. W., and Conolon, P. C.: Roentgenologic manifestations of primary hepatoma with particular reference to some unusual cholecystographic findings. A.J.R. *87*:777, 1962.

181. Sandy, R. E.: Cholecystography in the presence of polycystic disease of the liver. Radiology *85*:895, 1965.

182. Conlon, P. C., and Brust, R. W.: Cholecystography as an aid in the localization of upper abdominal masses. A.J.R. *88*:756, 1962.

INTRAVENOUS CHOLANGIOGRAPHY

by Robert N. Berk, M.D.

5

The introduction of sodium iodipamide (Bil-igrafin) in Germany in 1953 and in the United States shortly thereafter provided a unique radiologic modality for the diagnosis of diseases of the bile ducts. From then until the introduction of sonography, computed tomography, cholescintigraphy, and transhepatic and endoscopic cholangiography 20 years later, intravenous cholangiography (IVC) was the only preoperative method available for evaluation of the bile ducts.

Because iodipamide has six iodine atoms per molecule, the concentration of iodine that is achieved when iodipamide is excreted in bile is great compared with that of the oral contrast agents, which are excreted at the same rate but have only three iodine atoms per molecule. Since radiographic opacification depends on the number of iodine atoms in the path of the x-ray beam, the concentration of iodine with iodipamide is adequate for opacification of the bile ducts directly, and further concentration of the contrast material by the gallbladder is unnecessary.

The pharmacodynamics of the IVC contrast materials are discussed in Chapter 3. As noted in that chapter, it is regrettable that the biliary excretion of these agents is inexorably associated with the simultaneous flow of a relatively large volume of water into the bile (choleresis). This automatically dilutes the contrast agents and establishes an obligatory maximum concentration of the contrast material that can be achieved in bile. Consequently, an inherent limitation is imposed on the degree of radiographic opacification of the bile ducts that is possible with the contrast material. The radiographic density of the bile ducts during IVC with Cholografin (meglumine iodipamide) is at most only one-half of that achieved in the kidney during intravenous pyelography with the renal contrast materials. Consequently, opacification of the biliary tree with IVC agents is relatively poor.

It would be a monumental advance if a new contrast material were developed for intravenous use that could safely achieve iodine concentrations in bile that are ten- or one hundred-fold greater than those now possible with Cholografin. In the absence of such an agent or until new techniques, such as digital radiography, prove capable of nullifying this prerequisite, the use of IVC will continue to be limited. Indeed, it appears certain that, unless some such change occurs, IVC will become obsolete. Many authorities believe that it already is![1-4] Study of the biliary tree is so much more convenient and reliable with sonography, cholescintigraphy, computed tomography, and endoscopic and retrograde cholangiography that these innovations will inevitably replace IVC entirely. In addition to providing better images of the bile ducts, these new techniques also have the enormous advantage of allowing evaluation of the bile ducts in the presence of jaundice, when visualization with IVC would be impossible. At the University of California San Diego Medical Center, the number of IVCs performed between 1976 and 1980 declined by 94 per cent, and this has been the experience at medical centers across the United States.[1]

Information concerning the performance and interpretation of IVC is available largely as a result of the monumental achievements of Wise. Much of what follows in this chapter is taken from his classic contributions to the subject.

INDICATIONS FOR INTRAVENOUS CHOLANGIOGRAPHY

The various *potential* uses of IVC in clinical practice are listed in Table 5–1. Although there is uniformity of opinion concerning whether or not some of these are valid, others are the subject of considerable controversy.

163

Table 5–1. POTENTIAL USES OF INTRAVENOUS CHOLANGIOGRAPHY

Postcholecystectomy patients with recurrent symptoms
Patients with an acute abdomen when acute cholecystitis is part of the differential diagnosis
Patients in whom oral cholecystography is unlikely to be successful for whatever reason
Patients with cholelithiasis diagnosed by oral cholecystography, for the preoperative evaluation of the common duct
Patients with a normal oral cholecystogram, for the detection of abnormalities of the common duct
Patients with first-day nonvisualization of the gallbladder on oral cholecystography, to avoid the need to perform a second-day examination
Patients with second-day nonvisualization of the gallbladder on oral cholecystography when extrabiliary causes of the nonvisualization cannot be excluded or in whom further evidence of gallbladder disease is desired

The list becomes drastically abbreviated when the new modalities for evaluation of the bile ducts (sonography, cholescintigraphy, computed tomography, and endoscopic and retrograde cholangiography) are available.

IVC is used in the evaluation of postcholecystectomy patients with recurrent symptoms. In these patients, sonography is safer, simpler, and more reliable than IVC for the detection of bile duct stones when they cause obstruction and dilatation.[2] However, an IVC may disclose choledocholithiasis without obstruction or a gallstone in a cystic duct remnant.

IVC has poor sensitivity relative to endoscopic and transhepatic cholangiography, although compared with these procedures the IVC is less invasive and easier to perform. Goodman and coworkers used interpretations obtained by chart review to classify 128 IVCs according to the degree of common duct visualization.[3] Only 55 per cent of the studies had sufficient opacification of the duct to allow interpretation, whereas 23 and 22 per cent were suboptimal and nondiagnostic, respectively. The IVC diagnoses were verified when possible by comparison with the findings of transhepatic, endoscopic, or operative cholangiography; choledochotomy; or autopsy. In these cases the diagnostic error rate was 40 per cent, largely owing to overlooked gallstones. Osnes and colleagues reported similar results.[4]

Consequently, while the IVC is indicated in some symptomatic postcholecystectomy patients in whom the sonogram is normal, in those patients who have persistent complaints

or abnormal liver function studies, transhepatic or endoscopic cholangiography must be performed instead of or in addition to the IVC. In these circumstances the latter procedures are required to exclude a remediable bile duct abnormality with acceptable accuracy.

IVC is used to establish or exclude the diagnosis of acute cholecystitis in patients with acute abdominal pain. Sonography and cholescintigraphy have largely replaced the IVC for this purpose. The results of a prospective study designed by Sherman and associates to compare IVC with sonography for the diagnosis of acute cholecystitis were so obviously in favor of sonography that the investigators decided it was improper to continue the investigation.[5] The increased accuracy and other advantages of sonography and the use of cholescintigraphy for the diagnosis of acute cholecystitis will be discussed in subsequent chapters.

Even when the IVC is done for this purpose, opinions vary on when and in whom the examination should be performed. The premise is that the gallbladder will not fill with contrast material in patients with acute cholecystitis because the cystic duct is obstructed. Consequently, the diagnosis can be established on IVC when the common duct, but not the gallbladder, is opacified. If both the common duct and the gallbladder are visualized, the diagnosis of acute cholecystitis can be excluded.

Numerous optimistic reports on the use of IVC for the diagnosis of acute cholecystitis have appeared, beginning with that of Glenn and coworkers in 1954.[6-10] Johnson, McLaren, and Weens found no false-positive or false-negative examinations in a study of 220 patients with acute abdominal symptoms.[7] All of their patients in whom there was common duct opacification without visualization of the gallbladder had acute cholecystitis at surgery. Similarly, 100 per cent of those cases in whom both the common duct and the gallbladder opacified were shown not to have acute gallbladder disease. These investigators emphasized that false-positive examinations can be avoided only if the radiographs are made up to four hours after injection of contrast material. Forty per cent of their cases showed no opacification of the biliary tree at all, so that the IVC provided useful information in less than two-thirds of the cases. Harrington and colleagues reported 211 consecutive cases in which IVC was performed as an emergency procedure in patients with acute abdominal pain.[9] There were no false-positive or false-negative results in the series, but again there was no opacification of the biliary tree in a large proportion of the cases (40 per cent).

In a later report Thorpe and associates obtained opacification in 96 per cent of their 55 patients with acute abdominal pain.[11] Radiographs were obtained on all patients up to 24 hours after the injection of the contrast material. At least 85 per cent of the IVCs were considered diagnostically helpful, whereas 38 per cent significantly altered the admitting diagnosis. The lower incidence of complete nonvisualization of the biliary tree compared with the early reports probably represents improvement in radiographic technique over the years. Unless radiographs of superb technical quality are available, opacification of the common duct may be overlooked, and some studies will be incorrectly classified as having complete nonvisualization of the biliary tree.

Wise also reported a high degree of diagnostic accuracy in 123 patients with visualized bile ducts and nonvisualization of the gallbladder on IVC who subsequently had surgery.[12] The biliary tract was abnormal in 99 per cent of patients. Of these, 10 per cent had a normal gallbladder (false positives for gallbladder disease). However, all of these patients had primary common duct or pancreatic disease, and most needed surgery. Only one case (1 per cent) had a false-positive examination for biliary tract disease.

It is interesting to note that there is an impacted stone or edema actually obstructing the cystic duct in only a minority of instances of nonfilling of the gallbladder during IVC in patients with an intact gallbladder.[13] The nonfilling of the gallbladder in most of these cases must be due to functional resistance to flow through the cystic duct, intermittent obstruction caused by stones, or the fact that the study was terminated at two hours.

Most authors emphasize the importance of obtaining four- and 24-hour radiographs during IVC if the gallbladder fails to visualize earlier, yet no one except Halasz[14] reported false-positive results because of failure to do so. Furthermore, there are no data concerning to what extent the accuracy of the procedure is diminished if delayed films are not made. Halasz reported three patients who had an incorrect diagnosis of acute cholecystitis made on the basis of false-positive IVC.[14] Nonvisualization of the gallbladder at 12, 14, and 18 hours after injection of the contrast material served as the (mis)diagnostic criterion. There-fore, the examination should be continued for 24 hours after the injection of contrast material, or false-positive examinations will occur. There is delayed opacification of some apparently normal gallbladders for reasons that are obscure. This requirement interferes with the use of IVC as an emergency procedure, since one day is required before the gallbladder can be assumed to be obstructed. However, the absence of acute cholecystitis can be demonstrated promptly when the gallbladder is opacified on earlier radiographs. In some cases, a 24-hour radiograph reveals contrast material in the cecum and ascending colon when the biliary tree did not visualize earlier. This indicates that the contrast material has been excreted properly by the liver and is apparently accurate presumptive evidence that the gallbladder is obstructed.

IVC is warranted in patients with suspected acute cholecystitis only when the diagnosis cannot be established with reasonable certainty on the basis of clinical and laboratory findings. The surgeon caring for the patient must decide how firm the clinical diagnosis of acute cholecystitis is and whether confirmation on cholangiography is necessary.[15] IVC is not indicated if the patient has had previously verified radiologic evidence of biliary disease, if gallstones can be seen on a plain abdominal radiograph or a sonogram, if a tender mass is palpable in the right upper quadrant of the abdomen, or if the patient is jaundiced. The symptoms of biliary colic must not be confused with those of acute cholecystitis. In the former, IVC is unnecessary. These patients can be studied more accurately and conveniently by oral cholecystography or sonography when the colic has subsided. Patients with an established diagnosis of acute cholecystitis should not have IVC merely to evaluate the common duct prior to surgery. This can best be accomplished by operative cholangiography, which should be performed routinely during cholecystectomy.

IVC should be performed immediately after the patient is admitted to the hospital only if it is deemed necessary to use the examination to establish the diagnosis of acute cholecystitis in a patient in whom emergency surgery is contemplated. If a decision for delayed or elective surgery has been made, IVC is not indicated at all in this circumstance; sonography or oral cholecystography will suffice at a later time. If cholecystectomy is to be done within 24 to 72 hours after admission, the radiographic procedure should be performed promptly, but only during regular working hours. A clear distinction should be made between immediate and prompt cholangiography. The necessity for technical excellence often makes the reliable performance of IVC on an immediate basis difficult. When the procedure is performed at night, technicians who are unfamiliar with the examination and busy with other patients are prone to produce unsatisfactory radiographs.

The major indication for emergency surgery is perforation of the gallbladder or impending perforation. The diagnosis of this complication usually can be established on the basis of clinical findings with or without sonography, and IVC is not only unnecessary but delays surgical treatment. Otherwise, emergency surgery should be avoided, because most errors in diagnosis occur under these circumstances. Twenty per cent of 238 cases studied by Halasz with a diagnosis of acute cholecystitis ultimately were found to have other conditions, so that an orderly work-up of these patients is necessary to avoid a mistaken diagnosis.[14]

The principal arguments in favor of cholecystectomy performed promptly (24 to 72 hours after administration), rather than as an emergency, are (1) the patient's condition can be optimized prior to surgery with the use of nasogastric suction, antibiotics, anticholinergics, narcotics, and intravenous fluids; (2) co-existing diseases can be identified and treated; and (3) diagnostic evaluation of the patients with IVC, cholescintigraphy, sonography, intravenous pyelography, or other studies can proceed in a more careful manner. Few surgeons delay cholecystectomy beyond 72 hours anymore, since this has been shown not to reduce the operative mortality and morbidity and only prolongs the patient's hospital stay unnecessarily.[16]

IVC, therefore, is a useful procedure for the diagnosis of acute cholecystitis only when it is performed under optimal circumstances so that radiographs of excellent technical quality can be obtained. Even so, there will be a high incidence of apparent nonvisualization of the biliary tree, in which case the examination will fail to provide diagnostic information. A 24-hour radiograph must be included in the examination if the gallbladder does not visualize earlier, or false-positive results will occur. Consequently, it should be recognized that, in patients with suspected acute cholecystitis, the procedure requires 24 hours before that diagnosis can be established. Sonography and scintigraphy have numerous advantages compared

with IVC and for the most part have replaced the IVC for use in these cases.

IVC is indicated for the evaluation of the biliary tree in patients in whom opacification of the gallbladder cannot be expected on oral cholecystography (Fig. 5–1). Like most other indications for IVC, sonography has preempted the IVC for use in patients with impaired liver function, vomiting, acute pancreatitis, and so on in whom successful oral cholecystography is unlikely. Even when sonography is unavailable, it is usually advisable to delay the radiographic examination in these patients until the problem is resolved, if possible, so that an oral cholecystogram can be performed. The oral examination has a lower incidence of toxic reactions, takes less time and money, and is more accurate. IVC fails to demonstrate gallstones in the gallbladder in 13 to 45 per cent of patients with proved cholelithiasis,[12, 17] so that a normal IVC cannot be taken as reliable evidence that the patient does not have gallstones. Gallstones are missed on IVC because the gallbladder often is not well opacified and there is incomplete mixing of radiopaque and nonopaque bile on examinations that are discontinued after two hours. The accuracy would no doubt be improved if radiographs or upright spot films of the gallbladder were made 24 hours after the injection of the Cholografin.

Once cholelithiasis has been detected by oral cholecystography or sonography, IVC is not indicated to evaluate the common duct prior to surgery. Operative cholangiography serves this function much more accurately and more easily and should be performed routinely during cholecystectomy. Also, *IVC rarely is indicated to evaluate the common duct in patients who have been shown to have a normal gallbladder* on oral cholecystography or sonography (see Chapter 4). If obstruction of the common duct is not extensive enough to prevent opacification of the gallbladder by oral cholecystography, diseases of the pancreas may be present and may even cause compression of the common duct, but the abnormality is rarely sufficient to be evident on IVC. Dilatation of the common duct may occur in this situation but usually is not marked because the cystic duct is patent and the gallbladder is present. Finally, *an IVC is not indicated in an effort to detect common duct stones in patients with a normal oral cholecystogram or sonogram*, because choledocholithiasis is exceedingly rare in the absence of gallstones in the gallbladder. In

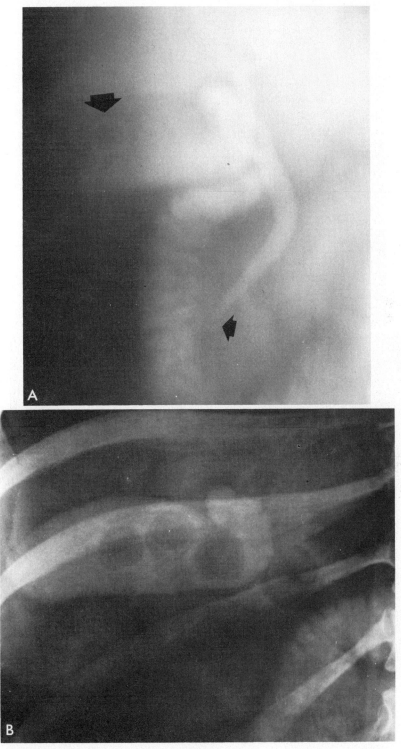

Figure 5–1. Intravenous cholangiograms in four patients with nonvisualization of the gallbladder on second-day oral cholecystography. *A,* Gallstones are visible in the gallbladder and common duct (arrows). Note contrast material in the second portion of the duodenum. *B,* Gallstones are visible in the gallbladder.

Illustration continued on following page

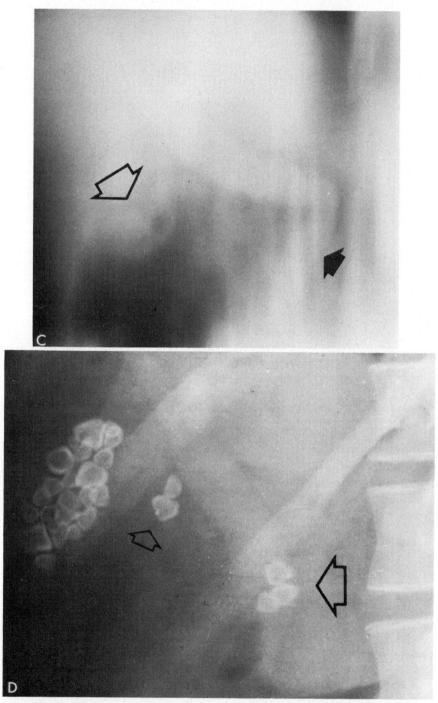

Figure 5–1 *Continued* *C*, There is partial obstruction of the common duct due to a stone impacted at the papilla of Vater (closed arrow). Note dilatation of the common duct and gallstones in the gallbladder (open arrow). *D*, Radiopaque gallstones causing partial obstruction are visible in the common duct (large arrow) and in the gallbladder. Two radiopaque stones are impacted in the cystic duct (small arrow), preventing opacification of the gallbladder.

Wise's series of 241 patients operated on for diseases of the biliary tract, only three (1.2 per cent) had stones in the common duct in the presence of a normal gallbladder.[12]

Some radiologists are accustomed to performing an IVC on patients who have nonvisualization of the gallbladder on oral cholecystography after a single dose of contrast material.

In this way an immediate diagnosis can be established, and the need for a second-dose cholecystogram the following day is avoided. Sonography serves this purpose much better. Furthermore, as noted previously, a normal IVC is not reliable to exclude the presence of gallstones in the gallbladder. Even without sonography, there are simpler and safer methods to spare the patient the second-day examination. Oragrafin calcium can be given if the patient fails to have adequate opacification of the gallbladder after the first dose of Telepaque (reinforcement cholecystography). Most patients have improved gallbladder opacification sufficient for diagnosis on radiographs made five hours later. Failure of the gallbladder to visualize on the five-hour radiograph is reliable evidence of gallbladder disease, and no further examination is indicated.[18, 19] It is best to avoid the dilemma altogether by using the single-visit technique for oral cholecystography proposed by Burhenne and others[20, 21] (see Chapter 4).

Mujahed, in a series of 5000 cases, has shown that failure of the gallbladder to opacify on a second-day cholecystogram is reliable evidence of gallbladder disease when extrabiliary causes of nonvisualization are excluded.[17] In his series of 152 patients who had surgery after consecutive nonvisualization, all had gallbladder disease. *Therefore, an IVC is not indicated in these patients* because further evidence of gallbladder disease is unnecessary. Wise claims that 10 per cent of patients with nonvisualization of the gallbladder on oral cholecystography have a normal IVC and probably do not have gallbladder dis-

ease.[12, 22, 23] However, his data are difficult to evaluate because they do not take into consideration whether one or two oral cholecystograms were performed. IVC may be necessary to confirm the diagnosis of biliary tract disease when impaired liver function or other extrabiliary problems cannot be excluded as the cause of nonvisualization on oral cholecystography. Again, however, this purpose is accomplished better by sonography.

RELATION BETWEEN VISUALIZATION AND LIVER FUNCTION

One of the uses of IVC in patients with an intact gallbladder is to visualize the biliary tree in patients whose liver function is reduced to within a specific range, in whom excretion of the intravenous contrast materials is still possible but elimination of the oral agents is impaired. Consequently, if the patients are selected properly, opacification is impossible by oral cholecystography and yet IVC is successful. In some of these cases it is unnecessary to resort to transhepatic or endoscopic cholangiography to study the biliary tree.

Since liver function is a concatenation of different processes, this range is sometimes difficult to identify by individual laboratory tests. However, Wise found a reasonably accurate correlation between the serum bilirubin concentration and the chance of opacifying the biliary tree on IVC using Cholografin (Table 5–2A).[12] Whether the serum bilirubin concentration is constant or changing when the examination is performed has a major bearing

Table 5–2. RELATION BETWEEN SERUM BILIRUBIN CONCENTRATION AND VISUALIZATION OF BILE DUCTS BY INTRAVENOUS CHOLANGIOGRAPHY

Serum Bilirubin (mg/100 ml)	No. with Visualization	No. without Visualization	Total	Percentage with Visualization
A. Data from Wise using Cholografin[12]				
0–1	838	69	907	93
1–2	107	24	131	82
2–3	16	24	40	40
3–4	7	15	22	32
>4	5	49	54	9
B. Data from Robbins et al. using Cholevue[24]				
2–3	4	1	5	80
3–4	2	0	2	100
4–5	2	0	2	100
5–6	3	2	5	60
6–7	1	1	2	50
7–8	0	2	2	0

Table 5–3. RELATION BETWEEN SERUM ALKALINE PHOSPHATASE AND VISUALIZATION OF BILE DUCTS ON INTRAVENOUS CHOLANGIOGRAPHY

Alkaline Phosphatase* (Bodansky Units)	No. with Visualization	No. without Visualization	Total	Percentage with Visualization
A. Data from Wise[12]				
Normal	452	17	469	96
Abnormal	107	163	270	39
B. Data from Atkins and Berk (unpublished)				
0–5	12	2	14	86
5–7	3	3	6	50
7–9	1	3	4	25
9–11	4	2	6	67
>11	2	5	7	29

*Normal less than 5.

on this relationship. Patients whose serum bilirubin is decreasing at a rapid rate are much more likely to have successful visualization of the biliary tree than those in whom the bilirubin concentration is fixed or rising.

Robbins and coworkers reported data suggesting that successful IVC in the presence of greater impairment of liver function may be possible with the intravenous contrast agent Cholevue instead of Cholografin[24] (Table 5–2B) (see Chapter 3). The number of patients in their series is small, and in view of the drastic reduction in the number of IVCs being performed it is unlikely that additional information will ever be forthcoming to confirm this observation.

There is a relationship between both the serum alkaline phosphatase and the serum glutamic oxaloacetic transaminase (SGOT) and the possibility of visualizing the biliary tree with Cholografin (Tables 5–3 and 5–4). However, the correlation is more approximate and the exceptions are more frequent than in the relationship between opacification and serum bilirubin concentration.

Fuchs and Preisig reported a high incidence of visualization of the biliary tree in the presence of liver disease in 45 patients using a prolonged intravenous infusion technique.[25] Twenty-two of their 45 patients had a serum bilirubin of between 2 to 4 mg per cent. All of the patients failed to have opacification during conventional cholangiography performed earlier with 40 ml of Biligrafin given over 30 minutes. The prolonged infusion technique consists of giving 40 ml of Biligrafin diluted in 500 ml of normal saline over a period of ten hours (overnight in the patient's hospital room). Theoretically, optimal concentration of contrast material in bile for a prolonged period might be achieved even in the presence of impaired liver function, provided that the plasma level of the agent is maintained to assure maximal biliary excretion (see Chapter 3). Using this technique, Fuchs and Preisig were able to obtain visualization of the biliary tree in 75 per cent of the patients in their series (Table 5–5).[25] These same investigators reported a series of 30 patients with an overall success rate of about 40 per cent (Figs. 5–2, 5–3, and 5–4). If it ever becomes possible to intensify faint images of the bile duct with

Table 5–4. RELATION BETWEEN SGOT AND VISUALIZATION OF BILE DUCTS ON INTRAVENOUS CHOLANGIOGRAPHY*

SGOT†	No. with Visualization	No. without Visualization	Total	Percentage with Visualization
8–40	13	2	15	87
40–100	7	8	15	47
>100	2	3	5	40

*Data from Atkins and Berk (unpublished).
†Serum glutamic oxaloacetic acid in units/ml. Normal value is less than 40 units/ml.

Table 5–5. **PROLONGED DRIP-INFUSION CHOLANGIOGRAPHY***

	Extrahepatic Biliary Disease (24 Patients)†	Parenchymal Liver Disease (21 Patients)†	Total (45 Patients)
Bile ducts visualized	18	12	30
Gallbladder visualized	10	14	24
Radiologic diagnosis possible	19 (79%)	16 (76%)	35 (75%)

*Data from reference 25.
†Four patients had prior cholecystectomy.

digital radiography, this drip-infusion IVC could assume considerable importance.

EFFECT OF COMBINED ADMINISTRATION OF CONTRAST MATERIALS

It has been shown that any of the iodinated organic anions that share some portion of the hepatic transport process may compete with each other for excretion in bile (see Chapter 3). When Cholografin and Telepaque are given simultaneously by intravenous infusion in dogs, the biliary excretion of Cholografin is markedly diminished.[26] However, other experiments in dogs suggest that ingestion of Telepaque 14 hours before IVC or the administration of Oragrafin just before IVC does not impair radiographic opacification of the biliary tree owing to the additive effect of the simultaneous excretion of both agents. Finby and Blasberg studied 75 postcholecystectomy patients, comparing cholangiography with Cholografin and Oragrafin.[27] For the combination studies, Oragrafin was given first in an attempt to visualize the common duct, followed four hours later by Cholografin. Large doses of Oragrafin (6 to 12 gm) in combination with Cholografin (20 to 40 ml) were used. Good visualization was found in 68 per cent of those given Cholografin alone, compared with only 17 per cent receiving the combination, suggesting that Oragrafin interfered with the excretion of Cholografin in patients having the combined study. Unfortunately, the patient sample was highly selective in that those included in the combination group were patients in whom the common duct could not be seen after an initial dose of Oragrafin. If the common duct was opacified with Oragrafin, the patient was not included in the study. In addition, patients in whom the common duct was not opacified with the combination of agents did not have subsequent cholangiography with cholografin alone to serve as controls. Additional clinical studies are necessary to clarify whether the combination of the contrast agents interferes with opacification of the bile ducts.

Finby and Blasberg reported a much higher incidence of reactions in their patients receiving Oragrafin and Cholografin than in those given Cholografin alone.[27] In view of the availability of sonography for use after first-dose impaired opacification of the gallbladder, the problem is moot because it should rarely be necessary to use combinations of oral and intravenous contrast materials.

TECHNICAL ASPECTS

Preparation of the Patient

Because of the uricosuric effect of Cholografin and the associated hazard of precipitating uric acid crystals in the renal tubules,[28] it is important that liquids be given freely prior to IVC. Johnson and Wise showed that the incidence of minor reactions is significantly reduced when patients are examined in a well-hydrated state and are not fasting.[29] In their cases, the degree of opacification of the ducts was at least as satisfactory when patients were permitted food and liquid as when they were not. For these reasons a liquid breakfast should be administered, but the meal should not include fat; fat in the diet stimulates the enterohepatic recirculation of bile salts, which increases bile flow. This additional bile flow dilutes the Cholografin in the bile unnecessarily and, theoretically at least, decreases the degree of radiographic opacification (see Chapter 3).

A cathartic, given the night before the examination, is useful to eliminate fecal material in the colon that might otherwise obscure the biliary tree.

Wise gives a 1-ml test injection of Cholo-

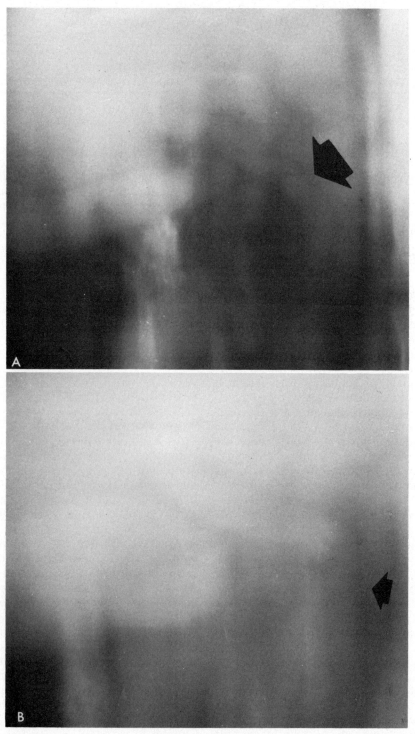

Figure 5–2. Successful visualization of the gallbladder and common bile duct in two patients with elevated serum bilirubin concentrations by the 12-hour infusion technique. *A,* Normal gallbladder and bile duct (arrow) in a patient with cirrhosis of the liver. Serum bilirubin concentration, 6 mg per cent. *B,* Partial obstruction of the common bile duct owing to choledocholithiasis (arrow). Serum bilirubin concentration, 8 mg per cent.

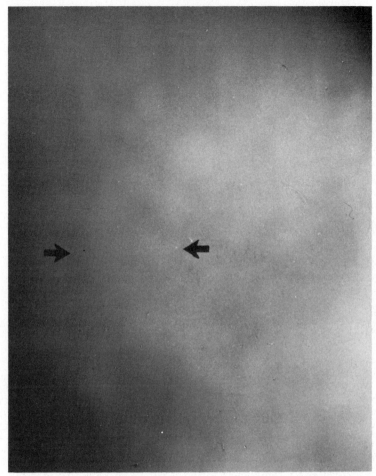

Figure 5–3. Faint common bile duct opacification by the 12-hour infusion technique in a patient whose serum bilirubin concentration was 8 mg per cent. There is marked dilatation of the common duct (arrows) owing to choledocholithiasis with obstruction.

grafin and waits three minutes before administering the remainder of the dose.[23] He and Martinez and colleagues[30] recommend the use of an antihistamine, given intramuscularly, prior to the examination in an effort to reduce the incidence of side effects (see Chapter 3).

Morphine may serve to increase the radiographic density of the bile ducts.[12] Morphine causes contraction of the sphincter of Oddi and produces a pharmacologic obstruction to the flow of bile, thereby increasing the amount of contrast material retained in the duct. The drug should not be used routinely because the delayed emptying and dilatation of the common duct associated with its use cannot be distinguished from partial obstruction of the duct due to an anatomic abnormality.[12]

Dose and Duration of Injection of Cholografin

The numerous combinations of dose and duration of infusion of Cholografin that have been studied in an attempt to improve opacification of the biliary tree and reduce toxicity during IVC have been reviewed and analyzed in detail in Chapter 3. Because of major problems associated with the performance and interpretation of these studies and because of insurmountable obstacles that interfere with valid comparisons of the results of different authors, it is virtually impossible to reach a final conclusion as to which of the various techniques is the best for use in daily practice.

Unless better data become available, it

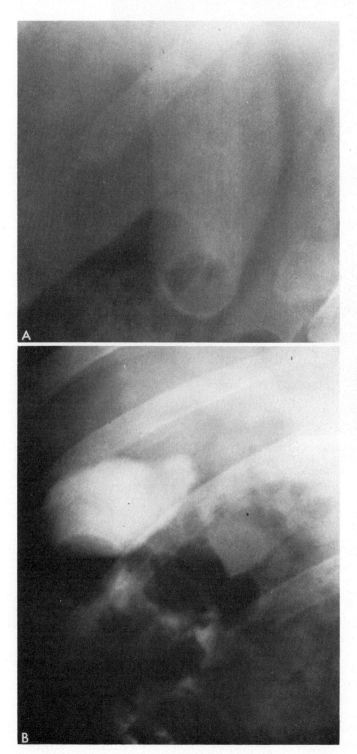

Figure 5–4. Opacification of the gallbladder in two patients with elevated serum bilirubin concentrations by the 12-hour infusion technique. *A*, Single gallstone in the gallbladder in a patient with a serum bilirubin concentration of 4 mg per cent. *B*, Normal gallbladder in a patient with cirrhosis; serum bilirubin concentration, 5 mg per cent.

would appear that the optimal method for performing IVC is to limit the amount of Cholografin used to 20 ml in most patients. An infusion given over 10 to 15 minutes is most convenient and facilitates control of toxicity, if it should occur. If larger doses of Cholografin are used, they should be infused over longer periods (see Chapter 3).

Radiographic Technique

As with other radiographic procedures in which contrast material is introduced, a plain film should be the first step in the examination. This not only provides a preliminary view of the anatomic area involved and detects the presence of barium in the colon that would interfere with the examination but gives the technologist an opportunity to adjust the technical factors, collimation, and the patient's position to ensure optimal technical quality for the subsequent radiographs. The plain abdominal radiograph should include the right upper quadrant of the abdomen and should be made on an 11 × 14 film with the patient supine, 15 degrees in the right posterior oblique projection. Dunn favors the prone oblique position in an effort to increase filling of the common bile duct with contrast material.[31] The patient should be made comfortable and should be instructed to stay in the same position for the remainder of the examination. This may be difficult for the patient, but it is essential if collimation and technical factors are to be constant throughout the study. To optimize the radiographic density of the contrast material, the radiographs must be made using low kilovoltage (60 to 70 kVp). The x-ray beam should be collimated carefully to include only the area of the gallbladder and main bile ducts to minimize scattered radiation.

After the injection of Cholografin, serial radiographs of the right upper quadrant should be made at 30-minute intervals. When the common duct is first opacified (usually on the 30-minute radiograph), the initial tomographic sections should be made. At least three cuts should be made, 1.0 cm apart, approximately in the midline of the body. Three cuts are necessary to determine whether future sections should be made more anteriorly or farther posteriorly. Often the common duct does not lay in a horizontal plane but is inclined inferiorly and posteriorly, so the entire duct is rarely visualized ideally in one section. Adjustments

in technique and collimation should be made after the initial tomograms, so that the second series of tomographic sections made one hour after injection, when there is maximum visualization of the common duct, are of optimal quality and in the proper plane. The second set of tomograms should include six sections, made at .50-cm intervals (Fig. 5–5). There is no uniformity of opinion concerning the value of tomography when the bile duct is not visible on conventional radiographs. It is rare to identify the duct on tomography when it is not seen at least to some extent on conventional radiographs. However, this does occur occasionally, particularly in the presence of gas and fecal material in the colon. The tomograms can be omitted if the examination is being performed to establish the diagnosis of acute cholecystitis, provided that the common duct is well seen on the conventional radiographs.

If the patient has had a cholecystectomy, radiographs should be made every 30 minutes for two hours, with tomograms made at 30 minutes and one hour. If the tomograms are satisfactory, the examination can be terminated. If the gallbladder is intact and is opacified, additional radiographs and upright spot films of the gallbladder should be made at two and/or four hours, depending on the degree of visualization of the gallbladder. If the gallbladder fails to opacify by two hours, additional films must be made at four hours and, if necessary, at 24 hours after injection of the contrast material.

Occasionally, conventional radiographs and tomograms made in the lateral projection are useful for optimal visualization of the common hepatic and common bile ducts.[32] Those ducts that lay in an antero-posterior plane are seen in profile on lateral projections, rather than *en face* as in the frontal views. Consequently, calculi can be identified more readily.

All radiographs must be carefully evaluated by the radiologist and the technologists as they are processed to ensure that the proper number and sequence of radiographs are made and to make certain that they are of excellent quality.

THE NORMAL INTRAVENOUS CHOLANGIOGRAM

The cystic duct is about 4 cm long and runs backward, downward, and to the left from the neck of the gallbladder, where it joins the

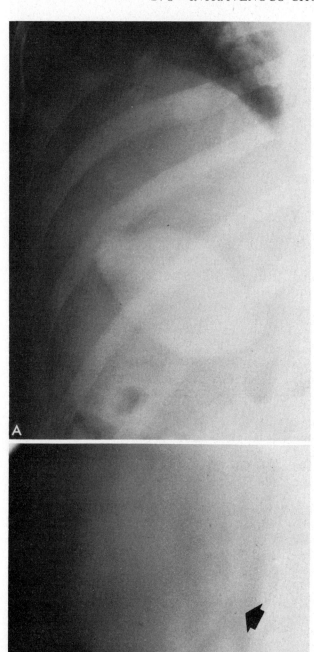

A

B

Figure 5–5. Hepatic cyst diagnosed on intravenous cholangiography. *A*, Ninety minutes after injection of Cholografin, there is opacification of a normal gallbladder. *B*, Posterior tomographic section shows opacification of the wall of the cyst compared with the fluid in the lumen (total body opacification effect) (arrows).

common hepatic duct to form the common bile duct.[33] The mucosa of the cystic duct is thrown into a series of crescentic folds that project into the duct in regular succession, constituting the spiral valves of Heister.[33] The common bile duct is about 7 cm long and descends along the right border of the lesser omentum in front of the portal vein and to the right of the hepatic artery. In the middle third, the common bile duct arcs gently downward and backward behind the first portion of the duodenum, so that the distal third is directed posteriorly and inferiorly in a groove on the right border of the head of the pancreas. The distal third of the duct normally tapers in diameter from above downward (Fig. 5–6).

Based on measurement of the common bile duct on IVC in 96 normal patients with an intact gallbladder, Wise determined the average normal diameter of the bile duct to be 5.5 mm, with a range of 2 to 15 mm.[12] This is not necessarily the widest diameter of the duct but the width of the duct as measured at the level of insertion of the cystic duct. This varies considerably, and it is not uncommon for the two ducts to lay adjacent to one another enclosed in a common outer coat for a short distance before uniting. The average normal diameter as determined on IVC is significantly larger than estimated with sonography, 5.5 and 4.0 mm, respectively, presumably because of radiographic magnification, the fact that different portions of the duct are measured with the two techniques, and because of distention of the bile duct caused by the choleresis associated with IVC.[34]

Wise determined that, in normal patients, maximum opacification of the common bile duct during IVC occurs 45 to 60 minutes after injection of the contrast material.[12] This normal time-density relationship indicates proper drainage of the duct. Consequently, when the duct empties normally, the density of the common duct at 120 minutes should not exceed that noted at 60 minutes. The gallbladder usually begins to fill at one hour, although visualization occasionally is delayed until four hours or even 24 hours in apparently normal patients.

Several radiographic findings that may be

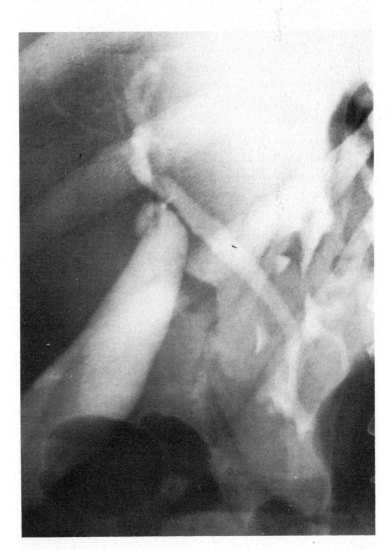

Figure 5–6. Normal intravenous cholangiogram. Ninety-minute radiograph showing the gallbladder and common bile duct. Note excretion of the contrast by the right kidney.

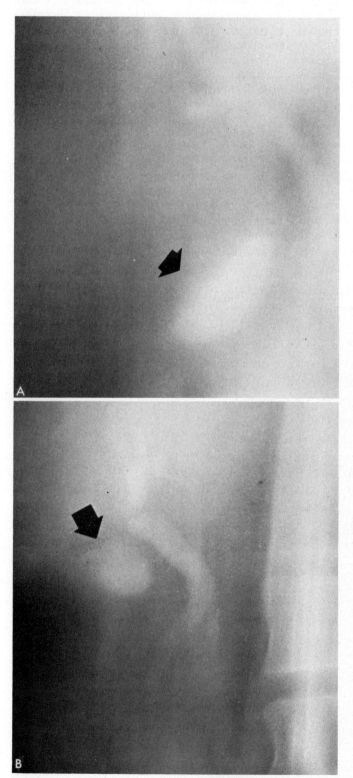

Figure 5–7. *A, B,* Tomograms made during an intravenous cholangiogram in two patients in which contrast material in the duodenal bulb (arrows) simulates opacification of the gallbladder.

seen in the course of a normal IVC may cause errors in interpretation. A round collection of contrast material lateral to the common bile duct, due to reflux of contrast material into the duodenal bulb, may simulate opacification of the gallbladder (Figs. 5–7 and 5–8).[35, 36] Differentiation from contrast material in the gallbladder is based on the variability of the contrast material in the duodenum compared with that in the gallbladder. Opacification of the gallbladder persists and becomes progressively more dense on serial radiographs; on the other hand, contrast material in the duodenum is transient, does not progressively increase in density, and sometimes can be seen to be continuous with contrast material in the second portion of the duodenum. Contrast material in the duodenal cap usually disappears when the patient's position is changed.

A second finding that must not be incorrectly interpreted involves the left costal cartilages. With the patient in a slight right posterior oblique projection, faint visualization of the left costal cartilages may simulate the common duct, since the cartilages are tubular and in the oblique position are parallel to the common duct (Fig. 5–9). However, the costal cartilages are wider than the common duct and often more than one can be identified. Occasionally, the costal cartilages can be seen inserting into the body of the sternum. Rarely, a bifid xiphoid may simulate an opacified gallbladder containing a calculus (Fig. 5–10).

Another potential pitfall is to mistake incomplete mixing of radiopaque and nonopaque bile in the gallbladder for cholelithiasis (Fig. 5–11) (see Chapter 4).[36] Rapid filling of the gallbladder with contrast-laden bile during IVC does not allow time for thorough mixing with the nonopaque bile already in the gallbladder. Consequently, the latter appears as a radiolucency in the gallbladder. On upright or decubitus radiographs, incomplete mixing produces stratification of the bile in the gallbladder with opaque and nonopaque layers interspersed. Radiolucent bile is variable in size

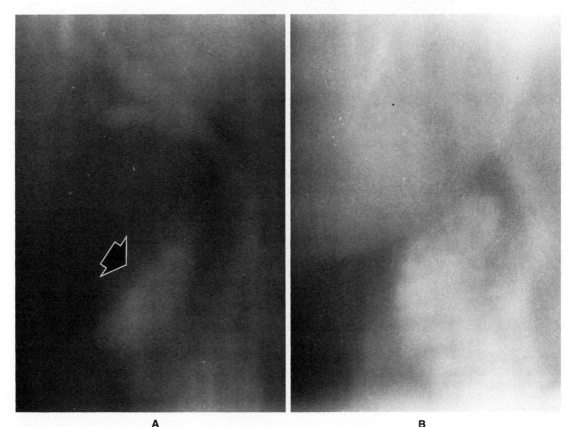

A **B**

Figure 5–8. Tomograms made at different times in the same patient during intravenous cholangiography. *A,* Contrast material in the duodenal cap (arrow) simulates opacification of the gallbladder. *B,* It is apparent that the contrast material is in the duodenum, not the gallbladder.

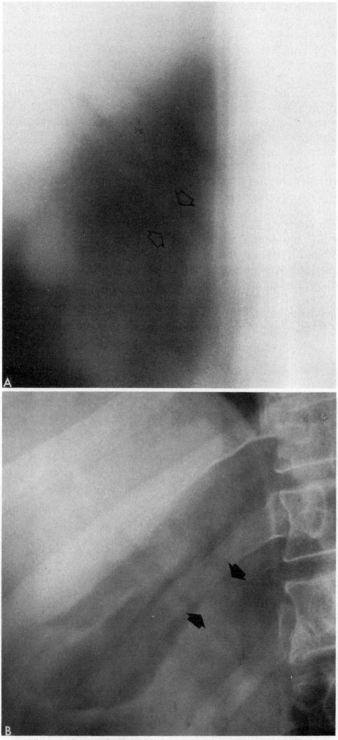

Figure 5–9. Faint visualization of the left costal cartilages simulates opacification of the common duct. *A, B,* Tomogram and radiograph in the same patient demonstrating a tubular density parallel to the common duct. *A,* Common duct (closed arrow); quadrate lobe of liver (open arrow). *B,* Common duct (arrows). *C, D,* Left costal cartilages simulate the common duct in another patient. *C,* The common duct (arrows). *D,* The costal cartilage (arrows).

Illustration continued on opposite page

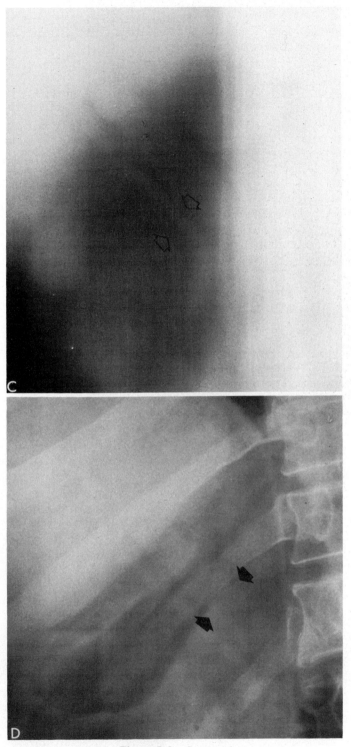

Figure 5–9 *Continued*

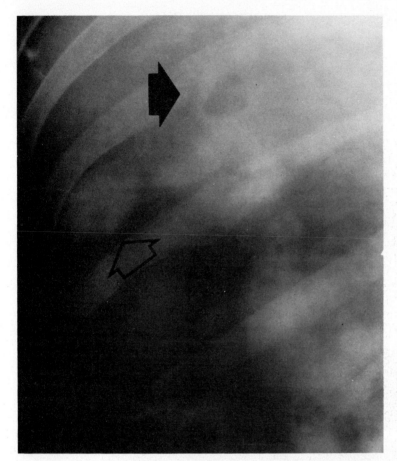

Figure 5–10. A bifid xiphoid simulates opacification of the gallbladder with a single stone on intravenous cholangiography (closed arrow). The radiograph, made 90 minutes after injection of Cholografin, shows faint opacification of the gallbladder (open arrow) and contrast material in the duodenum.

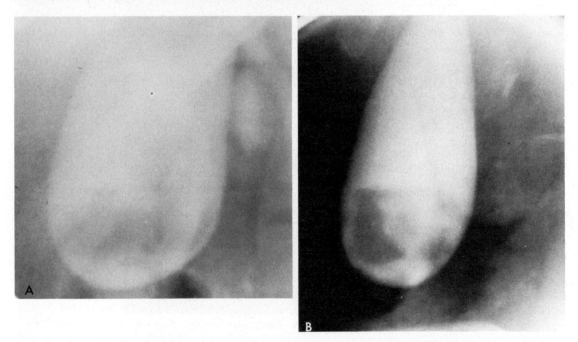

Figure 5–11. *A–C,* Upright spot films made 120 minutes after injection of Cholografin for intravenous cholangiography in three separate patients. There is incomplete mixing of the contrast material and nonopaque bile in the gallbladder. Gallstones are also present in the fundus of the gallbladder in *C. D,* Supine tomogram in another patient shows incomplete mixing of bile.

Illustration continued on opposite page

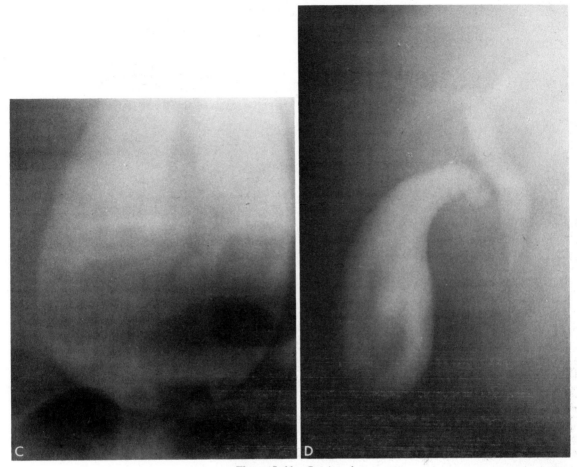

Figure 5–11 *Continued*

and shape compared with gallstones and does not persist on delayed radiographs (Fig. 5–12). Sonography or oral cholecystography performed at a later date is occasionally necessary to exclude gallstones with certainty.

A final area of difficulty concerns the sphincter of Oddi. When this contracts, it may produce an abrupt termination in the distal portion of the common duct with a concave defect on the cholangiogram that is indistinguishable from a gallstone (pseudocalculus sign).[37] This is more common during operative and postoperative cholangiography, but it may be visible during intravenous studies. When the defect is due to contraction of the sphincter, it is transient, whereas a defect due to a gallstone persists and is associated with dilatation and poor drainage of the common duct. If the defect persists, glucagon can be used to relax the sphincter so that a gallstone in the duct

can be identified or excluded on subsequent radiographs.

EXAMINATION OF THE POSTOPERATIVE PATIENT

Many authorities believe that the only remaining indication for IVC in current practice is the detection of common duct stones in patients with recurrent symptoms after cholecystectomy, in whom sonography is normal and whose clinical and laboratory findings do not warrant transhepatic or endoscopic cholangiography. In 77 patients with choledocholithiasis proved at surgery who had opacification of the common duct on IVC, Wise made the diagnosis correctly on the cholangiogram in 92 per cent of cases.[12] These results have not been confirmed by recent investigators who, as

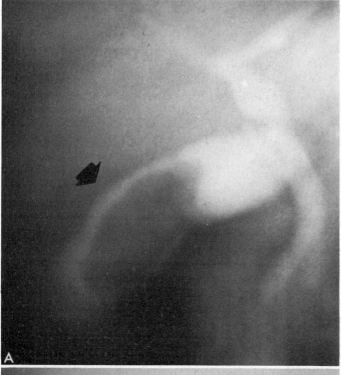

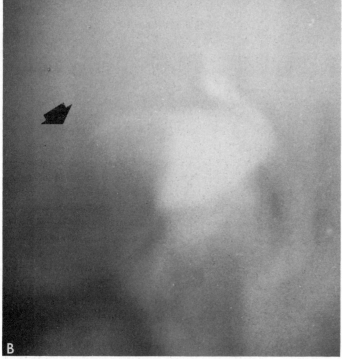

Figure 5–12. *A, B,* Tomograms in different patients made during intravenous cholangiography. There is a single, large stone (arrow) in each case, which must be differentiated from incomplete mixing of bile. A gallstone is persistent and constant in size and shape.

noted earlier, provided data to show poor sensitivity of the IVC to identify stones in the common duct.[2, 3] These workers also emphasize the shortcomings of the IVC concerning the frequency with which no diagnosis is possible because of inadequate opacification of the common duct.

The radiographic findings of stones in the common duct on IVC include identification of the gallstones directly as radiolucent defects in

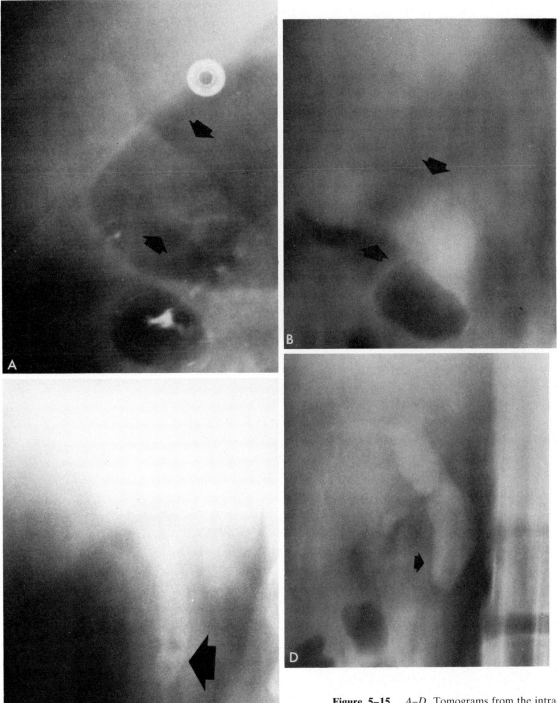

Figure 5–15. *A–D,* Tomograms from the intravenous cholangiograms in four postcholecystectomy patients, showing stones in the common bile duct (arrows). A cystic duct remnant is evident in *D.*

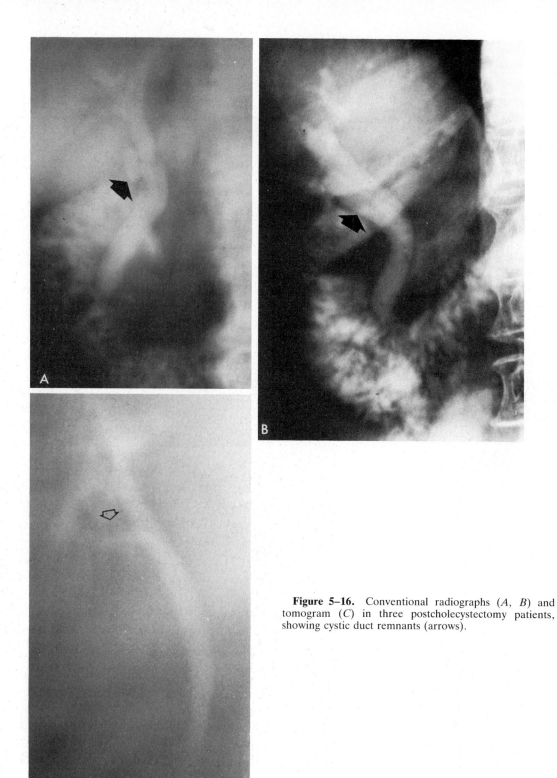

Figure 5–16. Conventional radiographs (*A, B*) and tomogram (*C*) in three postcholecystectomy patients, showing cystic duct remnants (arrows).

alization of the duct may be delayed. However, this also occurs in patients with impaired liver function, so it is of limited value in the recognition of obstruction.

Wise showed that dilatation of the common duct did not occur following cholecystectomy in 13 cases in which duct measurements were obtained before cholecystectomy and from two to 56 months after cholecystectomy.[12] Edmunds and coworkers measured the size of the common duct in 60 patients after cholecystectomy at intervals up to at least five years after surgery, and their data concurred with that of Wise.[39] These results and those of recent investigators who used sonography to determine the diameter of the duct[40, 41] indicate that when dilatation of the common duct is noted after cholecystectomy on IVC or sonography the presence of ductal obstruction should be suspected. If the patient's symptoms warrant it, transhepatic or endoscopic cholangiography is indicated.

A cystic duct remnant is a frequent occurrence after cholecystectomy and in the absence of stones should not be considered of clinical importance (Fig. 5–16). Wise noted that 68 cystic duct remnants were encountered in a total of 224 postcholecystectomy surgical explorations, indicating a 30 per cent incidence.[12] Of these, 11 (16 per cent) contained calculi at surgery. The stones were detected on the IVC in only two patients (18 per cent). Thus, the accuracy of the diagnosis of remnant calculi by IVC is poor (Figs. 5–17 and 5–18).

IVC may be useful in some patients who have persistent biliary-like symptoms following cholecystectomy (postcholecystectomy syndrome).[42-44] Whereas some patients with this syndrome have retained calculi in the common bile duct or fibrosis of the sphincter of Oddi, others fall into a nebulous category of functional disorders termed biliary dyskinesia (see Chapter 4). In most of these cases the preoperative diagnosis of symptomatic gallbladder disease was incorrect, which explains the continuation of symptoms after surgery. Occasionally another diagnosis, such as peptic ulcer or pancreatitis, has been overlooked. The concept of fibrosis of the sphincter of Oddi is not universally accepted. However, several authorities believe that partial obstruction of the common bile duct due to fibrotic changes at the sphincter does occur and that the condition can produce clinical symptoms (Fig. 5–19).[12] The passage of stones, surgical manipulation, and inflammation have all been implicated in the etiology. In a series of 33 postcholecystectomy patients found at surgery to have partial obstruction of the common duct due to fibrosis of the sphincter, a correct preoperative diag-

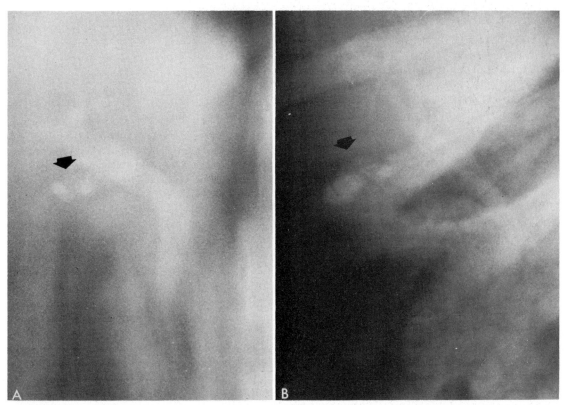

Figure 5–17. Tomogram (A) and conventional radiograph (B) from the intravenous cholangiograms in two postcholecystomy patients, showing gallstones in cystic duct remnants (arrows).

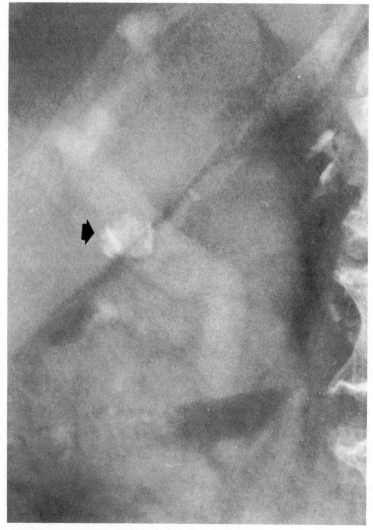

Figure 5–18.   Radiograph from the intravenous cholangiogram in a postcholecystectomy patient, showing a radio-paque calculus in a cystic duct remnant (arrow). There is also a radiolucent calculus in the common bile duct with dilation.

nosis was made in 88 per cent based on evidence of ductal obstruction (abnormal time-density relationship) on IVC.[12] The recent availability of endoscopic techniques to measure the pressure of the sphincter of Oddi and to treat patients with fibrosis of the sphincter with endoscopic papillotomy promises to bring additional understanding to this confused subject.

Opacification of the common duct on IVC rarely occurs in patients with a choledochoduodenostomy or choledochojejunostomy because the duct empties rapidly in the presence of an anastomosis. Occasionally, however, the examination is successful and the common duct is visualized (Fig. 5–20).

CARCINOMA OF THE GALLBLADDER AND BILE DUCTS

As discussed in Chapter 4, the diagnosis of carcinoma of the gallbladder or bile ducts is rarely made by oral cholecystography or IVC because obstruction of the cystic and common ducts occurs early in the course of these diseases. It was also pointed out in that chapter that there is an increased incidence of carcinoma of the gallbladder in the presence of porcelain gallbladder (Fig. 5–21). Clemett and Gould reported a case of polypoid carcinoma of the gallbladder demonstrated by IVC in which oral cholecystography showed nonvisualization.[45] An oval, partially calcified mass

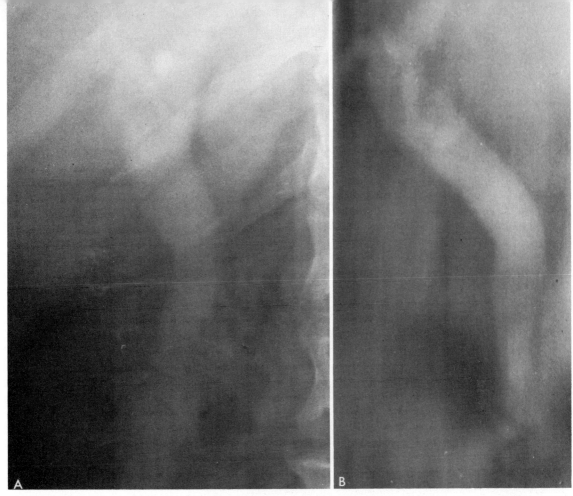

Figure 5–19. *A, B,* Intravenous cholangiogram in two postcholecystectomy patients, showing dilation of the common bile duct. At surgery, fibrosis and narrowing of the sphincter of Oddi were identified in both cases.

Figure 5–20. Intravenous cholangiogram in a patient with a choledochojejunostomy performed because of a stricture of the common duct following a cholecystectomy. The common duct is not dilated. Contrast material is visible in the jejunal loop. The arrow indicates the anastomosis.

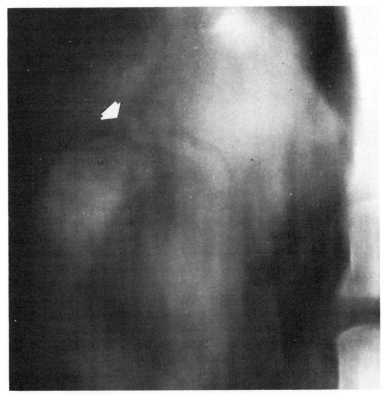

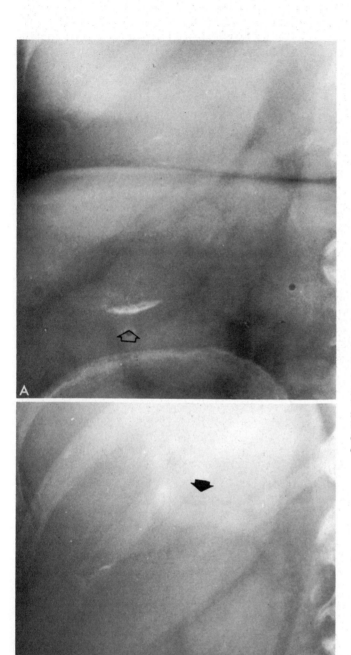

Figure 5–21. *A*, Plain abdominal radiograph in a patient with carcinoma of the gallbladder. Note calcification in the gallbladder wall (open arrow). *B*, Intravenous cholangiogram shows a normal common duct (arrow) with nonvisualization of the gallbladder. At surgery there was diffuse infiltration of the gallbladder wall and obstruction of the cystic duct owing to carcinoma of the gallbladder. Calcification in the gallbladder was also present.

was identified on IVC (Fig. 5–22). Carcinoma of the gallbladder is much more likely to be identified by sonography, because visualization of the gallbladder with this procedure does not depend on the presence of adequate liver function.

BILIARY ASCARIASIS

The giant roundworm *(Ascaris lumbricoides)* is a common human parasite with a worldwide distribution. In areas where it is endemic, biliary complications are common. In Africa it has been conservatively estimated that 60 million people harbor the parasite. The definitive hosts are man and the pig, and in man the adult ascarids mainly inhabit the small intestine, from which they can migrate into the biliary tree. The females lay ova that can remain viable for many years, so that repeated infection occurs from contaminated vegetables, water, and soil.

Cremin and Fisher from the Groote Schuur Hospital in South Africa reviewed the IVC in 126 cases referred because of possible biliary ascariasis.[46] Fifty-nine (47 per cent) were considered to be normal. Sixty-one (48 per cent) showed a worm in the common bile duct. Six (5 per cent) demonstrated nonvisualization, which was taken as positive in conjunction with other clinical or roentgenologic evidence of ascariasis infestation.

The worm was usually seen as a long, radiolucent filling defect in a dilated common bile duct (Fig. 5–23). Identification of the worm in many cases was not obvious, and a more frequent appearance was two parallel lines of contrast material outlining the worm. The worms frequently were multiple and some-

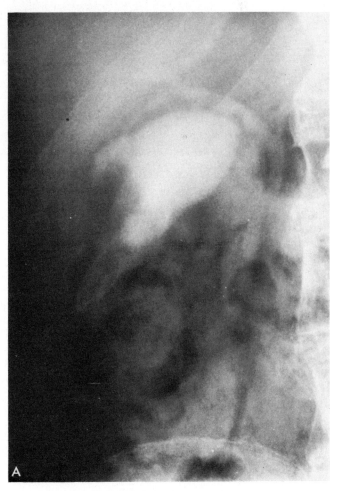

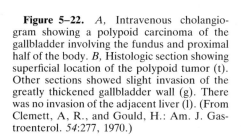

Figure 5–22. *A,* Intravenous cholangiogram showing a polypoid carcinoma of the gallbladder involving the fundus and proximal half of the body. *B,* Histologic section showing superficial location of the polypoid tumor (t). Other sections showed slight invasion of the greatly thickened gallbladder wall (g). There was no invasion of the adjacent liver (l). (From Clemett, A, R., and Gould, H.: Am. J. Gastroenterol. *54:*277, 1970.)

Illustration continued on following page

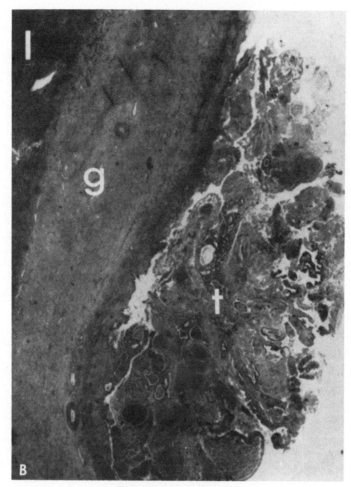

Figure 5–22 *Continued*

times were also present in the major intrahepatic ducts. In none of the cases was an ascarid identified in the gallbladder.

Clinically, jaundice is not a feature of the disease, since spasm of the sphincter of Oddi associated with the worm is intermittent and bile can flow into the duodenum.

VISUALIZATION OF THE GALLBLADDER BY UROGRAPHIC CONTRAST MEDIA

Heterotopic Excretion

Contrast materials for intravenous pyelography and angiography are excreted mainly by the kidney and, to a lesser extent, via the liver and small intestine. Factors that determine the pathway of excretion of the biliary contrast agents are discussed in Chapter 3. Hepatic

excretion of the urographic compounds sufficient to cause visualization of the gallbladder occurs (1) when there is severe impairment of kidney function; (2) when there is unilateral renal damage or unilateral ureteral obstruction, but normal renal function; and (3) when large quantities of the contrast agents are used (Fig. 5–24).[47-52] Becker and colleagues gave sodium diatrizoate to anephric dogs and observed vicarious excretion by the intestine as well as excretion by the liver with filling of the gallbladder.[50] An increased number of circulatory passages through the liver, with additional hepatic extraction, was suggested as the cause. This also may be the situation when heterotopic excretion occurs in the presence of unilateral ureteral obstruction. The administration of large quantities of contrast material increases the possibility of liver uptake and subsequent filling of the gallbladder. Kohler and Edgren noted filling of the gallbladder in

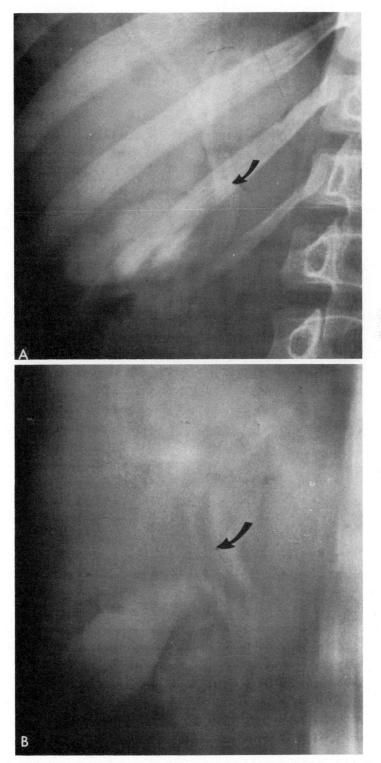

Figure 5–23. Intravenous cholangiogram in two patients with ascariasis (arrow) involving the common duct. *A*, Conventional radiograph. The worms are also visible in the right and left hepatic ducts. *B*, Tomogram in another patient showing a worm in the common duct. (Courtesy of B. J. Cremin and M. B. Fischer.)

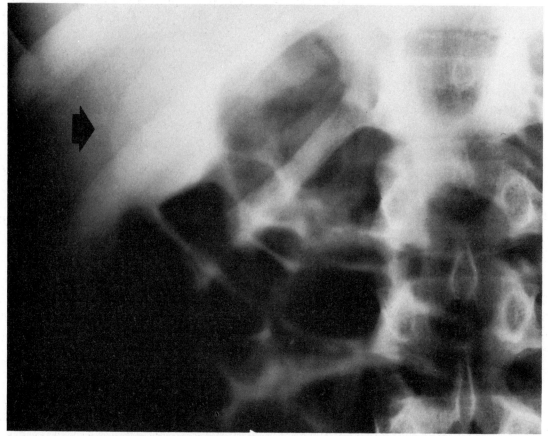

Figure 5–24. Radiograph showing heterotopic excretion of diatrizoate by the liver with opacification of the gallbladder (arrow) during intravenous pyelography in a patient with right ureteral obstruction due to a calculus.

26 of 127 patients (16 per cent) studied with Isopaque, whereas it occurred in only 4 per cent of those given Urografin.[48] The reason for this difference between the two contrast agents is unclear. Radiographs made 24 hours after angiography would be likely to show a high incidence of gallbladder opacification owing to heterotopic excretion of the angiographic contrast material because of the large amounts of contrast material often used.

Infusion Tomography of the Gallbladder

Genereaux and Tchang demonstrated hydrops of the gallbladder following infusion of urographic contrast material in conventional radiographs and with tomograms (Fig. 5–25).[55] In their case, the wall of the distended gallbladder appeared radiopaque relative to the mucus-filled gallbladder as a result of the total-body opacification effect of the contrast material. Rubushka, Love, and Moncada used the same technique to diagnose acute cholecystitis by demonstrating abnormal thickening of the gallbladder wall (Fig. 5–26).[56] It must be recognized that the gallbladder wall is visible during infusion tomography in from 14 to 42 per cent of normal patients and that the mere visualization of the wall cannot be accepted as the sole criterion for the presence of an abnormality.[57, 58] The gallbladder should not be considered abnormal unless the wall is at least 2 to 3 mm in thickness.

After an initial plain abdominal radiograph, tomographic scout films are made at a level approximately one-third of the distance from the anterior abdominal wall, with the patient either supine or prone. A dose of 2.2 ml/kg (1 ml/lb) of methylglucamine diatrizoate is infused over four to ten minutes. Tomography is begun at the end of the infusion.

In the Rabushka, Love, and Moncada study of 21 patients with suspected gallbladder disease, 18 had an opacified gallbladder wall outlining a radiolucent distended gallbladder,

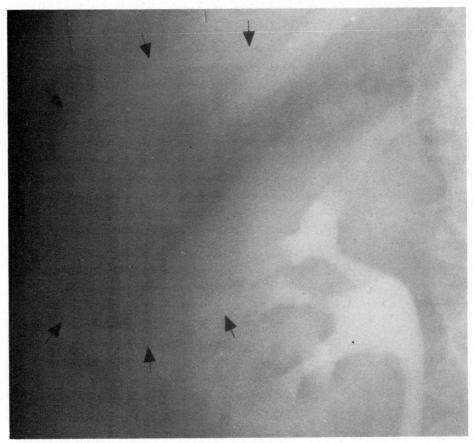

Figure 5–25. Tomogram of the right upper quadrant made after the rapid intravenous injection of a large dose of diatrizoate. The gallbladder wall is opacified (arrows). Distention of the gallbladder suggests the presence of hydrops, which was confirmed at surgery.

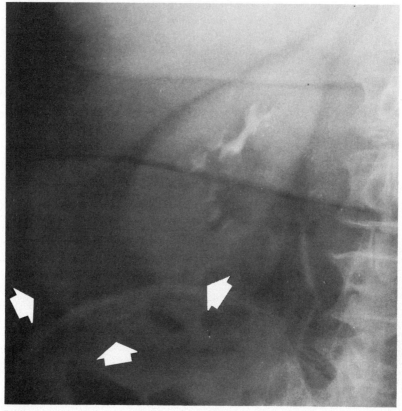

Figure 5–26. Radiograph made after the injection of diatrizoate shows opacification of a thickened gallbladder wall (arrows). The diagnosis of acute cholecystitis was made and confirmed at surgery.

permitting a diagnosis of acute cholecystitis.[56] Infusion tomography failed to reveal the gallbladder in two cases: in one, surgery revealed a normal gallbladder with cirrhosis of the liver; in the other, a small gallbladder was found embedded in the liver. An irregularly thickened gallbladder was demonstrated in one patient with carcinoma of the gallbladder. In 50 routine infusion pyelograms, tomographic sections demonstrated the gallbladder only once, and in this case the gallbladder wall was 1 mm thick.

Love reported his initial experience using infusion tomography in patients with suspected acute cholecystitis, impaired liver function or vomiting that precluded oral cholecystography, possible acalculous cholecystitis, or tumors.[57] Of 27 patients with histologic evidence of acute cholecystitis, 25 (96 per cent) had a positive study. A false-negative result occurred in a patient with gangrenous cholecystitis. No false-positive results were reported. In patients with chronic cholecystitis, 64 per cent had a positive infusion tomogram. If these preliminary data

are confirmed, the detection of a thickened gallbladder wall on infusion tomography appears to be an accurate indication of the presence of acute cholecystitis.[47-48] The examination can be done quickly (less than one hour compared with four hours or more for IVC), and the study does not depend on liver function. The value of the technique in the diagnosis of chronic acalculous cholecystitis remains to be determined. However, the procedure is unlikely to gain popularity for the diagnosis of either acute or chronic cholecystitis because sonography and cholescintigraphy offer numerous advantages compared with the infusion technique.

References

1. Berk, R. N., Ferrucci, J. T., Fordtran, J. S., Cooperberg, P. L., and Weissman, H. S.: The radiological diagnosis of gallbladder disease: an imaging symposium. Radiology *141*:49, 1981.
2. Graham, M. F., Cooperberg, P. L., Cohen, M. M., and Burhenne, H. J.: Ultrasonographic screening of

the common hepatic duct in symptomatic patients after cholecystectomy. Radiology *138*:137, 1981.

3. Goodman, M. W., Ansel, H. J., Vennes, J. A., Lasser, R. B., and Silvus, S. E.: Is intravenous cholangiography still useful? Gastroenterology *79*:642, 1980.

4. Osnes, M., Larsen, S., Lowe, P., Gronseth, K., Lotveit, T., and Nordshus, T.: Comparison of endoscopic retrograde and intravenous cholangiography in the diagnosis of biliary calculi. Lancet *2*:230, 1978.

5. Sherman, M., Ralls, P. W., Quinn, M., Halls, J., and Keats, J. B.: Intravenous cholangiography and sonography in acute cholecystitis: prospective evaluation. Am. J. Roentgenol. *135*:311, 1980.

6. Glenn, F., et al.: Intravenous cholangiography. Ann. Surg. *140*:600, 1954.

7. Johnson, H. C., McLaren, J. R., and Weens, H. W.: Intravenous cholangiography in the differential diagnosis of acute cholecystitis. Radiology *74*:790, 1960.

8. Sparkman, R. S., and Ellis, P. R.: Intravenous cholecystocholangiography in emergency abdominal diagnosis. Ann. Surg. *143*:416, 1956.

9. Harrington, O. B., et al.: Intravenous cholangiography in acute cholecystitis. Arch. Surg. *88*:585, 1964.

10. Ehrlich, E. W., Debras, J., and Howard, J. M.: Intravenous cholecystography as an immediate aid in differential diagnosis of acute pancreatitis and acute cholecystitis. Ann. Surg. *156*:287, 1962.

11. Thorpe, C. D., et al.: Emergency intravenous cholangiography in patients with acute abdominal pain. Am. J. Surg. *125*:46, 1973.

12. Wise, R. E.: Intravenous Cholangiography. Springfield: Charles C Thomas, 1962.

13. Eckelberg, M. E., Carlson, H. C., and McIlrath, D. C.: Intravenous cholangiography with intact gallbladder. Am. J. Roentgenol. *110*:235, 1970.

14. Halasz, N. A.: Counterfeit cholecystitis. Am. J. Surg. *130*:189, 1975.

15. Hermann, R. E.: Acute cholecystitis. J.A.M.A. *234*:1261, 1975.

16. Jarvinen, H. J., and Hastbacka, J.: Early cholecystectomy for acute cholecystitis: a prospective randomized study. Ann. Surg. *191*:501, 1980.

17. Mujahed, Z.: Nonopacification of the gallbladder and bile ducts. Radiology *112*:297, 1974.

18. Beseman, E. F.: Can ipodate calcium save the patient one day in hospitalization? Am. J. Roentgenol. *110*:226, 1970.

19. Crummy, A. B.: Five-hour reinforcement cholecystography. Gastrointest. Radiol. *1*:91, 1976.

20. Burhenne, H. J., Morris, D. C., and Graeb, D. A.: Single-visit oral cholecystography for inpatients. Radiology *140*:501, 1981.

21. Burhenne, H. J., and Obata, W. G.: Single visit oral cholecystography. N. Engl. J. Med. *292*:627, 1975.

22. Wise, R. E.: Pitfalls in roentgenographic diagnosis of gallbladder disease. Lahey Clin. Found. Bull. *15*:109, 1966.

23. Wise, R. E.: Current concepts of intravenous cholangiography. Radiol. Clin. North Am. *14*:521, 1966.

24. Robbins, A. H., et al.: Successful intravenous cholecystocholangiography in the jaundiced patient using meglumine iodoxamate (Cholevue). Am. J. Roentgenol. *126*:70, 1976.

25. Fuchs, W. A., and Preisig, R.: Prolonged drip-infusion cholangiography. Br. J. Radiol. *48*:539, 1975.

26. Goergen, T., Goldberger, L. E., and Berk, R. N.: The combined use of oral cholecystopaque media and iodipamide. Radiology *111*:543, 1974.

27. Finby, N., and Blasberg, G.: A note on the blocking of hepatic excretion during cholangiographic study. Gastroenterology *46*:276, 1964.

28. Postlehwaite, A. E., and Kelley, W. N.: Uricosuric effect of radiocontrast agents. A study in man of four commonly used preparations. Ann. Intern. Med. *74*:845, 1971.

29. Johnson, J. H., and Wise, R. E.: Intravenous cholangiography: a study of reactions to iodipamide methylglucamine. Lahey Clin. Found. Bull. *13*:245, 1964.

30. Martinez, L. O., et al.: Present status of intravenous cholangiography. Am. J. Roentgenol. *113*:10, 1971.

31. Dunn, F. H.: Personal communication.

32. Wise, R. E.: The lateral view in cholangiography. Radiol. Clin. North Am. *8*:139, 1970.

33. Gray, H.: *In* Gos, E. M. (ed.): Anatomy of the Human Body, 27th ed. Philadelphia: Lea & Febiger Co., 1958, pp. 1306–07.

34. Cooperberg, P. L., Lim, D., Wong, P., Cohen, M. M., and Burhenne, H. J.: Accuracy of common duct size in the evaluation of extrahepatic biliary duct obstruction. Radiology *135*:141, 1980.

35. Epstein, B. S., and Smulewicz, J.: Duodenal reflux during cholangiography simulating a reformed gallbladder. Am. J. Roentgenol *89*:837, 1963.

36. Berk, R. N.: Radiology of the gallbladder and bile ducts. Surg. Clin. North Am. *53*:973, 1973.

37. Martinez, L. O., and Cohen, G.: The pseudocalculus sign in intravenous cholangiography. South. Med. J. *65*:1066, 1972.

38. Scholz, F. J., Larsen, C. R., and Wise, R. E.: Intravenous cholangiography: recurring concepts. Semin. Roentgenol. *11*:197, 1976.

39. Edmunds, R., et al.: The common duct after cholecystectomy. Arch. Surg. *103*:79, 1971.

40. Mueller, R. P., Ferrucci, J. T., Simeone, J. F., Wittenberg, H., vanSonnenberg, E., Polansky, A., and Isler, R. J.: Postcholecystectomy bile duct dilatation: myth or reality. Am. J. Roentgenol. *136*:355, 1981.

41. Belsito, A. A., Marta, J. B., Cramer, G. G., and Dickinson, P. B.: Measurement of biliary tract size and drainage time, comparison of endoscopic and intravenous cholangiography. Radiology *122*:65, 1977.

42. Berlin, H. S., Poppel, M. H., and Stein, J.: Intravenous cholangiography: pitfalls in interpretation. Radiology *67*:840, 1956.

43. Cohn, E. M., et al.: The use of Cholografin in the post-cholecystectomy syndrome. Ann. Intern. Med. *42*:59, 1955.

44. Greenstein, A. J., and Dreiling, D. A.: The normal intravenous cholangiogram following cholecystitis: a clue to the cystic duct stump syndrome. Am. J. Gastroenterol. *59*:134, 1973.

45. Clemett, A. R., and Gould, H.: Polypoid carcinoma of the gallbladder demonstrated by intravenous cholangiography. Am. J. Gastroenterol. *54*:277, 1970.

46. Cremin, B. J., and Fisher, M. B.: Biliary ascariasis in children. Am. J. Roentgenol. *126*:352, 1976.

47. Frey, A., Ranniger, K., and Roth, F. J.: Gallbladder visualization following hepatic arteriography for hemangioma. Digest. Dis. *19*:477, 1974.

48. Kohler, R., and Edgren, J.: Gallbladder filling by urographic sodium metrizoate. Acta Radiol. *12*:184, 1972.

49. Arendt, J., and Zgoda, A.: Heterotopic excretion of intravenously injected contrast media. Radiology *68*:238, 1957.

50. Becker, J., et al.: Vicarious excretion of urographic contrast media. Radiology *90*:243, 1968.

51. Chamberlain, M. J., and Sherwood, J.: Extrarenal

excretion of diatrizoate in renal failure. Br. J. Radiol. *39*:755, 1966.

52. Cockerill, E. M., and Kurlander, G. J.: Extrarenal excretion of urographic contrast material in renal failure. J. Urol. *100*:6, 1968.

53. Frey, A. A., Ranninger, K., and Roth, F. J.: Gallbladder visualization following hepatic arteriography for hemangioma. Digest. Dis. *19*:477, 1974.

54. Genereaux, G. P., and Tchang, S. P. K.: Diatrizoate-induced total body opacification in the diagnosis of obstructive cholecystopathy. J. Can. Assoc. Radiol. *21*:242, 1970.

55. Genereaux, G. P., and Tchang, S. P. K.: Hydrops of the gallbladder: unusual roentgenographic demonstration. J. Can. Assoc. Radiol. *21*:39, 1970.

56. Rabushka, S. E., Love, L., and Moncada, R.: Infu-sion tomography of the gallbladder. Radiology *109*:549, 1973.

57. Love, L.: Infusion tomography of the gallbladder. Semin. Roentgenol. *11*:181, 1976.

58. Katzberg, R. W., Glasler, C. M., Booker, J. L., Mullins, J. D., and Kopp, D. T.: Infusion tomography and the total body opacification effect: Appraisal in the diagnosis of acute cholecystitis. Radiology *134*:297, 1980.

59. Karp, W., Herlin, T., and Owman, T.: Infusion tomography and ultrasonography of the gallbladder in the diagnosis of acute cholecystitis. Gastrointest. Radiol. *4*:253, 1979.

60. Escobar-Prieto, A., et al.: Infusion tomography of the gallbladder. Surg. Gynecol. Obstet. *141*:130, 1975.

BILIARY ULTRASONOGRAPHY

by George R. Leopold, M.D.

6

Although modern ultrasonography plays a role in the evaluation of many organ systems, there is no area where its impact is more keenly felt than in the assessment of the biliary tree.[1] Speed of examination, noninvasiveness, and proven accuracy combine to make it the preferred initial diagnostic study in nearly all patients presenting with complaints of potential biliary origin. Even when such complaints arise from other right upper quadrant organs, the sonographic study often provides a precise diagnosis or is helpful in selecting subsequent diagnostic studies.[2] This chapter will examine in detail the pertinent technical, anatomic, and pathologic findings that are responsible for its popularity.

GALLBLADDER

Scanning Techniques

Recognition of the gallbladder on ultrasonographic images is not difficult. It is well known that fluid-filled structures are by far the easiest structures to demonstrate with this technique. If the patient is being studied for cholelithiasis, a 12-hour fast is requested prior to the examination. This allows the gallbladder time to distend and further facilitates its recognition in addition to providing important information about the rigidity of its wall.

The choice of ultrasonic instrument for such evaluation is the subject of considerable debate between those who prefer static scanning and those who favor real-time. Although there are advantages and disadvantages to both, we prefer real-time because of its simplicity and rapidity. It is clear that a superb diagnostic study can be performed with either type of equipment, and the key to such an examination is ensuring that all segments of the gallbladder have been examined. Those favoring real-time point out that the thousands of images per-

formed during the examination statistically improve the likelihood of finding pathology,[3] but it should be noted that meticulously performed static scanning produces results of similar high accuracy.

Far more important than the type of ultrasound instrument used is the choice of transducer. Since the gallbladder in most patients is close to the skin, it is often possible to use frequencies as high as 5.0 MHz to achieve the penetration desired. The advantage of higher frequency transducers lies in their improved spatial resolution. In very large patients, it may be necessary to resort to 3.5 MHz, whereas in children and slender adults it may be possible to increase the frequency to 7.0 or 7.5 MHz. Resolution can be optimized by choosing a transducer whose focal zone lies at the same depth as the gallbladder. In most cases this will be a short- or medium-focus transducer. A long-focus transducer, which is designed for looking at structures further away from the skin surface, definitely should not be used. Being able to change transducers at will is at present a characteristic that is commonly found in static scanners but only rarely in real-time instruments.

The examination itself consists of recording a sufficient number of images to document that the organ has been demonstrated in its entirety (Fig. 6–1). In addition to transverse and sagittal views in the supine position, images made with the patient in a partial left lateral decubitus position are also required. This position has the advantage of folding the liver over the gallbladder and allowing the air-filled gastric antrum and duodenum to fall away. More importantly, small stones that previously were near the neck of the gallbladder and undetectable may roll down to the dependent fundus and become visible. Since the area of the gallbladder neck is often the site of impacted stones, it is an important area to demonstrate,

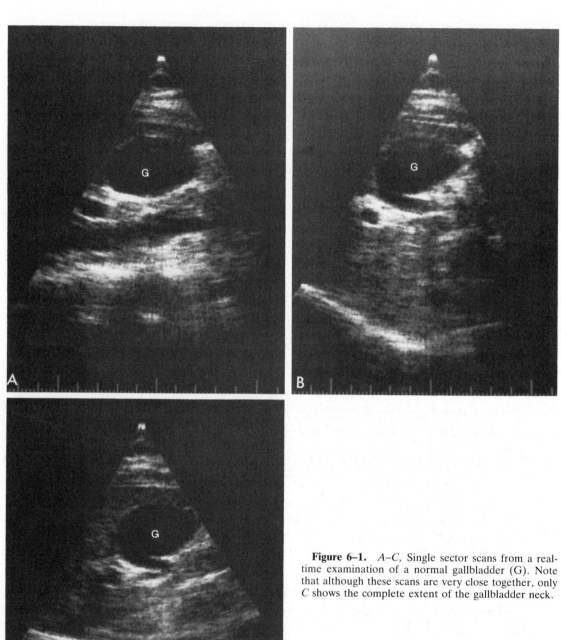

Figure 6–1. *A–C,* Single sector scans from a real-time examination of a normal gallbladder (G). Note that although these scans are very close together, only *C* shows the complete extent of the gallbladder neck.

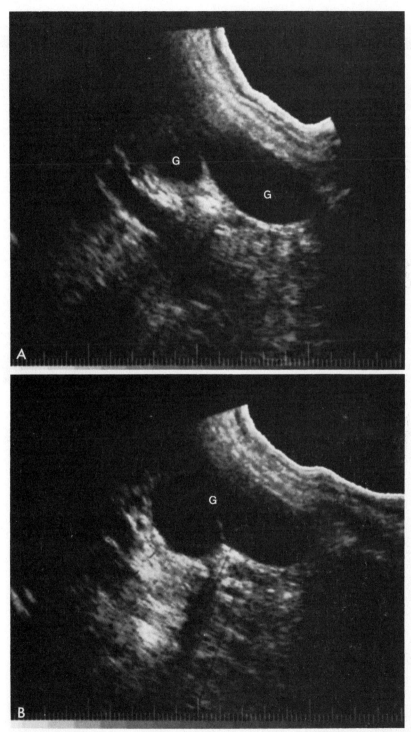

Figure 6–2. Single sector scans of gallbladder several millimeters apart. *A,* There appears to be a complete septation of the gallbladder. *B,* The apparent septation is merely a prominent fold.

whether using real-time or static scanning. Knowledge of the anatomy of this area is crucial to assure that the whole of this critical region has been examined. The gallbladder lies in the plane whose continuation is the main interlobar fissure of the liver. On sagittal or nearly sagittal scans, this plane may be recognized as an echogenic line connecting the gallbladder with the undivided portion of the right portal vein.[4] Failure to visualize this structure means that the gallbladder neck has not been completely imaged and the examination is incomplete.

Although it is true that ultrasound examinations of the pancreas and retroperitoneal structures are sometimes precluded by bowel gas, this is rarely, if ever, the case with gallbladder examinations. Even when excessive abdominal distention is present, the gallbladder can be demonstrated by utilizing the decubitus position and the overlying right lobe of the liver as a sonic window.

Since patients with inflammatory disease of the gallbladder are often capable of localizing their pain to the organ, the ultrasound examiner should make note of this important finding, specifically questioning the patient as to the presence or absence of tenderness in the area of the gallbladder as determined from the scans.[5]

Anatomic Variations

Anatomic variations in the gallbladder are reasonably common. They include septations and foldings of the organ. The most usual of the latter is the familiar phrygian cap, in which the fundus of the gallbladder is folded upon itself. When folds involve the gallbladder, a partial scan of the fold may suggest an internal septation (Fig. 6–2). This is particularly common in the neck of the gallbladder, where a junctional fold or incisura may cause confusion in diagnosis[6] (Fig. 6–3).

Ultrasonographers should bear in mind that true duplication of the gallbladder does exist but is quite rare. Agenesis of the gallbladder is even rarer in humans although common in some lower animal species.

Of the positional anomalies, intrahepatic gallbladder is the most commonly noted. This may appear as a cystic intrahepatic lesion at the junction of the right and left lobes. The diagnosis can usually be made by carefully scanning and noting that the gallbladder is not present in its normal location. If doubt still exists, nuclear medicine studies can be used to document the biliary origin of the lesion. When intrahepatically located, the gallbladder lies in the main interlobar fissure between the right and left lobes.

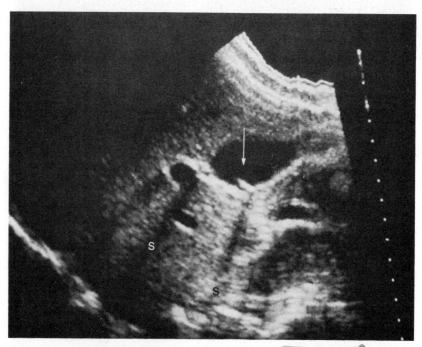

Figure 6–3. This scan of the gallbladder shows a prominent incisura or junctional fold (arrow) near the gallbladder neck. Note that there is an acoustic shadow (S) arising from it as well as from the more proximal portion of the gallbladder neck.

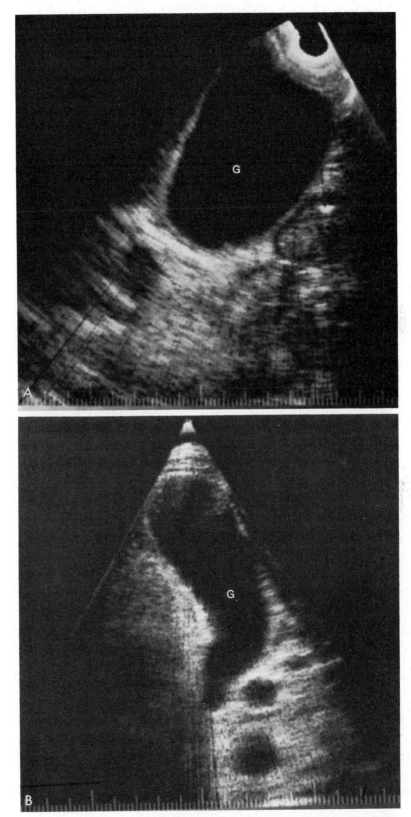

Figure 6–4. Scans of the gallbladder showing marked distention *(A)* and response to a fatty meal *(B)*. There was no clinical or laboratory evidence of gallbladder disease.

Gallbladder Size

Since enlargement of the gallbladder is a common finding in many pathologic conditions, it would be desirable to have absolute measurement criteria. Although some authors have suggested that an anteroposterior measurement of 4 cm or greater is abnormal, we have frequently observed normal fasting patients whose gallbladder distends beyond that dimension. This overlap between large normal gallbladders and mildly obstructed ones makes size a poor normal/abnormal discriminator in the individual case (Fig. 6–4). To make matters worse, a gallbladder wall that has become stiffened by a previous inflammatory process may be incapable of dilating significantly when obstruction of the cystic or common duct does develop.

Situations in which gallbladder enlargement may be the only sonographic abnormality present include hydrops (usually due to cystic duct obstruction) and Kawasaki's syndrome. The latter disorder, also known as the mucocutaneous lymph node syndrome, characteristically occurs in children. Whereas some of these cases have been treated surgically, others have been managed conservatively with success. At present, surgery should probably be reserved for those suffering from the complications of hydrops and not merely acute distention.[7]

At times, it is helpful to re-examine gallbladder size following the administration of a fatty meal or one of the cholecystokinin derivatives. If the gallbladder shrinks quickly in response to such stimuli, it can be assumed not to be obstructed. Failure to contract, however, cannot be used as absolute evidence of obstruction, since reaction to these pharmacologic agents varies greatly.

Cholelithiasis

The accuracy of ultrasonography in the detection of cholelithiasis has been proved to be in excess of 95 per cent.[8-13] Such studies have led many to believe that ultrasonography is the procedure of choice in making this diagnosis. At our own institution, the number of oral cholecystograms performed has shown a rapid and dramatic fall over the past several years.

Gallstones are recognized on ultrasonography as echo densities that nearly always occupy the dependent portion of the gallbladder and move rapidly to the new dependent point when the patient's position is changed (Fig. 6–5).

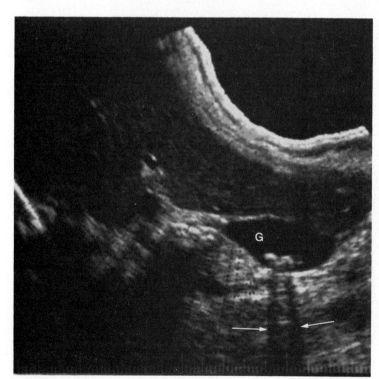

Figure 6–5. This gallbladder scan in the decubitus position shows a collection of gallstones in its most dependent portion. Acoustic shadowing (arrows) is noted from some of the stones.

Although it is true that some stones (pure cholesterol) do float and may form a layer between stratified layers of bile of differing component specific gravities, the vast majority of such cases occur when ultrasonic scanning is done with oral cholecystographic material present in the gallbladder.[14] The contrast agents used apparently have a higher specific gravity than the stones, causing a flotation effect. Occasionally stones are said to "float," when in fact it is only the anterior margin of a large stone that is being imaged. Decubitus views will easily solve this problem.

The most characteristic sonographic finding associated with gallstones is the presence of an acoustic shadow emanating directly from the observed intraluminal echodense focus. Shadowing is believed to result from the virtually complete reflection of the beam that occurs when its anterior edge is struck. Although it was first believed that the degree of calcification of the gallstone might be related to shadow-producing ability, it has now been demonstrated conclusively that composition of the stone is not a determining factor.[15-17] All stones, in fact, can be shown to shadow in the *in vitro* situation. Clearly, the technical features involved in performing the study are most important in shadow presence or absence. These include transducer frequency, focal characteristics of the transducer, position of the stone along the axial length of the beam, and size of the stone. In general, the greater the proportion of the beam "stopped" by the stone, the greater the likelihood of producing an acoustic shadow.[18] Thus, a small stone in the extreme near or far field of the beam may not produce a shadow, but it will if it lies near the focal zone of the transducer (where the transverse diameter of the beam is at its minimum). Since higher frequency transducers have narrower beams near their focal zones, it is easy to explain their improved rate of displaying shadowing. As the demonstration of shadowing is of critical importance in making this diagnosis, every effort should be made to elicit this feature. Using the methods outlined previously, shadowing can often be demonstrated from individual calculi as small as 1 mm in diameter. When a group of even smaller calculi is present, their aggregate mass often produces a shadow, which is also easy to recognize.

Care must be taken to avoid false-positive shadows. Such findings are often present near the neck of the gallbladder and have been attributed by some to the fibrous and convoluted nature of the valves of Heister (Fig. 6–3). More recently, others have pointed out that such shadows may not result from a discrete anatomic structure but rather originate from any area where cystic and solid areas are

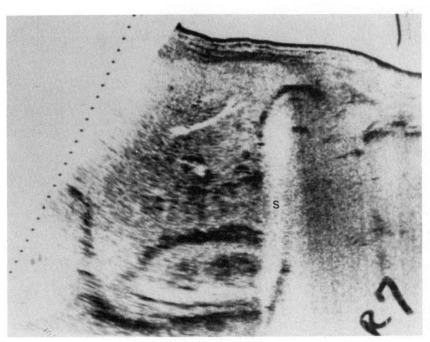

Figure 6–6. Sagittal scan of the right upper quadrant showing a prominent shadow (S) emanating from the gallbladder bed.

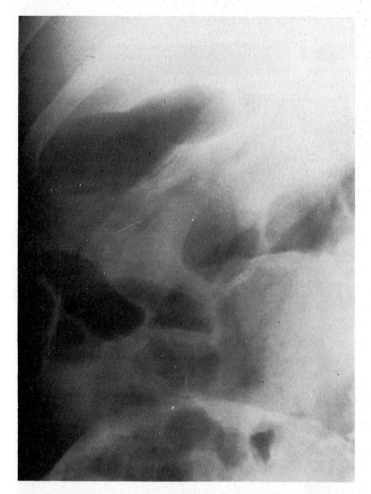

Figure 6–7. Plain film of the abdomen of the patient in Figure 6–6. The gallbladder wall and lumen contain gas, establishing the diagnosis of emphysematous cholecystitis. (Courtesy of Dr. Enrique Schwarz, Flossmoor, Ill.)

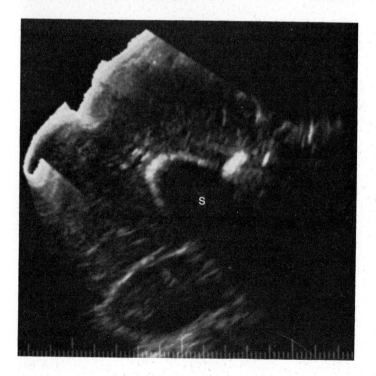

Figure 6–8. Prominent acoustic shadow (S) coming from the gallbladder fossa.

immediately adjacent (e.g., liver and gallbladder).[19] When the ultrasound beam strikes such areas tangentially, refractive effects occur that bend the beam, producing an edge shadow. Loops of bowel, particularly the duodenum and hepatic flexure of the colon, are often intimately related to the gallbladder and produce shadows of their own, which can cause confusion in diagnosis.

Shadowing from the gallbladder or gallbladder fossa occurs in at least two other conditions that ultrasonically may simulate a contracted or stone-filled viscus. Emphysematous cholecystitis, usually seen in elderly diabetics and believed to be a result of small vessel ischemia rather than being primarily infectious, is one such disorder. Although gas production is seen first in the wall of the gallbladder, the lumen soon becomes filled as the disorder progresses. Such patients are acutely ill at the time of the ultrasound examination. Sonography will show an acoustic shadow arising from the gallbladder fossa (Figs. 6–6 and 6–7). Some have stated that the shadow produced from gas collections, such as emphysematous cholecystitis, or the duodenum looks different from that produced by calculi. These observers state that stones produce a "clean" shadow because of great reflectivity, whereas that seen behind gas collections tends to be "dirty" because a greater portion of the incident beam is scattered rather than reflected.[20] Although this may occasionally be helpful, we have been misled often enough to rate it as only a minor diagnostic criterion.

Another disorder that produces a similar ultrasonic appearance is porcelain gallbladder, wherein the gallbladder wall has calcified, usually as a result of long-standing obstruction of the cystic duct (Figs. 6–8 and 6–9). Such gallbladders usually do contain stones, and these patients have a slightly increased potential for developing carcinoma of the gallbladder.

Ultrasonic experience with milk of calcium bile, also a condition resulting from long-standing obstruction of the cystic duct, is very limited. In a single case seen by us, the dependent portion, which correlated with the density seen on plain film, produced a marked acoustic shadowing (Fig. 6–10). (It should be noted that plain films are of great assistance in clarifying the situation in emphysematous cholecystitis, porcelain gallbladder, and milk of calcium bile.)

Cholecystitis

Since gallstones are present in a great number of individuals (10 to 25 per cent at autopsy) who are asymptomatic, their detection alone on ultrasonograms does not confirm the diagnosis of acute cholecystitis. Other findings must be present before the ultrasonographer may advance this diagnosis.[2, 5]

Focal Tenderness

Finding localized tenderness by palpation in the upper right quadrant on deep inspiration (Murphy's sign) has long been recognized as a predictor of gallbladder disease. Sonography provides an excellent way to extend physical diagnosis, since it is possible for the examiner to precisely locate the gallbladder. If the patient's tenderness is discretely localized to the gallbladder, a diagnosis of acute cholecystitis is virtually certain. It is important that the pain be localized to the gallbladder, since in a recent series only one-third of patients referred with upper right quadrant pain and a suspicion of cholecystitis actually proved to have this disorder.[2] (Interestingly, ultrasonography was often able to indicate causes other than gallbladder disease responsible for these symptoms.)

Wall Thickness

Numerous articles have pointed out that thickening of the gallbladder wall is frequently observable on ultrasonograms of patients with acute cholecystitis (Fig. 6–11).[21-25] Most regard a wall thickness greater than 2 mm as pathologic. Such measurements should be made on the anterior wall of the gallbladder where it abuts the liver, since the posterior wall is often more difficult to define because of acoustic enhancement and adjacent bowel. Although it is undoubtedly true that wall thickening does occur in many of these individuals, it should be kept in mind that a number of other disorders unrelated to cholecystitis can produce similar findings. This is a regular occurrence in patients with ascites, perhaps related to the hypoproteinemia that such individuals usually have.[26] Patients with right heart failure may also show marked edema of the gallbladder wall but no findings to suggest gallbladder

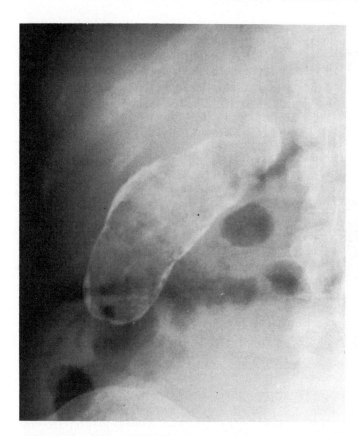

Figure 6–9. Plain film of the abdomen of the patient in Figure 6–8. A porcelain gallbladder (calcified wall) is evident.

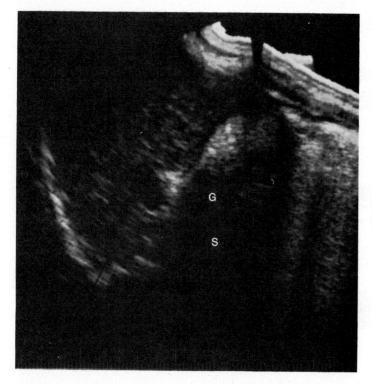

Figure 6–10. The anterior aspect of the gallbladder shows echogenic material. Posteriorly, the echo-free area produces marked attenuation of the beam and profound posterior acoustic shadowing (S). A plain film demonstrated milk of calcium bile.

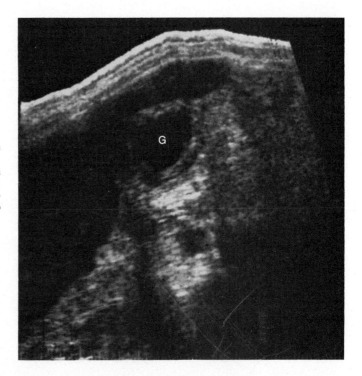

Figure 6–11. Transverse section of the gallbladder showing marked wall thickening. Although this could represent cholecystitis, in this patient it is the result of viral hepatitis. The patient had no clinical evidence of cholecystitis, and the gallbladder wall returned to normal thickness on follow-up scans.

dysfunction. We have also encountered a number of patients with active viral hepatitis who demonstrated significant wall thickening, which resolves as the clinical situation improves.[27] The etiology of the thickening in this case is obscure, although it is known that the virus is excreted in the bile of such individuals.

Perhaps the most common reason for apparent wall thickening is not related to any pathologic findings. Normal patients who have been incompletely fasted will regularly show a wall thickness of greater than 2 mm, so that an accurate history of dietary intake prior to the examination is essential (Fig. 6–12). This is particularly noticeable in infants, in whom prolonged fasting prior to examination is not possible.

Pericholecystic Fluid Collections

This recently described finding is a helpful sign when present but probably occurs only in severe cases of acute cholecystitis[29] (Figs. 6–13 and 6–14). At times, frank perforation of the gallbladder wall with a surrounding pericholecystic abscess is found, but in other cases only gray murky fluid will be present. Whether this represents perforations that are as yet too minute to be seen or simply edema of the gallbladder wall is not clear. Caution is advised

in using this sign in the presence of generalized peritoneal fluid, since such collections can invest the gallbladder and mimic this sign (as well as produce wall thickening, as noted previously).

Nonvisualizing Gallbladder

Numerous authors have noted that failure to visualize the gallbladder in a fasting patient has a very high correlation with disease— usually a shrunken gallbladder filled with stones[8, 29] (Fig. 6–15). Given the resolution of modern equipment, total nonvisualization is becoming a rare phenomenon. In most instances, careful attention to detail will show shadowing coming directly from the gallbladder fossa, thus adding to the certainty of the diagnosis. Although the possibility of encountering a patient with congenital absence of the gallbladder does exist, it is an extremely rare anomaly and therefore is of limited clinical significance.

Other Methods

Recently, radionuclide examination of the biliary tree using technetium-labelled deriva-

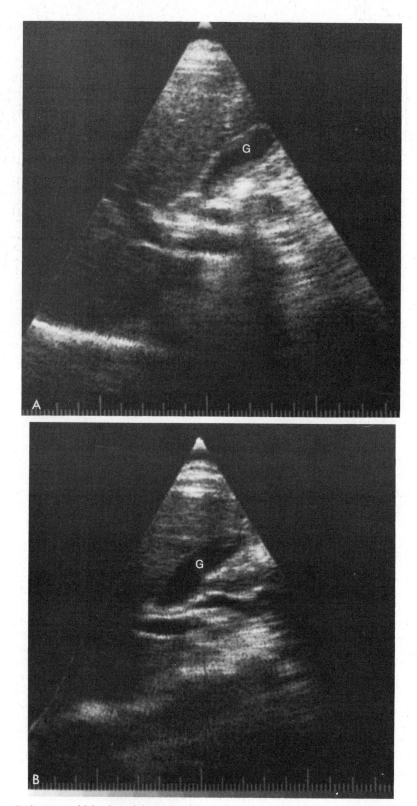

Figure 6–12. *A,* Apparent thickening of the gallbladder wall in a patient who was not fasting. *B,* Same patient after a 12-hour fast. The gallbladder wall is thin (normal).

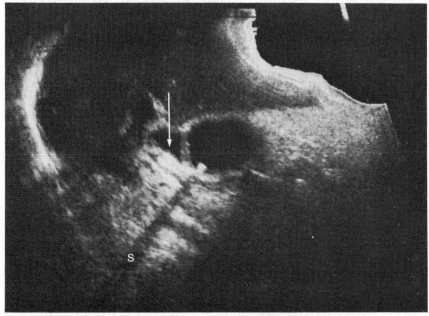

Figure 6–13. Scan shows thickening of the gallbladder wall, a gallstone with shadowing (S), and a small collection of fluid (arrow) adjacent to the gallbladder neck.

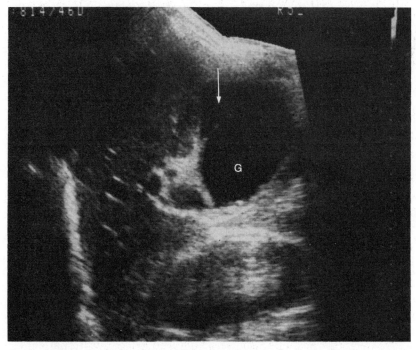

Figure 6–14. Scan near Figure 6–13 shows additional pericholecystic fluid collection. At surgery, there was perforation of the gallbladder and a pericholecystic abscess.

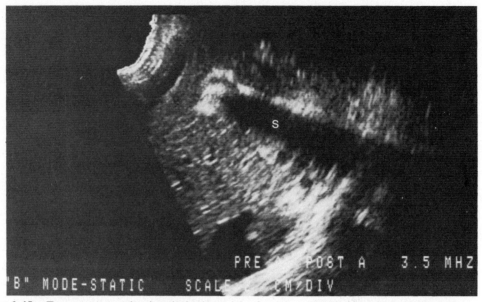

Figure 6–15. Transverse scan showing shadowing originating from within the liver in a patient with a contracted gallbladder. The intrahepatic origin is helpful in distinguishing this condition from shadowing produced by bowel adjacent to the liver.

tives of iminodiacetic acid (HIDA, PIPIDA, and so on) has been suggested as an initial screening technique for the diagnosis of acute cholecystitis.[30] This technique is well covered in other sections of this text and will not be dealt with at length here. Basically, demonstration of the gallbladder in such studies within one hour of intravenous administration of the isotope is presumptive evidence of patency of the cystic duct. Accuracy in the diagnosis of acute cholecystitis in excess of 95 per cent has been documented by some. In cases of chronic cholecystitis, accuracy drops to 50 per cent or less. In addition, others have reported that patients with alcoholic liver disease and those on hyperalimentation regimens may present as false positives (nonfilling of the gallbladder[31]). False-negative results have also occurred in patients who have anomalous connections between the biliary tree and the gallbladder, which permit the isotope to enter even when the cystic duct is obstructed by stone and/or edema.[32]

Both ultrasonography and biliary scintigraphy are excellent tests for the detection of acute cholecystitis. The choice between the two will ultimately be made by the clinicians who refer patients. This choice is based on the cost of the study, availability of the technique, and past experience with each method. At our institution, ultrasonography is the procedure of choice, but, given different circumstances, others might well begin the work-up with scintigraphy. As with many situations in diagnosis, algorithmic approach may be possible on a local level but is difficult to formulate on a wider basis.

Acalculous Cholecystitis

It is estimated that approximately 5 per cent of patients with acute cholecystitis will not have calculous disease.[33] Obstruction of the cystic duct is believed to be caused by edema in such cases. Obviously an ultrasonogram can be normal in these patients, although important secondary findings, such as localized tenderness and wall thickening, may point to the correct diagnosis. If the ultrasonogram is normal but a strong clinical suspicion of gallbladder disease still exists, further evaluation is indicated. If the patient is acutely ill and is already hospitalized, scintigraphy is indicated because of the acute desire to decrease hospitalization. Clinical experience in this situation is limited, however, and there are apparently some patients whose gallbladder will be visualized in this circumstance (false negative).

If the patient is neither acutely ill nor hospitalized, the normal ultrasonogram can be followed by conventional oral cholecystography to determine patency of the cystic duct. In most situations this will be more cost effective than scintigraphy, and there is no loss of accuracy.

Other Echo Sources Within the Gallbladder

Sludge

In many patients with obstruction of the biliary tree or prolonged fasting, the gallbladder will be seen to contain a dependent layer of low level echoes that moves very slowly with change in patient position (in contrast to the rapid movement of stones) (Fig. 6–16). No acoustic shadowing arises from this material. Usually termed "sludge," this substance was at first believed to represent extremely viscid bile.[34] Experimental work has shown, however, that viscosity alone cannot be the source of these echoes and that particulate matter of some sort must be responsible for their generation. The nature of this material is now known to be a mixture of calcium bilirubinate granules and cholesterol crystals.[35, 36] It is also known that not all individuals will exhibit this response to prolonged fasting. It is interesting to speculate that these individuals have an increased risk of developing gallstones, but this hypothesis remains to be proved.

Differentiation between sludge and stones is ordinarily not difficult, since shadowing and rapid positional change are not present in the former. When the two entities coexist, the relatively greater echogenicity of the calculi is easily demonstrated (Fig. 6–17).

Polypoid Lesions

Polyps are present within the gallbladder in a variety of conditions including cholesterolosis (Fig. 6–18), adenomyomatosis (Fig. 6–19), and carcinoma (Fig. 6–20). These generally appear as echogenic foci attached to the wall of the gallbladder and do not cast an acoustic shadow.[37, 38]

Gallbladder Carcinoma

Cancer of the gallbladder is a devastating disease that appears almost exclusively in patients over 50 years of age. Symptoms occur late in the course of the disease, so that it is often in a very advanced state at the time of diagnosis. Over 80 per cent of these patients will also have gallstones, and the sex predilection is predominantly female, as with gallstones. These facts have led some to suspect that gallstones may be etiologic in this disorder. This malignancy is at least twice as common as cholangiocarcinoma, the other major malignancy of the biliary tree.

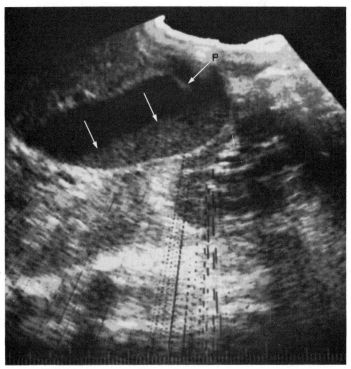

Figure 6–16. Sagittal scan of the gallbladder showing a layer of sludge (arrows) posteriorly. Note the absence of acoustic shadowing. A phrygian cap (P) is also noted.

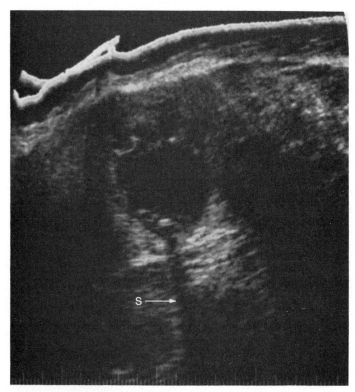

Figure 6–17. This patient exhibits a mixture of stones and sludge. Note that the stone has an acoustic shadow and is more echogenic than the surrounding sludge.

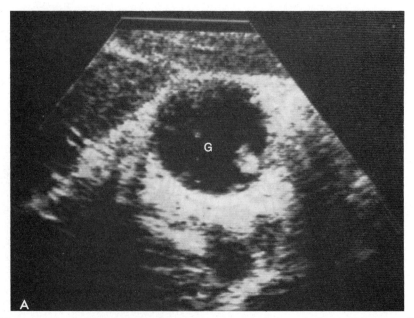

Figure 6–18. *A,* Scan shows nondependent echogenic foci attached to gallbladder wall.

Illustration continued on opposite page

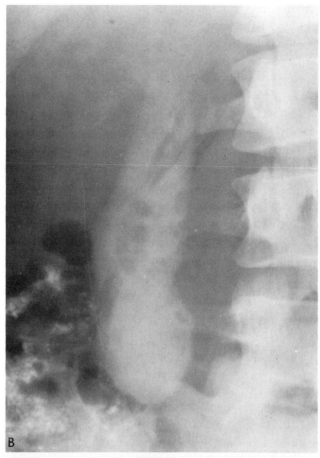

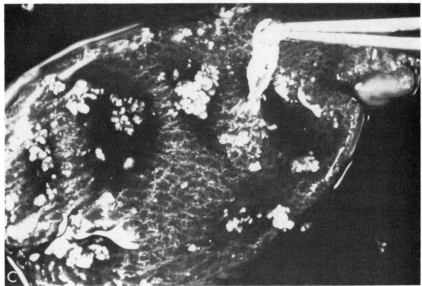

Figure 6–18. *Continued.* *B*, Oral cholecystography. Numerous filling defects are present. *C*, Gross specimen. Numerous cholesterol polyps are present. (Courtesy of Dr. Edward Stewart, Milwaukee, Wis.)

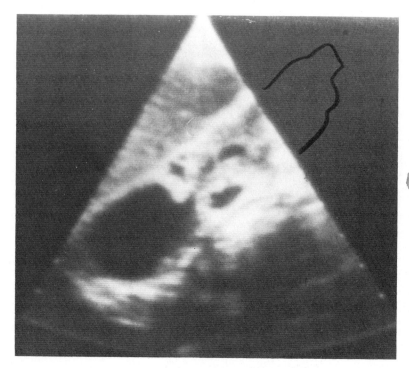

Figure 6–19. Scan of a patient with surgically proved adenomy-omatosis. The mural thickening and sinuses within are apparent. (Courtesy of Dr. Peter Cooper-berg.)

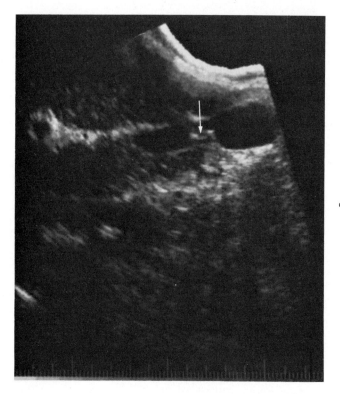

Figure 6–20. This innocent-looking gallblad-der mass (arrow) proved to be an early carcinoma.

Unfortunately, 90 per cent of these patients are dead within one year of diagnosis regardless of therapy employed. Of the patients who survive, nearly all are individuals whose lesion was a polyp confined to the gallbladder found incidentally at the time of cholecystectomy for symptomatic cholecystitis. It is this finding that clearly points out the role of the ultrasonographer in treating this disorder.

Ultrasonographically, the most common appearance of gallbladder carcinoma is a large mass in the porta hepatis producing bile duct obstruction, often with liver metastases already present.[39-42] Gallstones and shadowing are frequently seen within the mass (Fig 6–21). Such patients are inoperable. A second appearance said to correlate with carcinoma is diffuse or focal thickening of the gallbladder wall. This finding is relatively unusual and difficult to differentiate from the numerous other causes of wall thickening. Finally, as mentioned previously, gallbladder carcinoma may present as an intraluminal polyp. Since this is a curable form of the disease, close attention must be paid to this finding. Although a small gallbladder polyp might be safely observed in a younger patient (i.e., considered benign), it must be regarded as potentially malignant in older patients if there is to be any hope of cure. Indeed, the appearance of a first attack of cholecystitis in an older patient by itself should alert clinician and ultrasonographer alike to the possibility of gallbladder carcinoma. Confusion sometimes arises when sludge assumes a very focal, globby nature, and it may simulate a polyp (Fig. 6–22). Similarly, an encrusted stone may adhere to the wall of the gallbladder and mimic a polyp if shadowing is not demonstrable.

BILIARY TREE

The addition of ultrasonography as a noninvasive technique for imaging the biliary tree has been well received by clinicians. Such studies are now routinely performed in the evaluation of nearly all patients with upper right quadrant pain. In most patients presenting with jaundice, the test is capable of pinpointing the pathology (or site of pathology). Although the literature classically divides this entity into medical and surgical jaundice, we prefer to think in terms of dilated and nondilated biliary systems.[43] This results from the observation that there are situations when sur-

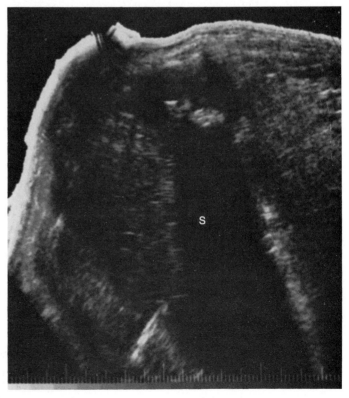

Figure 6–21. Transverse scan of large porta hepatis mass containing a shadowing gallstone. At surgery, an inoperable gallbladder carcinoma was discovered.

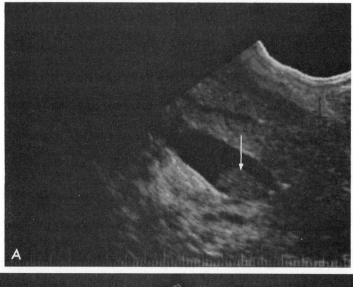

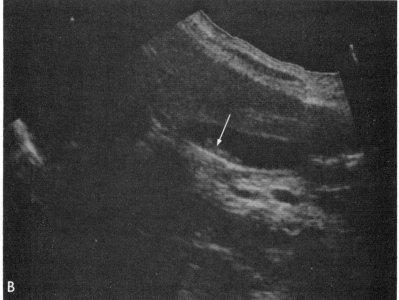

Figure 6–22. *A,* Scan showing polypoid "mass" (arrow) mimicking carcinoma or other pathology. *B,* Change in position. The "mass" is a focus of sludge and eventually redistributes itself to a new position.

gery is indicated and the bile duct caliber is normal; similarly, the bile ducts can be quite large and still not be obstructed.

At first, only dilatation of the intrahepatic portions of the biliary tree could be detected by ultrasonography. With increased knowledge of cross-sectional anatomy and steadily improving equipment, however, it soon became apparent that the extrahepatic segments could also be studied easily.

Because of anatomic considerations, we believe that it is convenient to divide the biliary tree into three distinct divisions, each requiring specific scanning maneuvers for optimum demonstration. This segmental approach to bile duct analysis should be applied routinely to patients undergoing abdominal sonography.

Intrahepatic Bile Ducts

In the normal fasting individual, the intrahepatic portions of the biliary tree are so small that they cannot be distinguished from other structures on routine sonography. When dilatation occurs, however, even very minimal changes are readily apparent. Since the bile ducts accompany the portal vein radicles, no special scanning technique is necessary to demonstrate them. As with most liver imaging, the best images result from single sector scans made with suspended respiration.

Since the bile ducts are not the only tubular structures present within the liver, the ultrasonographer must know the distinguishing criteria. The chief sources of confusion are the systemic and portal veins, since the arteries and lymphatics (like the bile ducts) are ordinarily invisible. The systemic veins—except for the largest branches—are easily identified by the absence of high-amplitude echoes at the interface between the vessel and surrounding liver. In addition, real-time studies reveal that these tubular structures converge upward toward the inferior vena cava. The major sources of confusion, then, are the portal veins. Although many authors allude to differences in course and caliber of these two systems, it should be remembered that corrosion cast studies have shown that the two (biliary and portal) systems are, in fact, almost identically paired. In fact, duplication of tubular systems is helpful in recognizing bile duct distention. This phenomenon has led to the popularity of the terms "shotgun"[44] and "parallel channel"[45] for the sign that is frequently present.

Fortunately for the ultrasonographer, distinction is usually made possible by the acoustic differences of the fluid contained within each set of tubes. Bile is a thin, watery liquid with essentially no protein content. As a result, the ultrasound transmitted through it undergoes very little attenuation and shows up on the far side of the bile duct as "acoustic enhancement" or "increased through transtransmission"[46] (Fig. 6–23). This phenomenon occurs behind most cystic structures when studied ultrasonographically. This explanation of enhancement behind bile ducts may be oversimplistic, since recent experimental evidence suggests that other factors, including refractive changes, may contribute to this phenomenon.[47] In any event, it is not observed behind blood-filled tubes (Fig. 6–24). Probably the solid elements within normal blood are at least partly responsible for the absorption that takes place. Whatever physical factors are operative, it is usually quite simple to see very minimal bile duct distention by recognizing the telltale ray of increased echogenicity radiating from its posterior margin. The only circumstance in which this finding fails is when the bile duct obstruction is long-standing and the bile has become inspissated. It is likely that the more solid nature of the bile accounts for this discrepancy.

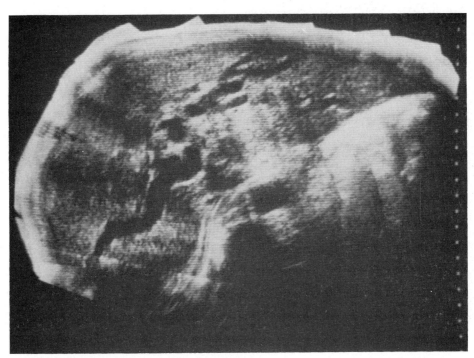

Figure 6–23. Transverse scan of the liver in a patient with marked intrahepatic dilatation. Note the areas of acoustic enhancement posterior to the dilated bile ducts.

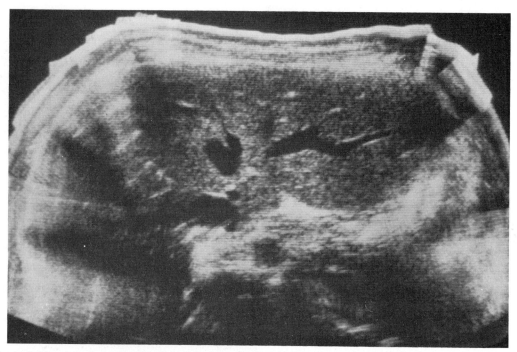

Figure 6–24. A patient with dilatation of the hepatic veins. Unlike the patient in Figure 6–23, there is no posterior acoustic enhancement.

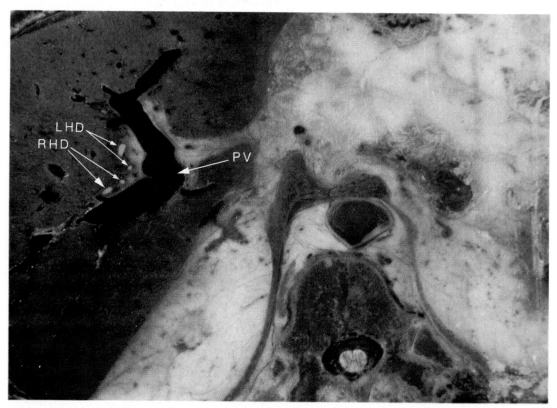

Figure 6–25. Cadaver specimen in which the portal veins (PV), hepatic artery, and bile ducts have been injected. Note the close relationship between the right (RHD) and left hepatic ducts (LHD) and the corresponding branches of the portal vein.

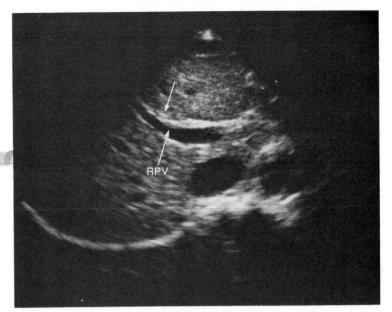

Figure 6–26. Scan of a normal patient showing the right portal vein (RPV) and the slit-like right hepatic duct just ventral to it (compare with Figure 6–25).

Although dilatation of the intrahepatic bile ducts most often results from distal obstruction, there are occasional patients with Caroli's disease (congenital cystic dilatation) who may present with similar findings. Ultrasonically, it is quite difficult to distinguish between these two situations.[48]

The main right and left hepatic bile ducts deserve separate consideration. The former courses along the ventral aspect of the right portal vein, whereas the latter is situated lateral to the left portal vein (Fig. 6–25). In both cases, these biliary branches are actually extra-hepatic in location (as are the portal vein branches). On sonograms, however, they appear to be intrahepatic and are therefore discussed in this section. Their importance lies in the fact that they are easy to demonstrate and are very sensitive indicators of extrahepatic obstruction (Fig. 6–26). Dilatation of these segments occurs well in advance of intrahepatic dilatation (Fig. 6–27). Filly and coworkers have called attention to the fact that on sagittal scans of the right lobe of the liver the undivided right portal vein is the dominant central feature.[18] On high quality scans, the right he-

Figure 6–27. Patient with extrahepatic bile duct obstruction. The dilated right hepatic duct (arrow) is evident. This appearance is often termed the "double barrel" or "shotgun" sign.

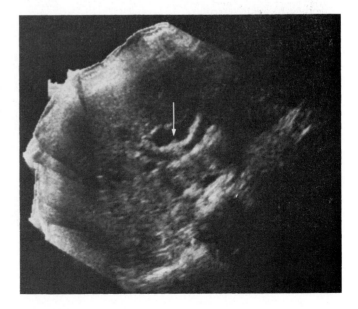

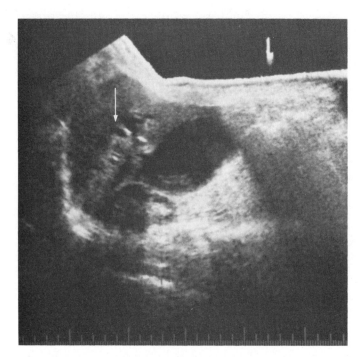

Figure 6–28. Sagittal scan of the right lobe of the liver in a patient with the "too many tubes" sign. Posterior enhancement is seen behind several of the minimally dilated bile ducts.

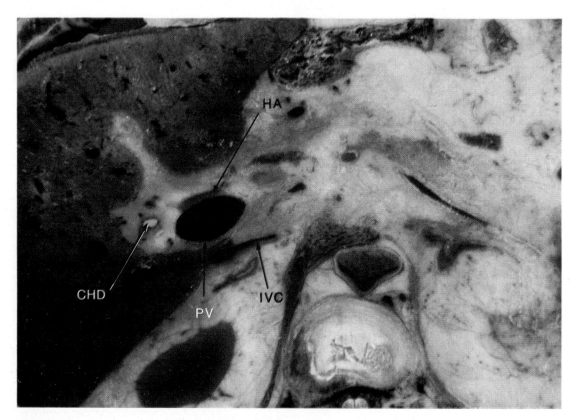

Figure 6–29. Cadaver section demonstrating the relationship of the portal vein (PV), common hepatic duct (CHD), and hepatic artery (HA) within the hepatoduodenal ligament. IVC = inferior vena cava.

patic duct may be seen as a tiny circular structure just ventral to the right portal vein. When enlargement occurs, these two structures become equal in size. As dilatation becomes more progressive, many circular structures appear in the area that originally showed only the right portal vein (Fig. 6–28). This phenomenon has been referred to as the "too many tubes" sign. Careful examination of these tubes will reveal that most of them display posterior acoustic enhancement, as previously discussed.

Extrahepatic Biliary Tree

Approximately 20 per cent of patients presenting with obstruction of the biliary tree will show changes only in the extrahepatic biliary tree. Many of these individuals will not manifest clinical jaundice.[49, 50] Analysis of these segments is therefore critical and requires detailed knowledge of the pertinent anatomy.[51] It is helpful to divide this analysis into two segments, the proximal duct, usually referred to as the common hepatic duct, and the distal duct or common bile duct.

The Common Hepatic Duct (CHD)

This segment of the extrahepatic biliary tree extends from the junction of the right and left hepatic ducts to the insertion of the cystic duct. The CHD is contained within a fold of peritoneum known as the hepatoduodenal ligament. The hepatoduodenal ligament forms the inferior border of the foramen of Winslow, the entrance to the lesser peritoneal sac. It also contains the main portal vein and hepatic artery. In most patients the portal vein lies posterior to the hepatic artery and the CHD (Fig. 6–29). The hepatic artery usually is situated ventral and medial to the portal vein, although in some patients who supply some or all of the right lobe of the liver from the superior mesenteric artery it lies posterior to the vein. The CHD is situated ventral and lateral to the vein.

Since the portal vein is an easily recognized landmark paralleling the CHD, it seems logical that a scan plane along the long axis of the vein increases the chance of seeing this segment of the biliary tree. By approaching this scan plane with the transducer angled toward the patient's head, the CHD may be imaged just anterior to the portal vein (Fig. 6–30). The precise plane is found more quickly with real-time scanning but with experience can easily be found by trial and error static studies. As noted by Behan and Kazam,[52] placing the patient in a partial right anterior oblique position seems to make the CHD easier to find. Probably the decubitus position helps by folding the liver lobes around the porta hepatis and allowing the air-filled loops of bowel to fall away.

Using this technique, Cooperberg and associates have reported success in visualizing the CHD in nearly all patients.[53, 54] A measurement (lumen) of 4 mm has been suggested as the top normal figure for this segment of the bile duct. In patients who have undergone previous cholecystectomy, a measurement of

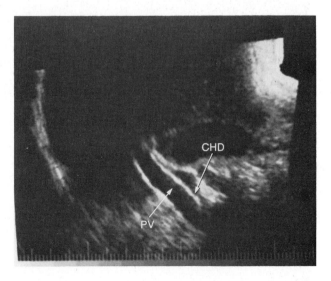

Figure 6–30. Oblique scan of a normal patient that projects the common hepatic duct (CHD) just anterior to the portal vein (PV).

7 mm is probably acceptable. In practice, the examiner's eye soon becomes adept at separating normal from abnormal by simple visual comparison with the adjacent portal vein. (It should be noted that measurements of the lumen using this technique as well as those given hereafter for the distal common bile duct are considerably smaller than figures derived from radiographic studies. This results from the fact that most radiographic measurements have been made after the administration of a choleretic agent. In addition, some radiographic magnification is unavoidable.[55]

An additional anatomic point worth considering in this view is the appearance of the right hepatic artery as it passes between the CHD and the portal vein. The circular lucency thus produced should be recognized as a normal anatomic structure and should not be confused with primary pathology of the CHD (Fig. 6–31).

CHD Pathology

The primary abnormality of the CHD detected by ultrasonography is dilatation. Although this frequently indicates distal obstruction, it should be remembered that dilatation can exist without obstruction (as in the postoperative state). Equally important, a bile duct of normal caliber may harbor significant pathology requiring surgical or percutaneous intervention.[56]

As ultrasonic equipment has improved, it has become possible to demonstrate many different types of pathology of the CHD. Congenital dilatations of the duct (choledochal cyst, choledochocele, choledochal diverticulum) are easily demonstrated since they represent various types of enlargement of the normal duct system[57] (Fig. 6–32). Although such patients are usually symptomatic (pain, jaundice), we have discovered some who were totally asymptomatic and had their lesions discovered during ultrasonography performed for other reasons.

Although ultrasonic imaging can demonstrate stones within the CHD (Figs. 6–33, 6–34, and 6–35), the reliability of finding them is much less than when calculi are in the gallbladder. Ultrasonography succeeds under the conditions in which the stones and the bile duct are large (such as intravenous cholangiography). When a stone is visualized on ultrasonography, it is usually safe to assume that it is

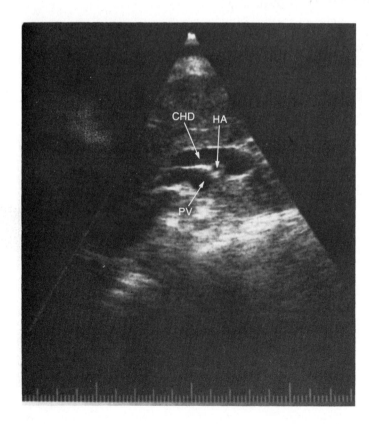

Figure 6–31. This oblique scan shows a dilated common hepatic duct (CHD). The hepatic artery (right branch) (HA) crosses between the common hepatic duct and the portal vein (PV) at this point.

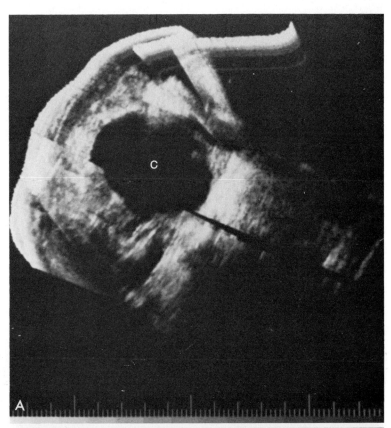

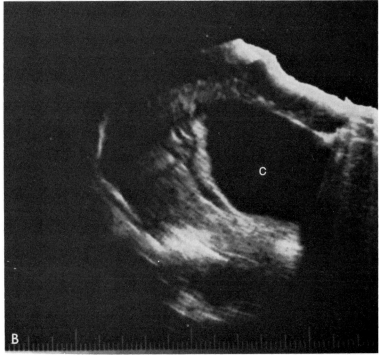

Figure 6–32. Transverse *(A)* and sagittal *(B)* scans of a child with a large choledochal cyst.

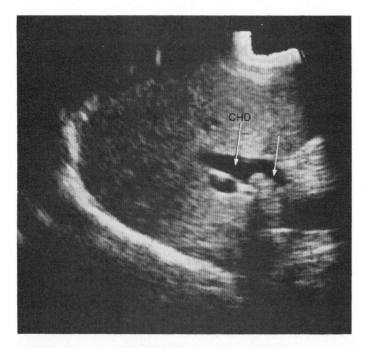

Figure 6–33. Oblique scan showing a dilated common hepatic duct (CHD) and a distal calculus (arrow).

not the one responsible for the obstruction, since that stone is usually impacted at the distal duct and is not surrounded by bile. On occasion, a stone impacted in the cystic duct produces obstruction of the proximal CHD (Mirizzi syndrome), and this occurrence can be recognized ultrasonically.[58]

We have also seen patients appear to have mechanical obstruction of the extrahepatic bile ducts on the basis of sludge (Fig. 6–36). Whether this material is identical to the sludge that forms in the gallbladder remains to be clarified. There is a peculiar form of inflammatory disease of the biliary tree termed "ori-

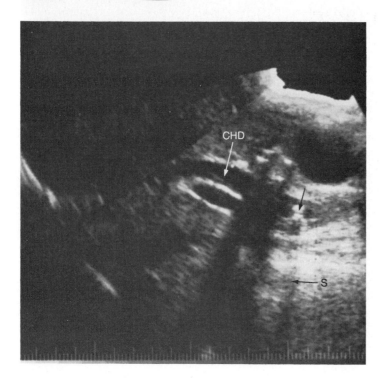

Figure 6–34. Oblique scan demonstrates shadowing (S) from a calculus (arrow) in the common hepatic duct (CHD). Several stones are seen in the gallbladder as well.

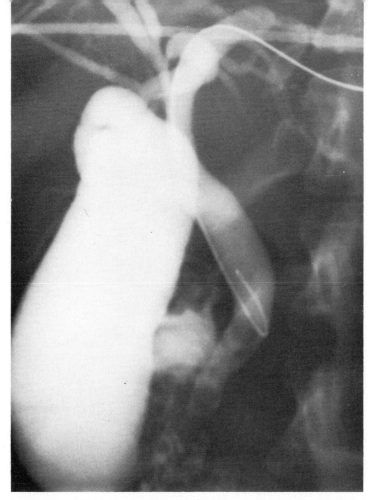

Figure 6–35. Cholangiogram of the patient in Figure 6–34. There are numerous calculi distal to the one actually visualized.

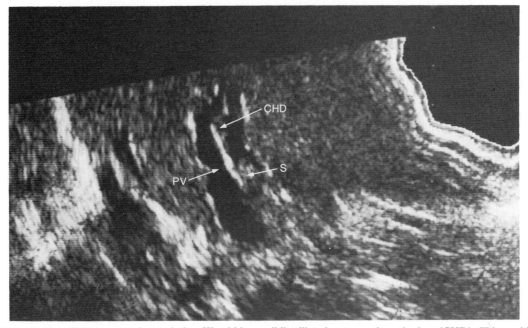

Figure 6–36. Oblique scan shows sludge (S) within a mildly dilated common hepatic duct (CHD). This could be easily confused with tumor. PV = portal vein.

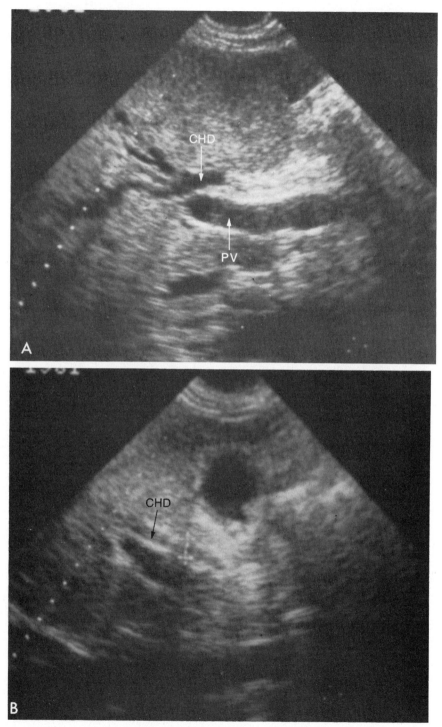

Figure 6–37. *A*, Oblique scan shows minimal dilatation of common hepatic duct (CHD) and abrupt cut-off. PV = portal vein. *B*, More distal scan shows echogenic material filling the common hepatic duct (arrow).

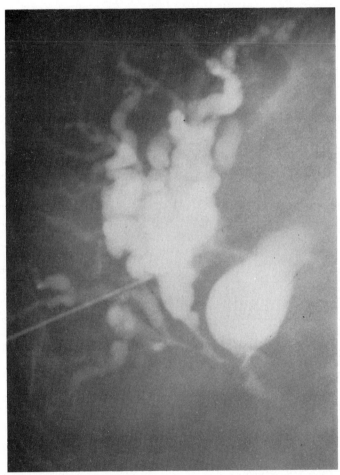

Figure 6–38. Cholangiogram shows constriction by tumor at the junction of the right and left hepatic ducts (cholangiocarcinoma).

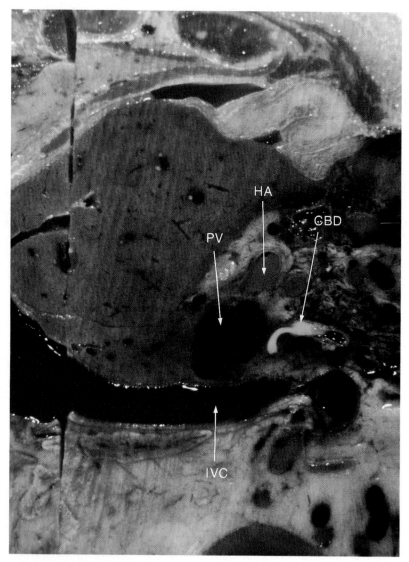

Figure 6–39. Sagittal cadaver section showing the bend in the common bile duct (CBD) as it leaves the hepatoduodenal ligament and begins its caudad and posterior course toward the head of the pancreas. PV = portal vein; HA = hepatic artery; IVC = inferior vena cava.

ental cholangiohepatitis" in which the accumulation of large amounts of sludge-like material in the extrahepatic biliary tree is common (with or without stones).[59] It has been pointed out that even massive bile duct dilatation in this circumstance may be overlooked by the ultrasonographer, since the altered consistency of the bile duct may be difficult to recognize in contrast to the normal surrounding structures.

Finally, cholangiocarcinoma, the most common malignancy of the bile ducts, may often be recognized as solid intraluminal masses. These tumors are usually situated in the CHD near the junction of the right and left hepatic ducts. If the lesion is located precisely at the junction (Klatskin tumor), equal dilatation of the right and left systems occurs (Figs. 6–37 and 6–38). The more distal bile duct is of normal caliber. When the tumor is eccentrically placed, either system may be preferentially dilated. In situations in which a high bile duct obstruction is present, it is mandatory to perform further radiologic studies of the intrahepatic bile ducts. Only with a detailed analysis of these structures can the surgeon adequately assess palliative bypass procedures and the best means of achieving them.

The Common Bile Duct (CBD)

Anatomic Considerations

Careful study of percutaneous and operative cholangiograms will reveal that there is an abrupt bend or knee in the extrahepatic bile duct in most patients (Fig. 6–39). This change in course usually occurs just distal to the insertion of the cystic duct. It is at this point that the bile duct exits the hepatoduodenal ligament and ceases to be parallel to the portal vein and hepatic artery. Its course is then caudad and dorsal, passing behind the duodenum to enter the substance of the head of the pancreas. In many patients this segment of the biliary tree (or at least a portion of it) lies in a parasagittal plane that passes through the inferior vena cava. Ultrasonic scans in this plane—an easily recognizable landmark—should be the starting point in identification of the CBD (Fig. 6–40). Decubitus positions seem to have no real advantage over the routine supine examination. On high quality transverse scans, the normal CBD can be identified within the head of the pancreas (Figs. 6–41 and 6–42), but recognition is far easier in

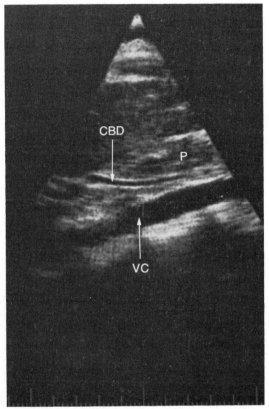

Figure 6–40. Sagittal sector scan showing the common bile duct (CBD) in its entirety. The vena cava (VC) is directly posterior to hhe duct. The pancreatic head (P) is also well seen.

sagittal planes. Although the gastroduodenal artery is also seen in this sagittal plane and is sometimes a source of confusion, it may be distinguished from the CBD by its course over the ventral surface of the pancreas.

Since the CBD is covered by duodenum, it is not surprising that the frequency with which it is visualized on ultrasonic scans is far less than that of the CHD. It is unusual to completely demonstrate the CBD, occurring in no more than 10 per cent of cases. On the other hand, careful attention to scanning technique will permit visualization of short segments of the CBD in approximately 60 per cent of studies (Fig. 6–43). Fortunately for ultrasonographers, as dilatation of this segment becomes progressively greater its recognition becomes easier (Figs. 6–44 and 6–45).

CBD Pathology

As with the CHD, the most common abnormality detected is dilatation. The normal CBD

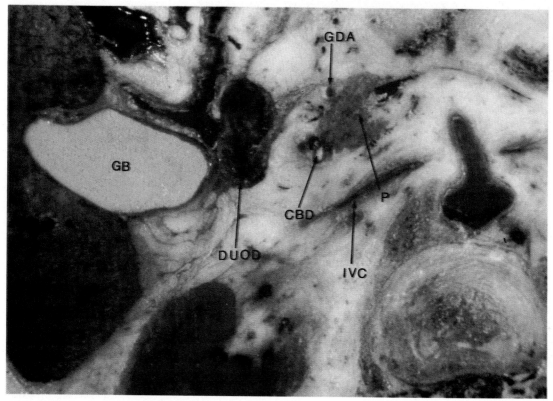

Figure 6–41. Transverse cadaver section showing the location of the common bile duct (CBD) within the pancreas. GB = gallbladder; Duod. = duodenum; GDA = gastroduodenal artery; P = pancreatic head; IVC = inferior vena cava.

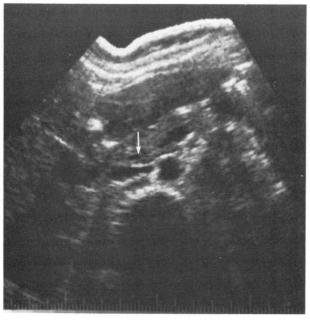

Figure 6–42. Transverse section in a normal patient. The common bile duct (CBD) (arrow) is seen in cross section within the head of the pancreas.

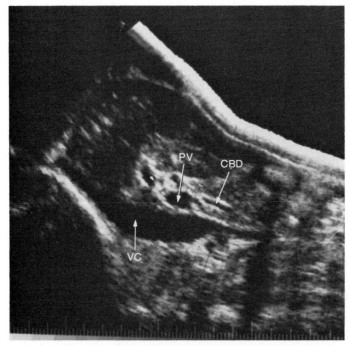

Figure 6–43. Sagittal scan showing only a short segment of the common bile duct (CBD). This is enough, however, to verify that no dilatation is present. PV = portal vein; VC = vena cava.

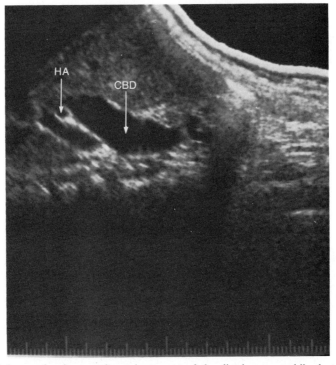

Figure 6–44. Sagittal scan showing massive enlargement of the distal common bile duct (CBD). HA = hepatic artery.

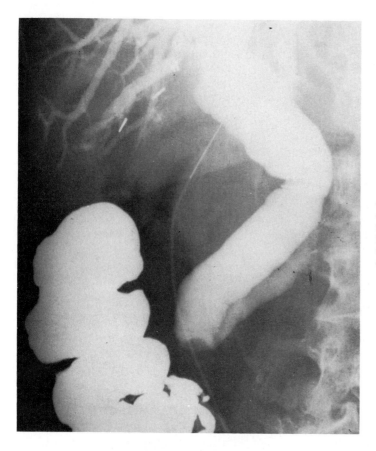

Figure 6–45. Operative cholangiogram on the patient in Figure 6–44. There is a distal stone, which cannot be detected on the sonogram. Although ultrasonography is accurate in defining the level of obstruction, it is very nonspecific in defining the cause of obstruction.

should not exceed 6 mm in diameter, although a measurement of 10 mm may be accepted in patients with previous cholecystectomy.[60, 61] Whether this increase occurs subsequent to cholecystectomy or existed at the time of surgery remains a subject for debate.[62, 63]

In situations in which the CBD measurement is borderline, there may be some utility in administering a fatty meal or cholecystokinin or one of its derivatives. In the normal individual, this stimulus causes relaxation of the sphincter of Oddi, allowing the diameter of the CBD to decrease (or at least remain constant). Increase in diameter following such administration is thought to indicate a mechanical obstruction. This hypothesis needs to be tested in a larger series before being uniformly applied.

The types of pathology seen in this segment of the biliary tree are similar to those described for the CHD. Obstruction at this level is far more likely to be caused by pancreatic mass or enlargement of the peripancreatic nodes. Even though a dilated duct may be traced directly to a mass in the pancreatic head, the ultrasonographic image cannot distinguish be-

tween carcinoma and focal pancreatitis. Enlargement of the extrahepatic biliary tree does occur in response to diffuse pancreatitis, and, at times, serial studies of the bile ducts may provide valuable information about the course of the disease.

References

1. Berk, R., and Leopold, G.: The present status of imaging of the gallbladder. Invest. Radiol. *13*:477, 1978.
2. Laing, F., Federle, M., Jeffrey, B., et al.: Ultrasonic evaluation of patients with right upper quadrant pain. Radiology *140*:449, 1981.
3. Cooperberg, P., Pon, M., Wong, P., et al.: Real time high resolution ultrasound in the detection of biliary calculi. Radiology *131*:789, 1979.
4. Callen, P., and Filly, R.: Ultrasonographic localization of the gallbladder. Radiology *133*:687, 1979.
5. Worthen, N., Uszler, J., and Funamura, J.: Cholecystitis: prospective evaluation of sonography and [99m]TC-HIDA cholescintigraphy. A.J.R. *137*:973, 1981.
6. Sukov, R., Sample, W., Sarti, D., et al.: Cholecystosonography—the junctional fold. Radiology *133*:435, 1979.
7. Slovis, T., Hight, D., Philippart, A., et al.: Sonography in the diagnosis and management of hydrops of

the gallbladder in children with mucocutaneous lymph node syndrome. Pediatrics 65:789, 1980.

8. Leopold, G., Amberg, J., Gosink, B., et al.: Gray scale ultrasonic cholecystography: a comparison with conventional radiographic techniques. Radiology 121:445, 1976.

9. Cooperberg, P., and Burhenne, H.: Real time ultrasonography. Diagnostic technique of choice in calculous gallbladder disease. N. Engl. J. Med. 302:1277, 1980.

10. Wolson, A., and Godberg, B.: Gray scale ultrasonic cholecystography. A primary screening procedure. J.A.M.A. 240:2073, 1978.

11. Crade, M., Taylor, K., Rosenfield, A., et al.: Surgical and pathologic correlation of cholecystosonography and cholecystography. A.J.R. 131:227, 1978.

12. Lee, J., Melson, G., Kochlcr, R., et al.: Cholecystosonography: accuracy, pitfalls, and unusual findings. Am. J. Surg. 139:223, 1980.

13. McIntosh, D., and Penney, H.: Gray scale ultrasonography as a screening procedure in the detection of gallbladder disease. Radiology 136:725, 1980.

14. Scheske, G., Cooperberg, P., Cohen, M., et al.: Floating gallstones: the role of contrast material. J. Clin. Ultrasound 8:227, 1980.

15. Carroll, B.: Gallstones: in vitro comparison of physical, radiographic, and ultrasonic characteristics. A.J.R. 131:223, 1978.

16. Good, L., Edell, S., Soloway, R., et al.: Ultrasonic properties of gallstones. Gastroenterology 77:258, 1979.

17. Purdom, R., Thomas, S., Kereiakes, J., et al.: Ultrasonic properties of biliary calculi. Radiology 136:729, 1980.

18. Filly, R., Moss, A., and Way, L.: In vitro investigation of gallstone shadowing with ultrasound tomography. J. Clin. Ultrasound 7:255, 1979.

19. Sommer, F., Filly, R., and Minton, M.: Acoustic shadowing due to refractive and reflective effects. A.J.R. 132:973, 1979.

20. Sommer, F., and Taylor, K.: Differentiation of acoustic shadowing due to calculi and gas collections. Radiology 135:399, 1980.

21. Handler, S.: Ultrasound of gallbladder wall thickening and its relationship to cholecystitis. A.J.R. 132:581, 1979.

22. Sanders, R.: The significance of sonographic gallbladder wall thickening. J. Clin. Ultrasound 8:143, 1980.

23. Marchal, G., Crolla, D., Baert, A., et al.: Gallbladder wall thickening: a new sign of gallbladder disease. J. Clin. Ultrasound 6:177, 1978.

24. Engel, J., Deitch, E., and Sikkema, W.: Gallbladder wall thickness: sonographic accuracy and relation to disease. A.J.R. 134:907, 1980.

25. Raghavendra, B.: Ultrasonographic features of primary carcinoma of the gallbladder: report of five cases. Gastrointest. Radiol. 5:239, 1980.

26. Fiske, C., Laing, F., and Brown, T.: Ultrasonographic evidence of gallbladder wall thickening in association with hypoalbuminemia. Radiology 135:713, 1980.

27. Shlaer, W., Leopold, G., and Scheible, F.: Sonography of the thickened gallbladder wall. A.J.R. 136:337, 1981.

28. Bergman, A., Neiman, H., and Kraut, B.: Ultrasonographic evaluation of pericholecystic abscesses. A.J.R. 132:201, 1979.

29. Harbin, W., Ferrucci, J., Wittenberg, J., et al.: Nonvisualized gallbladder by cholecystosonography. A.J.R. 132:727, 1979.

30. Weissman, H., Frank, M., Rosenblatt, R., et al.: Role of ^{99m}Tc-IDA cholescintigraphy in evaluating biliary tract disorders. Gastrointest. Radiol. 5:215, 1980.

31. Shuman, W., Gibbs, P., Rudd, T., et al.: PIPIDA scintigraphy for cholecystitis: false positives in alcoholism and total parenteral nutrition. A.J.R. 138:1, 1982.

32. Reimer, D., and Donald, J.: Technetium 99m-HIDA visualization of an obstructed gallbladder via an accessory hepatic duct. A.J.R. 137:610, 1981.

33. Howard, R.: Acute acalculous cholecystitis. Am. J. Surg. 141:194, 1981.

34. Conrad, M., Janes, J., and Dietchy, J.: Significance of low level echoes within the gallbladder. A.J.R. 132:967, 1979.

35. Filly, R., Allen, B., Minton, M., et al.: In vitro investigation of the origin of echoes within biliary sludge. J. Clin. Ultrasound 8:193, 1980.

36. Allen, B., Bernhoft, R., Blanckaert, N., et al.: Sludge is calcium bilirubinate associated with bile stasis. Am. J. Surg. 141:51, 1981.

37. Simeone, J., Mueller, P., and Ferrucci, J.: Significance of nonshadowing focal opacities at cholecystosonography. Radiology 137:181, 1980.

38. Rice, J., Sauerbrei, E., Semogas, P., et al.: Sonographic appearance of adenomyomatosis of the gallbladder. J. Clin. Ultrasound 9:336, 1981.

39. Yum, H., and Fink, A.: Sonographic findings in primary carcinoma of the gallbladder. Radiology 134:693, 1980.

40. Allibone, G., Fagan, C., and Porter, S.: Sonographic features of carcinoma of the gallbladder. Gastrointest. Radiol. 6:169, 1981.

41. Dalla Palma, L., Rizzatto, G., Pozzi-Mucelli, R., et al.: Grey scale ultrasonography in the evaluation of carcinoma of the gallbladder. Br. J. Radiol. 53:662, 1980.

42. Yeh, H.: Ultrasonography and computed tomography of carcinoma of the gallbladder. Radiology 133:167, 1979.

43. Leopold, G.: Ultrasonography of jaundice. Radiol. Clin. North Am. 17:127, 1979.

44. Weill, F., Eisenscher, A., and Zeltner, F.: Ultrasonic study of the normal and dilated biliary tree. The "shotgun" sign. Radiology 127:221, 1978.

45. Conrad, M., Landay, M., and Janes, J.: Sonographic "parallel channel" sign of biliary tree enlargement in mild to moderate obstructive jaundice. A.J.R. 130:279, 1978.

46. Laing, F., London, L., and Filly, R.: Ultrasonographic identification of dilated intrahepatic bile ducts and their differentiation from portal venous structures. J. Clin. Ultrasound 6:90, 1978.

47. Robinson, D., Wilson, L., and Kossoff, G.: Shadowing and enhancement in ultrasonic echograms by reflection and refraction. J. Clin. Ultrasound 9:181, 1981.

48. Mittelstaedt, C., Volberg, F., Fischer, G., et al.: Caroli's disease: sonographic findings. A.J.R. 134:585, 1980.

49. Weinstein, B., and Weinstein, D.: Biliary tract dilatation in the nonjaundiced patient. A.J.R. 134:899, 1980.

50. Zeman, R., Taylor, K., Burrell, M., et al.: Ultrasound demonstration of an icteric dilatation of the biliary tree. Radiology 134:689, 1980.

51. Hoevels, J.: Topographic relation of the portal vein to extrahepatic bile ducts. A combined portographic-

cholangiographic study in 25 cadavers. Fortsch. Rontgenstr. *129*:217, 1978.

52. Behan, M., and Kazam, E.: Sonography of the common bile duct: value of the right anterior oblique view. A.J.R. *130*:701, 1978.

53. Cooperberg, P.: High resolution real time ultrasound in the evaluation of normal and obstructed biliary tract. Radiology *129*:477, 1978.

54. Cooperberg, P., Li, D., Wong, P., et al.: Accuracy of common hepatic duct size in the evaluation of extrahepatic biliary obstruction. Radiology *135*:141, 1980.

55. Sauerbrei, E., Cooperberg, P., Gordon, P., et al.: The discrepancy between radiographic and sonographic bile duct measurements. Radiology *137*:751, 1980.

56. Beinart, C., Efremidis, S., Cohen, B., et al.: Obstruction without dilatation: importance in evaluating jaundice: J.A.M.A. *245*:353, 1981.

57. Kangarloo, H., Sarti, D., Sample, W.: Ultrasono-graphic spectrum of choledochal cysts in children. Pediatr. Radiol. *9*:15, 1980.

58. Dewbury, K.: The features of the Mirizzi syndrome on ultrasound examination. Br. J. Radiol. *52*:990, 1979.

59. Scheible, F., and Davis, G.: Oriental cholangiohepatitis: preoperative radiographic and ultrasonographic diagnosis. Gastrointest. Radiol. *6*:269, 1981.

60. Sample, W., Sarti, D., Goldstein, L., et al.: Grey scale ultrasonography of the jaundiced patient. Radiology *128*:719, 1978.

61. Parulekar, S.: Ultrasound examination in common bile duct size. Radiology *133*:703, 1979.

62. Mueller, P., Ferrucci, J., Simeone, J., et al.: Post cholecystectomy bile duct dilatation: myth or reality? A.J.R. *136*:355, 1981.

63. Graham, M., Cooperberg, P., Cohen, M., et al.: The size of the normal common hepatic duct following cholecystectomy: an ultrasonographic study. Radiology *135*:137, 1980.

COMPUTED TOMOGRAPHY OF THE GALLBLADDER AND BILE DUCTS

by Robert E. Koehler, M.D.
and Robert J. Stanley, M.D.

7

Computed tomography (CT) has made major contributions to the evaluation of the gallbladder and biliary tree since its clinical application in abdominal disease in 1975. Like ultrasonography, this noninvasive method provides information that was previously obtainable only by more invasive studies such as intravenous or percutaneous transhepatic cholangiography or angiography. Experience in numerous centers has now established that both CT and ultrasonography are accurate in detecting biliary tract disease, and in some situations CT can provide more specific information regarding the etiology and extent of disease than can be determined sonographically. For these reasons there is a growing tendency to use CT to confirm or alter the clinical impression in patients with jaundice or other indications of liver or biliary tract disease.

TECHNIQUE

To evaluate the liver and biliary tract, contiguous transverse images are ordinarily obtained at 1-cm intervals with 10 mm collimation (slice thickness) from the diaphragm to the level of the third portion of the duodenum. All scans are reviewed on the video console, varying the window level and width to optimize detection of structures that may differ only slightly in attenuation value from surrounding tissues. The density of the liver is assessed quantitatively and in relation to the density of the spleen.

If the findings are sufficient to explain the nature of the underlying disease, the study is terminated at this point. When no hepatobiliary abnormalities are detected on initial precontrast scans or when it is desirable to obtain better visualization of mildly dilated bile ducts or other suspected abnormalities, urographic contrast material is administered intravenously. Infusion of 150 ml of a 60 per cent solution of sodium iothalamate over approximately a 10-minute period is usually adequate. This causes contrast enhancement of the vascular structures in the liver and porta hepatis and of the parenchyma of the liver and pancreas. It also improves the visibility of the intra- and extrahepatic portions of the unenhanced biliary tree. Selected scans can be repeated with thin collimation (e.g., 2 to 5 mm) for improved spatial and contrast resolution.

It is sometimes useful to administer urographic contrast material as a rapid bolus intravenous injection. In such cases, 30 to 60 ml of a 67 per cent sodium iothalamate solution is injected through a 19-gauge needle into a large vein over 10 to 30 seconds. Bolus injection is particularly useful for more precisely displaying and evaluating focal hepatic lesions and the major blood vessels in and around the liver and biliary tree. Several scans obtained in rapid succession over the two minutes following injection yield information on the pattern of contrast enhancement, which may be helpful in determining the specific nature of an hepatic mass.[1-5]

Developmental efforts are proceeding on new organ-specific contrast agents that are concentrated in the liver. One such agent that shows promise is ethiodized oil emulsion (EOE-13).[6, 7] This radiopaque material is taken up by the reticuloendothelial cells of the liver and spleen and has been shown to significantly improve the visibility of lymphomatous or metastatic deposits in both of these organs. Continuing studies are aimed at determining the safety and clinical utility of this and other experimental contrast agents.

An important principle to keep in mind when interpreting any CT study is partial volume averaging. The shade of gray represented in any picture element, or pixel, in a CT reconstruction represents an average of the attenuation of the x-ray beam by all of the tissue within the volume represented by that pixel. Unless a structure occupies the entire thickness (Z axis) of the slice, the displayed density will include contributions from under-

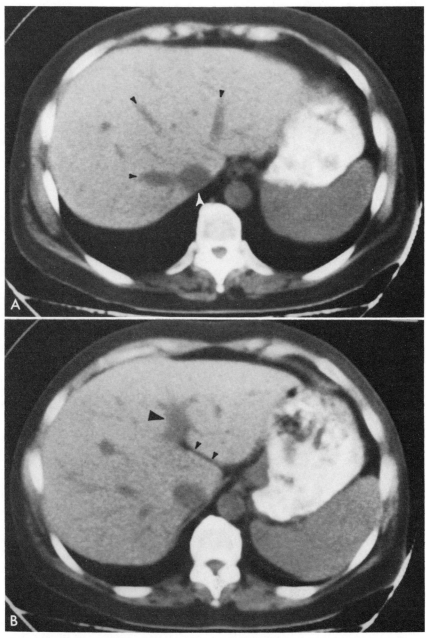

Figure 7–1. Four scans at descending levels in a patient with a normal CT appearance of the liver. *A,* Hepatic veins (black arrowheads) converge on the inferior vena cava (white arrowhead). *B,* At this level, the portal vein (large arrowhead) and the fissure for the ligamentum venosum (small arrowheads) are evident.

Illustration continued on opposite page

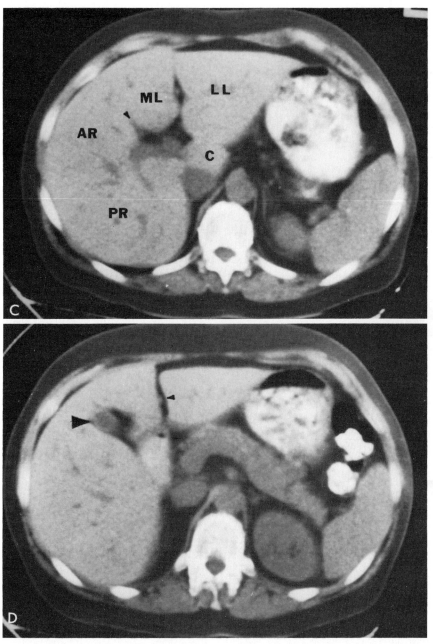

Figure 7–1. *Continued.* *C,* The major hepatic lobes and segments are indicated. LL = lateral segment of left lobe; ML = medial segment of left lobe; AR = anterior segment of right lobe; PR = posterior segment of right lobe; C = caudate lobe. Note the fat in cleft for the falciform ligament, which separates the medial and lateral segments of the left lobe, and the fat in a crevice of the gallbladder fossa (arrow), which lies along the plane dividing right and left lobes. *D,* At the lowest level the gallbladder (large arrowhead) is visible and the vena cava is no longer intrahepatic. Note the falciform ligament (small arrowhead) at this and the next higher level.

lying and overlying tissue within the slice plane. The thinner the structure compared with the slice thickness, the more the displayed density of that structure will resemble that of the surrounding tissue. This is one reason why small intrahepatic bile ducts running trans- versely, parallel to the plane of the CT slice, are often not visible. The problems presented by partial volume averaging can be minimized by the administration of intravenous contrast material to improve relative contrast and by the use of thinner slice collimation.

ANATOMY

Liver

Accurate CT evaluation of patients with known or suspected disease of the biliary tract requires a thorough knowledge of the normal CT appearance of the liver, bile ducts, gallbladder, and associated vascular structures. The liver occupies the right and mid portions of the upper abdomen, and considerable variation exists in its normal size and shape (Fig. 7–1). The right lobe is nearly always larger than the left, which may be congenitally quite small. Riedel's lobe, an infrequent variation in the shape of the right lobe generally found in women, is recognized by a fusiform widening of the inferior aspect of the right lobe, which may extend inferior to the right kidney. In some patients, the lateral segment of the left lobe is quite thin, measuring only 1.5 cm from front to back. Radionuclide images in livers of this shape are sometimes falsely interpreted as showing a focal defect in the left lobe. Correlation of the radionuclide findings with CT can clarify this situation and obviate further investigation.

In classical anatomic descriptions, the liver was considered to be divided into right and left lobes by the fissure for the ligamentum teres anteriorly and the fissure for the ligamentum venosum and gastrohepatic ligament posteriorly. However, investigations using injected corrosion casts have shown that, from the standpoint of vascular and ductal anatomy, the right and left lobes are usually separated by a plane extending from the gallbladder fossa to the sulcus for the inferior vena cava.[8] There is no corresponding fissure visible on the surface of the liver, and this division is not directly identifiable by CT. The fossae for the gallbladder and vena cava are visible, however, so it is not usually difficult to determine the division of right and left lobes.

The right and left lobes are each further subdivided into two segments. The right intersegmental fissure, not apparent on CT, divides the right lobe into anterior and posterior segments. The left intersegmental fissure corresponds to the fissure of the ligamentum teres, the classically described division between right and left lobes. It contains fat and is almost always visible. This fissure divides the left lobe into a medial segment, classically the quadrate lobe, and a lateral segment. The normally obliterated umbilical vein runs in the free margin of the falciform ligament and, when enlarged and serving as a collateral venous pathway in patients with portal hypertension, may be quite prominent on CT scans through this level. The major hepatic veins run within the fissures between lobes and segments, in

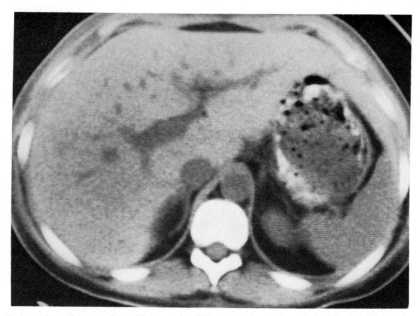

Figure 7–2. In anemic patients such as this one, the CT attenuation value of the blood is lower than usual, and the veins in the liver contrast sharply with the adjacent normal parenchyma. These unusually lucent but otherwise normal vascular structures should not be confused with dilated bile ducts.

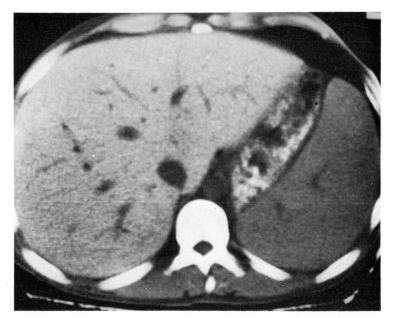

Figure 7–3. Abnormally high liver attenuation value (80 HU) in a patient with hemochromatosis. The liver is considerably more dense than the spleen and vascular structures.

contrast to the branches of the hepatic artery and portal vein, which run through the centers of the lobes and segments.

The caudate lobe can be considered to be separate from the left and right lobes. It is bounded posteriorly by the inferior vena cava and anteriorly by the portal vein and fissure of the ligamentum venosum. Arterial and portal venous branches from both right and left lobes supply the caudate lobe, and hepatic veins from this region usually drain directly into the inferior vena cava. This separate anatomic status may account for the relative sparing of the caudate lobe in some diffuse parenchymal diseases of the liver.

The CT attenuation (shade of gray) of the liver is quite homogeneous except for the lower density vascular structures within it. The density is normally slightly higher than that of the spleen, kidneys, and pancreas and tends to be in the range of 50 to 70 Hounsfield units (HU). Intravenous administration of iodinated contrast material increases the attenuation value in a dose-related fashion, often to a value of 120 HU or more.

Vascular Structures

In normal patients, the blood in the portal and hepatic veins is sufficiently lower in density than the surrounding hepatic parenchyma so that the veins are visible on CT. This density difference is accentuated by a reduction in the attenuation value of the blood in anemic patients (Fig. 7–2) or by an increase in the attenuation value of the liver, as in patients with hemochromatosis (Fig. 7–3) or some hepatic storage diseases. The density relationship between liver and blood can be transiently reversed by the bolus injection of contrast material, which increases the density of the blood more than that of the liver. The density relationship is also reversed in patients with diffuse fatty infiltration of the liver, in which case the normal veins stand out as structures of density higher than the surrounding liver even without the aid of a contrast agent (Fig. 7–4). Although the large vascular structures within the liver are usually visible either without contrast administration or immediately after a bolus injection, they can become less visible or even isodense with the surrounding parenchyma during the late equilibrium phase after contrast injection. For these reasons, intravenous contrast agents are commonly employed in an attempt to differentiate slightly dilated intrahepatic biliary ducts, which do not enhance, from arteries or veins of similar size.

The portal vein originates with the confluence of the splenic and superior mesenteric veins and runs cephalad and to the right within the hepatoduodenal ligament. It closely approaches, and in some patients touches, the inferior vena cava, which lies behind it. Hepatic veins are often seen on CT as well, although the confluence of the hepatic veins with the vena cava is occasionally obscured by

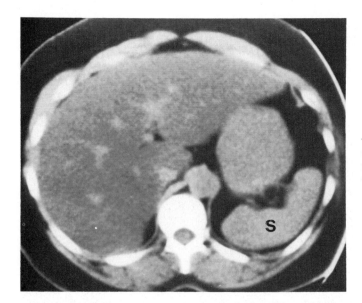

Figure 7–4. Fatty infiltration of the liver. The liver has a lower attenuation value than the blood vessels within it and is less dense than the spleen (S), a reversal of the normal density relationships.

artifact owing to cardiac motion. Portal vein branches grow larger as they approach the porta hepatis, whereas hepatic veins increase in diameter as they approach the diaphragm and their junction with the inferior vena cava.

In most patients, the hepatic artery and its branches follow a course similar to that of the portal venous system. Although the arteries are considerably smaller than the veins, the extrahepatic portions of the hepatic arterial supply are usually visible even without contrast enhancement. Intrahepatic arterial branches, however, are rarely seen on CT without the aid of a bolus injection of contrast material. The hepatic artery arises from the celiac axis and enters the hepatoduodenal ligament, where it lies anterior and medial to the main portal vein. In about 25 per cent of patients a replaced or accessory right hepatic artery arises separately from the superior mesenteric artery and is visible as it passes transversely between the inferior vena cava and portal vein to enter the medial surface of the right hepatic lobe.[9, 10] Infrequently, an hepatic artery arising normally from the celiac axis passes between the portal vein and vena cava. Similarly, in occasional patients a replaced hepatic artery passes ventral to the portal vein.[11]

Bile Ducts

The intrahepatic portions of the biliary tree follow the pathways of the hepatic arteries and portal veins. When they are of normal caliber, the intrahepatic bile ducts are too small to be seen with currently available CT equipment. Even when the bile is densely opacified by intravenously administered cholangiographic contrast material, the normal ducts are visible only in the immediate periportal area, and contrast materials of this type have found only limited application in CT of the biliary tract.

In approximately one-third of normal patients, the common hepatic duct or common bile duct can be seen in cross section as a circular, water-density structure from 2 to 6 mm in diameter (Fig. 7–5). The common hepatic duct lies anterior to the main portal vein, just lateral to the hepatic artery. The duct passes behind the first portion of the duodenum and descends along the medial wall of the second portion of the duodenum in the posterolateral aspect of the head of the pancreas.

Gallbladder

On transverse scans the gallbladder appears as an oval or elliptical structure containing bile of a density near that of water but often slightly denser than bile in the biliary tree owing to reabsorption of water by the gallbladder mucosa. It lies in a fossa on the inferior surface of the liver, which demarcates the fissure that divides the left and right hepatic lobes. Occasionally the gallbladder lies in an intrahepatic or other ectopic position, and anatomic variants of this sort can be worked out rather

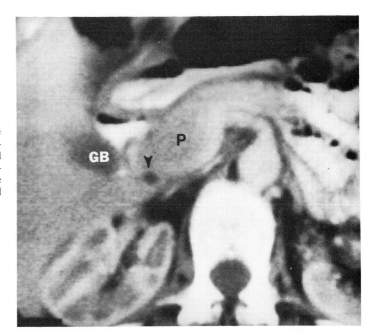

Figure 7–5. The normal common bile duct (arrowhead) lies between the posterior portion of the pancreatic head (P) and the adjacent duodenum. This duct measured 5 mm in diameter. The neck of the gallbladder (GB) is lateral to the duodenal bulb.

precisely with CT. Occasionally the normal gallbladder extends below the lower margin of the liver and appears as a round, water-density structure surrounded by fat. The gallbladder wall can usually be seen and, if the gallbladder is distended, does not ordinarily measure more than 2 mm in thickness.

BILIARY OBSTRUCTION

The CT diagnosis of biliary obstruction is based primarily on the demonstration of dilated intrahepatic and/or extrahepatic bile ducts. With present-day equipment, any portion of the intrahepatic biliary tree visible on CT in the absence of biliary air or cholangiographic contrast material can be assumed to be dilated. The extrahepatic bile duct is considered dilated if it is 9 mm or more in diameter.[12-17] Ducts of 7 or 8 mm diameter are of borderline size and raise the suspicion of obstruction. Those less than 7 mm are considered normal in caliber. When there is uncertainty as to the ductal size on CT, it is useful to administer urographic contrast material intravenously and perform slices with thin collimation, e.g., 5 mm.

Unfortunately, there is not a direct relationship between the caliber of the biliary tree and the presence or absence of clinically significant obstruction. In patients with significant dilatation of the biliary tree in whom the obstruction is later relieved surgically or by spontaneous passage of a calculus, the bile duct may remain somewhat more dilated than normal for the remainder of the patient's life. In such patients, the CT findings can falsely suggest the presence of biliary obstruction. In patients with little or no clinical or biochemical evidence of biliary obstruction in whom CT shows a dilated bile duct but no tumor, calculus, or other obstructing lesion, one must be skeptical about the presence of obstruction. In this situation, percutaneous cholangiography can be used to determine how readily bile passes from the dilated bile duct into the duodenum and whether a stricture is present in the distal common bile duct.

Conversely, occasional patients with calculi or other obstructing lesions of the biliary tract have a duct of normal caliber. This is a problem, primarily in patients in whom the obstruction is early or of low grade and in whom there is intermittent obstruction by calculi. Again, when there is discordance between the clinical and CT findings, one should not hesitate to proceed with more invasive means of imaging the biliary tract to clarify the situation.

Despite the lack of direct correlation between ductal caliber and ductal obstruction, CT has proved to be useful and accurate in establishing this diagnosis. In a prospective study of 103 patients with abnormalities of liver function suggesting biliary tract obstruction, obstruction was correctly identified in 45

(96 per cent) of the 47 patients later proved to have obstructive jaundice.[12] In the same series, a 2-cm common bile duct was incorrectly thought to indicate obstruction in one patient in whom percutaneous cholangiography subsequently showed that bile passed freely from the dilated duct through the ampulla of Vater into the duodenum.

Level of Obstruction

Once the presence of biliary obstruction has been ascertained, attention should be directed to determining the level of obstruction. This is important in pinpointing the etiology of the obstruction and in determining whether a surgical or other drainage procedure is advisable. It is helpful to categorize the level of obstruction as either intrahepatic, junctional, suprapancreatic, pancreatic, or ampullary.

Intrahepatic obstruction may result in ductal dilatation in only a portion of the liver.[18] With adequate function of the unobstructed portion of the liver, the serum bilirubin level remains normal, and an elevated serum alkaline phosphatase level may be the only biochemical clue to the presence of obstructive disease.

By analyzing the appearance and caliber of the extrahepatic bile duct on sequential transverse scans, it is ordinarily possible to determine the level of extrahepatic obstruction fairly accurately.[19] Obstruction at the junctional level causes dilatation of the main right and left hepatic ducts with an obliterated or nondilated common duct. With obstruction in the suprapancreatic region, the dilated common hepatic duct is evident anterior to the portal vein on one or two scans, and a duct of normal size may be seen at the level of the pancreatic head. If the dilated portion of the duct extends to or into the pancreas, the intrapancreatic portion of the duct is the likely site of obstruction. With ampullary obstruction, a dilated duct is seen all the way into the pancreatic head, and the dilated segment may extend 7 or 8 cm below the bifurcation. Lesions that obstruct the duct in its ampullary or pancreatic segment may also obstruct the main pancreatic duct, and one should look carefully for pancreatic ductal dilatation as a clue to the level and nature of the obstruction. The gallbladder is usually distended, with obstruction below the junction of the cystic and common ducts. Prior gallbladder disease can, of course, prevent distention, so the caliber of the gallbladder should not be relied upon too heavily to predict the level of obstruction.

Cause of Obstruction

There are many CT findings to consider in the determination of the cause of biliary ductal obstruction. Accurately placing the level of obstruction will suggest the correct etiology in many cases.[20] Intrahepatic obstruction affecting some segments of the liver more than others is often due to primary or secondary liver tumor, cholangiocarcinoma, or sclerosing cholangitis. In sclerosing cholangitis the intrahepatic ducts often have a peculiar and somewhat characteristic appearance. The degree of dilatation is usually mild, and some hepatic segments are more affected than others. The branching pattern is distorted and irregular, and the ducts do not taper normally as they near the periphery of the liver. These findings, coupled with the absence of a mass, often make it possible to suggest this diagnosis on the basis of the CT findings (Fig. 7–6).

Obstruction at the junction of the main right and left ducts suggests a complication of prior biliary surgery, cholangiocarcinoma, or an invasive gallbladder carcinoma (Fig. 7–7). Common duct obstruction at the suprapancreatic level is usually due to cholangiocarcinoma (Fig. 7–8), periportal lymph node enlargement by metastatic tumor, or lymphoma (Fig. 7–9), or to upward extension of pancreatic carci-

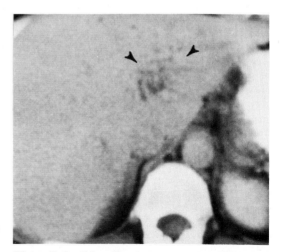

Figure 7–6. Sclerosing cholangitis. Minimal, focal dilatation of small branches of the biliary tree (arrowheads) in the left lobe produces a distorted cluster of ducts unlike that seen in simple biliary obstruction.

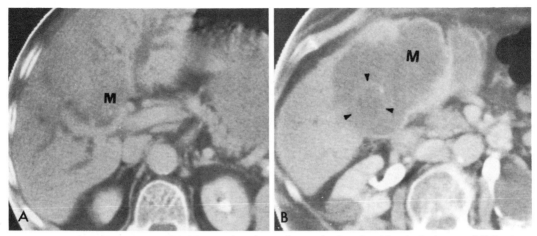

Figure 7–7. Carcinoma of the gallbladder causing obstruction at the junctional level. *A,* A mass (M) lies between the dilated right and left hepatic ducts. *B,* At a lower level the collapsed bile duct is not seen. The mass (M) extensively infiltrates the liver, and the gallbladder (arrowheads) is faintly visible within it. Renal cysts are present bilaterally.

noma. Obstruction at the pancreatic level suggests pancreatic carcinoma, stricture due to chronic pancreatitis (Fig. 7–10), or obstructing calculi (Fig. 7–11). Obstruction at the level of the ampulla is usually due to ampullary tumor or calculi (Fig. 7–12).

One should note the degree of dilatation of the intrahepatic biliary radicles. Mild to mod-

erate dilatation is nonspecific, but marked dilatation of intrahepatic ducts usually indicates a malignant basis for the obstruction. A prominent transversely oriented portion of the common duct on one or more CT slices has been proposed as a sign suggesting an underlying tumor,[20] but we have not found this finding to be particularly helpful or specific. It has been

Text continued on page 252

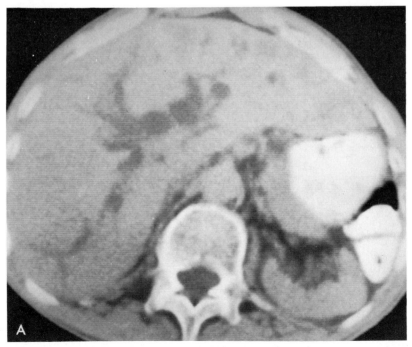

Figure 7–8. Scans at three levels in a patient with common hepatic duct obstruction due to cholangiocarcinoma. *A,* Marked dilatation of intrahepatic duct. Note obvious difference between CT attenuation value of bile within the ducts and that of aortic blood. This difference is useful in distinguishing dilated intrahepatic ducts from normal intrahepatic portal veins.

Illustration continued on following page

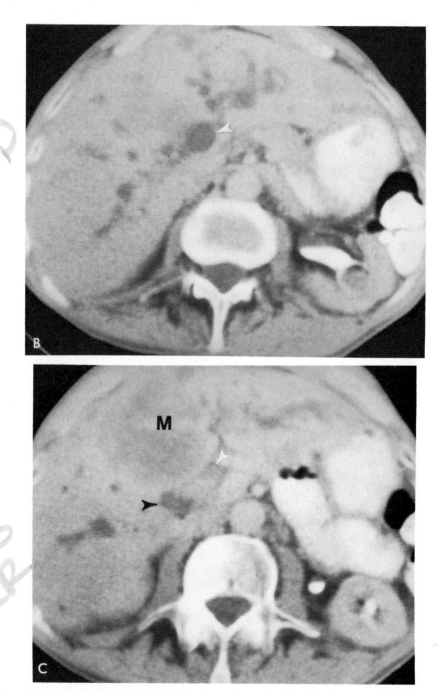

Figure 7–8. *Continued   B,* Common hepatic duct (arrow) exceeds 1.5 cm in diameter. *C,* at a slightly lower level the bile duct (area marked by white arrow) is no longer visible, abruptly obliterated 2 cm below the junction. No mass is evident. The neck of the gallbladder (black arrow) is seen at this level, as is a large metastatic lesion (M) in the medial segment of the left lobe.

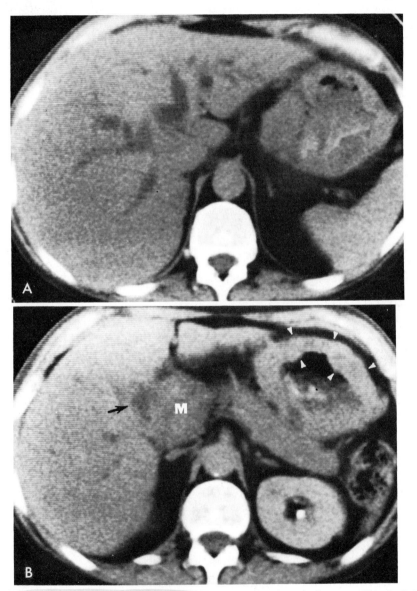

Figure 7–9. Common hepatic duct obstruction by lymphoma. *A*, Intrahepatic ducts are dilated. *B*, There is a mass (M) in the porta hepatis, which obstructs the common hepatic duct. Arrow indicates the gallbladder neck. Note thickened gastric wall (arrowheads), indicating gastric lymphoma.

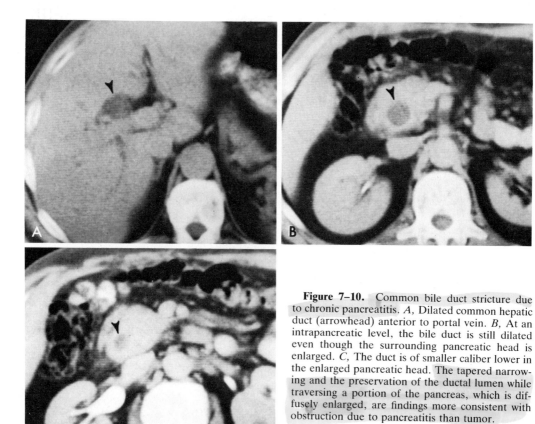

Figure 7–10. Common bile duct stricture due to chronic pancreatitis. *A*, Dilated common hepatic duct (arrowhead) anterior to portal vein. *B*, At an intrapancreatic level, the bile duct is still dilated even though the surrounding pancreatic head is enlarged. *C*, The duct is of smaller caliber lower in the enlarged pancreatic head. The tapered narrowing and the preservation of the ductal lumen while traversing a portion of the pancreas, which is diffusely enlarged, are findings more consistent with obstruction due to pancreatitis than tumor.

Figure 7–11. Obstruction of distal common bile duct by calculi. At the level of the pancreatic head the duct is dilated and stones (arrowheads) are layered along its dependent wall. The tiny lucent structure just anterior to bile duct is the normal pancreatic duct. There is a left renal cyst (C).

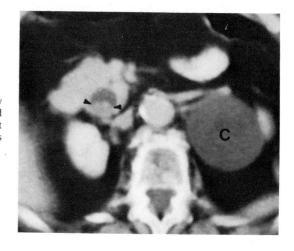

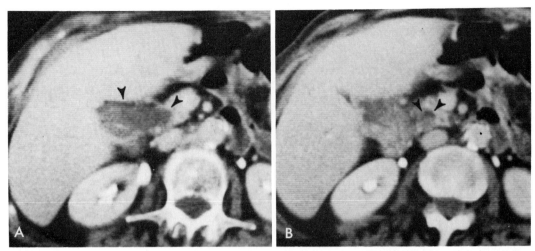

Figure 7–12. Common bile duct obstruction by calculi. *A,* Dilated, transversely oriented portion of common duct (arrowheads) passes from the porta hepatis toward the pancreatic head. *B,* Stone in dilated duct. The crescentic lucency (arrowheads) represents bile outlining the intraluminal stone. This crescentic configuration of the bile is a common CT finding when ductal calculi are partially obstructing the lumen.

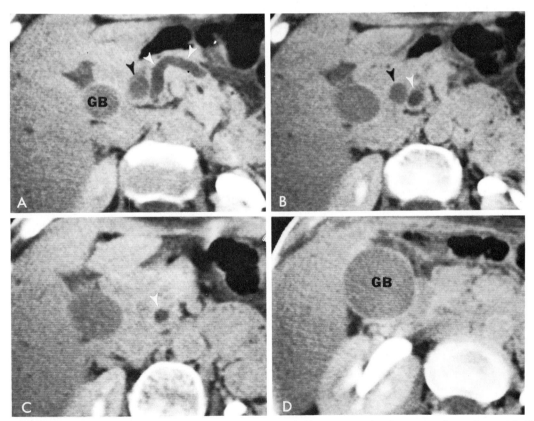

Figure 7–13. Scans at four descending levels in a patient with ductal obstruction by pancreatic carcinoma. *A,* Both the bile duct (black arrowhead), seen in cross section, and the pancreatic duct (white arrowheads), seen longitudinally, are dilated above the tumor. *B,* Both dilated ducts now seen in cross section. *C,* At the level of the tumor, the bile duct is obliterated, whereas the pancreatic duct is still patent. *D,* Still lower, both ducts are obliterated. Note the loss of the retropancreatic fat planes, owing to tumor infiltration, and the distended gallbladder (GB).

seen in cases of obstruction due to stone as well as tumor (Fig. 7–12) and can occur normally.[21]

It is important to note the shape of the bile duct as it passes through the transition from dilated to nondilated. Obstruction by tumor is usually accompanied by an abrupt transition over a distance of 1 or 2 cm (Fig. 7–13), and the shape of the ductal lumen at this level may be distorted or irregular. Ductal stricture due to chronic pancreatitis typically causes a longer, tapered transitional segment, with consecutive slices showing a circular duct of smaller and smaller caliber (Fig. 7–10).

One should search carefully for findings indicating the presence of a mass. Enlargement of the head of the pancreas, of course, suggests a tumor arising in that area. In patients with pancreatic carcinoma there may also be obliteration of the fat planes surrounding the pancreas, particularly posteriorly (Fig. 7–13). Cholangiocarcinoma or metastatic tumor in the suprapancreatic region tends to obliterate the visible margins of the undersurface of the liver, the portal vein, and the superior portion of the pancreatic head. There may also be other findings in the abdomen to suggest the presence of tumor such as masses in other abdominal organs or metastatic deposits in the liver (Fig. 7–8). Biliary obstruction with lymphoma is usually due to ductal compression by a mass of enlarged periportal lymph nodes. Often there is also splenomegaly and enlargement of retroperitoneal or mesenteric nodes.

Obviously, one should look carefully for stones in the bile duct. With the superior contrast resolution afforded by CT, biliary calculi are visibly calcified in most patients.[22] They appear as single or multiple filling defects in the dependent portion of the duct (Figs. 7–11 and 7–12), which have a density usually exceeding that of the surrounding bile. In searching for an impacted stone in the ampulla, it is useful to obtain scans before oral contrast material is given so as not to obscure a small calcification with contrast material in the adjacent duodenum or within a duodenal diverticulum projecting into the substance of the pancreatic head (Fig. 7–14).

The pancreas should be examined for evidence of pancreatic duct dilatation as a sign that the cause of the obstruction lies at that level. CT findings may also suggest chronic pancreatitis as evidenced by pancreatic calcifications, pseudocyst, or focal or diffuse pancreatic enlargement or atrophy. It is also im-

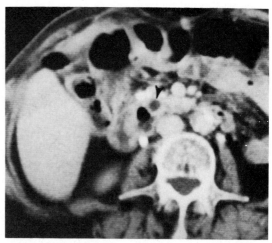

Figure 7–14. Duodenal diverticulum. In this patient with a calculus impacted in the ampulla of Vater (1.5 cm inferior to the plane of this scan), the mildly dilated common bile duct (arrowhead) is seen in close proximity to a gas-containing duodenal diverticulum, which lies partially within the substance of the pancreas. If the diverticulum were to be filled with dense oral contrast material, confusion could arise in the diagnosis of a distal common bile duct stone.

portant to examine the gallbladder for signs of cholecystitis, calculi, or tumor.

Assuming equipment with scan time of five seconds or less and considering CT findings in conjunction with the clinical history, one can expect to be able to correctly predict the etiology of biliary obstruction, including histologic tumor type when the obstruction is neoplastic, in about 70 per cent of patients.[12] In most of the remaining cases of obstruction due to neoplasm, CT findings accurately indicate the presence of a tumor but are not sufficiently specific to predict its histologic type.

NONOBSTRUCTIVE JAUNDICE

In evaluating the jaundiced patient, when the CT findings do not indicate ductal obstruction it is important to search for abnormalities that may indicate the presence of diffuse or focal disease of the liver parenchyma. Scans through the liver should be examined carefully with a narrow window width for signs of focal areas of low density, which might indicate liver abscess or neoplasm. Liver abscesses have a density lower than that of the surrounding parenchyma but higher than that of water or bile, ordinarily falling in the 20- to 40-HU range. When contrast material is injected intravenously, enhancement of the rim of the abscess is sometimes detectable, but there is no change in the CT attenuation number of the central portion. Most primary and secondary liver tumors are also of lower density than the liver parenchyma. When the clinical suspicion of tumor is high and abnormalities are not visible on precontrast scans, it may be useful to obtain additional scans through the liver at rapid intervals following the bolus injection of intravenous contrast material.

CT will often reveal liver abnormalities in patients with diffuse parenchymal disease of the liver. The size of the liver and spleen can be readily determined and can be quantitated if necessary.[22, 24] Fatty infiltration of the liver causes a decrease in the attenuation value of the parenchyma such that the density of the liver becomes less than that of the spleen (Fig. 7–4).[25-27] When fatty replacement of the liver is severe, there is a reversal of the normal contrast relationship between the liver parenchyma and the portal and hepatic venous branches within it such that the vessels stand out as branching structures of a density higher than that of the surrounding liver. Occasional patients with biochemical abnormalities indicating hepatic dysfunction are found to have a liver with a CT attenuation value that is abnormally high. This usually indicates the presence of hemochromatosis in which hepatic iron deposition significantly alters density of the liver on CT (Fig. 7–3).[28]

Cirrhosis is often suggested by morphologic changes in the liver. Characteristically, there is an alteration in the relative size of the various hepatic lobes and segments (Fig. 7–15). The right lobe diminishes in size, whereas the left lobe becomes larger than normal. Enlargement of the caudate lobe is particularly common. Measurement of the ratio of the width of the caudate lobe to that of the right lobe has been suggested as a diagnostic tool.[29] To perform such a measurement, vertical (parasagittal) lines are drawn tangential to the medial tip of the caudate lobe and the lateral aspect of the portal vein. The ratio of the width of the caudate lobe, expressed as the distance between these two lines, and the width of the right lobe, expressed as the distance from the lateral aspect of the portal vein to the lateral aspect of the right hepatic lobe, averages 0.37 in patients with a normal liver. When this C/RL ratio exceeds 0.65, cirrhosis can be diagnosed with 96 per cent confidence. An infrequent cause of a falsely predictive high ratio is a neoplasm in the caudate lobe. In such a case, the associated morphologic changes of cirrhosis, such as atrophy of the right lobe, would be absent.

Portal hypertension produces abnormalities on CT in many patients.[30] Splenomegaly is usually present and is easily detected. Dilatation of the splenic and portal veins can also be seen, as can varices in the splenic hilus, gastrohepatic ligament, and paraesophageal region. A dilated umbilical vein may also be evident in the falciform ligament.

GALLBLADDER DISEASE

It is unlikely that CT will become the primary radiologic method for evaluating patients suspected of having gallbladder disease. Oral cholecystography, ultrasonography, and, more recently, radionuclide studies accomplish this task satisfactorily at present. Nonetheless, CT sometimes reveals previously unsuspected abnormalities of the gallbladder during studies performed for other reasons, and it is sometimes useful for evaluating patients with known or suspected gallbladder disease in whom the results of other imaging tests are confusing. CT also plays a role when there is a discrepancy between clinical and radiologic findings.

The great majority of gallstones can be seen by CT[31-33] including many calculi not visible by conventional radiographic plain film technique (Fig. 7–16). Calcium bilirubinate stones, and most mixed stones contain sufficient calcium to be visible as densities surrounded by more lucent bile. Pure cholesterol stones are more difficult to see with CT but can sometimes be recognized as filling defects that are lower in attenuation value than the surrounding bile. In a recent prospective series[12] that included 23 patients proved to have calculi within the gallbladder, gallstones were detected by CT in 19 patients, by ultrasound in 19, and by the combined studies in all 23.

Uniform thickening of the gallbladder wall has been described as a sonographic abnormality in patients with acute or chronic cholecystitis,[34-36] and a similar finding can be detected by CT (Fig. 7–17).[31] The thickness of the gallbladder can usually be estimated fairly accurately from CT because of the density difference between the tissue of the wall itself and the lower density bile within the lumen. It should be kept in mind, however, that diffuse gallbladder wall thickening can also

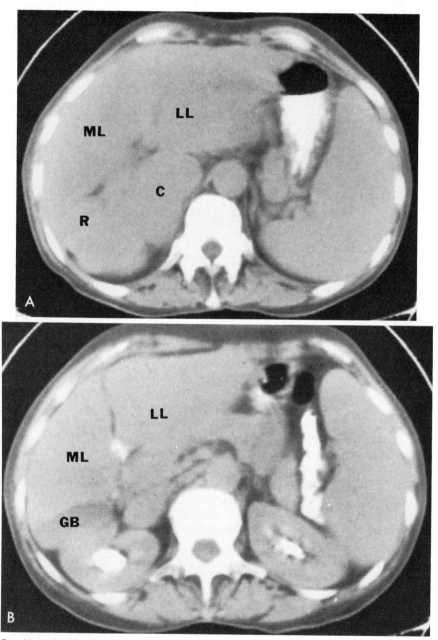

Figure 7–15. Alteration in the relative size of the hepatic lobes and segments in a patient with micronodular cirrhosis. *A*, Caudate lobe (C) and medial and lateral segments of left lobe (ML, LL) are enlarged, whereas right lobe (R) is quite small. *B*, Note the unusual position of the gallbladder (GB) resulting from these changes in liver morphology. The spleen is enlarged.

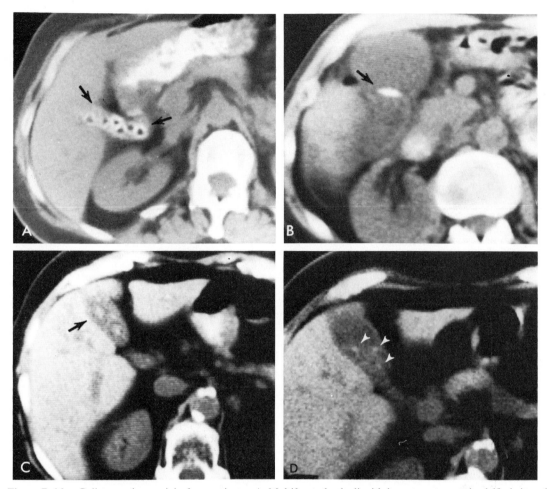

Figure 7–16. Gallstones (arrows) in four patients. *A*, Multifaceted calculi with lucent centers and calcified rims. *B*, Tiny, radiodense, calcium bilirubinate stones lying in the dependent portion of the gallbladder. *C*, Stones of various sizes, each of which has a calcified central nidus and lucent outer layer. *D*, Several stones, which are nearly isodense with the surrounding bile. Without the faint calcification in some areas of the stones, they might escape detection by CT.

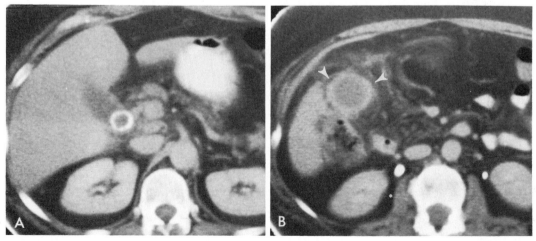

Figure 7–17. Cholelithiasis with cholecystitis. *A*, Calculus in the neck of the gallbladder. *B*, The gallbladder wall (arrows) is uniformly thickened. Also note the increased density of the pericholecystic fat, reflecting the inflammatory process.

develop in the absence of cholecystitis in patients with significant hypoalbuminemia.[37] Chronic cholecystitis may be accompanied by calcification of the gallbladder wall. The risk of gallbladder carcinoma is increased in patients with chronic calcific cholecystitis, and a careful search should be made for signs of tumor when the gallbladder wall is calcified. Gas can be detected in the gallbladder wall or lumen in patients with emphysematous cholecystitis. This severe form of acute cholecystitis is due to cystic duct obstruction and infection with gas-forming clostridial or coliform organisms and usually occurs in elderly diabetic individuals.

Pericholecystic inflammatory disease occasionally occurs as a result of spread of infection through an inflamed or necrotic gallbladder wall to the adjacent tissues. CT findings of pericholecystic inflammatory disease include a mass adjacent to the gallbladder. If the mass is phlegmonous in nature, it is of soft tissue density and strands of inflammatory reaction may reach from it toward adjacent organs or the abdominal wall (Fig. 7–18). When a frank abscess is present, a low density, fluid-containing region is usually visible within the inflammatory mass and is ordinarily in direct contact with the gallbladder.

CT has been used in the evaluation of the gallbladder that does not opacify after administration of oral cholecystographic contrast material. In one such study[38] of ten patients, eight were shown to have cholelithiasis, four had

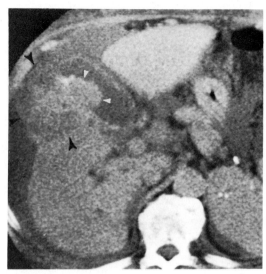

Figure 7–19. Carcinoma of the gallbladder. Polypoid mass projects into gallbladder lumen (white arrowheads) and extends into adjacent right hepatic lobe (black arrowheads). A few small calcified gallstones, seen at this level and at lower levels, were confirmed at operation. Ascites is also present.

gallbladder wall thickening, two had opacification of the common duct but not of the gallbladder, indicating cystic duct obstruction, and one patient was shown to have obstruction of the distal common bile duct. Experience in this area is limited, and ultrasonography will remain more applicable for this sort of problem in the foreseeable future.

CT is very useful in the diagnosis and staging of carcinoma of the gallbladder (Fig. 7–19). In one study of 27 patients with gallbladder carcinoma,[39] all had abnormal CT findings and the correct diagnosis was made prospectively in 20 (74 per cent) of the 27. Common CT abnormalities in this disease include, in decreasing order of frequency, a focal low density area in the liver adjacent to the gallbladder, mass in the region of the gallbladder, gallstones, biliary tract obstruction (usually at the level of the junction of the right and left hepatic ducts), gallbladder wall thickening, intraluminal mass in the gallbladder, liver metastases, and enlarged regional lymph nodes.[40, 41] Gallbladder wall thickening due to carcinoma is usually focal or discontinuous, but occasional cases exhibit uniform thickening, which can mimic the appearance of cholecystitis. CT abnormalities can be particularly difficult to interpret in patients who have both gallbladder wall thickening due to cholecystitis and metastatic liver disease from some other source.

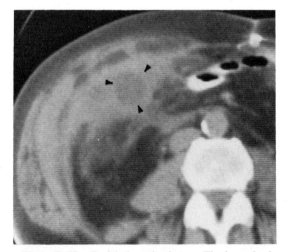

Figure 7–18. Pericholecystic abscess. The irregular inflammatory mass surrounds the gallbladder (arrowheads) and obliterates the normal fat between the gallbladder and the anterior abdominal wall.

CYSTIC DISEASE

Choledochal Cyst

Although experience with the CT evaluation of congenital or developmental anomalies of the biliary tree is limited, the clarity with which rapid, rotary CT scanners can image the normal and abnormal bile ducts indicates that the potential for noninvasive imaging of this type of disease is strong. Choledochal cysts of the Alonso-Lej type I have been clearly defined with CT.[42, 43] In this entity both intra- and extrahepatic cystic dilatation can be present. Intrahepatic dilatation is limited to the central portion of the left and right main hepatic ducts. This is in contrast to the picture of acquired obstruction, in which there is generalized dilatation of the intrahepatic bile ducts with gradually decreasing caliber in the periphery (Fig. 7–20).

When the dilatation is only extrahepatic, the diameter of the dilated segment is usually out of proportion to the remainder of the biliary tree and the transition point from dilated to normal is usually abrupt. Jaundice may be present in uncomplicated choledochal cysts without accompanying dilatation of the intrahepatic ducts. If a known or suspected choledochal cyst appears to have a superimposed pattern of generalized obstructive dilatation of the intrahepatic ducts, a secondary complication such a choledochocarcinoma should be suspected, especially in view of the association of malignancy with this anomaly.

In some patients one cannot be certain that the cyst communicates with the biliary tree. The intravenous use of meglumine iodipamide (Cholografin, Squibb) may help to resolve this question by showing enhancement of the bile within the cyst on CT scans obtained 30 to 60 minutes after infusion.

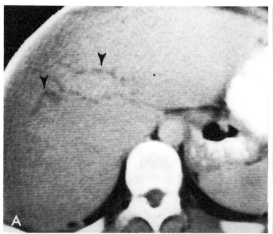

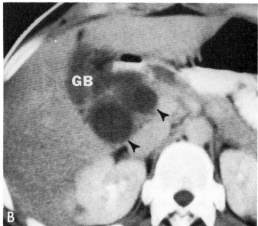

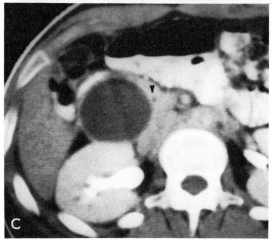

Figure 7–20. Choledochal cyst. *A,* Intrahepatic ducts (arrows) are only minimally dilated. *B,* At the level of the junction, the right and left main hepatic ducts (arrows) are grossly dilated. The neck of the gallbladder (BG) is displaced anteriorly and to the right. *C,* Cystic dilatation of the common bile duct. Note pancreatic duct (arrowhead) of normal caliber.

Caroli's Disease

Congenital cystic dilatation of the intrahepatic bile ducts, Caroli's disease,[44] is a rare condition thought to be inherited as an autosomal recessive trait. Caroli classified the disease into two forms: (1) a pure form, unassociated with cirrhosis and portal hypertension and having a high incidence of cholangitis and calculus formation; and (2) a form associated with congenital hepatic fibrosis in which the predominant clinical features are those of portal hypertension. In the latter type, complications of bile stasis may be latent or may occur late in the course of the illness.

CT findings in Caroli's disease have been reported in only a few patients,[45, 46] and one such patient was studied in our department during an episode of acute cholangitis. CT demonstrated multiple low-density branching tubular structures, characteristic of dilated bile ducts communicating with focally ectatic areas (Fig. 7–21). As with choledochal cysts, intravenous meglumine iodipamide may be of use in confirming communication of the cystic spaces with the biliary tree.

CONCLUSION

Experience to date would suggest that CT and ultrasonography have comparable sensitivity in detecting the presence of biliary obstruction but that CT appears to be somewhat more accurate in defining the level and underlying etiology. Because of its nonionizing nature and lower cost, it would seem reasonable to employ ultrasonography as the screening procedure for evaluating patients suspected of having obstructive biliary tract disease. When the intra- and extrahepatic ducts are well seen sonographically and are normal in caliber, no further radiologic evaluation is needed in most patients. CT plays a major role in those patients in whom (1) sonographic abnormalities indicate ductal dilatation but do not clearly establish the level and etiology of the obstruction, (2) sonographic findings are equivocal, or (3) there is strong clinical suspicion of biliary obstruction despite normal findings on sonography. In patients who are obese and in those with prior biliary-enteric bypass procedures, one can anticipate the likelihood of an unsatisfactory sonographic examination, and these patients are better suited for CT as the first procedure. We currently reserve percutaneous transhepatic or endoscopic retrograde cholangiography for patients in whom both examinations fail or are equivocal or for patients in whom a fluoroscopically guided biliary drainage procedure is planned. In selected patients with ductal obstruction high in the porta hepatis, we also employ percutaneous transhepatic cholangiography to help the surgeon decide whether or not to attempt a surgical biliary-enteric bypass procedure.

In evaluating gallbladder disease, CT has its major role in the detection and staging of carcinoma of the gallbladder, and it is probably the best test for evaluating patients with this often difficult diagnostic problem. There are also major advantages to using CT to assess

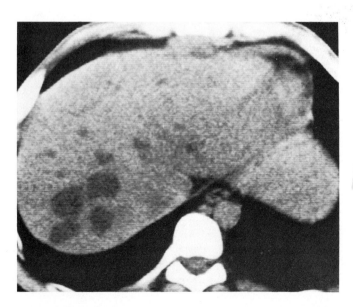

Figure 7–21. Round, low density defects in the posterior portion of the right hepatic lobe in a patient with Caroli's disease. Percutaneous cholangiography confirmed that these were focally ectatic bile ducts. Repeat CT scanning after intravenous cholangiographic contrast material would have had similar diagnostic value.

the extent of pericholecystic inflammatory disease. CT plays an ancillary role in the study of cholecystitis and calculous gallbladder disease, but one should be familiar with the appearances of these conditions since they are commonly encountered in patients studied for other reasons.

References

1. Araki, T., Itai, Y., Furui, S., and Tasaka, A.: Dynamic CT densitometry of hepatic tumors. A. J. R. *135*:1037, 1980.
2. Burgener, F. A., and Hamlin, D. J.: Contrast enhancement in abdominal CT: Bolus vs infusion. A. J. R. *137*:351, 1981.
3. Itai, Y., Furui, S., Araki, T., Yashiro, N., and Tasaka, A.: Computed tomography of cavernous hemangioma of the liver. Radiology *137*:149, 1980.
4. Johnson, C. M., Sheedy, P. F., Stanson, A. W., Stephens, D. H., Hattery, R. R., and Adson, M. A.: Computed tomography and angiography of cavernous hemangiomas of the liver. Radiology *138*:115, 1981.
5. Marchal, G. J., Baert, A. L., and Wilms, G. E.: CT of noncystic liver lesions: bolus enhancement. A. J. R. *135*:57, 1980.
6. Vermess, M., Doppman, J. L., Sugarbaker, P., Fisher, R. I., Catterji, D. C., Luetzeler, J., Grimes, G., Girton, M., and Adamson, R. H.: Clinical trials with a new intravenous liposoluble contrast material for computed tomography of the liver and spleen. Radiology *137*:217, 1980.
7. Vermess, M., Bernardino, M. E., Doppman, J. L., Fisher, R. I., Thomas, J. L., Velasquez, W. S., Fuller, L. M., and Russo, A.: Use of intravenous liposoluble contrast material for the examination of the liver and spleen in lymphoma. J. Comput. Assist. Tomogr. *5*:709, 1981.
8. Michels, N. A.: Newer anatomy of the liver and its variant blood supply and collateral circulation. Am. J. Surg. *112*:337, 1966.
9. Kuhns, L. R., and Borlaza, G.: Normal roentgen variant. Aberrant right hepatic artery on computed tomography. Radiology *135*:392, 1980.
10. Noon, M. A., and Young, S. W.: Aberrant right hepatic artery: A normal variant demonstrated by computed tomography. J. Comput. Assist. Tomogr. *5*:411, 1981.
11. Grant, J. C. B.: An Atlas of Anatomy, 5th ed. Baltimore: Williams & Wilkins Co., 1952, p. 144.
12. Baron, R. L., Stanley, R. J., Lee, J. K. T., Koehler, R. E., Melson, G. L., Balfe, D. M., and Weyman, P. J.: Prospective comparison of the evaluation of biliary obstruction with computed tomography and ultrasound. Radiology. (in press).
13. Graham, M. F., Cooperberg, P. L., Cohen, M. M., and Burhenne, H. J.: Ultrasonographic screening of the common hepatic duct in symptomatic patients after cholecystectomy. Radiology *138*:137, 1981.
14. Huabek, A., Pedersen, J. H., Burcharth, F., Gammelgaard, J., Hancke, S., and Willumsen, L.: Dynamic sonography in the evaluation of jaundice. A. J. R. *136*:1071, 1981.
15. Mueller, P. R., Ferrucci, J. T., Simeone, J. F., Wittenberg, J., vanSonnenberg, E., Polansky, A., and Isler, R. J.: Postcholecystectomy bile duct dilatation: myth or reality? A. J. R. *136*:355, 1981.
16. Sauerbrei, E. E., Cooperberg, P. L., Gordon, P., Li, D., Cohen, M. M., and Burhenne, H. J.: The discrepancy between radiographic and sonographic bile-duct measurements. Radiology *137*:751, 1980.
17. Zeman, R. K., Dorfman, G. S., Burrell, M. I., Stein, S., Berg, G. R., and Gold, J. A.: Disparate dilatation of the intrahepatic and extrahepatic bile ducts in surgical jaundice. Radiology *138*:129, 1981.
18. Thomas, J. L., and Bernardino, M. E.: Segmental biliary obstruction: its detection and significance. J. Comput. Assist. Tomogr. *4*:155, 1980.
19. Pedrosa, C. S., Casanova, R., and Rodriguez, R.: Computed tomography in obstructive jaundice: The level of obstruction. Radiology *139*:627, 1981.
20. Pedrosa, C. S., Casanova, R., Lezana, A. H., and Fernandez, M. C.: Computed tomography in obstructive jaundice: The cause of obstruction. Radiology *139*:635, 1981.
21. Jacobson, J. B., and Brodey, P. A.: The transverse common duct. A. J. R. *136*:91, 1981.
22. Itai, Y., Araki, T., Furui, S., Tasaka, A., Atomi, Y., and Kuroda, A.: Computed tomography and ultrasound in the diagnosis of intrahepatic calculi. Radiology *136*:399, 1980.
23. Henderson, J. M., Heymsfield, S. B., Horowitz, J., and Kutner, M. H.: Measurement of liver and spleen volume by computed tomography. Radiology *141*:525, 1981.
24. Moss, A. A., Friedman, M. A., and Brito, A. C.: Determination of liver, kidney, and spleen volumes by computed tomography: An experimental study in dogs. J. Comput. Assist. Tomogr. *5*:12, 1981.
25. Piekarski, J., Goldberg, H. I., Royal, S. A., Axel, L., and Moss, A. A.: Difference between liver and spleen CT numbers in the normal adult: Its usefulness in predicting the presence of diffuse liver disease. Radiology *137*:727, 1980.
26. Mulhern, C. B., Arger, P. H., Coleman, B. G., and Stein, G. N.: Nonuniform attenuation in computed tomography study of the cirrhotic liver. Radiology *132*:399, 1979.
27. Nishikawa, J., Itai, Y., and Tasaka, A.: Lobar attenuation difference of the liver on computed tomography. Radiology *141*:725, 1981.
28. Long, R. J., Doppman, J. L., Nienhus, A. W., and Mills, S. R.: Computed tomographic analysis of beta-thalassemic syndromes with hemochromatosis: pathologic findings with clinical and laboratory correlations. J. Comput. Assist. Tomogr. *4*:159, 1980.
29. Harbin, W. P., Robert, N. J., and Ferrucci, J. T.: Diagnosis of cirrhosis based on regional changes in hepatic morphology. Radiology *135*:273, 1980.
30. Clark, K. E., Foley, W. D., Lawson, T. L., Berland, L. L., and Maddison, F. E.: CT evaluation of esophageal and upper abdominal varices. J. Comput. Assist. Tomogr. *4*:510, 1980.
31. Havrilla, T. R., Reich, N. E., Haaga, J. R., Seidelmann, F. E., Cooperman, A. M., and Alfidi, R. J.: Computed tomography of the gallbladder. A. J. R. *130*:1059, 1978.
32. Moss, A. A., Filly, R. A., and Way, L. W.: In vitro investigation of gallstones with computed tomography. J. Comput. Assist. Tomogr. *4*:827, 1980.
33. Stanley, R. J., and Sagel, S. S.: Computed tomography of the liver and biliary tract. *In* Berk, R. N., and Clemett, A. R. (eds.): Radiology of the Gallbladder and Bile Ducts. Philadelphia; W. B. Saunders Co., 1977, pp. 370–373.
34. Engel, J. M., Deitch, E. A., and Sikkema, W.: Gallbladder wall thickness: sonographic accuracy and relation to disease. A. J. R. *134*:907, 1980.

35. Finberg, H. J., and Birnholz, J. C.: Ultrasound evaluation of the gallbladder wall. Radiology *133*:693, 1979.

36. Handler, S. J.: Ultrasound of gallbladder wall thickening and its relation to cholecystitis. A. J. R. *123*:581, 1979.

37. Ralls, P. W., Quinn, M. F., Juttner, H. U., Halls, J. M., and Boswell, W. D.: Gallbladder wall thickening: patients without intrinsic gallbladder disease. A. J. R. *137*:65, 1981.

38. Toombs, B. D., Sandler, C. M., and Conoley, P. M.: Computed tomography of the nonvisualizing gallbladder. J. Comput. Assist. Tomogr. *5*:164, 1981.

39. Itai, Y., Araki, T., Yoshikawa, K., Furui, S., Yashiro, N., and Tasaka, A.: Computed tomography of gallbladder carcinoma. Radiology *137*:713, 1980.

40. Ruiz, R., Teyssou, H., Fernandez, N., Carrez, J. P., Gortchakoff, M., Manteau, G., Ter-Davtian, P. M., and Tessier, J. P.: Ultrasonic diagnosis of primary carcinoma of the gallbladder: A review of 16 cases. J. Clin. Ultrasound *8*:489, 1980.

41. Yeh, H. C.: Ultrasonography and computed tomography of carcinoma of the gallbladder. Radiology *133*:167, 1979.

42. Araki, T., Itai, Y., and Tasaka, A.: CT of choledochal cyst. A. J. R. *135*:729, 1980.

43. Nakata, H., Nobe, T., Takahasi, M., Maeda, T., and Koga, M.: Choledochal cyst. J. Comput. Assist. Tomogr. *5*:99, 1981.

44. Caroli, J., Soupault, R., Kossakowski, J., et al.: La dilatation polykystique congenitale des voies biliaires intra-hepatiques: essai de classification. Sem. Hôp. Paris *34*:128, 1958.

45. Araki, T., Itai, Y., and Tasaka, A.: Computed tomography of localized dilatation of the intrahepatic bile ducts. Radiology *141*:733, 1981.

46. Kaiser, J. A., Mall, J. C., Salmen, B. J., and Parker, J. J.: Diagnosis of Caroli disease by computed tomography: report of two cases. Radiology *132*:661, 1979.

CHOLESCINTIGRAPHY

by Heidi S. Weissmann, M.D.

8

In the recent past, there was no need for a textbook dealing with radiology of the gallbladder and bile ducts to reserve an entire chapter for cholescintigraphy. However, during the time that great strides were being made in other imaging procedures for the radiologic evaluation of the biliary system, dramatic advances were also being made in the development of hepatobiliary radiopharmaceuticals, with a transition from iodine-131 rose bengal (I-131 RB) to technetium-99m iminodiacetic acid (Tc-99m IDA).[1-7] The diagnostic impact that Tc-99m IDA cholescintigraphy has had on hepatobiliary diagnosis is indicated by the fact that over 2000 Tc-99m IDA examinations were requested and performed in the first four years that this procedure was available at Montefiore Hospital and Medical Center. This provides fitting testimony to the clinical utility of and necessity for cholescintigraphy. The majority of studies have been performed for suspected acute cholecystitis. The second most common indication has been the postoperative evaluation of the patient following such procedures as cholecystectomy, biliary-enteric anastomosis, and Billroth I and II and Whipple resections. Other indications include suspected biliary leakage, chronic cholecystitis, cholestasis, and the further elucidation of defects identified on the Tc-99m sulfur colloid liver scan.

I-131 ROSE BENGAL IMAGING: ITS BEGINNING AND END

For nearly two decades, I-131 RB remained the only radiotracer, selectively taken up and excreted by the hepatocytes,[8] to be commercially available on a widespread basis. Its primary clinical niche became evaluation of the jaundiced patient.[9-11] However, I-131 RB imaging was fraught with technical problems, which eventually contributed to its decline as a clinically useful modality. As advances in the technology of other nonnuclear imaging procedures were occurring, rose bengal hepatobiliary imaging was becoming obsolete.

Although the rate of liver uptake and excretion of rose bengal is acceptable, the clinical application remained severely limited by the iodine-131 label (I-131). It has a high photon energy peak of 364 keV, which is suboptimal for Anger camera imaging. It has a long physical half-life of 8.1 days and significant particulate (beta) emission, which increases patient exposure and limits acceptable doses at the microcurie (μCi) range. Considering these physical factors, optimal visualization of the biliary system never could be achievable with the Anger camera. The development of I-123 RB represented a significant improvement. Iodine-123 has a lower gamma photon energy peak of 159 keV and a shorter physical half-life of 13.3 hours and is a pure gamma emitter.[12] However, since it is cyclotron produced, its relatively short half-life meant that an institution had to be near a cyclotron facility. This significantly limited its clinical availability.

Technetium-99m (Tc-99m), on the other hand, has an ideal physical half-life of six hours and is a pure gamma emitter. This enables the administration of multi-millicurie (mCi), instead of microcurie, doses, which results in a commensurate increase in the number of photon-emitting events capable of being detected by the Anger camera. It also has an ideal photon energy peak of 140 keV. These factors result in a significant improvement in the quality of the nuclear image. Additionally, Tc-99m is obtained from a molybdenum-99 generator that can be stored and "milked" on site in any nuclear medicine facility. Thus, it is the most ideal radionuclide currently available. The successful labeling of Tc-99m with a molecule

I wish to express my sincere appreciation and gratitude to Mrs. Edith Costabile for her diligence and assistance "above and beyond the call of duty" in the preparation of this manuscript.

such as iminodiacetic acid (IDA) represents a major breakthrough for hepatobiliary scintigraphy. IDA is readily taken up by the hepatocytes and excreted into the bile, and it can be distributed commercially in kit form.

COMPARISON OF THE AVAILABLE Tc-99m IDA DERIVATIVES

Dimethyliminodiacetic acid (HIDA), a structural analog of lidocaine, was the first IDA derivative successfully labeled with Tc-99m.[13-17] Since the development of Tc-99m HIDA in 1975, numerous other IDA molecules have been produced by commercial companies including DEIDA (diethyliminodiacetic acid, Amersham Labs, Arlington Heights, IL), PIPIDA (paraisopropyl iminodiacetic acid, Medi-Physics Corp., Emeryville, CA), BIDA (parabutyl iminodiacetic acid), and DISIDA (diisopropyl iminodiacetic acid, both from New England Nuclear Corp., North Billerica, MA) (Fig. 8–1).

Tc-99m HIDA (initially made available by Merck Frosst Laboratories, Dorval, Quebec) consistently yields excellent biliary visualization when the bilirubin level is normal or slightly elevated. In situations in which it is the only available IDA analog, acceptable visualization may be achievable when the bilirubin level is as high as 5 to 8 mg/100 ml. The limitation of Tc-99m HIDA is that it has an

alternate excretory pathway of significant magnitude. Of all the IDA molecules, it has the greatest degree of kidney excretion (about 15 per cent in the normal individual). As hepatocyte function becomes more and more compromised, usually reflected by progressive hyperbilirubinemia, an even greater portion is eliminated from the body via the renal route with proportionately less by the hepatobiliary system. Enhanced hepatobiliary excretion with concomitant diminution in the renal excretory component has been achieved by increasing the length and complexity of the alkyl chain of the benzene ring. Thus, the longer-chain molecules are capable of biliary visualization in cases of more extreme hyperbilirubinemia.

Tc-99m PIPIDA, although relatively similar to HIDA in function, has the advantage of affording a better chance of visualizing the biliary tract when the bilirubin level reaches the low teens.[18,19] Its major disadvantage is that the degree of visualization of the common duct is poorer than that obtainable with the other IDA analogs, even in anicteric patients. This qualitative difference probably does not alter the diagnostic accuracy of the procedure, particularly in cases of suspected acute cholecystitis.

Although Tc-99m BIDA has the advantage of affording less renal excretion, its usefulness is hampered by its significantly slower rate of hepatic uptake and excretion. In the early days of Tc-99m IDA cholescintigraphy, it held

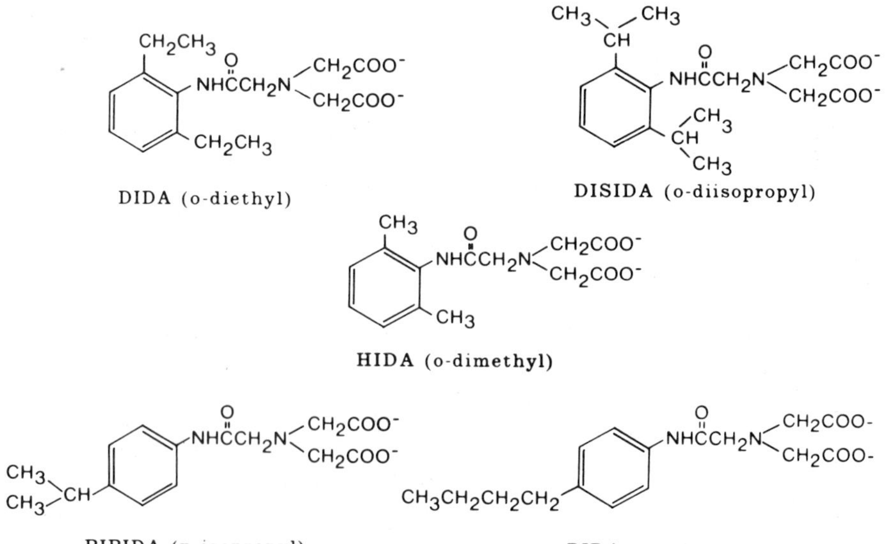

Figure 8–1. Chemical structures of the Tc-99m IDA derivatives that have been utilized for clinical evaluation. (Reprinted with permission from Loberg, Nunn, and Porter. *In* Nuclear Medicine Annual 1981. New York: Raven Press, 1981.)

promise for the evaluation of patients with bilirubin levels greater than 10 mg/100 ml and occasionally 20 mg/100 ml.[20] However, with the development of a newer derivative, Tc-99m DISIDA, there is no longer any reason to have to deal with the problems created by the slower, poorer hepatobiliary kinetics of Tc-99m BIDA. The blood clearance of Tc-99m BIDA is slower, especially when the bilirubin level exceeds 5 mg/100 ml. Additionally, the hepatic uptake is lower and the rate of washout is slower at all levels of hyperbilirubinemia. In a cross-over study comparing these two radio-tracers, in the first hour Tc-99m BIDA failed to visualize the gallbladder in three cases and dilated ducts in two, whereas Tc-99m DISIDA succeeded.[20] Conceivably, these structures might have been visualized with Tc-99m BIDA if more delayed scintiphotos had been obtained.

Of all the IDA agents currently available, Tc-99m DISIDA appears to be the best overall analog.[20-24] In the lower bilirubin range, it equals (and possibly even excels) the degree of common duct visualization obtained when compared with Tc-99m HIDA. Additionally, it is far superior to the other IDA derivatives when the bilirubin range is between 15 and 30 mg/100 ml.[20, 21, 23]

The newest available derivative, Tc-99m DEIDA, comes closest quantitatively to Tc-99m DISIDA. Comparison of these two analogs reveals the only significant difference to be a higher hepatic uptake relative to background for Tc-99m DISIDA. No significant difference in the degree of blood retention or rate of liver washout has been identified.[23] For the most part, DISIDA and DEIDA appear to be comparable in actual clinical practice. However, Tc-99m DISIDA has occasionally proved more effective in obtaining biliary visualization when marked hyperbilirubinemia is present.[23, 24]

Thus, all of the IDA analogs appear to have diagnostic merit in the evaluation of suspected acute cholecystitis, whereas Tc-99m DISIDA has a distinct advantage in cases of marked hyperbilirubinemia, followed closely by Tc-99m DEIDA.

TECHNIQUE

Patient Preparation

It is preferable to have the patient fast for four to six hours prior to the intravenous injection of 1 to 5 mCi of Tc-99m IDA. This eliminates the possibility of interference with normal gallbladder filling by physiologic post-prandial gallbladder contraction. It has been shown in two patient series[25, 26] that the endogenous release of cholecystokinin, in response to the presence of food in the proximal small intestine, can result in failure to visualize a normal gallbladder. In the earlier study, utilizing Tc-99m pyridoxylidene-glutamate, gallbladder visualization in normal volunteers was reduced from 100 per cent in the fasting group to 47 per cent in the nonfasting group,[25] and evaluation of normal nonfasting patients with Tc-99m IDA resulted in only 36 per cent gallbladder visualization.[26] Thus, it is strongly recommended that patients be kept NPO. The unexpected emergency is the only situation in which this could conceivably pose a problem. In actual fact, however, since anorexia, nausea, and/or vomiting frequently is a prominent symptom in the acutely ill patient referred for study, this has not been a problem. As a rule, the individual who is thought to have acute cholecystitis typically has been anorectic for several hours prior to presentation in our department.

Routine pretreatment of all patients with cholecystokinin (CCK) has been advocated by some investigators.[27, 28] Others have recommended its utilization when the gallbladder fails to visualize in one to one and one-half hours.[29] The temporal response of the gallbladder to the slow, intravenous administration of CCK (40 Ivy dog units) (CCK-PZ GIH research units, Karolinska Institute, Stockholm, Sweden) or sincalide (the terminal octapeptide of CCK; 0.2 to 0.4 mg/kg; Kinevac, Squibb, New Brunswick, NJ) is significantly different from its response to the postprandial release of CCK. Endogenously released CCK induces gallbladder emptying with a half-time of about 45 minutes, which therefore interferes with subsequent gallbladder filling with labeled bile. Exogenously administered CCK induces gallbladder contraction at five minutes and has a half-time of 12 minutes.[30] In selected cases, the technique of intravenous CCK pretreatment results in facilitation of subsequent gallbladder filling and, therefore, visualization. Theoretically, this occurs in patients who have gallbladders filled with viscous bile or sludge, in which case stimulating the gallbladder to contract and empty a portion of its contents aids in enhancing subsequent gallbladder filling. This appears to have been more critical in the days of I-131 RB, when biliary visualization was much less optimal.[27, 28] With Tc-99m IDA cholescintigraphy, we have found it preferable to obtain delayed views when necessary (see Additional Views) rather than pretreating with CCK.[31] Both methods, delayed views and CCK pretreatment, are directed at the same patient population.[31] Patients who would ordinarily exhibit delayed gallbladder visualization revert to normal with CCK pretreatment. Our preference for the former is based on several facts. Most of the patients studied have normal cholescintigrams; therefore, routine pretreatment means unnecessary pharmacologic intervention in the majority of cases. The use of CCK markedly decreases the sensitivity of this study to detect chronic cholecystitis, and the occasional case of acute cholecystitis exhibiting delayed gallbladder visualization (rather than nonvisualization) would be completely missed (see Acute Cholecystitis). Additionally, delayed views have often serendipitously revealed the presence of nonbiliary pathology as the cause of the patient's acute symptomatology[32] (see Serendipitous Detection of Nonbiliary Pathology).

Routine Imaging Procedures

The usual dose of Tc-99m IDA is between 3 and 5 mCi. As little as 1 mCi has been successfully used in anicteric adults, and doses larger than 5 mCi may be helpful in cases of severe hyperbilirubinemia. The appropriate activity of pertechnetate is injected into a commercially available kit of IDA. Prior to the intravenous administration of Tc-99m IDA, patients are positioned supine under the Anger camera. A large field-of-view scintillation camera is preferable but not absolutely necessary. The patient should be positioned so that the liver, common bile duct, gallbladder, duodenum, and jejunum are imaged (Fig. 8–2). The anterior view is routinely performed, with each scintiphoto consisting of 500,000 counts. Views in varying positions are obtained in specific clinical situations (see Additional Views).

Although the exact imaging sequence employed may vary from institution to institution, there are two general principles to keep in mind when selecting a protocol best suited to one's own practice. The procedure should be monitored as it is progressing. Tc-99m IDA cholescintigraphy is a dynamic study of hepatobiliary function. This means that if a question arises at a specific point in time, the answer may be lost if it is not worked out immediately. Later the labeled bile may have progressed away from the area of concern or may be obscured by other structures that subsequently come into view. Thus, in the interest of greatest accuracy and reliability, the images should be examined as they are obtained. Second,

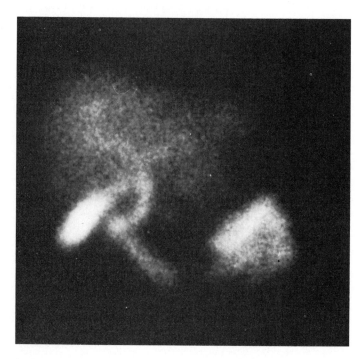

Figure 8–2. This scintiphoto was obtained 20 minutes after the intravenous injection of Tc-99m HIDA. It illustrates the structure routinely visualized in the field of view including the left, right, common hepatic, and common bile ducts; duodenum; jejunum; cystic duct region; and gallbladder.

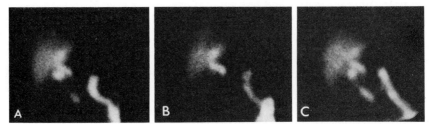

Figure 8–3. This figure illustrates the value of obtaining serial scintigrams with sufficient frequency to indicate the manner in which structures are filling and emptying. On the scintiphoto obtained at 30 minutes, a structure is visualized that could either be the gallbladder or the region of the junction of the first and second portions of the duodenum. This structure has completely emptied and therefore is not visualized on the scintiphoto obtained at 45 minutes *(B)*; it is then observed to fill at one hour *(C)*. In *C*, the continuity between this structure and the second portion of the duodenum is better visualized as well. The manner in which the structure in question rapidly fills, empties, and refills in a short period of time indicates that the structure is definitely the duodenum and that the gallbladder is not visualized.

images should be taken with sufficient frequency in the first 30 to 45 minutes to indicate how structures are filling and emptying. For example, the gallbladder fills progressively with time, whereas the duodenum tends to repeatedly fill and empty (Fig. 8–3). Our "routine" imaging sequence includes a scintiphoto at one minute to visualize the blood pool phase (see Serendipity), followed by scintiphotos every five minutes for the first half hour. Then, images are obtained at 45 and 60 minutes. The majority of studies are terminated within one to one and one-half hours with visualization of the liver, common duct, gallbladder, and intestine (Fig. 8–4). If there is nonvisualization of any of these structures, delayed views—up

to four hours—are obtained. In these cases, the study is terminated earlier if there is no significant persistence of hepatic activity when the intestinal activity is excluded from the field of view by a lead shield.

Evaluation of the contractile response of the gallbladder can be achieved by administering an oral fatty meal (Liposperse, Summit Medical Products, NY) and imaging between 30 and 60 minutes after ingestion. However, since lack of contraction may be due to variable intestinal absorption, the results are meaningful only when the gallbladder does, in fact, respond. Intravenous stimulation with CCK 40 Ivy dog units or sincalide (0.2 to 0.4 mg/kg) is a more reliable method of examination.[31, 33] If the

Figure 8–4. Normal Tc-99m IDA cholescintigram. The hepatic parenchyma, gallbladder, common bile duct, and intestine are all well visualized within 30 minutes. (Reprinted with permission from Weissmann et al.: Semin. Nucl. Med. *9*:25, 1979.)

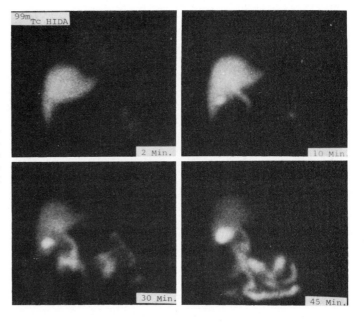

baseline and post-stimulation images are recorded in digital form on a computer, subsequent playback and quantitative evaluation of the degree of gallbladder contraction can be obtained.

Additional Views

Usually, the anterior image is all that is required to provide the necessary diagnostic information. However, on occasion additional views may be indicated. For example, if the differential diagnosis in an acutely ill patient rests between acute cholecystitis and hepatic abscess, the cholescintigram would be the best single test to perform. With advance knowledge of the clinical concern of space-occupying disease within the liver, the imaging protocol should be altered to include right anterior oblique, right lateral, and posterior views during the hepatocyte phase (see Serendipity). These views are also obtained, in the absence of pertinent history, if an abnormal or suspicious area is noted on the anterior scintiphoto. Although the hepatic parenchymal phase of the Tc-99m IDA cholescintigram generally corresponds to the Tc-99m sulfur colloid study, the former does not replace the latter. For example, cholescintigraphy cannot identify the presence of a colloid shift or visualize splenic morphology.

Determination of whether or not the gallbladder is visualized is essential to cholescintigraphic interpretation. Occasionally, right renal activity or positioning of the gallbladder immediately anterior to the duodenal sweep may pose a diagnostic problem. These are two specific instances in which obtaining images at frequent intervals during the first 45 minutes as well as monitoring the study as it is progressing proves to be extremely useful. Identification of activity in the upper right quadrant, secondary to renal excretion, is usually noted when Tc-99m HIDA is the analog employed.[34] Typically, renal activity is evident in the upper right quadrant during the first ten minutes of the study and then becomes less apparent. Usually, this is not a source of confusion because the gallbladder appears later and will become more intense with time. Thus, identification of the initial time of visualization and the sequence of filling and emptying of the structure in question is extremely useful. Additionally, utilizing the one-minute blood pool scintiphoto as a "road map" has proved helpful. Correlation with this view can

reveal if the area of activity in the upper right quadrant corresponds to the location of the right kidney. On occasion, a right lateral or posterior view may be required to solve the dilemma. Since the gallbladder is anterior and the kidney is posterior, when the structure in question is more apparent on the posterior than the anterior scan, it is confirmed to be the right kidney. Similar identification of the location of the region of interest on the lateral view is useful.

In the majority of cases, the gallbladder and duodenum are clearly discerned as separate structures. However, on occasion, the gallbladder may overlie the duodenal sweep. This should be considered when the lateral margin of the second portion of the duodenum has an irregular, unusual contour or when the proximal portion of the sweep consistently appears to be significantly increased in activity. When suspected, the left anterior oblique view is most helpful. Right anterior oblique and right lateral views also may be useful. Another worthwhile maneuver is to have the patient drink a small amount of water. This has a twofold effect. It dilutes the duodenal activity and aids in its progression distal to the region in question. Only rarely will the question remain unanswered such that it is necessary to resort to sonographic assistance. In these instances, the patient's skin surface can be marked over the area in question, and ultrasonography can then be performed to determine whether or not the gallbladder is situated directly under the area marked.[35] Gallbladder nonvisualization is documented and the suspicion of acute cholecystitis confirmed when the gallbladder is identified to be distant to the area of concern. It should be emphasized that such maneuvers are required in the rarest of instances.

The main diagnostic limitation of cholescintigraphy is the degree of anatomic resolution that can be achieved. At best, only an estimation of actual size can be obtained when structures such as the common bile duct appear enlarged. This can be accomplished with the aid of a "snake" marker that alternates 1.0 cm of lead with 1.0 cm of cobalt-57. In this way, the width of the common bile duct can be approximated to within about 0.5 cm. It is important to stress that this represents an estimation of size and does not have the millimeter accuracy of sonography. The apparent size of a structure is related to the degree of activity within that structure at a given point in time. Therefore, a structure with a high specific activity may appear larger than it actually is, whereas a structure with a low specific activity may appear smaller than it actually is. For this reason, impressions of the presence of pathologic changes such as dilatation should be based on demonstration that the suggested abnormality is persistent with time. A dilated and functionally obstructed common bile duct is almost invariably present when the duct consistently appears equal to or greater than 1 cm and there is delay in the excretion of Tc-99m IDA into the intestine beyond one hour.[36] One cannot accurately estimate the size of the common duct if it appears normal or is not visualized on the cholescintigram, particularly when significant hyperbilirubinemia exists.[36]

Delayed views between one and one-half and four hours are routinely obtained in four specific instances. First, when there is nonvisualization of the gallbladder despite prompt hepatic uptake and visualization of the common duct and intestine in the first hour, it is imperative that later views be evaluated for delayed gallbladder visualization; the importance of this is discussed hereafter (see Acute Cholecystitis). Second, delayed views are required when there is absent or delayed visualization of the intestine (see Acute Cholecystitis: Nonvisualization of Gallbladder and Bile Ducts with Absent or Delayed Excretion into the Intestine; Biliary Atresia; and Chronic Cholecystitis: Delayed Biliary-to-Bowel Transit). Third, delayed views are called for in all postoperative cases. For example, a post-cholecystectomy study may appear entirely normal within the first 60 minutes, with only the more delayed views identifying the presence of a cystic duct remnant. A similar situation may occur in cases in which a bile leak is present. Since this frequently may be an unsuspected cause of a patient's poor postoperative clinical condition, delayed images are routinely obtained in any postoperative patient regardless of the type of recent biliary or biliary-enteric surgery (see Postoperative Evaluation). Fourth, in any case in which biliary leakage is suspected, regardless of the etiology (post-traumatic, postoperative, or spontaneous), delayed views are necessary (see Bile Leak Detection).

ACUTE CHOLECYSTITIS

Evaluation of the patient with acute onset of abdominal pain is a diagnostic problem that frequently confronts the clinician. When the clinical presentation is typical for acute cholecystitis, including localized pain and tenderness in the upper right quadrant, a positive Murphy sign, fever, and a leukocytosis, no additional imaging work-up is necessary. However, most of the acutely ill patients do not present quite so typically. It is in these less clear-cut clinical situations that accurate assessment of cystic duct patency is extremely important. In the United States, cholelithiasis and its associated complications are the most common cause for abdominal surgery and the fourth most common indication for surgical hospitalization of adults. Over 500,000 operations are performed annually in the United States for gallbladder disease. A significant percentage of these cases are related to acute inflammatory disease of the gallbladder.[37] It is estimated that 20,000,000 Americans have cholecystitis and cholelithiasis.[38] It is true that cholelithiasis is the imaging hallmark of chronic cholecystitis, since more than 90 per cent of patients with cholelithiasis do have chronic cholecystitis. Gallstones are accurately and readily detected by oral cholecystography and ultrasonography. However, in view of the prevalence of cholelithiasis in our population, documenting its presence in a patient presenting with acute abdominal pain is insufficient to determine that the stones are the etiology of the patient's acute clinical presentation. Cholelithiasis is not a *sine qua non* for acute cholecystitis. Identification of cystic duct obstruction is a much more suitable imaging finding, because more than 95 per cent of cases of acute cholecystitis are associated with cystic duct obstruction at some point in the development of the disease.[38a] Since cholescintigraphy is the most sensitive and reliable imaging modality available for evaluating cystic duct patency, it is the diagnostic procedure of choice for suspected acute cholecystitis.

Prior to the advent of technetium-99m IDA cholescintigraphy, radiographic evaluation depended on the use of iodinated contrast material, including oral cholecystography[39] and intravenous cholangiography.[40] More recently, ultrasonography[41] and, to a lesser extent, computed tomography[42] have proved to be of diagnostic value in this area. Although it is true that each of these imaging procedures may contribute useful information in a work-up of suspected cholecystitis, each has significant shortcomings that limit their applicability in the acute clinical situation.

Technetium-99m IDA cholescintigraphy has many advantages that make it the procedure of choice for suspected acute cholecystitis. It is a rapid, safe, and simple procedure that provides functional as well as anatomic information about the hepatobiliary system. There are no absolute contraindications. Pregnancy is the only relative contraindication. Cholescintigraphy has proved to be more accurate and reliable than other modalities previously and currently in use.[29, 43-49] For example, evaluation of 323 consecutive patients revealed an overall accuracy of 97.6 per cent, a false-positive rate of 0.58 per cent, and a false-negative rate of 4.8 per cent.[44]

Limitations of Other Imaging Procedures

Oral Cholecystography

Iodinated contrast agents, such as iopanoic acid (Telepaque), that require oral ingestion may be associated with side effects. The most frequently observed include nausea, vomiting, and diarrhea. Fortunately, the more severe side effects, such as bronchospasm, laryngospasm, pulmonary edema, delayed hypotension, renal failure, and acute anaphylaxis, are rare.[50, 51]

Through the years, the excellent diagnostic accuracy of oral cholecystography (OCG) when the gallbladder visualizes has been established.[39] However, a significant limitation of OCG is that visualization of a normally functioning gallbladder requires oral ingestion, intestinal absorption, and hepatic conjugation of the iodinated contrast in addition to patency of the cystic duct. Also, its clinical utility is limited in the face of hyperbilirubinemia. For all these reasons, there are many causes of gallbladder nonvisualization that are unrelated to the presence of cholecystitis. These include failure to take the tablets, vomiting, esophageal or gastric obstruction, malabsorption, diarrhea, and hepatitis, to name a few.[39, 52] Another limiting factor in OCG is the time it takes to perform the procedure. OCG requires a minimum of 12 hours,[53] and one-fourth of all patients studied will require a double-dose examination, which delays the diagnosis up to 48 hours.[52] It is imperative that acute cholecystitis be diagnosed promptly to maintain the lowest possible morbidity and mortality. The incidence of complications, with particular concern for gallbladder perforation, has been observed to peak approximately 72 hours after the initial onset of symptoms. Therefore, the rapid diagnosis of acute cholecystitis is imperative.[37, 54, 55] All of these factors render oral cholecystography inadequate for the evaluation of suspected acute cholecystitis.

Intravenous Cholangiography

Intravenous cholangiography (IVC) has significant advantages over OCG because it does not require oral ingestion, intestinal absorption, hepatic conjugation, or the presence of a functioning gallbladder. However, its disadvantages far outweigh its advantages. Iodipamide is considered by many to be the most noxious radiographic contrast material available. It has a morbidity of 10 to 20 per cent, including numerous side effects that range in severity from nausea and vomiting to anaphylaxis. The hepatic and renal toxicity of the iodine-containing contrast agents has been established.[56-59] Therefore, any procedure that involves the use of iodinated contrast media must be performed with caution, if at all, in patients with hepatic or renal failure. The mortality rate of IVC has been reported to be 1 in 5000, which is two to six times greater than that of intravenous pyelography.[60, 61] Visualization of the biliary system decreases appreciably from 50 per cent to less than 10 per cent when the serum bilirubin level rises from 2 to 4 mg/100 ml. The chances of visualizing a normal patent biliary tree when the bilirubin level is above 4 mg/100 ml is exceedingly small.[62] Furthermore, the reported accuracy of intravenous cholangiography in the diagnosis of acute cholecystitis is severely limited.[62-64] In a representative series reported by Ekelberg, Carlson, and McIlwrath in which IVC was performed with tomography and delayed views, the false-positive rate ranged from 12 to 22 per cent, depending on the patient population evaluated. The former figure was derived from evaluation of those patients who had nonvisualization of the gallbladder despite common duct visualization and who were documented to have normal gallbladders at surgery. The latter figure was derived from the patient population with a normal functioning gallbladder visualized by OCG. Thus, failure to visualize the gallbladder on IVC, even though excellent visualization of the common bile duct is achieved, cannot reliably be equated with acute cholecystitis. Furthermore, when it was thought that diagnostic visualization of the entire biliary system had been obtained, cholelithiasis was accurately diagnosed in only 55 per cent and choledocholithiasis in only 45 per cent of cases.[64] Numerous other studies have appeared in the literature reporting similarly poor diagnostic results for IVC. For instance, a study concluded that IVC frequently presented misleading information. Almost half of the examinations were technically suboptimal, and in the remaining half IVC was correct only about 50 per cent of the time. Therefore, the conclusion of the study was that IVC left a lot to be desired as a diagnostic test.[64] Certainly studies such as these indicate that IVC should not be used as a gold standard for patient evaluation.

Ultrasonography

The advantages of ultrasonography include its excellent resolution and its ability to visualize many anatomic structures without requiring contrast administration or organ function. Thus, its accuracy and sensitivity in the detection of gallstones are superior to all available imaging modalities, even when they are only a few millimeters in diameter. This can be of value in patients suspected of having acute cholecystitis if the gallstones are specifically identified in the region of the neck of the gallbladder or cystic or common bile ducts. Other findings, such as a thickened gallbladder wall or pericholecystic collection, also can be useful. However, a word of caution is warranted. Simply documenting the presence of cholelithiasis by sonography should not be equated with confirming the presence of acute cholecystitis. It is estimated that 800,000 individuals, most of whom are asymptomatic, develop gallstones each year.[65, 66] With a total of 20,000,000 Americans estimated to have cholelithiasis, merely detecting the presence of gallstones floating within the gallbladder, even in the acutely ill patient, does not always mean that acute cholecystitis is present. In view of the epidemic proportions of cholelithiasis and chronic cholecystitis in the United States, there is a very real possibility that the chronic biliary disease detected by sonography may be an incidental finding in the patient who is presenting acutely secondary to another disorder such as penetrating ulcer disease, pancreatitis, pyelonephritis, appendicitis, and so on. This has been borne out by several prospective series of patients evaluated with ultrasonography and cholescintigraphy.[49, 67, 68] At our institution, over 40 per cent of patients who were studied for suspected acute cholecystitis in whom sonography demonstrated the presence of calculi had the diagnosis of acute cholecystitis as the cause of their acute presentation correctly excluded by demonstration of a normal Tc-99m IDA cholescintigram. This illustrates the major weakness of ultrasonography. It is a purely anatomic method of imaging that gives very limited information about function.

It is incapable of evaluating the functional patency of the cystic duct. The key imaging finding that correlates best with acute cholecystitis is cystic duct obstruction. Since identification of a stone specifically located in the cystic duct region is an infrequent observation in sonography, the diagnosis of acute cholecystitis usually cannot be unequivocally confirmed with this modality. In fact, it has been documented that the cystic duct region is one of the most difficult areas to evaluate with sonography because of the tortuosity of the cystic duct, the acoustic interference created by the valves of Heister and fat in the region, and the proximity of bowel loops in the area. It has been demonstrated that sonography is most likely to be falsely negative when a single calculus is situated in the cystic duct region.[69] This is the very stone that will result in a truly positive cholescintigram and the very stone that you want to identify when acute cholecystitis is present. Another problem with sonography, in this regard, is that cystic duct obstruction typically is a functional abnormality, secondary to edema and inflammation within the region and not necessarily directly related to the presence of an obstructing stone in the cystic duct at the time the patient is being studied. Thus, while an anatomic abnormality may not be sonographically identifiable, cholescintigraphy can clearly detect and document the presence of the functional abnormality.

An additional advantage of scintigraphy when compared with sonography is that it is much less operator and equipment dependent. The quality of each image, and therefore the entire study, does not depend on the expertise of the technologist or physician performing the study. This means that there is less opportunity for human error to be a factor in misdiagnosis, and there should be less interinstitution variability with regard to overall accuracy and reliability.

Despite the development of Tc-99m IDA imaging, it has recently been proposed by Laing and coworkers that ultrasound be the imaging procedure of choice to evaluate patients with suspected acute cholecystitis.[70] There are two main points upon which this proposal is based. First, only one-third of patients suspected of having acute cholecystitis actually have the disease.[40, 70-72] Not only can sonography rapidly detect the presence of gallstones, but the surrounding anatomic structures can also be evaluated. This may aid in determining the etiology of the acute illness in the remaining two-thirds of cases. Although it is true that the regional anatomy can be examined, this ability is not unique to sonography (see Serendipity). Nonbiliary pathology was detected cholescintigraphically in 14.5 per cent of patients studied for suspected acute cholecystitis. More importantly, the nonbiliary finding was related to the cause of the patient's acute clinical presentation and correctly directed the clinician in 9.5 per cent of the patients studied. Thus, cholescintigraphy is also capable of evaluating surrounding structures and detecting nonbiliary abnormalities with a significant frequency. Additionally, although it is true that being able to visualize the regional anatomy in any patient population studied for any clinical reason can prove useful, this should only be considered an added bonus for a modality and not a primary reason for using a specific procedure. Although it may be true that most patients thought to have acute cholecystitis actually do not have that abnormality, this is a retrospective observation obtained when a large series of patients is evaluated, and it should not be utilized as an argument to determine which procedure is best suited to solve the given clinical problem. It certainly does not help the referring physician, who firmly believes that acute cholecystitis is the most likely diagnosis in a specific patient, to utilize a procedure that is not as well suited to solve that specific clinical problem but is capable of visualizing the "regional anatomy." The procedure of choice to screen for a specific clinical problem is the one that comes closest to supplying the critical piece of information most needed to make the diagnosis in question. In the case of acute cholecystitis, that information concerns cystic duct obstruction or patency. The fact that scintigraphy is highly accurate in supplying this necessary, functional information better than any of the currently available morphologically oriented modalities, such as sonography, has been documented by many investigators.[44-49, 67, 68, 73] No one can question the fact that sonography has exquisite anatomic resolution that enables detection of gallstones, dilated ducts, and other morphologic abnormalities in a manner clearly unrivaled by the nuclide study. By the same token, the functional information with regard to ductal patency obtained by radionuclide imaging is unrivaled by ultrasound.

The advantage of obtaining functional versus anatomic information in cases of suspected acute cholecystitis is further emphasized when one considers the subpopulation of patients who will turn out to have acute acalculous cholecystitis. Acute acalculous cholecystitis has remained a particularly difficult diagnostic problem for the clinician and radiologist for many years. This may be an important factor contributing to the significantly higher morbidity and mortality observed in patients with this disorder. Frequently, the sonogram appears entirely normal in these patients because there is no apparent structural change in the gallbladder. Despite this, the vast majority of these patients do, in fact, have functional cystic duct obstruction, which can be detected and diagnosed by cholescintigraphy (see Acute Acalculous Cholecystitis).

The second major tenet upon which the philosophy of Laing and colleagues is based is that some patients exhibit focal gallbladder tenderness; when this is identified in conjunction with the presence of calculi, it is an extremely accurate means of diagnosing acute inflammatory disease of the gallbladder. However, when classic focal tenderness is present, the referring physician requires little or no imaging assistance to make the diagnosis. The services of a radiologist are most needed in the problem cases. Confirming the presence of focal pain and tenderness over the gallbladder is a subjective finding that requires meticulous attention to technique as well as the presence of a very reliable, cooperative patient. Although it may be useful when a patient can clearly communicate that pain is truly focal and localized to the gallbladder, the overall value of focal tenderness remains controversial. Numerous articles have been written that describe completely different sonographic criteria for diagnosing acute cholecystitis and do not mention identification of focal pain.[74, 75]

The fact that identification and evaluation of focal gallbladder tenderness in the presence of cholelithiasis is highly subjective on the part of the technologist and physician as well as the patient is indicated by noting that misinterpretation of this finding has resulted in misdiagnosing patients who actually have chronic cholecystitis as having acute cholecystitis.[70, 76]

An additional point that has been stressed by proponents of the use of sonography for the diagnosis of acute cholecystitis is the rapidity with which the procedure can be completed. Here again, the question of priority has to be considered. Evaluation of cost effectiveness, which includes wasted time, is in vogue. However, this should not be allowed to color sound clinical and imaging judgment. The majority of cholescintigrams are completed within one hour. Even though it is true that some studies require imaging up to two to four hours, I daresay that a clinician and patient would prefer a procedure that may take longer but has a much greater specificity and predictive value to a shorter method that has a significantly lower specificity and predictive value. Although numerous studies can be cited from many different institutions that indicate the predictive value of scintigraphy for acute cholecystitis to be far superior to that of sonography, the most convincing support for this statement can be found in papers that are clearly biased toward sonography and conclude that sonography is preferable. For instance, in Laing's article the predictive value (true-positive/true-positive + false-positive) of sonography in diagnosing acute cholecystitis is 77.3 per cent,[70] whereas the predictive value for scintigraphy has been shown by other studies to be 99.1 per cent.[44]

In conclusion, there can be no doubt that the sonographic demonstration of calculi is the best available imaging method for diagnosing chronic cholecystitis. However, ancillary findings, such as controversial focal tenderness, gallbladder size and shape, and gallbladder wall thickness, are indirect indicators of the possibility of acute cholecystitis and are less specific than cholescintigraphic detection of cystic duct obstruction.

Other Advantages of Tc-99m IDA Cholescintigraphy

Radionuclide hepatobiliary imaging is a safe, simple, and reliable procedure that has no associated morbidity or mortality. It does not require specialized equipment, such as that needed for cardiovascular nuclear medicine, nor does it require the technical expertise of sonography. The presence of overlying bowel gas, the configuration of the patient's rib cage, and the overall body habitus of the individual may pose technical problems for radiographic and sonographic procedures, but they are of no concern with cholescintigraphy.

Although it is true that most patients with acute cholecystitis have normal or slightly elevated bilirubin levels, Tc-99m IDA has the ability to visualize a patent biliary system in patients with severe hyperbilirubinemia up to 30 mg/100 ml (see Cholestasis). This is in marked contrast to the limitations of oral cholecystography and intravenous cholangiography in the presence of mild hyperbilirubinemia.

The Anger camera is capable of detecting much smaller concentrations of Tc-99m IDA in the gallbladder than the iodine concentration that must be achieved to document cystic duct patency with conventional radiography.[28] Therefore, since scintigraphy is more sensitive in documenting cystic duct patency, it is more accurate than iodine contrast studies in evaluating suspected acute cholecystitis. This is illustrated by the observed false-positive rate of 0.58 per cent for cholescintigraphy as compared with the observed false-positive rate of between 12 and 22 per cent for intravenous cholangiography.[44, 63]

Acute pancreatitis does not interfere with gallbladder visualization in cholescintigraphy as has been observed in cholangiography. Although the etiology is not really known,[77] a normal gallbladder will fail to visualize on IVC in 25 to 60 per cent of cases, even in the absence of jaundice.[72, 78-84] To date, this has not been noted to represent a significant problem for cholescintigraphy. With little exception, nonvisualization of the gallbladder with Tc-99m IDA in patients with acute pancreatitis has meant that cholecystitis is also present (Fig. 8–5).[85-87]

In comparison with OCG and IVC, the ability of the radionuclide study to visualize the liver parenchyma represents another advantage. Evaluation of the "hepatocyte phase," usually during the first 20 minutes after intravenous injection of Tc-99m IDA, has enabled the detection of space-occupying disease within the liver (see Technique and Serendipity).[32, 88] The importance of this is indicated by the fact that 5.8 per cent of the patients who were thought to have acute cholecystitis actually had abscesses, hepatomas, and metastases as the causes of their acute clinical presentation. These were correctly detected by cholescintigraphy.[32] Comparing Tc-99m IDA scanning with sonography, which also has the capacity to image hepatic morphology, analysis of the rate and degree of radiotracer uptake may, in the future, provide a means for evaluating hepatocyte function.[89-95] However, at the present time, this remains controversial.

Disadvantages of Tc-99m IDA Cholescintigraphy

As with other nuclear medicine imaging studies, Tc-99m IDA cholescintigraphy has the disadvantage of limited spatial resolution. This technical problem is significantly outweighed

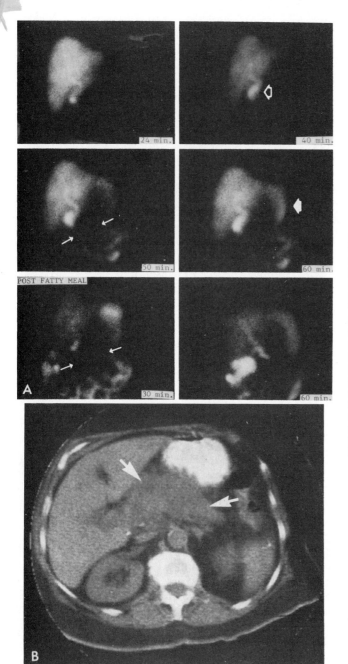

Figure 8–5. *A,* Acute cholecystitis and acute pancreatitis. Sequential scintiphotos show non-visualization of the gallbladder. There is a notable absence of bowel activity in its usual location. This persistent photon-deficient area (arrows) suggests that the bowel is being displaced by a mass. Additionally, the persistent "hold up" of activity in the second portion of the duodenal sweep (open arrowhead) suggests the presence of an inflammatory process in the region. The activity in the upper left quadrant appearing at 50 minutes represents gastric reflux (closed arrowhead). *B,* Computerized tomographic scan of the upper abdomen demonstrates a diffusely enlarged pancreas (arrows), which went on to abscess formation. A pancreatic abscess and an acutely inflamed gallbladder were found at surgery. (Reprinted with permission from Weissmann et al.: Semin. Nucl. Med. *9:*25, 1979.)

by the fact that, in certain specific clinical situations, the functional changes associated with the presence of disease occur earlier than the morphologic responses (see Acute Chole-cystitis: Nonvisualization of Gallbladder and Bile Ducts with Absent or Delayed Excretion Into the Intestine; Postcholecystectomy: "Complete" Ductal Obstructive Pattern; and Cholestasis: Acute Biliary Obstruction).

Radionuclide scanning does not have the anatomic resolution to detect the presence of calculi. Although it is true that their presence may be suggested, on occasion, by visualization of a photon-deficient area within the gallbladder or common bile duct, a cholescintigram should never be performed to visualize gallstones. This finding is infrequently observed in comparison with the incidence of cholelithiasis. Additionally, since identification of a persistent zone of photon deficiency is a nonspecific finding and since other abnormalities such as tumor or enlarged lymph nodes can result in the same pattern, when it is noted, further evaluation with a modality that has better anatomic resolution, such as sonography, is indicated. Scintigraphy should be performed to evaluate for patency and not to detect the presence of stones.

Cholescintigraphic visualization of the hepatobiliary system requires the preservation of some degree of hepatocyte function if the Tc-99m IDA molecules are to be taken up by the hepatocytes and transferred to the bile. At times, this can be a disadvantage for cholescintigraphy. Fortunately, with analogs such as DISIDA, function usually has to be severely depressed to compromise the diagnostic ability of the study (see Cholestasis). Additionally, certain specific clinical states that result in profound alteration of normal bile physiology, such as total parenteral hyperalimentation and chronic alcoholism, have recently been reported to pose a problem for cholescintigraphy.[96] On rare occasions, the presence of sepsis has also been noted to affect hepatocyte uptake and excretion.[44]

Spectrum of Cholescintigraphic Patterns in Acute Cholecystitis

As has been indicated, the diagnostic procedure of choice for suspected acute cholecystitis is Tc-99m IDA cholescintigraphy.[35, 43-49, 67] The primary diagnostic criterion is the presence or absence of gallbladder visualization, corresponding to cystic duct patency and obstruction, respectively. Usually this finding is readily apparent and easily interpreted. However, the radiologist should be aware of the spectrum of cholescintigraphic patterns that exists and their respective implications. The secondary parameters to be evaluated include the degree and rate of hepatic uptake, the presence or absence of ductal visualization, the time of gallbladder visualization, the presence or absence of intestinal activity, and the time at which labeled bile is first noted to progress from the biliary tree into the intestine.

Establishing the Diagnosis of Acute Cholecystitis

Identification of persistent nonvisualization of the gallbladder (up to four hours) in a fasting patient who otherwise demonstrates normal hepatocyte uptake and excretion into the duodenum (Fig. 8–6) confirms the diagnosis of acute cholecystitis with an extremely high degree of accuracy (Tables 8–1 and 8–2). Of 296 patients studied for suspected acute cholecystitis, 119 demonstrated this cholescintigraphic pattern. One hundred eighteen of these individuals were confirmed to have acute cholecystitis. In only one case was nonvisuali-

Figure 8–6. Acute cholecystitis. Persistent nonvisualization of the gallbladder despite prompt heaptic uptake and common duct visualization in this acutely ill patient was diagnostic of cystic duct obstruction. Hepatic uptake was identified within the first five minutes *(A)* with prompt visualization of the common duct in less than 20 minutes *(B)* and progressive excretion into the intestine within the first 60 minutes *(D)*. Throughout the four hours of imaging, there was no evidence of visualization of the gallbladder.

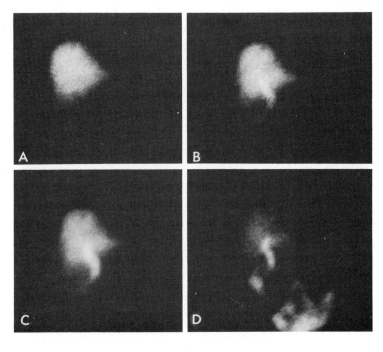

Table 8–1. ANALYSIS OF CHOLESCINTIGRAPHIC PATTERNS IN 143 CASES OF PROVED ACUTE CHOLECYSTITIS*

Nonvisualization of GB		118 (82.5%)
With normal CBD	103	
With medially displaced CBD	9	
With dilated CBD and delayed BBT	3	
With nonvisualization of CBD and normal BBT	3	
Visualization of GB		6 (4.2%)
<1 hr	1†	
At 1 hr	2†	
>1 hr	3	
Nonvisualization of GB and CBD		19 (13.3%)
With no bowel visualization	17	
With delayed bowel visualization	2	

*Reprinted with permission from Weissmann et al.: Radiology *138*:167, 1981.

†In one patient, administration of sincalide did not result in gallbladder contraction.

CBD = common bile duct
GB = gallbladder
BBT = biliary-to-bowel transit

zation due to the presence of chronic cholecystitis. In this individual, the acute symptomatology was secondary to the presence of a villous adenoma partially obstructing the common bile duct. Therefore, even though this cholescintigraphic finding has been observed in some cases of chronic cholecystitis,[97, 98] in the acute clinical setting it has not proved to be a diagnostic problem. When the patient is acutely ill, detection of the presence of cystic duct obstruction correlates with acute cholecystitis 99 per cent of the time. Certainly, documenting the presence of cystic duct obstruction is a more specific finding. It correlates much more closely with the presence of acute cholecystitis than does documenting the presence of gallstones, which was one of the major criteria used prior to the advent of Tc-99m IDA imaging. An important factor in the success of cholescintigraphy has been the routine performance of delayed views.[99] Chronic cholecystitis may create a partial functional cystic duct obstruction. Therefore, studies in some patients with chronic inflammatory gallbladder disease may fail to visualize their gallbladders within the first hour. Usually, however, when an acute inflammatory component is not superimposed on their chronic disease, they will go on to demonstrate delayed gallbladder visualization between one and four hours (Fig. 8–7) (see Chronic Cholecystitis: Delayed Gallbladder Visualization).[31, 44] Generally, the delayed views are obtained at one and one-half, two, and four hours. Evaluation of the 296 patients revealed that if the studies had been prematurely terminated (see Technique), the false-positive rate would have been unnecessarily high at 9.9 per cent, as compared with 0.58 per cent. Additionally, the specificity would have been unacceptably low at 87 per cent, as compared with 99.2 per cent (Table 8–3). Obtaining delayed views revealed subsequent gallbladder visualization and enabled us to accurately exclude acute cholecystitis in 14 patients as well as diagnose hepatocellular disease instead of gallbladder disease in two cases.[99]

The radiologist should be aware of a report recently published by Shuman and colleagues in which alcoholic individuals and patients on total parenteral nutrition were studied. Acute cholecystitis was not the sole indication for cholescintigraphic evaluation of these patients. This study revealed false-positive rates of 60 and 92 per cent, respectively. The fact that their clinical experience is so profoundly dif-

Table 8–2. RESULTS IN 296 PATIENTS STUDIED FOR ACUTE CHOLECYSTITIS*

		Nonvisualization of Gallbladder†	Visualization of Gallbladder
Acute cholecystitis		118	6
No acute cholecystitis		1	171
Accuracy	97.6%	False-positive	0.58%
Specificity	99.2%	False-negative	4.8%
Sensitivity	95.2%	True-negative	99.4%

*Reprinted with permission from Weissmann et al.: Radiology *138*:167, 1981.

†With visualization of the common bile duct or normal biliary-to-bowel transit time. Studies continued for four hours or until no significant activity remained in the liver, whichever came first.

Table 8–3. IDA RESULTS IN 296 STUDIES FOR ACUTE CHOLECYSTITIS

| | Nonvisualization of Gallbladder* | | Visualization of Gallbladder | |
	1 Hr	4 Hr	1 Hr	4 Hr
Acute cholecystitis	121	118	3	6
No acute cholecystitis	17	1	155	171

	1 Hr	4 Hr
Accuracy (%)	93.2	97.6
Specificity (%)	87.7	99.2
Sensitivity (%)	97.6	95.2
False-positive (%)	9.9	0.58
False-negative (%)	2.4	4.8
True-negative (%)	90.1	99.4

*With visualization of CBD or normal biliary-to-bowel transit time.

ferent from that observed by numerous other investigators deserves mention.[35, 43-49, 67] These other reports did not specifically single out these two patient populations. However, it should be noted, for example, that in our series of patients there was a significant number of individuals who had complicated medical and surgical histories, including alcoholism and the need for total parenteral nutrition, that did not pose a source of diagnostic error. Obviously, further evaluation of these factors is indicated. At this point, it appears warranted to emphasize the fact that, to date, we have not had a single case of gallbladder nonvisualization in which the gallbladder was subsequently documented to be normal. It should also be noted that it is the patient with nonvisualization of the gallbladder who is actively and rapidly worked up to a conclusion that is usually surgery. Thus, it is a false-positive cholescintigram that we would be most likely to discover. Furthermore, our experience has taught us that cholescintigraphy can be more accurate in diagnosing acute cholecystitis than surgical inspection. We have had three cases in which cholescintigraphy demonstrated gallbladder nonvisualization, and the gallbladder looked grossly normal to the surgeon's eye. Owing to the patient's symptomatology, lack of identification of other sources of pathology,

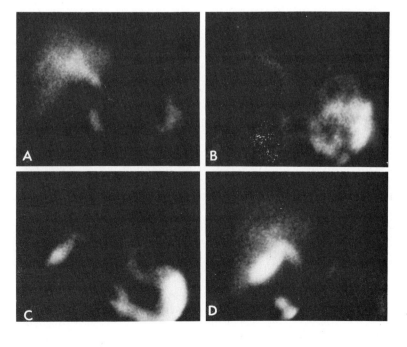

Figure 8–7. Chronic cholecystitis, delayed gallbladder visualization. Despite prompt hepatic uptake with visualization of the common duct and proximal small bowel in the first 30 minutes (A), there is persistent nonvisualization of the gallbladder through the first one and one-half hours (B). The gallbladder is first identified at two hours (C). This is better identified when a lead shield is utilized to exclude the counts from the small intestine as evidence by the scintiphoto obtained at two hours with the use of a lead apron (D). The presence of cholelithiasis was documented subsequently by sonography. Surgery confirmed the presence of gallstones and chronic cholecystitis.

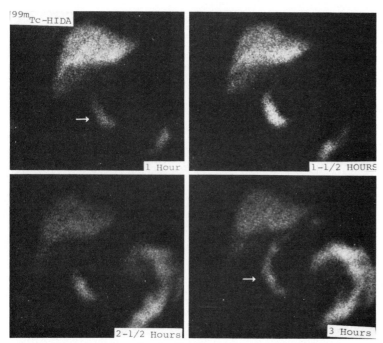

Figure 8–8. Acute cholecystitis and necrotizing pancreaticoduodenitis. The liver, common bile duct, and intestine were visualized within the first hour. Throughout the examination there was nonvisualization of the gallbladder. Additionally, persistence of activity in the second portion of the duodenal sweep was noted (arrows). This finding has demonstrated a correlation with the presence of inflammatory disease (e.g., pancreatitis) in the region. At surgery, necrotizing pancreaticoduodenitis, secondary to a recent Gelfoam embolization for variceal bleeding, was diagnosed and treated. The gallbladder appeared grossly normal, as did the intraoperative cholangiogram. Therefore, the gallbladder was not removed at that time. Postoperatively, the patient's condition worsened, and a plain film of the abdomen obtained eight days after the initial surgery revealed persistence of the iodine contrast within the gallbladder. Upon re-exploration, a gangrenous gallbladder was removed. This case, and others like it, suggest that the functional abnormality of cystic duct obstruction associated with acute cholecystitis may be detectable cholescintigraphically prior to the development of gross anatomic changes.

and the cholescintigraphic findings, these gallbladders were removed in two cases at the time of the initial operation and in the other case eight days after the initial operation. The pathologist clearly identified the presence of histologic changes indicative of acute cholecystitis in each case. Similarly, the limitations of gross surgical inspection of the gallbladder have been previously described by Nathan and associates.[100] This is illustrated by the study in Figure 8–8, which was performed on a patient who developed upper right quadrant pain ten days after the successful treatment of a varicele bleed by Gelfoam embolization. With the clinical suspicion of acute cholecystitis, the cholescintigram was performed. Throughout the study, there was no evidence of visualization of the gallbladder. In addition, persistence of activity in the second portion of the duodenal sweep suggested the presence of a functional abnormality that has demonstrated a correlation with the presence of inflammatory disease in the region (e.g., pancreatitis, Fig. 8–5). At surgery, necrotizing pancreaticoduodenitis was noted. The gallbladder appeared completely normal to the experienced surgeons as did the operative cholangiogram to the radiologist. Therefore, it was assumed that the pancreaticoduodenitis was the entire cause of the patient's acute problem. Postoperatively, the pa-

tient's condition worsened. Eight days after the initial surgery, a plain film of the abdomen demonstrated that the contrast media from the intraoperative cholangiogram was still present within the gallbladder. At that point, re-exploration was undertaken and revealed the presence of a gangrenous gallbladder. Thus, as cases such as this have demonstrated, cholescintigraphy is capable of detecting the functional abnormality of cystic duct obstruction associated with acute cholecystitis prior to the development of gross anatomic changes.

Table 8–1 summarizes the spectrum of cholescintigraphic patterns observed in the first 143 patients studied who were subsequently documented to have acute cholecystitis.

Gallbladder Nonvisualization

Nonvisualization of the gallbladder with normal visualization of the common bile duct is the most common cholescintigraphic pattern observed in patients with acute cholecystitis (Table 8–1, 73.3 per cent) (Fig. 8–6). As discussed previously, delayed views obtained to a maximum of four hours are important because chronic cholecystitis may otherwise simulate these findings. Of the 112 patients who exhibited this cholescintigraphic pattern with persistent gallbladder nonvisualization, nine additionally had the presence of acute gallbladder hydrops correctly suggested by identification of medial displacement of the common bile duct. This was commonly associated with the presence of a photon-deficient zone identifiable in the region of the gallbladder fossa (Fig. 8–9).

Three patients with persistent nonvisualization of the gallbladder demonstrated dilatation of the biliary radicles in conjunction with delayed biliary-to-bowel transit. Two of these individuals were subsequently confirmed to have choledocholithiasis. In addition to acute cholecystitis, the third patient had carcinoma of the head of the pancreas. The presence of a mass in the region of the pancreas was correctly suggested on the basis of the cholescintigram (Fig. 8–10).

Three individuals who had gallbladder nonvisualization secondary to acute cholecystitis also exhibited persistent nonvisualization of the common bile duct. Normal excretion into the intestine was present within the first hour. These patients did not have choledocholithiasis or other ductal abnormality. Nonvisualization of the common duct was most probably related to the fact that the ducts were "so normal" as to measure 3 to 4 mm in diameter at surgery.

Thus, the small, normal ducts were not scintigraphically visualized. This observation suggests a significant difference in the ability to presume the presence of cystic duct obstruction with cholescintigraphy as compared with intravenous cholangiography. On IVC, nonvisualization of the common bile duct precludes any diagnostic statement regarding cystic duct obstruction. Even though the observed incidence of this scintigraphic pattern is low, the correlation suggests that when the biliary-to-bowel transit time is normal, cystic duct obstruction can be presumed by cholescintigraphy if the gallbladder fails to visualize. The implication is that if enough Tc-99m IDA is taken up by the hepatocytes and excreted into the bile to visualize the intestine in less than one hour, regardless of whether or not the common duct is seen, then it can be assumed that enough radiotracer is being excreted by the liver to achieve gallbladder visualization when the cystic duct is patent.

Gallbladder Visualization

Gallbladder visualization reliably excludes the diagnosis of acute cholecystitis in most cases (99.4 per cent) (Table 8–2). Of the 177

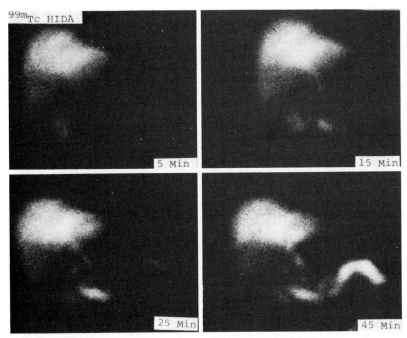

Figure 8–9. Acute cholecystitis with hydrops. Nonvisualization of the gallbladder with a medially displaced common duct and large photon-deficient area at the inferior aspect of the right lobe of the liver. Prompt hepatic uptake was noted at five minutes with a large photon-deficient zone overlying the region of the inferior right lobe of the liver, which persisted throughout the study. Its broad linear margin and visualization of a normal inferior liver contour suggest an extrinsic origin. In addition, at 15, 25, and 45 minutes, the common bile duct is extrinsically displaced medially. (Reprinted with permission from Weissmann et al.: Radiology *138*:167, 1981.)

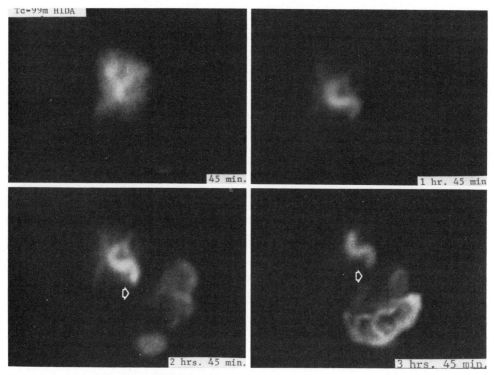

Figure 8–10. Acute cholecystitis with incidental discovery of a mass in the head of the pancreas resulting in obstruction of the common duct. Nonvisualization of the gallbladder with a dilated common bile duct and delayed biliary-to-bowel transit time. Despite prompt hepatic uptake within the first 5 minutes (not shown), there was delayed visualization of the dilated intrahepatic radicles and common duct, first noted at 45 minutes. The obstructed common duct is clearly seen at 1 hour 45 minutes, with no evidence of intestinal activity until 2 hours 45 minutes. Throughout the study (continued to 4 hours 45 minutes, not shown), a photon-deficient area persisted in the region of the head of the pancreas (arrowheads) with persistent nonvisualization of the second portion of the duodenal sweep. These findings correctly suggested the cause of the biliary obstruction as a mass (adenocarcinoma) in the head of the pancreas. (Reprinted with permission from Weissmann et al.: Radiology *138*:167, 1981.)

patients who demonstrated gallbladder visualization, 158 visualized within the first hour (Fig. 8–4). It was subsequently confirmed that 155 of these patients did not have acute cholecystitis. In 19 patients the gallbladders were visualized in a delayed fashion between one and four hours. In this group, hepatocellular disease was clearly felt to be the cause of the abnormal scintigraphic finding in the two individuals who exhibited delayed hepatocyte uptake and excretion with commensurately delayed gallbladder visualization. The remaining 17 patients had prompt hepatocyte uptake and excretion with disparately late visualization of the gallbladder; chronic cholecystitis was subsequently confirmed in 14 patients (Fig. 8–7). As these numbers indicate, one patient whose gallbladder was visualized in less than one hour (Fig. 8–11), two patients whose gallbladders were visualized at one hour, and three patients whose gallbladders were visualized at greater than one hour were subsequently confirmed to

have acute cholecystitis at surgery. Thus, visualization of the gallbladder results in an overall false-negative rate of 4.8 per cent. Fortunately, five out of these six patients had abnormally delayed gallbladder visualization at, or following longer than, one hour. Therefore, temporal visualization of the gallbladder in less than one hour for all intents and purposes excludes acute cholecystitis. Since 82.4 per cent of patients who had delayed gallbladder visualization had chronic cholecystitis,[44] identification of delayed gallbladder visualization makes the diagnosis of chronic cholecystitis most likely but does not definitely exclude the possibility of acute cholecystitis. This should not be surprising, since acute cholecystitis is most commonly, but not always, associated with complete cystic duct obstruction. Thus, a spectrum of cholescintigraphic patterns has been observed in acute cholecystitis ranging from the most common pattern of gallbladder nonvisualization to the less common pat-

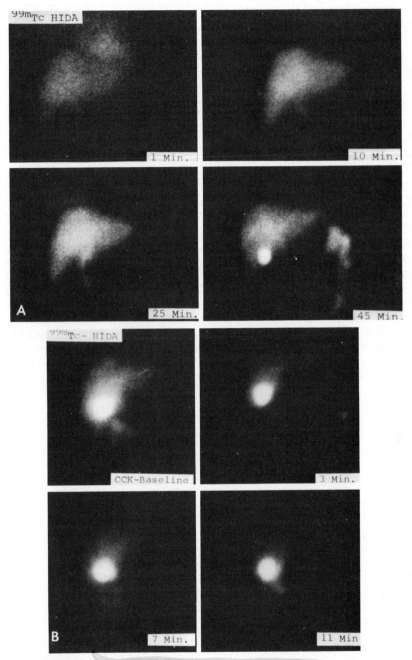

Figure 8–11. Acute acalculous cholecystitis. Uncommon cholescintigraphic pattern. Visualization of the gallbladder in less than one with failure to contract in response to sincalide administration. *A,* The study shows prompt hepatic uptake within the first 10 minutes, visualization of the common bile duct at 25 minutes, and gallbladder and intestinal activity at 45 minutes. *B,* After intravenous administration of sincalide, there is no evidence of gallbladder contraction. The gallbladder was monitored for 30 minutes (not shown), followed by repeat imaging for another 30 minutes after a double dosage of sincalide failed to demonstrate gallbladder contraction. (Reprinted with permission from Wiessmann et al.: Radiology *138*:167, 1981.)

terns of delayed visualization secondary to partial functional cystic duct obstruction (2.1 per cent), borderline visualization at one hour (1.4 per cent), and normal visualization in less than one hour (0.7 per cent). In the last two groups, two individuals had been given sincalide. Although it is true that the role of CCK or sincalide administration remains controversial,[28, 29, 100, 101] it fortunately provided a confirmatory clue to the possibility of the presence of a diseased gallbladder in two patients who received it who had acute cholecystitis with gallbladder visualization (Fig. 8–11). The reason for sincalide administration in both cases was the strong clinical suspicion of acute cholecystitis despite gallbladder visualization. In both instances the gallbladder failed to contract. Sonography was then recommended and demonstrated the presence of stones in the region of the neck of the gallbladder in the patient who had borderline gallbladder visualization at one hour. At surgery, acute calculous cholecystitis without cystic duct obstruction was confirmed. Ultrasound was normal in the individual whose gallbladder was visualized in less than one hour. This patient also had a normal IVC. Progression of her symptoms necessitated surgery, at which time the diagnosis of acute acalculous cholecystitis was made. This case has actually proved to be the exception for acute acalculous cholecystitis and definitely is not the rule (Fig. 8–11) (see Acute Acalculous Cholecystitis).

Nonvisualization of Gallbladder and Bile Ducts with Absent or Delayed Excretion into the Intestine

In the acutely ill patient, demonstration of prompt hepatic uptake with persistent nonvisualization of the biliary system and absent or delayed intestinal excretion to between two and four hours after the start of the procedure

Table 8–4. DEMONSTRATION OF CBD OBSTRUCTION IN PATIENTS STUDIED FOR SUSPECTED ACUTE CHOLECYSTITIS

27 of 323 patients studied had a pattern suggestive of virtually complete CBD obstruction

25 of 27 confirmed to have CBD obstruction
    22 by calculi
    3 by tumor

2 of 27 not confirmed to have CBD obstruction
    1 clinically passed CBD stone
    1 acute cholecystitis with ascending cholangitis

25/27 = 92.6 per cent specificity

Table 8–5. EARLY DIAGNOSIS OF ACUTE CBD OBSTRUCTION BY Tc-99m IDA CHOLESCINTIGRAPHY*

Normal Caliber Common Bile Duct	Dilated Intrahepatic and Common Ducts	Nonvisualization of Common Bile Duct
14 (70%)	4 (20%)	2 (10%)

*Ultrasonographic findings in 20 patients with cholescintigraphic pattern suggestive of significant common bile duct obstruction.

strongly suggests the possibility of a significant common bile duct obstruction (Fig. 8–12). The presence of common duct obstruction was confirmed in 25 of 27 patients who exhibited this cholescintigraphic pattern (92.6 per cent specificity) (Table 8–4). Thus, although the pattern is not pathognomonic, it certainly is strongly suggestive of common duct obstruction. In these cases, sonography has had an unacceptably high false-negative rate of 70 per cent (Table 8–5). Therefore, sonography has only proved useful when it has been positive and has confirmed the presence of obstruction. Sonography was performed in 20 of the 25 patients who had definite common duct obstruction. Fourteen (70 per cent) had normal caliber intrahepatic and common bile ducts identified sonographically. This indicates that cholescintigraphy can detect the functional abnormality associated with common duct obstruction before the morphologic response of dilatation has occurred; alternatively, the obstruction in these cases may be transient and intermittent and ductal dilatation may never occur. Therefore, when we identify this cholescintigraphic pattern, we indicate to the clinician that sonography will only be diagnostically helpful if it demonstrates the presence and cause of obstruction. If the sonogram is negative, we recommend that the patient undergo an endoscopic retrograde pancreaticoduodenogram (ERCP) or a percutaneous transhepatic cholangiogram (PTC) to definitively exclude the possibility of obstruction. This scintigraphic pattern may be the earliest and most sensitive "noninvasive" method for detecting acute common duct obstruction. One patient exhibited this pattern prior to a rise in bilirubin or alkaline phosphatase level, and a normal caliber common duct was visualized by sonography. Nonetheless, an intraoperative cholangiogram revealed the normal caliber common duct to be completely obstructed by a stone at the ampulla.[102]

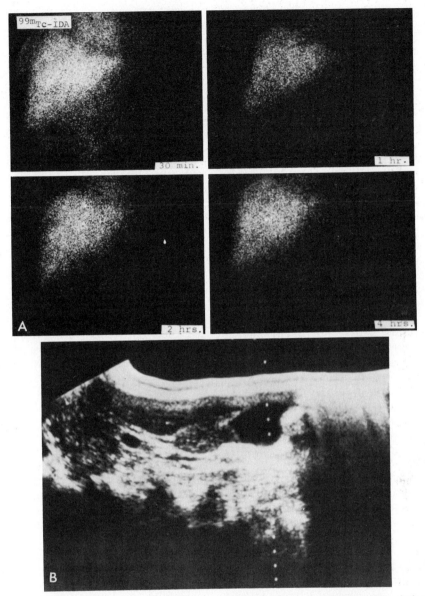

Figure 8–12. Early common bile duct obstruction in a patient suspected of having acute cholecystitis. *A*, The cholescintigram demonstrates hepatic uptake with persistent nonvisualization of the biliary tree and intestine throughout the four hours of examination. This cholescintigraphic pattern strongly suggests the presence of significant common bile duct obstruction. *B*, Ultrasonography demonstrated a normal caliber common duct without evidence of any abnormality. At surgery, the presence of a normal caliber bile duct was confirmed on the intraoperative cholangiogram, which revealed a stone in the region of the ampulla completely obstructing the flow of contrast.

Acute Acalculous Cholecystitis

Through the years, the diagnosis of acute acalculous cholecystitis has remained a problem. Accurate preoperative diagnosis is particularly important when one considers that it is associated with a mortality of about 6.5 per cent if it remains untreated. Early diagnosis and prompt surgical intervention can be effec-tive in decreasing this rate.[103] Even after appropriate surgical treatment, the morbidity and mortality remain particularly high in comparison with acute calculous disease.[103, 104] This may be related to the fact that diagnosis of this entity has remained difficult and elusive, such that patients may remain undiagnosed for an inordinately long period of time. The oral cholecystogram may reveal normal gallbladder visualization,[105] a functioning gallbladder with cholelithiasis,[105, 106] or a nonfunctioning gallbladder.[105] Likewise, sonography may reveal a "normal" gallbladder or may demonstrate the presence of nonexistent gallstones.

Initially, it appeared that diagnosis of acute acalculous cholecystitis would also be a significant source of error for cholescintigraphy. Theoretically, this is the main clinical subgroup in which the cystic duct would be most likely to be patent despite the presence of acute inflammation of the gallbladder. Additionally, as luck would have it, the first patient with acute acalculous cholecystitis to be studied scintigraphically at our institution was the first individual with acute disease to demonstrate visualization of the gallbladder in less than 60 minutes. As previously described, failure of the gallbladder to respond to the intravenous administration of sincalide was the only clue to the presence of gallbladder disease in this patient (Fig. 8–11). The sonogram and intravenous cholangiogram subsequently performed were normal. This case unnecessarily raised serious doubts as to the future value of cholescintigraphy in patients with this disorder. Now that we have much more experience with this disease entity, we can unequivocally state that this case has proved to be the exception rather than the rule. Between March 1978 and December 1980, preoperative Tc-99m IDA studies were performed on 15 patients with pathologically confirmed acute acalculous cholecystitis. The typical cholescintigraphic pattern of cystic duct obstruction, evidenced by persistent gallbladder nonvisualization despite normal hepatic uptake and excretion, was demonstrated in 12 cases. Thus, the presence of edema and inflammation results in functional obstruction of the cystic duct in most patients with acute acalculous cholecystitis. Two individuals in this group demonstrated the common duct obstructive pattern previously described. The etiology of this cholescintigraphic pattern in these patients is uncertain. It is possible that the inflammatory reaction in the region has created an ampullitis with intense spasm of the sphincter of Oddi, yielding a transitory functional common duct obstruction. Alternatively, the presence of a solitary common duct stone, which passed subsequent to the Tc-99m IDA cholescintigram, may be postulated. This hypothesis is not so implausible when one considers that a significant number of patients diagnosed as having acute acalculous cholecystitis actually exhibit evidence of having passed common duct stones.

The overall accuracy of 93.3 per cent[108, 108a] for the cholescintigraphic diagnosis of acute acalculous cholecystitis compares favorably with the accuracy observed in detecting the more common acute calculous disease.[28, 29, 43-49] Thus, the single patient who demonstrated gallbladder visualization despite the presence of acute acalculous cholecystitis truly was an exception. The significance of the observation that the gallbladder did not respond to sincalide administration remains to be established.[31] Previous reports regarding cholecystokinin cholecystography[109-111] indicate the controversy. Up to 25 per cent of cases that demonstrate lack of gallbladder response may have grossly normal gallbladders at surgery. However, lack of gallbladder contraction has been recommended to be useful in determining which patients with roentgenographically normal gallbladders and persistent symptomatology may benefit from cholecystectomy.[109-111] Their experiences have shown that histologic evidence of inflammatory disease has been present in the majority of instances.

In our series of patients with acute acalculous cholecystitis, the cholescintigram was the most useful imaging procedure for correctly detecting the presence of gallbladder disease. Of the eight sonograms performed in this group, four were normal and four revealed "calculi." Of three OCGs, two were normal and one demonstrated gallbladder nonvisualization. There was one normal IVC and one normal PTC. Thus, it appears that of all the available imaging modalities the cholescintigram remains the diagnostic procedure of choice for acute acalculous as well as acute calculous cholecystitis.

Interestingly, comparison of patients with surgically and pathologically confirmed acute acalculous cholecystitis before and after the introduction of Tc-99m IDA imaging to our

Table 8–6. FOUR NONBILIARY PHASES OF HIDA CHOLESCINTIGRAPHY*

Blood pool phase
1–5 min after injection

Hepatocyte phase
5–20 min after injection

Renal excretion phase
5–15 min after injection

Intestinal phase
30–60 min after injection

*Reprinted with permission from Weissmann et al.: Radiology 135:449, 1980.

Table 8–7. BLOOD POOL PHASE*

Cardiovascular
  Cardiac chamber enlargement, aneurysm, pericardial
    effusion
Altered perfusion patterns
  Hyper- or hypovascular lesions, redistribution of flow
Organomegaly
  Cardiac, splenic, or renal enlargement
Miscellaneous
  Ascites

*Reprinted with permission from Weissmann et al.:
Radiology *135*:449, 1980.

Table 8–8. HEPATOCYTE PHASE*

Focal space-occupying lesions
  Hepatoma, metastases, abscess, cyst, hematoma, etc.
Contour defect or displacement
  Intrahepatic, e.g., hepatoma
  Subcapsular, e.g., hematoma
  Extrahepatic, e.g., subphrenic collection, abnormality
    in adjacent organ

*Reprinted with permission from Weissmann et al.:
Radiology *135*:449, 1980.

institution revealed the length of time between admission and indicated surgery to have been decreased by half in the latter group. Additionally, there has been a considerable decrease in postoperative morbidity. This indicates that the clinical impact of cholescintigraphy on the evaluation of this disorder may be particularly significant.

The diagnostic problem associated with this entity has in actuality been minimal. In our series of patients studied for acute cholecystitis, it contributed 0.7 per cent (1/143) to the total false-negative rate of 4.2 per cent.[44]

Serendipitous Detection of Nonbiliary Pathology

Clearly, cholescintigraphy is performed to evaluate the biliary system. However, impor-

tant additional information can be obtained by evaluating the four nonbiliary phases of this study. These are the blood pool, hepatocyte, renal excretion, and intestinal phases (Table 8–6). In 9.5 per cent of cases, the serendipitous detection of previously unsuspected nonbiliary pathology correctly directed the patient's work-up away from the erroneously suspected acute cholecystitis and toward the true source of the patient's acute symptomatology.[32]

Blood Pool Phase (Table 8–7)

A static scintiphoto obtained one minute after the intravenous injection of Tc-99m IDA visualizes vascular structures including the heart, aorta, common iliac arteries, inferior vena cava, kidneys, liver, and spleen (Fig. 8–13). Therefore, an abnormality involving any one of these structures can potentially be de-

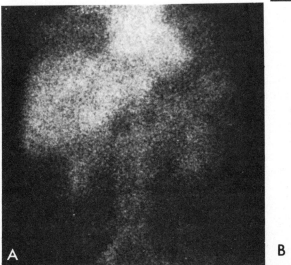
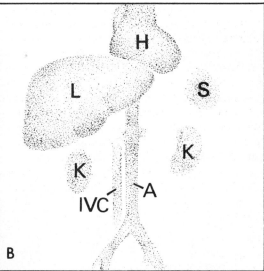

Figure 8–13. Blood pool phase. The scintiphoto *(A)* demonstrates the normal field of view of a 1-minute image. The structures visualized are illustrated *(B)*. A = aorta; H = heart; IVC = inferior vena cava; K = kidneys; L = liver; S = spleen. (Reprinted with permission from Weissmann et al.: Radiology *135*:449, 1980.)

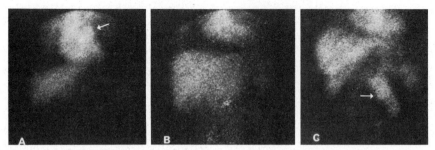

Figure 8–14. Cardiovascular abnormalities identified on the blood pool phase. *A,* Enlarged left atrium (arrow) secondary to mitral insufficiency. *B,* Pericardial effusion with wide separation between cardiac and hepatic activity. *C,* Abdominal aortic aneurysm (arrow). (Reprinted with permission from Weissmann et al.: Radiology *135*:449, 1980.)

tected (Fig. 8–14). (Unlike the Tc-99m sulfur colloid study, this is the only view that visualizes the spleen.)

Hepatocyte Phase (Table 8–8)

The hepatic parenchyma is best visualized early in the study prior to the onset of visualization of the biliary tree. This usually occurs during the first 20 minutes of the study. During this time, anterior, right anterior oblique, right lateral, and posterior views can be obtained to examine the liver for space-occupying disease.[32, 88] The most common source of confusion for the clinician suspecting acute cholecystitis has been unsuspected hepatic lesions including abscess, hepatoma, and metastasis (Fig. 8–15).

Even though hepatomas consist of a prolif-

eration of hepatocytes and Tc-99m IDA is actively taken up by these hepatic parenchymal cells, most hepatomas lack sufficient cellular differentiation to preserve this function. Of seven hepatoma cases, six were detected as a photon-deficient area within the liver, and only one demonstrated uptake and concentration of Tc-99m IDA. Case reports have appeared in the literature describing well-differentiated primary hepatomas that demonstrate active accumulation of various hepatobiliary radiotracers including rose bengal[112] and Tc-99m pyridoxylidene glutamate.[113] Also described is uptake of Tc-99m PIPIDA in pulmonary metastasis from a hepatoma.[114]

Renal Excretion Phase (Table 8–9)

The only advantage of using an IDA analog with considerable renal excretion, such as Tc-

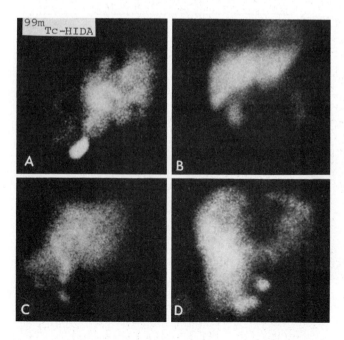

Figure 8–15. Abnormalities identified during the hepatocyte phase. *A,* Multiple focal lesions secondary to metastatic laryngeal carcinoma, which are noted to be extrinsically distorting the patent biliary tree. It should be noted in this case that sonography demonstrated the presence of hepatic metastases as well as gallstones. Having identified both abnormalities, sonography was unable to determine which was the cause of the patient's acute presentation, acute cholecystitis or necrotic, possibly infected, metastasis. Cholescintigraphy was able to exclude the possibility of acute cholecystitis by documenting cystic duct patency with visualization of the gallbladder. *B,* Hepatoma resulting in a contour defect at the dome of the right lobe of the liver. *C,* Large focal lesion involving the right lobe of the liver secondary to a hepatoma. *D,* Focal metastatic breast carcinoma.

Table 8–9. RENAL EXCRETION*

Nonvisualization of kidneys
  Azotemia, agenesis, post-nephrectomy, etc.
Enhanced or prolonged kidney visualization
  Primary: obstructive uropathy, e.g., calculi, etc.
  Secondary: hepatocellular disease, obstructive jaundice
Morphologic changes
  Mass, size alterations, etc.
Positional changes
  Axis shift or other displacement

*Reprinted with permission from Weissmann et al.: Radiology *135*:449, 1980.

Table 8–10. INTESTINAL PHASE*

Congenital variant
  Malrotation
Displacement by mass
  Renal, pancreatic, intra-abdominal abscess, etc.
"Hold up" or nonfilling of loop
  Pancreatic or duodenal disorders, ischemic bowel
    disease
Postoperative displacement
  Diversionary shunts
Gastric reflux

*Reprinted with permission from Weissmann et al.: Radiology *135*:449, 1980.

99m HIDA, is that renal abnormalities can occasionally be detected. The time interval during which the kidneys are best visualized corresponds to the hepatocyte phase, i.e., during the first 15 to 20 minutes.

Intestinal Phase (Table 8–10)

The possibility of an intra-abdominal mass should be considered whenever bowel displacement or persistent absence of intestinal activity is identified in a specific region (Fig. 8–16A). When suspected, it is important to obtain serial scintiphotos at 30- to 60-minute intervals to ensure that an apparent photon-deficient area is not secondary to the presence of normal intestinal loops not yet filled with labeled bile. Evaluating the location of the visualized bowel loops (Fig. 8–16B) as well as the rate of transit through the intestine (Fig. 8–16D) also is important.

The association of cholecystitis and pancreatic disease is known. Occasionally, the presence of a pancreatic mass or inflammatory changes can be suggested by findings observed on the Tc-99m IDA study. These findings include a persistent photon-deficient area in the region of the pancreas (Figs. 8–5 and 8–10), distal common bile duct obstruction (Fig. 8–10), persistent absence of activity in the region of the duodenal sweep (Fig. 8–10), or persistence of activity in the second or third portion of the duodenal sweep throughout the study (Fig. 8–5).[35, 44] Ischemic bowel disease has also been observed to be associated with the latter finding (Fig. 8–8).

CHRONIC CHOLECYSTITIS

The role of cholescintigraphy in evaluating patients with suspected chronic cholecystitis is limited. Tc-99m IDA imaging does not have the anatomic resolution to visualize the pres-

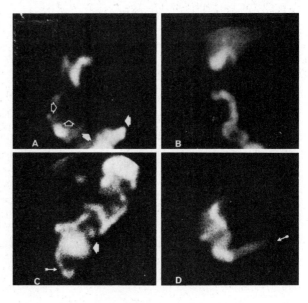

Figure 8–16. Abnormalities identified during the intestinal phase. *A,* Polycystic renal disease. A large photon-deficient area occupying the left abdomen displaces and depresses the bowel loops (solid arrowheads) and a smaller area in the right abdomen (open arrowheads), corresponding to the avascular nonfunctioning renal masses, which were identified on the earlier scintiphotos of this patient's study (not shown) during the blood pool and renal excretion phases. *B,* Malrotation. The proximal small bowel has an aberrant vertical course with the jejunum visualized in the right side of the abdomen. *C,* Right inguinal hernia. Activity is identified in the distal ileum (arrow), which is located in the scrotum below the level of bladder activity (arrowhead). *D,* Intestinal obstruction secondary to adhesions. There is persistent visualization of a distended loop of proximal small bowel with failure of Tc-99m HIDA to progress beyond a point of distal tapering (arrow). (Reprinted with permission from Weissmann et al.: Radiology *135*:449, 1980.)

ence of gallstones or a thickened gallbladder wall, which are the imaging hallmarks that correlate best with the presence of chronic inflammation of the gallbladder. Additionally, the majority of patients with chronic cholecystitis have functionally patent cystic and common bile ducts. Therefore, cholescintigraphy is not useful as a screening procedure for this disorder because up to 90 per cent of patients will have a completely normal cholescintigram.[98, 115] Cholescintigraphic evaluation of chronic cholecystitis is further complicated by the fact that the remainder of patients will exhibit a broad spectrum of cholescintigraphic patterns dependent upon whether or not there is partial or complete obstruction of the cystic and/or the common bile ducts.[115] Although some of these cholescintigraphic patterns correlate exceedingly well with chronic cholecystitis (e.g., delayed gallbladder visualization), none is truly pathognomonic. With regard to cystic duct patency, the spectrum ranges from normal, to faint, to delayed, and finally to complete nonvisualization of the gallbladder. Although it is true that some investigators have reported a fairly high percentage of patients with chronic cholecystitis who exhibited gallbladder nonvisualization,[29] it should be noted that their patient referral process skewed the results by specifically selecting those individuals who had extensively diseased gallbladders. It is self-evident that the more diseased gallbladders will have greater functional impairment, such as may be seen with patients who have small shrunken gallbladders or gallbladders packed with stones. The two main patterns to discuss are delayed gallbladder visualization and delayed biliary-to-bowel transit.

Delayed Gallbladder Visualization

The significance of first identifying gallbladder filling at one hour or longer in cases in

Table 8–11. DELAYED VISUALIZATION OF GALLBLADDER IN SUSPECTED CHOLECYSTITIS IN 37 PATIENTS ($\geq$1 HOUR)*

27 Chronic cholecystitis
1 Acute cholecystitis
1 Sclerosing cholangitis
8 Normal gallbladder
28/37 Cholecystitis = 75.6%

*Reprinted with permission from Weissmann, Sugarman, and Freeman: Nuclear Medicine Annual 1981. New York: Raven Press, 1981.

Table 8–12. DELAYED GALLBLADDER VISUALIZATION AS A SIGN OF CHRONIC CHOLECYSTITIS IN 37 PATIENTS*

Time of Visualization	No. with Cholecystitis/No. Studied	Correlation (%)
At 1 hr	6/13	47
Between 1 hr and 1½ hr	2/3	67
1½ hr	5/6†	83
>1½ hr	15/15‡	100

*Reprinted with permission from Freeman, Sugarman, and Weissmann: Semin. Nucl. Med. *11*:186, 1981.
†One case of sclerosing cholangitis.
‡One case of acute cholecystitis.

which hepatocyte uptake and common duct visualization were identified to be normal within the first 60 minutes has already been touched upon in the discussion of acute cholecystitis. Although this pattern of delayed gallbladder visualization can occasionally be observed in patients with acute cholecystitis, it is much more common secondary to the presence of chronic cholecystitis (Fig. 8–7). Evaluation of the first 37 patients with this cholescintigraphic finding revealed that cholecystitis was present in 75 per cent. Twenty-seven had chronic cholecystitis, and one had acute cholecystitis (Table 8–11). The most significant factor in correlating the presence of gallbladder disease with delayed gallbladder filling proved to be the time at which gallbladder visualization was first noted. The more delayed the visualization, the more likely it is that the patient has chronic cholecystitis (Table 8–12). It is hypothesized that the mechanism of delayed entry of labeled bile into the gallbladder is that the bile is taking the path of least resistance through the common duct into the intestine. There is a partial functional cystic duct obstruction secondary to the presence of excessively viscous bile, sludge, and/or stones within the gallbladder as well as chronic mucosal thickening and possibly some fibrosis. As a result, it takes longer to get enough labeled bile into the gallbladder to be detectable with the scintillation camera. This hypothesis is supported by work reported by Eikman and coworkers[27, 28] and Paré, Shaffer, and Rosenthall,[29] in which utilization of cholecystokinin as a premedicant for cholescintigraphy was reported. In 2 out of 20 patients who did not demonstrate gallbladder filling on an initial cholescintigram, visualization was achieved when they were pretreated with CCK. Delayed

Table 8–13. DELAYED BILIARY-BOWEL TRANSIT TIME IN SUSPECTED CHOLECYSTITIS IN 51 PATIENTS (≥1 HOUR)*

33 Chronic cholecystitis
2 Acute cholecystitis
16 Normal gallbladder

35/51 Cholecystitis = 69%

*Reprinted with permission from Weissmann, Sugarman, and Freeman: Nuclear Medicine Annual 1981. New York: Raven Press, 1981.

views were not obtained.[29] Theoretically, the administration of CCK prior to injection of Tc-99m HIDA compels the gallbladder to empty its viscous bile and/or sludge. This in turn makes it easier for the Tc-99m labeled bile to subsequently enter the gallbladder. A comparative study between the technique of obtaining delayed views and that of pretreating with CCK or sincalide has indicated that both methods are aimed at the same patient population. Patients who would otherwise exhibit delayed gallbladder visualization reverted to normal visualization when premedicated with sincalide.[31]

A variant of this cholescintigraphic pattern that has also been found to correlate with chronic cholecystitis is disparate gallbladder visualization. In these cases, even though the gallbladder visualizes in less than one hour, it appears to be disparately late in filling when compared with the much earlier time at which the common bile duct and intestine are first identified.

Delayed Biliary-to-Bowel Transit

Prompt hepatic uptake with visualization of the common bile duct and gallbladder in less than one hour in association with delayed excretion into the intestine also has been observed to be associated with the presence of chronic cholecystitis (Fig. 8–17) (Table 8–13).[35, 115] In a manner analogous to delayed gallbladder visualization, the more delayed the initial time of intestinal visualization, the more likely the patient is to have chronic cholecystitis (Table 8–14). However, it should be noted that the correlation between this pattern and the presence of chronic disease is not quite as strong as that of delayed gallbladder visualization. Although 85 per cent of patients who

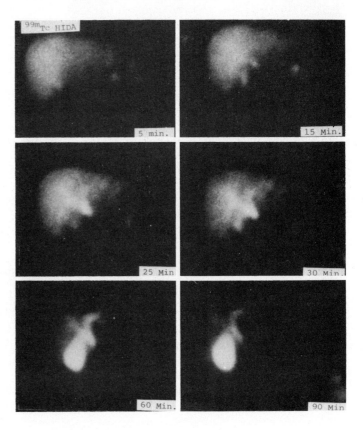

Figure 8–17. Chronic cholecystitis with delayed biliary-to-bowel transit. Serial scintiphotos demonstrate prompt hepatic uptake with visualization of the common bile duct and gallbladder within the first 30 minutes. Despite the fact that the common bile duct is visualized as early as 15 minutes, there is no evidence of intestinal excretion throughout the first one and one-half hours. A correlation between this cholescintigraphic finding of delayed biliary-to-bowel transit and chronic cholecystitis has been noted.

Table 8–14. DELAYED BILIARY-BOWEL TRANSIT TIME IN SUSPECTED CHOLECYSTITIS IN 51 PATIENTS*

At 1 hr	8/16†	= 50%
Between 1 and 1½ hr	2/3	= 67%
At 1½ hr	6/9	= 67%
Between 1½ hr and 2 hr	2/3	= 67%
Longer than 2 hr	17/20	= 85%

*Reprinted with permission from Weissmann, Sugarman, and Freeman: Nuclear Medicine Annual 1981. New York: Raven Press, 1981.

†No. with cholecystitis/total no.

first exhibit intestinal excretion from their normal-appearing common bile duct at two hours or longer do have chronic cholecystitis, this means that 15 per cent do not have gallbladder disease. Examination of the latter group of patients indicates that many other abnormalities can cause this pattern including other inflammatory foci such as pancreatitis, appendicitis, and duodenal ulcers; the presence of duodenal drainage tubes; prior vagotomies; starvation; hyperalimentation; and anesthesia or analgesic administration such as morphine. The etiology of this scintigraphic finding in patients with chronic cholecystitis may be related to the development of an associated "ampullitis," which may be caused by the repeated passage of small calculi through the common bile duct. Repeated acute and subacute episodes of cholecystitis have been noted to cause edema in the surrounding structures, and chronic changes, such as mucosal thickening and fibrosis, may develop in the ampullary region. When this occurs, transit of labeled bile through the cystic duct rather than the common duct may be the path of least resistance. The gallbladder will continue to fill while there is no evidence of transit through the common duct into the intestine. It is also possible that this cholescintigraphic pattern is an imaging manifestation of a functional abnormality that has been theorized to exist in some patients with chronic cholecystitis, in which bile stasis is thought to be a predisposing factor to the development of chronic gallbladder disease. Typically, administration of sincalide, CCK, or a fatty meal overcomes the minimal functional obstruction and promotes prompt excretion into the duodenum. Some of the other cholescintigraphic patterns that have been found to correlate with the presence of chronic cholecystitis include faint gallbladder visualization, identification of persistent photon-deficient areas within the gallbladder or common bile duct, poor contractile response to administration of CCK, and ductal dilatation.[115]

Instances of Chronic Cholecystitis in Which Cholescintigraphy May Be of Clinical Value

Although Tc-99m IDA imaging is not useful as a screening procedure for chronic cholecystitis, in specific clinical situations it can be extremely helpful. If a clinician is confronted with an acutely ill patient who he knows (from previous history and evaluation) has chronic cholecystitis, then cholescintigraphy may be useful. A normal study can demonstrate that superimposed acute cholecystitis is an unlikely cause of the patient's current problem and indicate the need for pursuing the other potential nonbiliary causes that are being considered. Tc-99m IDA imaging also may prove to be of value in those problem cases in which the clinical history is strong for the presence of chronic cholecystitis but other imaging methods have failed to be diagnostic. For example, if a two-day OCG suggests the presence of gallbladder disease by nonvisualization of the gallbladder but sonography fails to confirm the presence of pathology,[35] on rare occasions it has also proved helpful in identifying the occasional false-negative sonogram or OCG.

POSTOPERATIVE EVALUATION

Cholescintigraphy has proved to be quite useful in evaluating the postoperative patient, so much so that it has become one of the main diagnostic imaging modalities utilized by the surgeon to evaluate surgical results and complications. Evaluation of the postoperative patient is the second most common indication for cholescintigraphy at our institution.

Evaluation of the Post-Cholecystectomy Patient

In view of the high incidence of calculous biliary disease in the United States, it should not be surprising that the cholecystectomy is the most frequently performed abdominal operation.[116, 117] Each year, well over 500,000 gallbladders are removed with the intent of relieving the symptoms caused by gallbladder disease.[37, 116] Despite the relative ease and safety with which cholecystectomies are performed, the reported frequency of symptomatic cure only ranges from 50 to 88 per cent.[118-122] At best, post-cholecystectomy distress is observed in a significant percentage of patients. Clinicians have found cholescintigraphy to be a welcome addition to their diagnostic armamentarium in evaluation of these patients because of its ability to evaluate ductal obstruction as well as detect the presence of cystic duct remnants and biliary leakage.

Evaluation of Ductal Patency

If a post-cholecystectomy patient complains of upper right quadrant pain or has hyperbilirubinemia, the primary differential diagnosis is between extrahepatic biliary obstruction and hepatocellular disease. The former requires surgical intervention, whereas medical management is indicated in the latter. Typically, the patient's history, physical exam, liver biopsy, and biochemical tests are inconclusive.[123, 124] With hepatobiliary tracers such as the diisopropyl derivative, cholescintigraphy has been used to establish biliary patency in cases in which the bilirubin level has been as high as 30 mg/100 ml.[21] The main weakness of the procedure is its inability to specifically determine the cause of an obstruction when the presence of an obstruction has been identified. With its limited anatomic resolution, the presence of a stone, stricture, or tumor usually has to be inferred by the presence of a combination of scintigraphic findings. These parameters include ductal dilatation, absent or delayed biliary-to-bowel transit, and/or abnormal ductal time activity dynamics. It should be pointed out that, although cholescintigraphy's inability to visualize retained common duct stones is a limitation, procedures such as sonography and computed tomography, which have superior anatomic resolution, also have significant limitations in this regard.[125] Furthermore, although it is true that the identifiable functional changes are less specific, they appear to be more sensitive and reliable indicators of ductal obstruction.[102, 126]

The presence of obstruction usually does not represent an all or nothing phenomenon; it is a continuum of degrees of occlusion. Therefore, it is understandable that we have identified a spectrum of cholescintigraphic patterns in post-cholecystectomy patients that tends to correlate with the range of degrees of obstruc-

Table 8–15. SCINTIGRAPHIC FINDINGS IN POST-CHOLECYSTECTOMY PATIENTS*

Normal Tc-99m IDA
Dilated ducts with functional patency
Partial ductal obstructive pattern
  Dilated ducts with delayed B-BT
  Abnormal ductal time activity dynamics
  Nonvisualization of ducts with delayed B-BT
"Complete" ductal obstructive pattern
Persistent cystic duct remnant
Biliary leakage
Nonbiliary abnormality found in hepatic phase of study
Persistent photon deficiency in ducts

*Reprinted with permission from Weissmann et al.: Semin. Nucl. Med. *12*:27, 1982.

tion.[126] These are summarized in Table 8–15. The overall accuracy of cholescintigraphy was observed to be 94.4 per cent.[126] However, the reliability of each pattern will be described.

Normal Cholescintigram

Our experience has revealed that the presence of common duct obstruction can be excluded with 97 per cent accuracy when there is prompt hepatic uptake, visualization of a "normal" caliber common duct (appearing to be less than 1 cm in diameter when compared with a radioactive marker), and appearance of intestinal activity in less than one hour. In only one instance was the presence of a potentially significant abnormality overlooked. In that individual, THC visualized a distal common duct stricture.[126] Thus, even though it has been shown that stones can be present in normal caliber common ducts in 5 to 13 per cent of cases,[124, 127-129] it appears that, in the symptomatic post-cholecystectomy patient, retained stones are most likely to result in functionally detectable abnormalities even though their ductal caliber is unaltered (see Post-cholecystectomy: "Complete" Ductal Obstructive Pattern). The ability of this functional procedure to detect the presence of obstruction to bile flow prior to the development of morphologic changes appears to be a significant advantage of the cholescintigram when compared with the purely anatomic sonogram.[102, 126] Therefore, the reported 5 to 10 per cent "failure" rate for sonography in detecting partial extrahepatic obstruction because of the presence of normal caliber common bile ducts cannot be extrapolated to cholescintigraphy, in which dynamic, functional information is obtained that yields additional diagnostic parameters such as delayed biliary-to-bowel transit and abnormal ductal time activity dynamics. A similar observation was made in 1957 with intravenous cholangiography when it was observed that in only 14.5 per cent of cases was size able to be used as the sole criterion to indicate the presence or absence of obstruction. Additional criteria were required in the remaining 85.5 per cent of cases for the test to be diagnostic.[130]

Although some instances of surgically correctible extrahepatic obstruction may be so mild or intermittent as to have no significant effect on the flow of bile, in our experience it appears that this would be a rare exception in the symptomatic post-cholecystectomy patient. Scintigraphy seems to have fewer false-negative post-cholecystectomy cases than sonography. This appears to relate to the fact that in partial ductal obstruction the functional changes occur before the morphological changes.

Ductal Dilatation with Functional Patency

For many years, common duct dilatation was erroneously considered to be a normal compensatory phenomenon following cholecystectomy.[131, 132] However, through the decades, numerous studies have been performed that confirm that post-cholecystectomy common duct dilatation only occurs when there is pathologic obstruction to bile flow.[130, 133-138] Additionally, evidence has been presented that indicates that there is no causal relationship between bile duct exploration and postoperative common hepatic duct dilatation.[139] There-

fore, visualization of a dilated common duct after cholecystectomy indicates that the duct is abnormal. However, without the benefit of a normal preoperative study for comparison, the only thing that can be stated with certainty is that an obstruction was present at some time.[140] A common duct may never return to normal caliber even though the obstruction has been relieved. It frequently does not decrease significantly in size after common duct stones have been removed.[136, 139] Even after the performance of successful surgical drainage procedures, ductal dilatation has been reported to persist.[129] It has been shown that no correlation exists between post-cholecystectomy distress and common duct caliber.[136] Cholescintigraphic evaluation of a large series of post-cholecystectomy patients confirms that when a dilated common bile duct is the only identifiable abnormality, it usually represents residual enlargement from a previous obstruction (85 per cent) (Fig. 8–18). (A word of caution is indicated here. The term "dilatation" used in reference to cholescintigraphy does not have the same implication of precision as when it is applied to sonography. With nuclear imaging, the apparent size of a structure depends, in part, on the specific activity of radiotracer in that structure. Therefore, the impression of ductal dilatation on a cholescintigram should be based on persistence of this finding throughout the study. Even though a rough estimate of common duct size can be

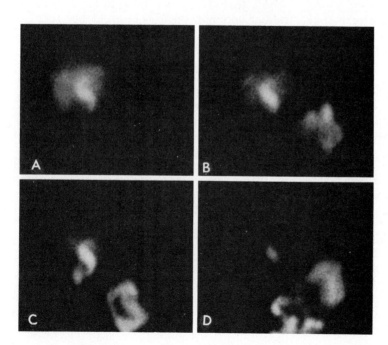

Figure 8–18. Dilated common duct with functional patency in a post-cholecystectomy patient. The dilated common bile duct is identified on the 15 minute scintiphoto *(A)*. Intestinal excretion is present within the first 30 minutes *(B)*. Additionally, normal ductal time activity dynamics are observed as evidenced by the fact that the common bile duct is less intense at 90 minutes *(D)* when compared with the 45-minute view *(C)*.

obtained with a cobalt-57 "snake" marker, approximating it to be "smaller or larger" than 10 mm, this type of anatomic measurement is more appropriately delegated to sonography.)

Although an obstructing lesion may be significant enough to result in ductal dilatation, normal bile flow dynamics will be preserved in 15 per cent of cases. This observation is consistent with the sphincteric physiology that has been described in the literature.[141-144] With an incomplete obstruction, net bile outflow is preserved because the maximum secretory pressure of the liver is able to overcome the obstruction.[142] It may be that a normal biliary-to-bowel transit time is preserved because sphincteric dilatation occurs, resulting in a decreased resistance to bile flow.

Therefore, it appears that when a cholescintigraphic pattern of ductal dilatation with normal biliary-to-bowel transit is observed, even though it is most likely to be a morphologically unobstructed common bile duct,[130, 145] further evaluation is indicated (e.g., PTC or ERCP). This is recommended because potentially serious sequelae may ensue if an abnormality such as retained common duct stones is overlooked. In the few cases in which scintigraphy demonstrated the presence of a dilated functionally patent duct in the presence of existing pathology, all patients had retained common duct stones.

In view of this limitation, it appears that if the ducts are dilated, noting the first time at which activity is identified in the duodenum is less significant than observing other findings such as the presence of persistent photon-deficient areas within the duct or abnormal time activity dynamics (see Partial Ductal Obstruction Patterns). Even though intestinal activity is identified in less than one hour, visualization of a duct that is persistently dilated to a specific point on multiple sequential images should suggest the presence of an obstructing lesion. Typically, the duct will appear enlarged and more intense in activity proximal to the level of obstruction than distally. This is even more significant when a persistent photo-deficient zone is noted within the duct at the level of presumed obstruction. Identification of a persistent photon-deficient zone is most common secondary to the presence of retained common duct stones; however, strictures, tumors, and enlarged lymph nodes can also have the identical appearance (Fig. 8–19).

Serial scintigraphy is useful. The only time that the isolated abnormal scintigraphic finding of ductal dilatation can be interpreted as pathognomonic of obstruction is when serial cho-

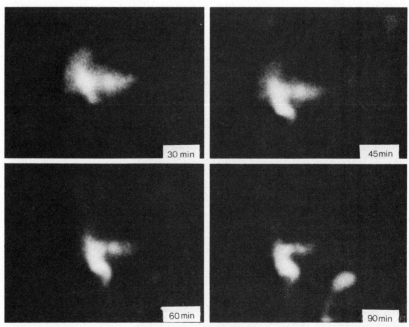

Figure 8–19. Dilated CBD with delayed biliary-to-bowel transit time. The markedly dilated ducts are quite apparent. No bowel activity was noted until 90 minutes. The persistent defect in the medial portion of the left hepatic duct was confirmed to be secondary to a stone on transhepatic cholangiography. (Reprinted with permission from Weissmann et al.: Semin. Nucl. Med. *12*:27, 1982.)

lescintigrams demonstrate a progression; for instance, visualization of a recent change from normal to dilated, or increased ectasia from one study to the next. If, when compared with a preoperative cholescintigram, the common duct appears to have increased in size, it should not be misdiagnosed as "compensatory dilatation." The presence of ductal pathology should be strongly suggested.

Partial Ductal Obstructive Patterns

The cholescintigraphic patterns that correlate with varying degrees of partial common duct obstruction include delayed biliary-to-bowel transit, abnormal ductal time activity dynamics, delayed ductal visualization, and complete absence of ductal and intestinal activity.

Visualization of dilated ducts in less than one hour with delay in bile transit from the common duct to the duodenum at greater than an hour correlates with the presence of obstructing pathology. Strictures, choledocholithiasis, and metastatic tumor have all been identified as etiologies of this cholescintigraphic pattern.[126]

Another finding that correlates strongly with the presence of partial common duct obstruction is the observation of abnormal time activity dynamics of dilated ducts. This may be identified in conjunction with normal biliary-to-bowel transit, delayed biliary-to-bowel transit, and/or delayed visualization of the di-

lated common bile duct. As discussed previously, when the common duct is dilated, the presence of duodenal activity within the first 60 minutes does not exclude the possibility of partial obstruction. The presence of abnormal ductal time activity dynamics is a much more significant diagnostic parameter. It is based on the fact that an unobstructed duct retains labeled bile for a significantly shorter period of time than does an obstructed duct. Hence, the degree of activity within a normal duct should decrease when the two-hour scintiphoto is compared with the one-hour scintiphoto (Fig. 8–18). If, instead, a duct appears more intense on the later scintiphoto, obstruction is most likely present (Fig. 8–20). This finding is similar to the time density retention concept that Wise, Johnston, and Salzman[130] reported and others confirmed[146, 147] for intravenous cholangiography. The reliability of this parameter is dependent upon two factors: an apparently normal blood clearance rate by the hepatocytes, and the absence of a safety valve, e.g., a gallbladder or fistula.[130] This parameter can also be utilized to detect the presence of partial intrahepatic obstruction. If the right or left hepatic duct demonstrates increased activity at one and one-half or two hours when compared with the one-hour view, then the diagnosis of a localized ductal obstruction should be made. To be able to make a valid comparison between serially obtained scintiphotos, it is essential that careful attention be paid to tech-

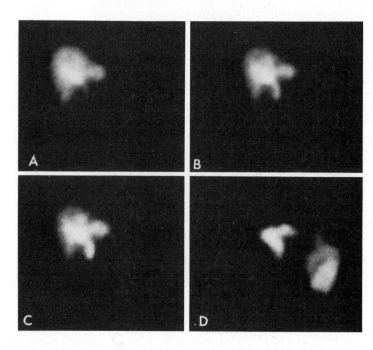

Figure 8–20. Post-cholecystectomy patient with partial common duct obstruction. Abnormal ductal time activity dynamics and delayed biliary-to-bowel transit. Activity within the common bile duct is most intense on the 2-hour view *(D)* when compared with the scintiphotos obtained at 45 minutes *(B)* and 60 minutes *(C)*. These findings were secondary to the presence of retained common duct stones.

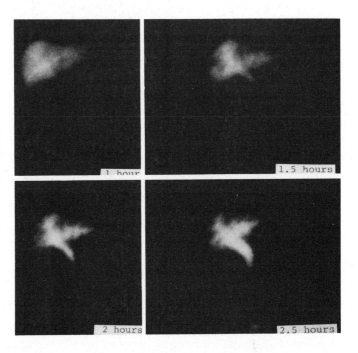

Figure 8–21. Post-cholecystectomy patient with partial functional common duct obstruction. Abnormal ductal time activity dynamics with delayed visualization of a dilated common bile duct. Up to one hour, no significant common duct activity was noted. Beginning with the one hour, and more so on the one and one-half hour view, a dilated common duct starts to visualize. The activity level in the duct at two and three hours appears progressively greater than that at 1 or 1½ hours. Retained common duct stones were identified at surgery. (Reprinted with permission from Weissmann et al.: Semin. Nucl. Med. *12*:27, 1982.)

nique. If images are obtained by setting for a fixed number of counts, care should be taken to keep the patient's position and degree of intestinal shielding unchanged. This is readily accomplished.[126] Then, if the intensity in ductal activity between one and one-half and two hours appears equal to or greater than that observed at one hour, it should be considered abnormal and indicative of partial ductal obstruction, regardless of the time that Tc-99m IDA is first identified to pass through the sphincter of Oddi into the duodenum.

Abnormal ductal time activity is an even stronger indication of partial obstruction when observed in conjunction with delayed biliary-to-bowel transit and/or delayed visualization of the common duct (Fig. 8–21).[126]

Nonvisualization of the ducts with delayed biliary-to-bowel transit is rare, having been identified in only 1 out of 125 cases. Nonetheless, its significance is described for completeness. In one individual, activity was first identified within the duodenum at 90 minutes, despite prompt hepatic uptake. Throughout the study, there was no evidence of common duct visualization. Subsequently, transhepatic cholangiography and surgery revealed the presence of carcinoma of the common hepatic duct with multiple levels of obstruction. The failure of cholescintigraphy to visualize the common duct was probably secondary to the presence of multiple levels of obstruction high within the biliary tree, which meant that proximal compensatory dilatation could not be scintigraphically detected. It should be noted that in many cases of high ductal obstruction at or above the level of the common hepatic duct proximal dilatation and normal-appearing distal ducts have been identified scintigraphically. Occasionally localized altered time activity dynamics and/or a persistent photon-deficient area has been identified separating the two regions.

"Complete" Ductal Obstructive Patterns

Persistent nonvisualization of the common bile duct with absent or markedly delayed visualization of the intestine (between two and four hours) strongly suggests the presence of virtually complete common bile duct obstruction. The significance of this cholescintigraphic pattern is comparable to that identified in patients who have been studied for suspected acute cholecystitis. Complete obstruction occurs when the pressure at which bile secretion and backflow into the blood and lymph reaches equilibrium. This occurs when the pressure necessary to bypass the existing obstruction is greater than the maximum secretory pressure of the liver.[142]

We have found that the scintigraphic findings observed after three to four hours have not altered our diagnostic impression of the presence of a significant common duct obstruction, since eventually some Tc-99m IDA may pass the obstruction in sufficient concentration to be detected. Therefore, whether or not some intestinal activity is noted between two and four hours or beyond does not obviate the need for further work-up for obstruction.[102, 126]

Similar to what we have observed in patients studied for suspected acute cholecystitis who exhibited this cholescintigraphic pattern, sonography is only useful in these cases if the findings are positive.[102] A patient with this obstructive cholescintigraphic pattern and a "normal" sonogram should be further evaluated with either ERCP or THC. This obstructive cholescintigraphic pattern is strongly suggestive, but not pathognomonic, of obstruction because other abnormalities that create functional obstruction have also been occasionally identified to result in this finding. These abnormalities have included cholangitis and ampullitis. The pattern becomes pathognomonic when it is combined with identification of dilated ducts in the region of the porta hepatis, which can be identified as Y-shaped or branching zones of photon deficiency.

A final point regarding this cholescintigraphic pattern is worth mentioning. A similar finding has recently been described in patients with intrahepatic cholestasis.[148] The patient population recorded in this study by Kuni, Klingensmith, and Fritzberg appears quite different clinically. They were being evaluated for cholestasis. They were not being studied for suspected acute cholecystitis or "post-cholecystectomy syndrome" and did not have pain as a feature of their clinical presentation.

Serial Evaluation of Ductal Obstruction

Serial scintigraphy has proved useful in evaluating the natural evolution of biliary pathology as well as the response to treatment. The performance of serial examinations in patients with ductal obstruction has confirmed our impression that the scintigraphic findings described in the preceding section represent a continuum of patterns that are indicative of varying degrees of occlusion. Changes identified have included a progression in the abnormal finding, such as more delayed excretion into the intestine, as well as a combination of an increasing number of abnormal findings. The progression identified has included a more prolonged delay in intestinal visualization, to ductal dilatation with delayed biliary-to-bowel transit, to abnormal time activity dynamics, to delayed visualization of dilated ducts, and finally to the complete obstructive pattern.

Detection of Cystic Duct Remnants

Since a cystic duct remnant can become a diseased gallbladder of small size, which can result in persistent or recurrent symptoms,[121, 122, 149-163] it is important to detect its presence. For instance, failure to appreciate the presence of a cystic duct remnant may result in incomplete surgery in a patient who is being treated for choledocholithiasis,[163] since remnant stones may become common bile duct stones.[121, 164] Cholescintigraphy has proved to be one of the most sensitive tests available for the detection of the presence of a cystic duct remnant (Fig. 8–22).[126] This is not surprising in view of the already well-established sensitivity of the cholescintigraphic method in being able to demonstrate cystic duct patency.[27, 28, 44-47] It has proved essential to obtain delayed views in all post-cholecystectomy patients, regardless of the completely normal appearance of the study in the first hour. This is done to demonstrate the presence of a cystic duct remnant or bile leak, which would otherwise remain undetected in a significant percentage of patients.[126] We continue the study as long as activity remains identifiable within the hepatobiliary system (when the intestinal activity is shielded) such that there could still conceivably be delayed visualization of either abnormality, with the maximum being four hours.

Evaluation of the Biliary Enteric Bypass Patient

The postoperative complications that result from gastrointestinal bypass surgery usually are obstruction and/or loss of integrity of the anastomosis. Cholescintigraphy provides a noninvasive means of evaluating anastomotic patency as well as a very sensitive method for detecting the presence of biliary leakage.

Limitations of Other Available Modalities

In the past, the upper gastrointestinal series was the primary method used for evaluating bypass patency. However, this is a nonphysiologic procedure that requires the flow of contrast retrograde to the normal flow of bile, and the diagnosis is inferred from an indirect sign. Failure to demonstrate the reflux of barium into the biliary tree is considered a harbinger of anastomotic obstruction.

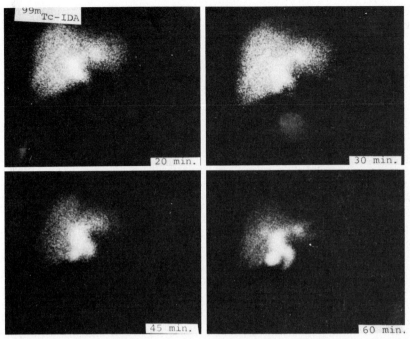

Figure 8–22. Cystic duct remnant. The presence of a cystic duct remnant was detected by cholescintigraphy in this patient who complained of recurrent upper right quadrant pain 26 years post-cholecystectomy. An IVC did not visualize the remnant. At surgery it was found to contain multiple stones.

To achieve sufficient iodine concentration for common duct visualization, the intravenous cholangiogram requires the presence of a competent sphincter of Oddi. Since the functioning sphincter has been bypassed in these patients, IVC cannot be utilized for biliary visualization.

If a cholangio-intestinal anastomosis has been performed involving the duodenum, then ERCP can be utilized. However, if the biliary enteric reconstruction involves a more distal loop of bowel, such as hepaticojejunostomy, or if there have been other alterations in the normal anatomy, such as Whipple resection (pancreaticoduodenectomy), then the anastomosis cannot be reached by the endoscope and ERCP is technically not feasible.

Sonographic evaluation is also difficult in these patients. Bypassing the sphincter of Oddi enables air to rise freely into the biliary radicles. Since air is a source of acoustic interference, this significantly interferes with sonography's ability to visualize the ductal system and liver parenchyma. In these patients, a reduction in the sensitivity of sonography to about 50 per cent has been reported. Additionally, if dilated biliary radicles are identified, the problems are the same as those described in the post-cholecystectomy patient. The presence of dilatation only indicates that

obstruction was present at some time, and it does not necessarily mean that the obstruction still exists. Thus, even though the obstructing lesion may have been successfully bypassed, the dilatation may remain permanently. This is where the advantage of cholescintigraphy as a functional imaging modality becomes evident.

Advantages of Cholescintigraphic Bypass Patency

Cholescintigraphy is the only noninvasive procedure available that is capable of accurately assessing anastomotic function in an antegrade "physiologic" manner regardless of the level of the cholangio-intestinal anastomosis (Fig. 8–23). If an individual has not had such reconstructive surgery, then the role of Tc-99m IDA imaging in evaluating cholestasis is a variable one (see Cholestasis).[126, 165] However, cholescintigraphy clearly has a distinct advantage in the evaluation of the jaundiced bypass patient. Not only can it be utilized to evaluate for bypass patency, but it is also capable of providing information about the integrity of the anastomosis. Tc-99m IDA cholescintigraphy is one of the most sensitive

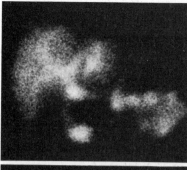
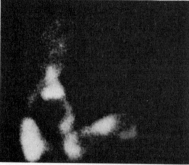

Figure 8–23. Patent biliary-enteric anastomosis. Free flow of the Tc-99m IDA through a choledochoduodenostomy in one patient *(A)* and a choledochojejunostomy in another patient *(B)* are clearly demonstrated. (Reprinted with permission from Weissmann et al.: Semin. Nucl. Med. *12*:27, 1982.)

Table 8–16. CHOLESCINTIGRAPHIC PATTERNS IN EVALUATING BILIARY ENTERIC ANASTOMOSES*

Normal intestinal excretion in <1 hr without ductal dilatation
Intestinal excretion in <1 hr with ductal dilatation
Intestinal excretion at 1 hr or longer
  Without evidence of ductal enlargement
  With ductal enlargement
  With ductal enlargement and abnormal time-activity dynamics
  With delayed visualization, dilated ducts, and abnormal time-activity dynamics
"Complete" ductal obstructive pattern
Biliary leakage

*Reprinted with permission from Weissmann et al.: Semin. Nucl. Med. *12*:27, 1982.

procedures available for detecting biliary leakage[126, 166] (see Bile Leak Detection).

To intelligently evaluate and interpret the studies performed on patients who have undergone reconstructive surgery, it is imperative that the case be discussed with the surgeon prior to imaging, because his surgical alterations result in a loss of the normal anatomic landmarks.

Cholescintigraphic Evaluation of Bypass Patency

The cholescintigraphic patterns that we have identified in patients who have undergone biliary enteric anastomoses are summarized in Table 8–16.

Patent Cholangio-Intestinal Anastomotic Patterns

The experience of several different investigators has indicated that identification of intestinal activity within the first hour after injection of Tc-99m HIDA or Tc-99m DISIDA confirms that a biliary enteric bypass is patent.[126, 167, 168] The advantages of cholescintigraphy in comparison with other available imaging procedures is illustrated by the patient whose study is shown in Figure 8–23B. This patient has sclerosing cholangitis, for which a choledochojejunostomy had been performed 30 months previously. He presented with progressive hyperbilirubinemia and alkaline phosphatasemia with a resultant differential diagnosis between anastomotic obstruction and progressive intrahepatic cholestasis. Since the former possibility would be amenable to surgical revision, it was necessary to evaluate his anastomosis. PTC was technically impossible because of the sclerosis of his intrahepatic ducts. ERCP was not feasible because he had a jejunal anastomosis. Ultrasonography was nondiagnostic because of the interference of the air in the biliary tree. However, in view of the sclerosis of his intrahepatic ducts, even if the biliary radicles could have been visualized, identification of a nondilated ductal system would not have excluded the possibility of anastomotic obstruction. Tc-99m HIDA imaging was diagnostic despite the presence of biliary cirrhosis with resultant abnormal liver chemistries. Demonstration of the free flow of labeled bile through the anastomosis into the jejunum within 30 minutes documented anastomotic patency. This confirmed that his rising alkaline phosphatase level was secondary to progression of the intrahepatic sclerosing cholangitis and that surgical revision would not be helpful. (It should be noted that cholescintigraphy was of diagnostic utility in this instance because it was able to successfully establish that the patient's bypass was patent. If, however, an obstructive pattern was identified, the procedure would not have been as useful. In view of this patient's underlying hepatic disease, failure to demonstrate intestinal visualization could not have been considered pathognomonic of obstruction.)

Identification of a dilated ductal system with visualization of intestinal activity in less than

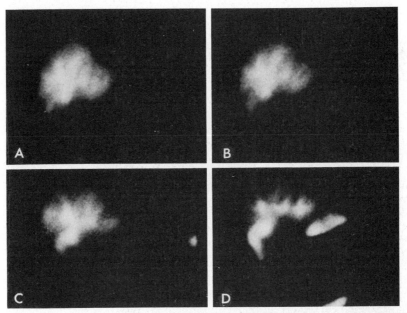

Figure 8–24. Patent choledochoduodenostomy. Dilated biliary radicles with free flow of Tc-99m IDA. Scintiphotos obtained at 10 *(A)*, 15 *(B)*, and 25 *(C)* minutes visualized the dilated biliary tree with progression of labeled bile through the choledochoduodenostomy anastomosis. At the end of the first hour *(D)*, most of the Tc-99m IDA had been excreted from the liver into the biliary tree and through the anastomosis into the intestine. The majority of the intestinal activity was shielded by a lead apron to better visualize the dilated intrahepatic biliary radicles. The bypass was performed for obstructing choledocholithiasis. Despite the success of the surgery in relieving the obstruction, the biliary tree remained ectatic. This case illustrates that a dilated biliary system is not necessarily an obstructed system.

one hour strongly suggests that the anastomosis was successful in bypassing the existing obstruction (Fig. 8–24).

Partial Obstructive Patterns

Observation of delayed intestinal excretion until one hour or longer as an isolated scintigraphic finding is suggestive of anastomotic obstruction. However, it is conceivable that a similar cholescintigraphic pattern could be identified in patients with significant hepatocellular compromise. Therefore, visualization of delayed transit into the bowel without associated ductal enlargement should be interpreted with caution in individuals who are known to have underlying hepatic parenchymal disease.

Persistent enlargement of the ductal system in association with delayed transit into the intestine indicates the likelihood of obstructed anastomosis and the need for additional evaluation. The presence of abnormal ductal time activity dynamics further reinforces the likelihood of obstruction. Additional identification of delayed visualization of dilated ducts is further evidence for the presence of significant common duct obstruction.

"Complete" Obstructive Patterns

As described in post-cholecystectomy patients, identification of prompt hepatic uptake with nonvisualization of the common duct and absent or markedly delayed excretion into the intestine is strongly suggestive of the presence of a significant common duct obstruction. However, if the liver chemistries are elevated and the hepatic uptake is slow and poor, secondary to compromised hepatic function, then a nonobstructive cholestatic etiology also has to be considered. Nonetheless, when we have observed this cholescintigraphic pattern with slow, poor uptake of Tc-99m IDA, the cause of the abnormality has remained ductal obstruction, with associated hepatocellular dysfunction secondary to progressive malignant obstruction.

Evaluation of Other Types of Gastrointestinal Anastomoses

Tc-99m IDA imaging is also useful in obtaining diagnostic information regarding the patency and integrity of other surgical anastomoses involving the gastrointestinal tract such as Billroth II, Billroth I, and Whipple resections. For instance, it is well suited for antegrade evaluation of afferent loop patency.[167, 169] In the presence of afferent loop or inlet-outlet obstruction, transit from the common bile duct into the "A" loop is normal; however, there is progressive accumulation of technetium-99m labeled bile within this proximal loop. This has been observed to be significant

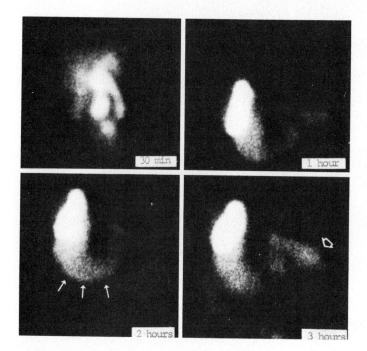

Figure 8–25. Afferent loop obstruction following Billroth II gastroenterostomy. The gallbladder and bile ducts are visualized on the 30-minute scintophoto. Starting at 1 hour, there is progressive filling of a very dilated afferent loop (arrows) to the level of the gastric pouch (open arrowhead). (Reprinted with permission from Weissmann et al.: Semin. Nucl. Med. *12*:27, 1982.)

when the activity persists within the dilated loop for more than two hours (Fig. 8–25).[167] Patency of the afferent loop is confirmed by normal filling and emptying of the proximal limb with no evidence of dilatation and progressive hold-up of activity. When diffuse hepatocellular disease is present, slow hepatic uptake with commensurately slow excretion into the bile ducts as well as afferent and efferent loops is identified.

BILE LEAK DETECTION

A significant reduction in morbidity and mortality can be achieved by the early detection of postoperative or post-traumatic biliary disruption. Cholescintigraphy has been observed to be an extremely sensitive method for detecting the presence of a bile leak, secondary to penetrating or nonpenetrating trauma, as well as its location and extent. Antegrade visualization of the route of bile flow can yield information of potential diagnostic significance. Additionally, the response to medical or surgical therapy can be successfully evaluated by serial scintigraphic examinations. Current methodology has important advantages over I-131 RB techniques[170-173] as well as the available radiographic procedures. In the past, rose bengal has been shown to be more sensitive than conventional contrast radiographic procedures in the detection of cholecysto-enteric fistulas, and Tc-99m IDA imaging is even

more sensitive than I-131 RB. The enhanced anatomic resolution afforded by the Tc-99m label enables delineation of the actual site and extent of a bile leak. Manipulations for detecting and quantitating the presence of a bile leak, such as measuring the presence of radioactivity in ascitic fluid after I-131 RB injection, are no longer necessary.[172] Although the use of I-131 RB has been documented to be more sensitive than conventional contrast radiography in the detection of biliary leakage, it is less sensitive and more limited when compared with radiographic procedures that utilize the injection of contrast directly into a fistula.[170] These roentgenographic studies currently in use are nonphysiologic. For instance, the percutaneous injection of contrast material into a fistula involves insertion of a catheter and injection under pressure. Hence, the contrast material is being forced to flow retrograde to the normal course of biliary drainage. Delineation of the entire extent of the tract may be obscured by the presence of debris within the fistula. The advantage of Tc-99m IDA scintigraphy is its ability to yield diagnostically significant physiologic information. It is capable of visualizing the actual aberrant course of bile flow in the antegrade direction. In comparison with intravenous cholangiography, it is not limited by the same technical factors that can interfere with the visualization of biliary extravasation by the routine radiographic techniques. External radiation detection devices such as the Anger camera are capable of detecting significantly smaller concentrations of radiotracer than the concentration of iodine that would have to accumulate to be detectable radiographically.[28] This translates into a much greater sensitivity for cholescintigraphy when compared with conventional radiography for the detection of biliary leakage. Additionally, the patient's body habitus, presence of overlying bowel gas, overlying costochondral calcification,[174] or lack of an external communication does not pose a technical problem for cholescintigraphy as it does for radiography. Sonography and computed tomography can identify the presence of a cystic collection or free fluid within the abdomen. However, they are unable to definitively establish the presence or absence of a communication with the biliary system. Taking all of these factors into consideration, it seems that Tc-99m IDA scintigraphy should be a sensitive technique for detecting biliary disruption, and this has been observed by numerous investigators to be true clinically.[126, 167, 175-178]

Further documentation of the sensitivity of cholescintigraphy in the detection of biliary extravasation is indicated by the fact that in the evaluation of a large series of patients no leak was overlooked.[126] Additionally, in one case, cholescintigraphy detected the presence of a bile leak with a subcapsular collection seven days prior to the onset of symptoms. This patient was studied immediately prior to discharge, after a "routine cholecystectomy," as part of a study evaluating the "normal" post-cholecystectomy patient. The presence of a persistent area of increased activity at the inferior aspect of the right lobe of the liver, which became more intense with time, was identified (Fig. 8–26). In view of the fact that the patient was completely asymptomatic, had no other objective evidence to indicate the presence of an abnormality, and had had his T-tube recently removed, the clinical significance of this observation was considered uncertain, and no treatment was administered. Seven days later, he returned to the emergency room complaining of nausea and severe upper right quadrant pain. He was febrile. Under ultrasonic guidance, a subcapsular bilious collection was successfully drained.

Examination of our postoperative patients revealed the ability of cholescintigraphy to detect the presence of biliary leakage with a wide variety of etiologies. These included pa-

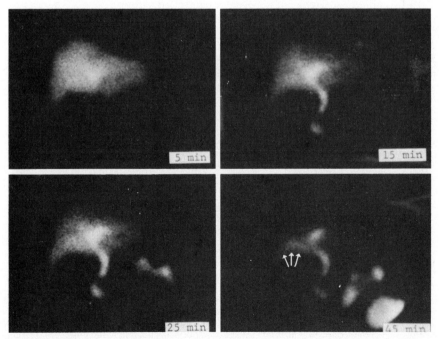

Figure 8–26. Post-cholecystectomy bile leak with a subcapsular collection identified seven days prior to the time that the patient became symptomatic. There is prompt hepatic uptake within the first 5 minutes, with visualization of the common duct and duodenum at 15 minutes. At this time, a blush of activity in the region of the inferior aspect of the right lobe of the liver began to be identified. It became more apparent with time as a contained collection of bile, seen at 45 minutes (arrows). This collection persisted and became more intense over the 4 hours of examination. A subcapsular collection of bile was drained under ultrasonographic guidance seven days after the cholescintigram.

tients with retained common duct stones that created "complete" common duct obstruction, cholangiocarcinoma, and metastatic invasion. When the collection is intrahepatic, it typically appears as a photon-deficient area initially, which becomes "isodense" and then more intense in activity than the surrounding hepatic parenchyma with time. Critical to the detection of bile leaks in the postoperative patients was the routine utilization of delayed views beyond one hour despite the "normal" appearance of the study within the first hour.

In cases in which surgical repair is considered, it will be necessary to obtain a better anatomical "road map" with the aid of procedures such as transhepatic cholangiography. However, it appears that, in many instances, cholescintigraphy's disadvantage of limited anatomic resolution is offset by its advantage of being a noninvasive "physiologic" means of visualizing biliary disruption. Antegrade visualization of biliary extravasation has the advantage of yielding information of potential prognostic significance.[126, 167, 175] Evaluation of the preferential route of bile flow has proved to be a useful indicator of the potential response to conservative management. If most of the bile is being excreted through the normal anatomic pathway, e.g., into the duodenum or through a patent anastomosis, with a much smaller proportion (which may only be detectable on the delayed views) taking the aberrant course, then it appears reasonable to conclude that the bile leak will respond to conservative therapy (Fig. 8–27). Serial scintigraphy has been useful in documenting the favorable response to therapy, e.g., external drainage.[126] If, on the other hand, the majority of bile is taking the aberrant course, then surgical intervention will most likely be necessary (Fig. 8–28). Thus, although the degree of cholescintigraphic resolution limits the ability to precisely locate the origin of the bile leak, it has the advantage of being one of the most sensitive methods available for detecting the presence of a bile leak and being able to estimate the relative proportion flowing normally versus that accumulating outside the liver, biliary tract, and intestine. Another type of information that has been considered to be of prognostic significance is documenting that an intrahepatic cavity (e.g., abscess) is freely communicating with the biliary system. In a reported case in which this was identified, the decision to avoid surgical intervention and allow time for normal drainage to occur via the biliary tract, following removal of a common duct stone, was based on the scintigraphic

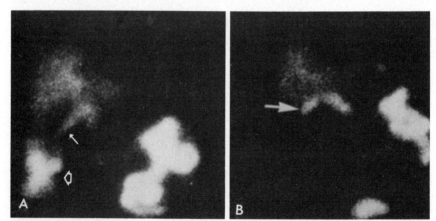

Figure 8–27. Choledochoduodenostomy with an anastomotic leak. *A*, Scintiphotos obtained during the first hour (not shown) demonstrated free flow of Tc-99m IDA into the intestine. On this view, obtained at 2½ hours, an abnormal tract of activity is identified extending laterally from the region of the anastomosis (arrow). It is leading to an abnormal collection of activity in the right mid abdomen (open arrowhead). The activity in the left was noted to be contiguous with the duodenum and filled progressively, correctly indicating activity within the jejunum. This patient was ten days post-cholecystectomy and choledochoduodenostomy for acute cholecystitis and choledocholithiasis. His clinical condition was quite poor. Since cholescintigraphy revealed the preferential route of bile flow via the anastomosis with the bile leak only detectable on the more delayed views, it was decided to treat the patient with conservative management. *B*, Cholescintigraphy performed 11 days after the institution of external drainage for treatment documented a significant improvement. This scintiphoto obtained at 3 hours demonstrates that there is only a small amount of activity extending from the anastomosis into the cavity that had formed previously (arrow). Therefore, evaluation of the preferential group of bile flow in this case correctly indicated that the patient would respond to conservative management.

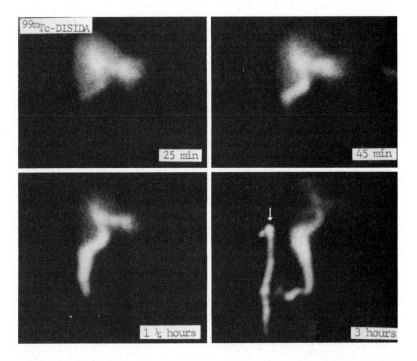

Figure 8–28. Biliary leakage following cholecystectomy. An abnormal tract of activity is seen along the inferior liver border on the 45-minute study. Subsequently, at 1½ hours, it proceeds inferiorly in a vertical band along the right lateral portion of the abdomen and finally drains outward to the skin on the 3-hour study. (A linear radioactive source demarcates the skin surface on the 3-hour view [arrow].) Cholescintigraphy demonstrated that the bile was preferentially taking the aberrant course, with no identifiable intestinal activity. Surgical repair was performed. The leak was secondary to accidental transsection of the right hepatic duct at cholecystectomy. (Reprinted with permission from Weissmann et al.: Semin. Nucl. Med. *12*:27, 1982.)

findings. This reasoning appeared to be correct in view of the fact that the patient reportedly did well.[176]

Cholescintigraphy is also well suited for the evaluation of patients who have had blunt abdominal trauma, since no external communication is required to obtain the study (Fig. 8–29).[175-179] The possibility of biliary tract injury should be considered in any patient who has had blunt (or penetrating) abdominal trauma. Post-traumatic bile cysts have been identified to occur weeks, months, and even years after the initial insult.[180-182] Typically, a patient who appears to have recovered from the initial injury will complain of intermittent abdominal pain, distention, fever, or jaundice. These signs and symptoms develop gradually over a period of weeks to months. Usually, these traumatic cysts are large and involve the right lobe of the liver. They may or may not

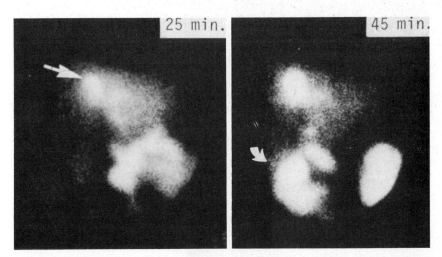

Figure 8–29. Post-traumatic bile cyst. This study was obtained 36 days after the patient was hit by a truck. The trauma was nonpenetrating. On the 25-minute view, a post-traumatic bile containing cyst is identified in the region of the right hepatic duct (arrow). It filled progressively with time, being more intense on the 45-minute view. (Incidentally, the gallbladder is visualized inferiorly [curved arrow].)

communicate with the biliary system. If a cyst that communicates with the system ruptures, free bile within the peritoneal cavity results. These findings can be detected by cholescintigraphy. Another situation in which the presence of free bile within the peritoneum has been detected cholescintigraphically has been secondary to perforation of the gallbladder.[178]

CHOLESTASIS

The Screening Procedure of Choice: Cholescintigraphy Versus Ultrasonography

Ultrasonography continues to be the best noninvasive imaging procedure for the evaluation of cholestasis, particularly in cases of chronic biliary obstruction. Not only is it a sensitive and accurate method for detecting ductal dilatation, but, when obstruction is present, the level and cause frequently can also be determined.[183-186] However, not all dilated ducts are functionally obstructed, and not all functionally obstructed ducts are dilated. Additionally, the accuracy and reliability of sonography is more apt to vary from institution to institution, because it is more dependent on physician and technician expertise as well as the quality of the available instrumentation. Thus, with the added ability to supply impor-

tant functional information concerning bile flow as well as being less operator dependent, cholescintigraphy has proved useful and even superior in evaluating cholestasis in selected cases. More commonly, sonography and scintigraphy have proved useful as complementary procedures, combining the anatomic with the functional information obtained by each.

When necessary, cholescintigraphy can be utilized as a screening procedure for cholestasis. This has been of greatest value when sonography has been overburdened with regard to patient scheduling. Tc-99m IDA imaging can accurately confirm the presence of pre- or intrahepatic ("medical") jaundice by documenting the presence of a normal patent biliary system. This obviates the need for additional imaging studies and indicates that the diagnostic work-up should progress along other lines, e.g., liver biopsy. Additionally, in some cases of extrahepatic ("surgical") jaundice, cholescintigraphy can confirm the presence of obstruction and identify the level of the abnormality.

Scintigraphic Patterns of Cholestasis

Tc-99m IDA analogs, such as the diisopropyl derivative, that enable visualization and documentation of the presence of patent biliary systems in patients with marked hyperbiliru-

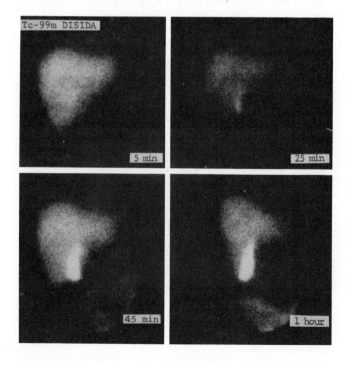

Figure 8–30. Nonobstructive jaundice. Normal Tc-99m DISIDA cholescintigram documenting a patent biliary system in a patient whose bilirubin level was 18.5 mg/100 ml. Prompt hepatic uptake is identified within the first 5 minutes, followed by normal visualization of the common bile duct, gallbladder, and intestine within the first 45 to 60 minutes.

Figure 8–31. Partial obstruction of the proximal common bile duct with a Courvoisier's gallbladder, secondary to metastatic carcinoma. Cholescintigraphy revealed the presence and proximal level of biliary obstruction. Delayed visualization of the dilated central intrahepatic ducts with obstruction at the level of the proximal common duct was demonstrated. The dilated cystic duct and Courvoisier's gallbladder filled progressively between 2 and 4 hours. The area in the mid gallbladder, which was initially photon deficient at 2 hours (open arrowhead), corresponds to the position of gallstones that were demonstrated sonographically. In this case, the presence and extent of ductal dilatation were not appreciated by ultrasound. Despite the fact that sonography revealed the presence of a mass in the head of the pancreas, gallbladder dilatation, and cholelithiasis, dilatation of the biliary radicles was not identified. Several attempts at percutaneous transhepatic cholangiography were unsuccessful. At laparotomy, pancreatic carcinoma with multiple metastases throughout the liver was noted.

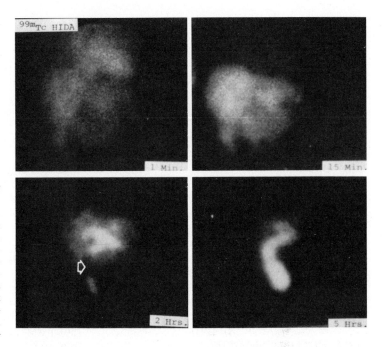

It was felt that the tremendous extent of the space-occupying metastatic disease prevented dilatation of the more peripheral hepatic ducts. This prevented opacification of the ductal system by transhepatic cholangiography as well as interfering with sonographic visualization.

binemia successfully eliminate the possibility of biliary obstruction when a normal cholescintigram is observed (Fig. 8–30).

Identification of a persistent photon-deficient area with proximal dilatation and a normal distal biliary tree indicates the presence and level of an obstructing lesion. In a clinical situation in which the nature of the abnormality is known, e.g., lymphoma or the presence of a known primary malignancy, obtaining this information may be all that is necessary to institute treatment.[18] In clinical situations in which the etiology of the abnormality is not as well defined, additional imaging studies are necessary. On occasion, cholescintigraphy can be useful in identifying the presence of a partial ductal obstruction when other modalities have failed. For instance, in patients who have an underlying disorder, such as sclerosing cholangitis or metastatic liver disease, that prevents ductal dilatation in response to obstruction, the degree of obstruction may not be fully appreciated with procedures such as sonography. By the same token, the nondilated obstructed ducts may make transhepatic cholangiography technically difficult (Fig. 8–31).[155]

The significance of the "complete" or virtually complete common duct obstructive pattern as a sensitive, early indicator of obstruc-

tion, consisting of prompt hepatic uptake with persistent nonvisualization of the biliary system and absent or delayed excretion into the intestine (Fig. 8–12), has already been discussed in this chapter. In those clinical situations, identification of this cholescintigraphic pattern usually provides strong evidence for the presence of a significant common duct obstruction. So much so that even if sonography appears normal, further evaluation with other procedures, e.g., PTC or ERCP, is indicated. However, in the clinical context of possible intrahepatic cholestasis, the situation is not as clear-cut. In intrahepatic cholestasis, the obstruction can occur at the canalicular level, e.g., drug-induced cholestasis, resulting in a similar cholescintigraphic pattern.[176] There is no diagnostic dilemma when intrahepatic cholestasis instead yields a pattern of poor hepatic uptake with slow visualization of the biliary system and commensurately slow excretion into the intestine. The main disadvantage of identifying this cholescintigraphic pattern when obstruction is present is that the level and cause of the occlusion are not identifiable, as they can be with CT, PTC, and/or ERCP. When hepatocellular function is severely compromised, there may be absent or minimal liver uptake and only persistent renal excretion identifiable. This pattern is observed much less frequently now that the newer IDA analogs are available, such as Tc-99m DISIDA, which has enabled visualization of a patent biliary system in patients whose bilirubin levels have been in the 20 to 30 mg/100 ml range.

Specific Cholestatic Problems Particularly Well Suited For Cholescintigraphic Evaluation

In evaluating patients with cholestasis, two main clinical areas have emerged in which cholescintigraphy has proved particularly useful: acute biliary obstruction and localized intrahepatic obstruction. At times in these clinical situations, cholescintigraphy has been the only procedure that accurately detected the presence and level of obstruction.

Acute Biliary Obstruction

A correlative diagnostic approach between ultrasonography and hepatobiliary scintigraphy is recommended for the evaluation of patients suspected of having acute biliary obstruction. In this clinical setting, the combination of the anatomic with the functional imaging procedure has proved useful. It has enabled detection of the normal caliber common bile duct, which is nonetheless significantly obstructed (Fig. 8–12). As previously discussed, cholescintigraphy can identify the functional abnormality associated with obstruction before the morphologic response of dilatation has occurred and occasionally before the bilirubin and other liver function tests have begun to rise (see Acute Cholecystitis: Nonvisualization of Gallbladder and Ducts with Absent or Delayed Excretion into the Intestine). Thus, scintiscanning has proved useful in evaluating the acutely ill patient by detecting the presence of acute common duct obstruction (Tables 8–4 and 8–5). Additionally, it has proved useful in evaluating patients who are post-cholecystectomy and who generally have a more protracted and less acute clinical history. In a significant percentage of these patients, scintigraphy has detected obstruction, whereas their sonograms appeared normal. In view of the extremely limited ability of sonography to visualize stones in a normal caliber common bile duct[184] and the fact that many of the post-cholecystectomy patients who had re-

current symptoms had retained common duct stones, it is not surprising that a combined approach utilizing sonography and scintigraphy appears to be most valuable for evaluating these individuals.

A combined approach has also been helpful when dilated ducts have been identified sonographically. Since dilatation does not automatically mean that obstruction is present, when sonography demonstrates dilated ducts but fails to determine a cause of obstruction, cholescintigraphic documentation of the presence of functional obstruction has proved helpful (see Postoperative Evaluation).

Localized Biliary Obstruction

Occasionally, sonographic detection of localized intrahepatic ductal obstruction may be difficult. The fact that cholescintigraphy is much less operator and instrument dependent than sonography has proved useful in some patients with localized intrahepatic ductal obstruction. Hepatobiliary scanning does not depend on obtaining the appropriate cross-sectional views to identify the localized dilated ducts. The advantage of the technical simplicity of scintigraphy is illustrated by the patient whose scintiphoto is shown in Figure 8–32. This cholescintigram was obtained in a 32-year-old woman with breast carcinoma that was metastatic to the liver. She was admitted because of recurrent fever and a rising alkaline phosphatase level. Hepatobiliary scintigraphy was the only procedure to accurately diagnose the cause of her problem as localized biliary obstruction. Both sonography and PTC visualized the normal common bile duct and right intrahepatic ducts as well as the metastatic mass. It was also thought that the left intrahepatic ducts were visualized and normal. Cholescintigraphy was the only procedure to identify localized obstruction of the left intrahepatic ducts by the large metastatic lesion.

CONGENITAL DISORDERS

Biliary Atresia

Since significant extrahepatic ductal obstruction in a jaundiced neonate is an indication for surgical intervention, it is of the utmost importance to distinguish neonatal hepatitis with a patent extrahepatic biliary system from bili-

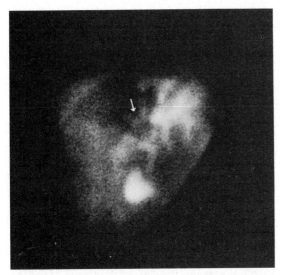

Figure 8–32. Localized intrahepatic ductal obstruction secondary to breast carcinoma metastatic to the liver. This scintiphoto was obtained at 1 hour. The large central photon-deficient area is secondary to the metastatic breast carcinoma. The normal common bile duct is visualized. The right intrahepatic ducts are not visualized since they are not obstructed and are of normal caliber. The dilated left intrahepatic biliary radicles are demonstrated, with the level of obstruction identified at the level of the margin of the metastasis (arrow). Ultrasonography and transhepatic cholangiography revealed a "normal biliary system." Both procedures visualized the normal common bile and right hepatic ducts as well as the metastatic mass. However, the obstructed left ducts were not visualized.

ary atresia or other surgically correctable abnormalities.[50] Irreversible hepatic damage ending in death results if successful treatment is not implemented within the first four months of life.[187] The need for even earlier diagnosis and treatment has been indicated by the significantly improved results achieved when surgery is performed before ten weeks of age.[187, 188] Thus, it is imperative that the diagnosis of biliary atresia be made as soon as possible. The clinical course, *in vitro* laboratory studies, and closed needle biopsy frequently are unable to distinguish biliary atresia from neonatal hepatitis.[189, 190] Thus, by documenting biliary patency, cholescintigraphy may be the only procedure capable of eliminating the performance of unnecessary surgery. The diagnosis of biliary atresia is accurately excluded when some degree of intestinal activity is identified (Fig. 8–33).

The value of I-131 RB imaging for the evaluation of neonatal jaundice has been well documented. For instance, in a representative series reported by Silverberg, Rosenthall, and Freeman,[191] the presence of biliary atresia was accurately excluded in 11 out of 15 infants with conjugated hyperbilirubinemia by the demonstration of the free flow of bile into the intestine. This is the one clinical situation in which the long physical half-life of I-131 (8.1 days) is

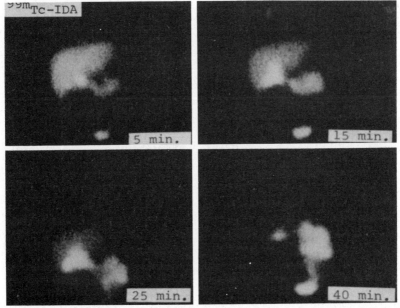

Figure 8–33. Neonatal hepatitis. Cholescintigraphic evaluation of a 3-week-old jaundiced infant documents complete patency of a normal biliary system with visualization of the liver, gallbladder, and intestine in the first 5 to 15 minutes. This unequivocally excludes the possibility of biliary atresia.

advantageous. It enables imaging to be performed over a 72- to 96-hour period. Identification of intestinal activity at any point during this study absolutely excluded the possibility of biliary atresia. However, in the remaining four neonates, absence of intestinal excretion on the delayed views was secondary to the presence of severe hepatitis. Thus, when an "obstructed" cholescintigraphic pattern is identified, obstruction cannot be distinguished from severe primary hepatic parenchymal disease. Hence, the false-positive rate can be significant, even as high as 20 per cent.[192, 193] This is unfortunate, because in view of the gravity of missing an obstruction, such neonates may be subjected to unnecessary surgery and intraoperative cholangiography. The diagnostic capability of rose bengal scanning has improved by additionally obtaining quantitative 72-hour stool analyses for I-131 RB activity. The activity recovered in the stool of patients with neonatal hepatitis should be greater than or equal to 10 per cent of the administered activity, whereas infants with biliary atresia will have a recovery rate of less than 5 per cent.[194] One of the major problems with this technique is the need for the staff of a neonatal nursery to be properly instructed and able to obtain stool specimens that do not have any urinary contamination.

It was hoped that Tc-99m IDA cholescintigraphy would eliminate the need for obtaining urine and stool specimens for quantitation, the thought being that the improved anatomic resolution of Tc-99m IDA imaging would enhance the ability to detect intestinal activity in cases of biliary patency. However, to date the role of Tc-99m IDA cholescintigraphy for evaluation of suspected biliary atresia remains controversial and uncertain.

Collier and associates[195] concluded that I-131 RB remained the agent of choice for evaluation of neonates with conjugated hyperbilirubinemia. They administered a dose of 50 μCi (1.85 mBq) of Tc-99m BIDA/kg. Three out of five patients with neonatal hepatitis failed to demonstrate intestinal activity within the first 20 hours. The six-hour physical half-life of Tc-99m, along with the small administered dose, restricted the useful imaging time for cholescintigraphy to about 24 hours. Thus, this is the one clinical situation in which the otherwise ideal short physical half-life of Tc-99m poses a problem. Bile flow into the intestinal tract more than one day after injection could not be detected, whereas in the same

three problem cases, I-131 RB documented intestinal activity between 48 and 160 hours after injection.

In a larger series, Madj, Reba, and Altman[192] concluded that Tc-99m IDA cholescintigraphy after three to seven days of phenobarbital therapy is the diagnostic procedure of choice for suspected biliary atresia. To minimize gallbladder contraction and the possibility of diluting the radiotracer excreted into the intestine, the 22 neonates were kept NPO from one hour before until two hours after Tc-99m PIPIDA injection. The administered dose of 1 mCi was significantly larger than that of Collier's series.[195] This may have been a significant factor in enabling more delayed images to be obtained. This is the primary clinical situation in which it is useful to routinely obtain delayed views beyond four hours to detect the presence of even the slightest amount of intestinal excretion. Phenobarbital was administered orally (5 mg/kg/day divided in two equal doses) for three to seven days in the 11 cases that failed to demonstrate small bowel activity. The Tc-99m PIPIDA cholescintigram was then re-

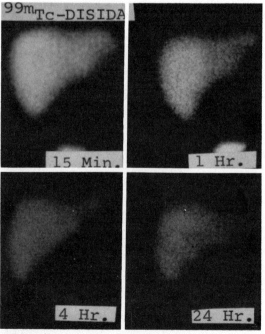

Figure 8–34. Biliary atresia. Cholescintigraphic evaluation of a jaundiced 5-week-old infant reveals excellent hepatic uptake with persistent absence of visualization of the biliary system and intestine over a 24-hour period. This study had been performed after seven days of phenobarbital administration. At laparotomy, the presence of biliary atresia was confirmed, and a Kasai procedure was performed.

peated. The six infants with persistent intestinal nonvisualization were subsequently confirmed to have biliary atresia (Fig. 8–34), whereas intestinal activity was evident on this repeat study in four out of the five infants with intrahepatic cholestasis. Thus, in only one neonate with hepatocellular dysfunction did the phenobarbital therapy fail to have an effect on the cholescintigraphic pattern. Reportedly, the blood clearance of Tc-99m PIPIDA by the liver in this infant was extremely poor, and this finding served to distinguish this case from the other neonates who had biliary atresia.

Another pharmacologic agent that is currently being investigated for use in conjunction with, or in place of, phenobarbital is cholestyramine. Whether or not this choleretic preparation will have any beneficial effect on cholescintigraphic imaging remains to be determined. Another area of active investigation is the quantitative evaluation of hepatocyte clearance, hepatobiliary transit, and excretion. Conceivably, mild to moderate hepatocellular disease may be distinguishable from obstructive jaundice by quantitative analysis because the primary target structures for these two disease processes are very different. In neonatal hepatitis, it is the hepatocyte that is primarily affected and the ductal system that is relatively spared, whereas in biliary atresia it is the ductal system that is primarily involved. Theoretically, early in the disease process patients with biliary atresia could be distinguished from those with hepatocellular disease by the relative preservation of hepatocyte clearance with parallel alterations in hepatobiliary transit time. This differentiation should become less pronounced as the obstruction persists because parenchymal damage occurs secondarily. Sufficient confirmation of these hypotheses remains to be obtained.

Cholescintigraphy can be utilized to evaluate anastomotic patency and the degree of improvement in hepatobiliary function in patients who have had bypass surgery performed for biliary atresia.

Choledochal Cysts and Other Biliary Ectasias

Several reports have appeared in the literature concerning I-131 RB demonstration of choledochal cysts.[196-200] Figure 8–35 illustrates a choledochal cyst identified in a patient who had undergone a diversionary choledochoenterostomy 20 years earlier. Her current admission was for suspected acute cholecystitis. Cholescintigraphy clearly visualized her choledochal cyst and documented patency of her anastomosis as well as demonstrated cystic duct obstruction evidenced by persistent nonvisualization of the gallbladder.[201] Other congenital ectasias, such as intrahepatic biliary duct dilatation (e.g., Caroli's disease), can be similarly demonstrated.

Figure 8–35. Choledochal cyst, patent bypass, and acute cholecystitis. This patient had a surgical diversionary shunt performed 20 years earlier for drainage of her choledochal cyst. At that time, the gallbladder was clearly shown to be arising from the choledochal cyst. She presented acutely and was studied cholescintigraphically for suspected acute cholecystitis. There was prompt hepatic uptake with visualization of the choledochal cyst (arrow) and patent anastomosis within the first 25 minutes. There was persistent nonvisualization of the gallbladder throughout the 4 hours of examination. At surgery the gallbladder was identified arising from the choledochal cyst, and acute cholecystitis was present.

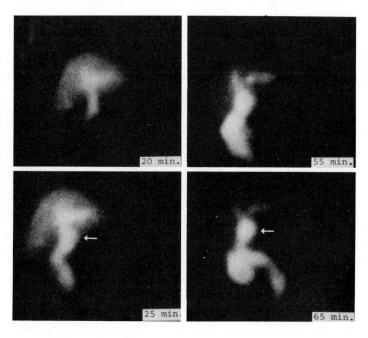

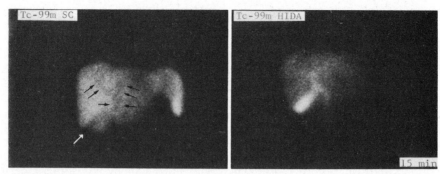

Figure 8–36. Elucidation of a defect observed on a Tc-99m sulfur colloid study with Tc-99m IDA. A small defect is identified on the colloid study in the region of the gallbladder fossa at the inferior aspect of the right lobe of the liver (white arrow). Also noted is a branching Y-shaped photon-deficient area in the region of the porta hepatis (black arrows). Cholescintigraphy confirms these photon-deficient zones to be related to the normal biliary system.

EVALUATION OF DEFECTS IDENTIFIED ON Tc-99m SULFUR COLLOID SCANS FELT TO BE BILIARY IN ORIGIN

For many years, I-131 RB imaging was performed to confirm that defects in the region of the portal hepatis or gallbladder fossa corresponded to the biliary system.[202] Since the improved resolution of Tc-99m IDA enhances the ability to visualize these biliary structures, it is utilized in a similar fashion for this purpose. Thus, identification of oblique or vertical linear bands of decreased activity in the interlobar fissure or porta hepatis or a concave defect in the region of the inferior aspect of the right lobe of the liver on the Tc-99m sulfur colloid study is subsequently followed by Tc-99m IDA imaging (Fig. 8–36).

References

1. Lin, T. H., Khentigen, A., and Winchell, H. S.: A 99mTc-labeled replacement for 131I-Rose Bengal in liver and biliary tract studies. J. Nucl. Med. *15*:613, 1974.
2. Kubota, H., Eckelman, W. C., and Poulose, P.: Technetium-99m-pyridoxyli-deneglutamate, a new agent for gallbladder imaging: Comparison with 131I–rose bengal. J. Nucl. Med. *17*:36, 1976.
3. Harvey, E., Loberg, M., and Cooper, M.: Tc-99m-HIDA: A new radiopharmaceutical for hepatobiliary imaging. J. Nucl. Med. *16*:533, 1975. (Abstract.)
4. Loberg, M., Cooper, M., Harvey, E., et al.: Development of new radiopharmaceuticals based on N-substitution of iminodiacetic acid. J. Nucl. Med. *17*:633, 1976.
5. Firnau, G.: Why do 99mTc chelates work for cholescintigraphy? Eur. J. Nucl. Med. *1*:137, 1976.
6. Wistow, B. W., Subramanian, G., Van Heertum, R. L., et al.: An evaluation of 99mTc-labeled hepatobiliary agents. J. Nucl. Med. *18*:455, 1977.
7. Chiotellis, E., Sawas-Dimopoulou, C., Koutoulidis, C., et al.: 99mTc-HIDA, a gallbladder imaging agent. Experimental aspects. Eur. J. Nucl. Med. *3*:41, 1978.
8. Rosenthall, L.: The Application of Radioiodinated Rose Bengal and Colloidal Radiogold in the Detection of Hepatobiliary Disease. St. Louis: Warren H. Green, 1969.
9. Eyler, W. R., Schuman, B. M., DuSault, L. A., et al.: The radioiodinated rose bengal liver scan as an aid in the differential diagnosis of jaundice. Am. J. Roentgenol. *94*:469, 1965.
10. Freeman, L. M., and Kay, C.: Radioactive rose bengal abdominal scanning in jaundiced patients. NY State J. Med. *66*:1778, 1966.
11. Whiting, E. G., and Nusynowitz, M. C.: Radioactive rose bengal testing in the differential diagnosis of jaundice. Surg. Gynecol. Obstet. *127*:729, 1968.
12. Serafini, A. N., Smoak, W. M., and Hupf, H. B.: Iodine-123-rose bengal. An improved hepatobiliary imaging agent. J. Nucl. Med. *17*:36, 1976.
13. Harvey, E., Loberg, M., and Cooper, M.: Tc-99m HIDA: A new radiopharmaceutical for hepatobiliary imaging. J. Nucl. Med. *16*:533, 1975. (Abstract.)
14. Loberg, M., Cooper, M., Harvey, E., and Callery, P., and Faith, W.: Development of new radiopharmaceuticals based on N-substitution of iminodiacetic acid. J. Nucl. Med. *17*:633, 1976.
15. Loberg, M., Fields, A., Harvey, E., and Cooper, M.: Radiochemistry of Tc-N-Ni-(2,6-dimethylphenylcarbamoylmethyl) iminodiacetic acid (Tc-99m HIDA). J. Nucl. Med. *17*:537, 1976. (Abstract.)
16. Callery, P. S., Faith, W. C., Loberg, M. D., Fields, A. T., Harvey, E. B., and Cooper, M. D.: Tissue distribution of technetium-99m and carbon-14 labeled N-(2,6 dimethylphenylcarbamoylmethyl) iminodiacetic acid. J. Med. Chem. *19*:962, 1976.
17. Ryan, J., Cooper, M., Loberg, M., Harvey, E., and Sikorsky, S.: Technetium-99m labeled N-(2,6-dimethylphenylcarbamoylmethyl) iminodiacetic acid (Tc-99m HIDA): A new radiopharmaceutical for hepatobiliary imaging studies. J. Nucl. Med. *18*:995, 1977.
18. Weissmann, H. S., Rosenblatt, R., Sugarman, L. A., and Freeman, L. M.: The role of nuclear imaging in evaluating the patient with cholestasis. Semin. Ultrasound *1*:134, 1980.
19. Porter, D. W., Loberg, M. D., Eacho, P. L., and

Weiner, M.: Comparison of hepatobiliary radiopharmaceuticals in an in vitro model. J. Nucl. Med. 20:642, 1979.

20. Hernandez, M., and Rosenthall, L.: A cross-over study comparing the kinetics of Tc-99m-labeled diisopropyl and p-butyl IDA analogs in patients. Clin. Nucl. Med. 5:159, 1980.

21. Weissmann, H. S., Badia, J. D., Hall, T., Sugarman, L. A., and Freeman, L. M.: Tc-99m diisopropyl iminodiacetic acid (DISIDA): The best overall cholescintigraphic radionuclide for the evaluation of hepatobiliary disorders. J. Nucl. Med. 21:18, 1980. (Abstract.)

22. Klingensmith, W. C., III, Fritzberg, A. R., Spitzer, V. M., and Kuni, C. C.: Clinical comparison of Tc-99m-diisopropyl-IDA and Tc-99m diethyl-IDA for evaluation of the hepatobiliary system. J. Nucl. Med. 21:18, 1980. (Abstract.)

23. Hernandez, M., and Rosenthall, L.: A crossover study comparing the kinetics of Tc-99m labeled diethyl- and diisopropyl-IDA. Clin. Nucl. Med. 5:352, 1980.

24. Green, A., Rosenberg, N., and Sheahan, M.: Multicenter trial of Tc-99m disofenin (di-isopropylphenylcarbamoylmethyl iminodiacetic acid): A new hepatobiliary agent for imaging jaundiced and unjaundiced patients. J. Nucl. Med. 21:18, 1980. (Abstract.)

25. Baker, R. J., and Marion, M. A.: Biliary scanning with Tc-99m pyridoxylideneglutamate—the effect of food in normal subjects: Concise communication. J. Nucl. Med. 18:793, 1977.

26. Klingensmith, W. C., Spitzer, V. M., Fritzber, A. R., et al.: The normal fasting and postprandial Tc-99m diisopropyl-IDA hepatobiliary study. J. Nucl. Med. 22:P7, 1981.

27. Eikman, E. A., Cameron, J. L., Colman, M., et al.: Radioactive tracer techniques in the diagnosis of acute cholecystitis. J. Nucl. Med. 14:393, 1973. (Abstract.)

28. Eikman, E. A., Cameron, J. L., Colman, M., et al.: Test for patency of the cystic duct in acute cholecystitis. Ann. Intern. Med. 82:318, 1975.

29. Paré, P., Shaffer, E. A., and Rosenthall, L.: Nonvisualization of the gallbladder by 99mTc-HIDA cholescintigraphy as evidence of cholecystitis. Can. Med. Assoc. J. 118:384, 1978.

30. Shaffer, E. A., McOrmon, P., and Duggan, H.: Quantitative cholescintigraphy: Assessment of gallbladder filling and emptying and duodenogastric reflux. Gastroenterology 79:899, 1980.

31. Freeman, L. M., Sugarman, L. A., and Weissmann, H. S.: Role of cholecystokinetic agents in 99mTc-IDA cholescintigraphy. Semin. Nucl. Med. 11:186, 1981.

32. Weissmann, H. S., Sugarman, L. A., Frank, M. S., and Freeman, L. M.: Serendipity in technetium-99m dimethyl iminodiacetic acid. Radiology 135:449, 1980.

33. Spellman, S. J., Shaffer, E. A., and Rosenthall, L.: Gallbladder emptying in response to cholecystokinin. Gastroenterology 77:115, 1979.

34. Brachman, M., Levy, R., Tanasescu, L., Ramonna, L., and Waxman, A.: Letter to the editor: Re: False negative gallbladder scintigram in acute cholecystitis. J. Nucl. Med. 22:291, 1981.

35. Weissmann, H. S., Frank, M., Rosenblatt, R., Goldman, M., and Freeman, L. M.: Cholescintigraphy, ultrasonography, and computerized tomography in the evaluation of biliary disorders. Semin. Nucl. Med. 9:25, 1979.

36. Rosenthall, L., Damtew, B., Kloiber, R., and Warshawski, R.: Difficulty of estimating biliary tract distension by radionuclide imaging. Diag. Imaging 50:154, 1981.

37. Schein, C. J.: Acute Cholecystitis. New York: Harper & Row, 1972.

38. Motolo, N. M.: Symposium on biliary tract disease: Foreword. Surg. Clin. North Am. 61:763, 1981.

38a. Byrne, J. J.: Acute cholecystitis. Am. J. Surg. 97:156, 1959.

39. Ochsner, S. F.: Performance and reliability of cholecystography. South. Med. J. 63:1268, 1970.

40. Thorpe, C. D., Olsen, W. R., Fischer, H., Doust, V. L., and Joseph, R.: Emergency intravenous cholangiography in patients with acute abdominal pain. Am. J. Surg. 125:46, 1973.

41. Wilson, R. L., and Shaub, M.: The use of ultrasound in suspected cholecystitis. Appl. Radiol. 7:119, 1978.

42. Stanley, R. J., and Sagel, S. S.: Computed tomography of the liver and biliary tract. In Berk, R. N., and Clemett, A. R. (eds.): Radiology of the Biliary Tract. Philadelphia: W. B. Saunders, 1977, pp. 352–375.

43. Weissmann, H. S., Frank, M., Bernstein, L. H., and Freeman, L. M.: Rapid and accurate diagnosis of acute cholecystitis with Tc-99m HIDA cholescintigraphy. Am. J. Roentgenol. 132:523, 1979.

44. Weissmann, H. S., Badia, J., Sugarman, L. A., Kluger, L., Rosenblatt, R., and Freeman, L. M.: Spectrum of cholescintigraphic patterns in acute cholecystitis. Radiology 138:167, 1981.

45. Cheng, T. H., Davis, M. A., Seltzer, S. C., Jones, B., Abbruzzese, A. A., Finberg, H. J., and Drum, E.: Evaluation of hepatobiliary imaging by radionuclide scintigraphy, ultrasonography and contrast cholangiography. Radiology 133:861, 1979.

46. Suarez, C. A., Block, F., Bernstein, D., Serafini, A., Rodman, G., Jr., and Zeppa, R.: The role of HIDA/PIPIDA scanning in diagnosing cystic duct obstruction. Ann. Surg. 191:391, 1980.

47. Szlabick, R. E., Catto, J. A., Fink-Bennett, D., and Ventura, V.: Hepatobiliary scanning in the diagnosis of acute cholecystitis. Arch. Surg. 115:540, 1980.

48. Freitas, J. E., Fink-Bennett, D., Thrall, D. M., Resinger, J. H., Calderon, H. C., Mirkes, S. H., and Shah, P. K.: Efficacy of hepatobiliary imaging in acute abdominal pain: Concise communication. J. Nucl. Med. 21:919, 1980.

49. Freitas, J. E., Mirkas, S. H., Fink-Bennett, D. M., et al.: Suspected acute cholecystitis: Comparison of hepatobiliary cholecystitis: Comparison of hepatobiliary imaging versus ultrasonography. (Submitted for publication.)

50. Canales, C. O., Smith, G. H., Robinson, J. C., Remmers, A. R., and Sarles, H. E.: Acute renal failure after the administration of iopanoic acid as a cholecystographic agent. N. Engl. J. Med. 281:89, 1969.

51. Hatfield, P. M., and Wise, R. E.: Radiology of the Gallbladder and Bile Ducts. Baltimore: Williams & Wilkins, 1976, p. 42.

52. Mujahed, Z., Evans, J. A., and Whalen, J. P.: The nonopacified gallbladder on oral cholecystography. Radiology 112:1, 1974.

53. Whalen, J. P., Rizzuto, R. J., and Evans, J. A.: Time of optimal gallbladder opacification with telepaque (iopanoic acid). Radiology 105:523, 1972.
54. Danley, R. B., Love, L., and Pickelman, J. R.: Rapid roentgenologic diagnosis of acute cholecystitis. Surg. Gynecol. Obstet. 143:602, 1976.
55. Barksdale, J. W., and Johnston, J. H.: Acute cholecystitis. Ann. Surg. 127:816, 1948.
56. Stillman, A. E.: Hepatotoxic reaction to iodipamide meglumine injection. J.A.M.A. 228:1420, 1974.
57. Craft, I. L., and Swales, J. D.: Renal failure after cholangiography. Br. Med. J. 2:736, 1967.
58. Canales, C. O., Smith, G. H., Robinson, J. C., Remmers, A. R., and Sarles, H. E.: Acute renal failure after the administration of iopanoic acid as a cholecystographic agent. N. Engl. J. Med. 281:89, 1969.
59. Bergman, L. A., Ellison, M. R., and Durea, G.: Acute renal failure after drip infusion pyelography. N. Engl. J. Med. 279:1277, 1968.
60. Danley, R. B., Love, L., and Pickelman, J. R.: Rapid roentgenologic diagnosis of acute cholecystitis. Surg. Gynecol. Obstet. 143:602, 1976.
61. Ansell, G.: Adverse reactions to contrast agents. Scope of the problem. Invest. Radiol. 5:374, 1970.
62. Wise, R. E., Johnston, D. O., and Salzman, F. A.: The intravenous cholangiographic diagnosis of partial obstruction of the common bile duct. Radiology 68:507, 1957.
63. Ekelberg, M. E., Carlson, H. C., and McIlrath, D. C.: Intravenous cholangiography with intact gallbladder. A.J.R. 110:235, 1970.
64. Goodman, M. W., Silvis, S. E., and Vennes, J. A.: Should intravenous cholangiograms be discontinued as a diagnostic procedure? Gastrointest. Endosc. 24:198, 1978. (Abstract.)
65. Schoenfeld, I. J.: Animal models of gallstone formation. Gastroenterology 3:189, 1972.
66. Ingelfinger, F. J.: Digestive disease as a national problem. V. Gallstones. Gastroenterology 55:102, 1968.
67. Samuels, B. I., Freitas, J. E., Bree, R. L., Schwab, R. E., and Heller, S. T.: Diagnosis of acute cholecystitis: A comparison of radionuclide hepatobiliary imaging and real-time ultrasonography. (Submitted for publication.)
68. Weissmann, H. S., Rosenblatt, R., Sugarman, L. A., and Freeman, L. M.: An update in radionuclide imaging in the diagnosis of cholecystitis. J.A.M.A. 246:1354, 1981.
69. Leopold, G. R., Amberg, J., and Gosink, B. B.: Gray scale ultrasonic cholecystography: A comparison with conventional radiographic techniques. Radiology 212:445, 1976.
70. Laing, F. C., Federle, M. P., Jeffry, R. B., and Brown, T. W.: Ultrasonic evaluation of patients with acute right upper quadrant pain. Radiology 140:449, 1981.
71. Johnson, H. C., Jr., McLaren, J. R., and Weens, H. S.: Intravenous cholangiography in the differential diagnosis of acute cholecystitis. Radiology 74:790, 1960.
72. Harrington, O. B., Beall, A. C., Jr., Noon, G., et al.: Intravenous cholangiography in acute cholecystitis. Use in differential diagnosis. Arch. Surg. 88:585, 1964.
73. Zeman, R. K., Burrell, M. I., Cahow, C. E., and Caride, V.: Diagnostic utility of cholescintigraphy and ultrasonography in acute cholecystitis. Am. J. Surg. 141:446, 1981.
74. Raghavendra, B. N., Feiner, H. D., Subramanyam, B. R., et al.: Acute cholecystitis: sonographic-pathologic analysis. A.J.R. 137:327, 1981.
75. Worthen, N. J., Uszler, J. M., and Funamura, J. L.: Cholecystitis: prospective evaluation of sonography and 99mTc-HIDA cholescintigraphy. A.J.R. 137:973, 1981.
76. Laing, F. C., Federle, M. P., Jeffrey, R. B., and Brown, T. W.: Letter to the editor—retort. Radiology 143:280, 1982.
77. Berk, R. N.: Oral cholecystography. In Berk, R. N., and Clemett, A. R.: Radiology of the Gallbladder and Bile Ducts. Philadelphia: W. B. Saunders, 1977, Chapter 4.
78. Weens, H. S., and Walker, L. A.: The radiologic diagnosis of acute cholecystitis and pancreatitis. Radiol. Clin. North Am. 2:89, 1964.
79. Silvani, H. L., and McCorkle, H. J.: Temporary failure of gallbladder visualization by cholecystography in acute pancreatitis. Ann. Surg. 127:1207, 1948.
80. Johnson, H. C., Jr., Minor, B. D., Thompson, J. A., and Weens, H. S.: Diagnostic value of intravenous cholangiography during acute cholecystitis and acute pancreatitis. N. Engl. J. Med. 260:158, 1959.
81. Weens, H. S., and Clements, J. L., Jr.: The radiologic diagnosis of acute cholecystitis. Semin. Roentgenol. 11:245, 1976.
82. Diaco, J. F., Miller, L. D., and Copeland, E. M.: The role of early diagnostic laparotomy in acute pancreatitis. Surg. Gynecol. Obstet. 129:263, 1969.
83. Kaden, V. G., Howard, J. M., and Doubleday, L. C.: Cholecystographic studies during and immediately following acute pancreatitis. Surgery 38:1082, 1955.
84. Stone, L. B., Easton, S. B., and Ferrucci, J. T.: Inflammatory disease of the pancreas. Curr. Prob. Radiol. 5:17, 1975.
85. Fonseca, C., Greenberg, D., Rosenthall, L., Arzoumanian, A., and Lisbona, R.: Tc-99m IDA imaging in the differential diagnosis of acute pancreatitis. Radiology 130:525, 1979.
86. Frank, M. S., Weissman, H. S., Chun, K. J., Sugarman, L. A., Brandt, L. J., and Freeman, L. M.: Visualization of the biliary tract with Tc-99m HIDA in acute pancreatitis. Gastroenterology 78:1167, 1980. (Abstract.)
87. Serafini, A. N., Al-Sheikh, W., Barkin, J. S., Hourani, M., Sfakianakis, G. N., Clarke, L. P., and Ashkar, F. S.: Biliary scintigraphy in acute pancreatitis. Radiology 144:591, 1982.
88. Floyd, J. L., Weiland, F. L., Hale, A. J., and Nusynowitz, M. L.: Hepatic imaging: A comparison of Tc-99m-sulfur colloid and PIPIDA in the detection of defects. Clin. Nucl. Med. 6:53, 1981.
89. Pors Nielsen, S., Trap-Jensen, J., Lindenberg, J., et al.: Scintigraphy and hepatography with Tc-99m diethyl-acetanilide-iminodiacetate in obstructive jaundice. J. Nucl. Med. 19:452, 1978.
90. Harvey, E., Loberg, M., Ryan, J., Dikorski, S., Faith, W., and Cooper, M.: Hepatic clearance mechanism of Tc-99m-HIDA and its effect on quantitation of hepatobiliary function: Concise communication. J. Nucl. Med. 20:310, 1979.
91. Cox, P. H., Tjen, HS, van der Pompe, W. B.: The clinical value of Tc-99m labelled diethyl-acetanilido-imino-diacetate complex for dynamic studies of hepatobiliary function. Nucl. Compact 9:67, 1978.
92. Sauer, J.: Funktionsszintigraphie der Leber mit Tc-99m-Diathyl-IDA (EHIDA). Function scintigraphy of the liver using Tc-99m diethyl-IDA (EHIDA). Nucl. Compact 9:97, 1978.
93. Welcke, U., Rodtke, J., Mahlstedt, J., and Joseph,

K.: Hepatobiliare Funktionsszintigraphie mit Dia-thyl-IDA (EHIDA) und HIDA. Nucl. Compact 9:74, 1978.

94. Reichelt, H. G.: Nuclearmedizinische Leber—und Gallenwegs—diagnostic mit dem hepatotropen, cholonphilen Radiopharmakon Tc-99m-Diathyl-IDA (EHIDA). Nucl. Compact 9:86, 1978.

95. Sialer, G., Lochel, H., Pfeiffer, F., and Horst, W.: Unterschungsergebnis mit einer Tc-99m markierten gallengangigen Substanz. Nucl. Compact 9:81, 1978.

96. Shuman, W. P., Gibbs, P., Rudd, T. G., and Mack, L. A.: PIPIDA scintigraphy for cholecystitis: False positives in alcoholism and total parenteral nutrition. A.J.R. 138:1, 1982.

97. Weissmann, H. S., Sugarman, L. A., and Freeman, L. M.: The value of the delayed view on Tc-99m dimethyl iminodiacetic acid (HIDA) cholescintigraphy. Paper presented at the 65th Scientific Assembly of the Radiological Society of North America, Chicago, IL, 1979.

98. Freitas, J. E., and Fink-Bennett, D. M.: Asymptomatic cystic duct obstruction in chronic cholecystitis. J. Nucl. Med. 21:17, 1980. (Abstract.)

99. Weissmann, H. S., Sugarman, L. A., Badia, J. D., and Freeman, L. M.: Improving the specificity and accuracy of Tc99m IDA cholescintigraphy with delayed views. J. Nucl. Med. 21:P17, 1980.

100. Nathan, M. H., Newman, A., Murray, D. J., et al.: Cholecystokinin cholecystography. A four year evaluation. Am. J. Roentgenol. 110:240, 1970.

101. Hedner, P., and Lunderquist, A.: The use of the C-terminal octapeptide of cholecystokinin for gallbladder evacuation in cholecystography. Am. J. Roentgenol. 116:320, 1972.

102. Weissmann, H. S., Rosenblatt, R. R., Sugarman, L. A., Badia, J. D., and Freeman, L. M.: Early diagnosis of acute common bile duct obstruction by Tc-99m-IDA (iminodiacetic cholescintigraphy). J. Nucl. Med. 21:P41, 1980.

103. Glenn, F.: Acalculous cholecystitis. Ann. Surg. 189:458, 1979.

104. Glenn, F., and Mannix, M.: The acalculous gallbladder. Ann. Surg. 144:670, 1956.

105. Munster, A. M., and Brown, J. R.: Acalculous cholecystitis. Am. J. Surg. 113:730, 1967.

106. Andersson, A., Bergdahl, L., and Boquist, L.: Acalculous cholecystitis. Am. J. Surg. 122:3, 1971.

107. Johnsson, P. E., and Andersson, A.: Postoperative acute acalculous cholecystitis. Arch. Surg. 111:1097, 1976.

108. Weissmann, H. S., Berkowitz, D., Fox, M. S., Gliedman, M. L., Rosenblatt, R., Sugarman, L. A., and Freeman, L. M.: The role of technetium-99m iminodiacetic acid (IDA) cholescintigraphy in acute acalculous cholecystitis. Radiology. (In press).

108a. Weissmann, H. S., Berkowitz, D., Fox, M., Rosenblatt, R., Sugarman, L. A., and Freeman, L. M.: Tc-99m iminodiacetic acid cholescintigraphic evaluation of acalculous cholescystitis. J. Nucl. Med. 22:P7, 1981. (Abstract.)

109. Goldstein, F., Grun, R., and Margulies, M.: Cholecystokinin cholecystography in the differential diagnosis of acalculous gallbladder disease. Digest. Dis. 19:835, 1974.

110. Nathan, M. H., MacFarland, J., et al.: Cholecystokinin cholecystography. Radiology 93:1, 1969.

111. Nora, P. F., McCarthy, W., and Sanez, N.: Cholecystokinin cholecystography in acalculous gallbladder disease. Arch. Surg. 108:507, 1974.

112. Shoop, J. D.: Functional hepatoma demonstrated with rose bengal scanning. Am. J. Roentgenol. 107:51, 1969.

113. Utz, J. A., Lull, R. J., Anderson, J. H., Lanbrech, R. W., Brown, J. M., and Henry, W.: Hepatoma visualization with Tc-99m pyridoxylidene glutamate. J. Nucl. Med. 21:747, 1980.

114. Cannon, J. R., Jr., Long R. F., Berens, S. W., and Caplan, G. E.: Uptake of Tc-99m PIPIDA in pulmonary metastases from a hepatoma. Clin. Nucl. Med. 5:22, 1980.

115. Weissmann, H. S., Frank, M., and Freeman, L. M.: Spectrum of 99mTc dimethyl iminodiacetic acid (HIDA) cholescintigraphic patterns in acute and chronic cholecystitis. Paper presented at the 64th Scientific Assembly of the Radiological Society of North America, Chicago, IL, 1978.

116. Glenn, F.: Critical sequelae in biliary tract disease. Am. J. Surg. 42:735, 1976.

117. Todd, G. J., and Reemtsma, K.: Cholecystectomy with drainage factors influencing wound infection in 1,000 elective cases. Am. J. Surg. 135:622, 1978.

118. Bodvall, B., and Oevergaard, B.: Computer analysis of postcholecystectomy biliary tract symptoms. Surg. Gynecol. Obstet. 124:723, 1967.

119. Hess, W.: Praktische Chirurgie, Heft 91: Nachoperationen an den Gallenwegen. Stuttgart: F. Enke. 1977.

120. Stefanini, P., Carboni, P., Patrassi, N., et al.: Transduodenal sphincteroplasty. Its use in the treatment of lithiasis and benign obstruction of the common duct. Am. J. Surg. 128:672, 1974.

121. Glenn, F., and McSherry, C.: Secondary abdominal operations for symptoms following biliary tract surgery. Surg. Gynecol. Obstet. 121:979, 1965.

122. Ehnmark, E.: The gallstone disease, a clinical-statistical study. Acta Chir. Scand. (Suppl. 57), 1939. (Thesis.)

123. Goldstein, L., Sample, W., Kadell, B., et al.: Grayscale ultrasonography evaluation and thin needle cholangiography in the jaundiced patient. J.A.M.A. 238:1041, 1977.

124. Bergdall, L., and Holmlund, D.: Retained bile duct stones. Acta Chir. Scand. 142:145, 1976.

125. Kazam, E., Schneider, M., and Rubenstein. W. A.: The role of ultrasound and CT in imaging the gall bladder and biliary tract. In Alavi, A., and Arger, P. H. (eds.): Multiple Imaging Procedures, Vol. 3, Abdomen. New York: Grune & Stratton, 1980.

126. Weissmann, H. S., Gliedman, M. L., Wilk, P. J., Sugarman, L. A., Badia, J., Guglielmo, K., and Freeman, L. M.: Evaluation of the postoperative patient with 99mTc-IDA cholescintigraphy. Semin. Nucl. Med. 12:27, 1982.

127. Sample, W. F., Sarti, D. A., Goldstein, L. T., et al.: Gray-scale ultrasonography of the jaundiced patient. Radiology 128:719, 1978.

128. Greenwald, R., Pereiras, R., Morris, S., et al.: Jaundice choledocholithiasis and a nondilated common duct. J.A.M.A. 240:1983, 1978.

129. Taylor, K., Rosenfield, A., and Spiro, H.: Diagnostic accuracy of gray scale ultrasonography for the jaundice patient. Arch. Intern. Med. 193:60, 1979.

130. Wise, R., Johnston, D., and Salzman, F.: The intravenous cholangiographic diagnosis of the partial obstruction of the common bile duct. Radiology 68:507, 1957.

131. Oddi, R.: D'une disposition a sphincter specale de l'ouverture du canal choledoque. Arch. Ital. Biol. 8:317, 1887.

132. Judd, E. S., and Mann, F. C.: Effects of removal of

the gallbladder; An experimental study. Surg. Gynecol. Obstet. *24*:347, 1917.

133. Bornhurst, R. A., and Hutzman, E.: New concept of intravenous cholangiography. NY State J. Med. *68*:3027, 1968.

134. Hughes, J., LoCurcio, S., Edmundo, R., et al.: The common duct after cholecystectomy. J.A.M.A. *197*:247, 1966.

135. Qvist, C.: The influence of cholecystectomy on the normal common bile duct. Acta Chir. Scand. *113*:30, 1957.

136. LeQuesne, L. P., Whitside, C. G., and Hand, B. W.: The common bile ducts after cholecystectomy. Br. Med. J. *1*:329, 1959.

137. Longo, M. Hodgson, J., and Ferris, D.: Size of the common bile duct following cholecystectomy. Ann. Surg. *165*:250, 1967.

138. Twiss, J. R., et al.: Post cholecystectomy oral cholangiography: A preliminary report. Am. J. Med. Sci. *227*:372, 1954.

139. Graham, M. F., Cooperberg, P. L., Cohen, M., et al.: Size of the normal common hepatic duct following cholecystectomy: an ultrasonographic study. Radiology *135*:137, 1980.

140. Bartlett, M. K., and Waddel, W. R.: Indication for common duct exploration, evaluation in 1,000 cases. N. Engl. J. Med. *258*:164, 1958.

141. Scott, G. W., Ferris, D. O., Hallenbeck, G. A. et al.: Resistance to flow through common bile duct in man. Bull. Soc. Intern. Chir. *4*:509, 1963.

142. Burgener, F. A., Fischer, H. W., and Adams, J. T.: Intravenous cholangiography in different degrees of common bile duct obstruction, an experimental study on dogs. Invest. Radiol. *10*:342, 1975.

143. Scott, G. W., Smallwood, R. E., and Rowlands, S.: Flow through the bile duct after cholecystectomy. Surg. Gynecol. Obstet. *140*:912, 1975.

144. Scott, G. W.: Measurement of the resistance to flow through the sphincter of Oddi in patients following cholecystectomy and choledochostomy. MS thesis, University of Minnesota, 1964.

145. Hicken, N. F., and McAllister, A. J.: Operative cholangiography as an aid in reducing the incidence of "overlooked" common bile duct stones: A study of 1,293 choledocholithotomies. Surgery *55*:753, 1964.

146. Bilsito, A., Marta, J., Cramer, G., et al.: Measurement of biliary tract size and drainage time. Radiology *122*:65, 1977.

147. Weissmann, H. S., Sugarman, L. A., and Freeman, L. H.: The clinicul role of technetium-99m iminodiacetic acid cholescintigraphy. *In* Freeman, L. M., and Weissmann, H. S. (eds.): Nuclear Medicine Annual 1981. New York: Raven Press, 1981.

148. Kuni, C. C., Klingensmith, W. C., and Fritzberg, A. R.: Evaluation of intrahepatic cholestasis with radionuclide hepatobiliary imaging. Paper presented at 67th Scientific Assembly of the Radiological Society of North America, Chicago, IL, 1981.

149. Beye, H. S.: Conditions necessitating surgery following cholecystectomy: An analysis of 66 cases and a discussion of certain technical problems concerned in removal of the gallbladder and in operations upon the common bile duct. Surg. Gynecol. Obstet. *62*:191, 1936.

150. Coulter, E. B.: Postcholecystectomy symptoms due to cystic duct and gallbladder remnants. West. J. Surg. *62*:539, 1954.

151. Adams, R., and Stranahan, A.: Cholecystitis and cholelithiasis: An analytical report of 1104 operative cases. Surg. Gynecol. Obstet. *85*:776, 1947.

152. Clute, H. M.: Cystic duct stones after cholecystectomy. Surg. Clin. North Am. *13*:603, 1933.

153. Garlock, J. H., and Hurwitt, E. S.: The cystic duct stump syndrome. Surgery *29*:833, 1951.

154. Hicken, N. F., White, L. B., and Coray, Q. B.: Incomplete removal of the cystic duct as a factor in producing postcholecystectomy complication. Surgery *21*:309, 1947.

155. Womack, N. A., and Credes, R. L.: The persistence of symptoms following cholecystectomy. Ann. Surg. *126*:31, 1947.

156. Gray, H. K., and Sharpe, W. S.: Biliary dyskinesis: Role played by a remnant of the cystic duct. Proc. Mayo Clin. *19*:164, 1944.

157. Colcock, B. P., and McManus, J. E.: Cholecystectomy for cholelithiasis: A review of 1356 cases. Surg. Clin. North Am. *35*:765, 1955.

158. Grimes, A. E., and Redd, H.: Residual cystic ducts, a factor in the postcholecystectomy syndrome, now visualized by a new contrast medium, with cases. J. Kentucky State Med. Assn. *53*:958, 1955.

159. Monteiro, A., and Tourinho, O.: Litiase do dieto cestico residual e sindrome de poscolecistectomia. Rev. Bras. Cir. *29*:275, 1955.

160. Peterson, F. R.: Re-formed gallbladder: A review of 42 cases. J. Iowa State Med. Soc. *36*:134, 1946.

161. Bauer, W. B. A. J.: Postcholecystectomy complications due to incomplete removal of gallbladder and cystic duct: Report of a so-called reformed gallbladder. Arch. Surg. *63*:612, 1951.

162. Morton, C. B.: Postcholecystectomy symptoms from cystic duct remnants. Ann. Surg. *139*:679, 1954.

163. Glenn, F., and Johnson, G.: Cystic duct remnant, a sequela of incomplete cholecystectomy. Surg. Gynecol. Obstet. *101*:331, 1955.

164. Bodvall, B., and Overgaard, B.: Cystic duct remnant after cholecystectomy: Incidence studied by cholegraphy in 500 cases and significance in 103 reoperations. Ann. Surg. *163*:382, 1966.

165. Weissmann, H. S., Rosenblatt, R., Sugarman, L. A., et al.: The role of nuclear imaging in evaluating cholestasis—an update. Semin. Ultrasound *1*:134, 1980.

166. Weissmann, H. S., Chun, K. J., Frank, H. S., et al.: Demonstration of traumatic bile leakage with cholescintigraphy and ultrasonography. Am. J. Roentgenol. *133*:843, 1979.

167. Rosenthall, L., Fonseca, C., Arzoumanian, A., et al.: ^{99m}Tc-IDA hepatobiliary imaging following upper abdominal surgery. Radiology *130*:735, 1979.

168. Zeman, R. K., Lee, C., Stahl, R. S., et al.: Ultrasonography and hepatobiliary scintigraphy in the assessment of biliary enteric anastomoses. Paper presented at the 67th Scientific Assembly and Annual Meeting of the Radiological Society of North America, 1981.

169. Weissmann, H. S., Rosenblatt, R., Goldman, M., et al.: Evaluation of the postoperative patient with Tc-99m dimethyliminodiacetic acid (HIDA) cholescintigraphy. J. Nucl. Med. *20*:686, 1979.

170. Zaw-win, B., Darwish, M., Dibos, P. E., and Razzak, I. A.: ^{131}I-rose bengal scanning in the detection of cholecystocolic fistula. Am. J. Gastroenterol. *68*:396, 1977.

171. Henderson, R. W., Lee, Y. C., and Telfer, N.: Demonstration of traumatic hepato-pleural cutaneous defect by ^{131}I-rose bengal. Clin. Nucl. Med. *3*:432, 1978.

172. Wiener, S. N., and Vyas, M.: The scintigraphic demonstration of bile leakage utilizing ^{131}I-rose bengal. J. Nucl. Med. *15*:1044, 1974.

173. Spencer, R. P., Marshall, M. K., and Glenn, W. L.: Use of ^{131}I-rose bengal to follow bile leakage. Am. J. Dig. Dis. *12*:1169, 1967.

174. Henzel, J. H., Blessing, W. D., and Deweese, M. S.: Intrahepatic biliary disruption, report of two cases occurring during use of balloon-tipped biliary catheters. Arch. Surg. *102*:218, 1971.

175. Weissmann, H. S., Chun, K. J., Frank, M. S., Koenigsberg, M., Milstein, D. M., and Freeman, L. M.: Demonstration of traumatic bile leakage with cholescintigraphy and ultrasonography. Am. J. Roentgenol. *133*:843, 1979.

176. Kuni, C. C., Klingensmith, W. C., Koep, L. J., and Fritzberg, A. R.: Communication of intrahepatic cavities with bile ducts: Demonstration with Tc-99m-diethyl-IDA imaging. Clin. Nucl. Med. *5*:349, 1980.

177. Klingensmith, W. C., Koep, L. J., and Fritzberg, A. R.: Bile leakage into a hepatic abscess in a liver transplant: Demonstration with ^{99m}Tc diethyliminodiacetic acid. Am. J. Roentgenol. *133*:889, 1978.

178. Brunetti, J. C., and Van Heertum, R. L.: Preoperative detection of gallbladder perforation. Clin. Nucl. Med. *5*:347, 1980.

179. Sty, J. R., Babbitt, D. P., and Squires, W.: Tc-99m IDA hepatobiliary imaging: A fractured liver. Clin. Nucl. Med. *4*:493, 1979.

180. Henson, S. W., Hallenbeck, G. A., Gray, H. K., and Dockerty, M. B.: Benign tumors of the liver. Surg. Gynecol. Obstet. *104*:302, 1957.

181. Brandberg, R.: Contribution to the study of traumatic injuries of the liver and uninjured capsule. Acta Chir. Scand. *9*:321, 1928.

182. Robertson, D. E., and Graham, R. R.: Rupture of the liver without tear of the capsule. Ann. Surg. *98*:899, 1933.

183. Taylor, K. J. W., Carpenter, D. A., and McCready, V. R.: Ultrasound and scintigraphy in the differential diagnosis of obstructive jaundice. J. Clin. Ultrasound *2*:105, 1974.

184. Kazam, E., Schneider, M., and Rubinstein, W. A.: The role of ultrasound and computed tomography in imaging the gallbladder and bile ducts. In Arger, P., and Alavi, A. (eds.): Diagnostic Studies in Abdominal Disease. New York: Grune & Stratton, 1980.

185. Malini, S., and Sabel, J.: Ultrasonography in obstructive jaundice. Radiology, *123*:429, 1977.

186. Perlmutter, G. S., and Goldberg, B. B.: Ultrasonic evaluation of the common bile duct. J. Clin. Ultrasound *4*:107, 1976.

187. Kasai, M., Watanabe, I., and Ohi, R.: Follow-up studies of long-term survivors after hepatic portoenterostomy for "noncorrectable" biliary atresia. J. Pediatr. Surg. *10*:173, 1975.

188. Altman, R. P.: The portoenterostomy procedure for biliary atresia: A five year experience. Ann. Surg. *188*:351, 1978.

189. Hays, D. M., Woolley, M. M., Snyder, W. H., Jr., et al.: Diagnosis of biliary atresia: relative accuracy of percutaneous liver biopsy and postoperative cholangiography. J. Pediatr. *71*:598, 1967.

190. Landing, B. H.: Editorial: Changing approach to neonatal hepatitis and biliary atresia. Pediatrics *53*:647, 1974.

191. Silverberg, M., Rosenthall, L., and Freeman, L. M.: Rose bengal excretion studies as an aid in the differential diagnosis of neonatal jaundice. Semin. Nucl. Med. *3*:69, 1973.

192. Majd, M., Reba, R. C., and Altman, R. P.: Hepatobiliary scintigraphy with Tc-99m-PIPIDA in the evaluation of neonatal jaundice. Pediatrics *67*:140, 1981.

193. Hayden, P. W., Rudd, T. G., and Christie, D. L.: Rose bengal sodium I-131 studies in infants with suspected biliary atresia. Am. J. Dis. Child., *133*:834, 1979.

194. Ghadimi, H., and Sass-Kortsak, A.: Evaluation of the radioactive rose-bengal test for the differential diagnosis of obstructive jaundice in infants. N. Engl. J. Med. *265*:351, 1981.

195. Collier, B. D., Treves, S., Davis, M. A., et al.: Simultaneous ^{99m}Tc-P-Butyl-IDA and ^{131}I-rose bengal scintigraphy in neonatal jaundice. Radiology *134*:719, 1980.

196. Tada, S., Yashukochi, H., Shida, H., Motegi, F., and Fukada, A.: A choledochal cyst demonstrated by I-131 rose bengal scanning—report of a case. Am. J. Roentgenol. *116*:587, 1972.

197. Rosenfield, N., and Griscom, N. T.: Choledochal cysts: Roentgenographic techniques. Radiology *114*:113, 1975.

198. Williams, L. E., Fisher, J. H., Courtney, R. A., and Darling, D. B.: Preoperative diagnosis of choledochal cyst by hepatoscintigraphy. N. Engl. J. Med. *283*:84, 1980.

199. Park, C. H., Garafola, J. H., and O'Hara, A. E.: Preoperative diagnosis of asymptomatic choledochal cyst by rose bengal liver scan. J. Nucl. Med. *15*:310, 1974.

200. Oshiumi, Y., Nakayama, C., Numaguchi, Y., Koga, I., and Matosura, K.: Serial scintigraphy of choledochal cysts using ^{131}I-rose bengal and ^{131}I-bromsulphalein. Am. J. Roentgenol. *128*:769, 1977.

201. Weissmann, H. S., Gold, M., Goldstein, R. D., Sugarman, L. A., and Freeman, L. M.: Choledochal cyst complicated by acute cholecystitis and bypass obstruction: Diagnostic role of Tc-99m HIDA cholescintigraphy. Clin. Nucl. Med. *6*:395, 1981.

202. Johnson, P. M.: The liver. In Freeman, L. M., and Johnson, P. M. (eds.): Clinical Scintillation Imaging. New York: Grune & Stratton, pp. 434, 451.

203. Loberg, M. D., Nunn, A. D., and Porter, D. W.: Development of hepatobiliary imaging agents. In Freeman, L. M., and Weissmann, H. S.: Nuclear Medicine Annual 1981. New York; Raven Press, 1981.

TRANSHEPATIC CHOLANGIOGRAPHY

9

by Joseph T. Ferrucci, Jr., M.D.,
Peter R. Mueller, M.D., and
Eric vanSonnenberg, M.D.

Following the introduction of the thin-walled, fine caliber "skinny" needle by Okuda and coworkers in 1974,[1] percutaneous trans-hepatic cholangiography was transformed from a greatly feared, dangerous technique into a widely accepted routine clinical procedure for direct bile duct opacification.[2-12] Previously, percutaneous cholangiography had seldom been performed except as an immediate pre-operative maneuver in densely jaundiced patients. At present it is often employed as an elective diagnostic procedure for investigation of obstructive liver chemistries or ultrasound/computed tomographic evidence of ductal dilatation and not infrequently is carried out prior to the onset of frank clinical jaundice.[12, 13]

Fine-needle percutaneous transhepatic cholangiography (FNPTC) has largely replaced the older, sheathed needle technique because of its improved rate of duct opacification and wider safety margin; its comparable results, ease of performance, general availability, and lower cost also compare favorably with endoscopic retrograde cholangiography (ERCP).[4, 6, 12, 14, 15] More recently, the role of FNPTC has been further expanded to that of an essential preliminary diagnostic step prior to insertion of percutaneous biliary drainage catheters and other related transcatheter therapeutic interventional measures.[16-28]

As FNPTC has evolved into a standard, commonly employed diagnostic procedure, certain important trends in its clinical utilization have emerged (Table 9–1). This chapter will emphasize technical and interpretive considerations for FNPTC based on the pertinent literature and the authors' personal experience with over 700 cases. Measures to restrict complications and enhance the accuracy of cholangiographic diagnosis will be emphasized.

TECHNIQUE

Technical considerations for FNPTC have been elucidated in a series of papers from this institution.[4, 6, 11, 12] A synopsis of the major technical points is presented in Table 9–2.

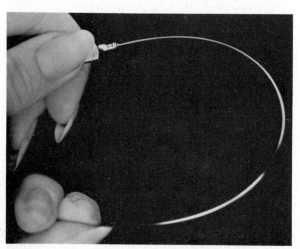

Figure 9–1. Fine caliber (22 gauge), thin-walled "Chiba," "skinny" flexible needle for percutaneous cholangiography. The flexibility of the needle minimizes the risks of laceration of hepatic parenchyma owing to respiratory excursions.

Table 9–1. FINE-NEEDLE PERCUTANEOUS TRANSHEPATIC CHOLANGIOGRAPHY (FNPTC) — TRENDS IN UTILIZATION: 1982

Clinical

Low threshold for performance
  Preicteric hyperbilirubinemia
  "Borderline" ducts by US/CT

"STAT" procedures, esp. acute cholangitis
  Immediate availability incl. nights, weekends

Routine preliminary step for transcatheter interventions
  Percutaneous drainage
  Endoprosthesis
  Balloon dilatation of strictures

Technical

No absolute contraindication
Routine antibiotic prophylaxis
No limit on number of needle passes
Tilt table essential
Selective puncture (L) hepatic duct common
Majority of FNPTCs now lead to drainage

The fine caliber, "skinny," "Chiba" needle is a thin-walled, 22-gauge (OD = 0.7 mm) needle, 15 cm in length with a 30-degree beveled noncutting tip (Figs. 9–1 and 9–2). Longer, 20-cm needles are also available for obese patients. The small caliber and flexibility of the needle allow it to deflect with respiratory excursions of the liver, minimizing the tearing effect on hepatic parenchyma as well as the risk of major puncture laceration of large vessels or ducts. The basic needle design is available through a variety of manufacturers.

Several modifications of the FNPTC needle have been developed, principally involving the use of a fitted 20-gauge cannula sheath to permit a single puncture cholangiogram and drainage or to accept a guide wire for a subsequent catheter exchange sequence.[29, 30] In general, these designs have not been effective and have not met with wide acceptance.

1. Patient Preparation

Patient preparation is detailed in Table 9–3. These measures apply for both diagnostic FNPTC and percutaneous biliary drainage (to be discussed in Chapter 12). Attention to bleeding parameters and prevention of sepsis are crucial concerns, since a high percentage of patients with biliary obstruction have infected bile and abnormalities of clotting function due to hepatic cellular dysfunction. Preventive measures for bleeding and sepsis are

Table 9–2. FINE-NEEDLE PERCUTANEOUS TRANSHEPATIC CHOLANGIOGRAPHY: TECHNIQUE SYNOPSIS

1. **Preparation**
   Bleeding parameters. IV antibiotics. Premedication. Sterile prep. Local analgesia. IV fluids. Blood pressure monitoring.

2. **Choice of Puncture Site**
   Lateral mid axillary line approach. Eighth to ninth intercostal space. Modify by assessment of hepatic size and configuration based on fluoroscopy and palpation. Avoid pleural recess. Can select puncture site and target with aid of metal markers.

3. **Needle Path**
   Toward opposite axilla. Horizontal, parallel to table. Needle tip directed toward margin of eleventh or twelfth intrathoracic vertebral body. Subsequent passes sequentially more caudad and shallow.

4. **Puncture Thrust**
   Rapid, continuous, during end-expiratory apnea and fluoroscopic control. Needle placement is "guided" not "blind." Remove stylet. Inject contrast.

5. **Contrast Injection**
   Under fluoroscopic control inject contrast and incrementally withdraw needle (2 to 3 cm) until ducts opacified. No prolonged attempt to aspirate bile.

6. **Fluoroscopic Observations**
   Veins, lymphatics, ducts. Subcapsular contrast deposition causes epigastric/substernal pain.

7. **Ducts Opacified**
   Rapid centrifugal flow of contrast. "Melting wax" appearance due to bile-contrast mixing. Frequent initial poor opacification of extrahepatic ducts in presence of high grade distal obstruction → periportal pseudo-obstruction.

8. **Positioning**
   Real versus pseudo-obstruction analyzed by combined semi-erect and left lateral decubitus positions to promote gravity mixing of contrast and bile in high pressure system.

9. **Filming**
   Spot and overhead radiography. Review films before removing needle. Obtain further films as needed.

10. **Ducts not Opacified**
   No diagnostic conclusions warranted. Should make at least 15 to 20 passes varying cephalo-caudad and antero-posterior course of needle path.

11. **Post-Procedure**
   Chest film (R/O pneumothorax), Hct.
   1. Normal, sclerosed ducts → aspirate and remove needle.
   2. Obstructed ducts → surgery pending → aspirate and remove needle → catheter drainage elected → leave fine needle → proceed with catheter procedure.

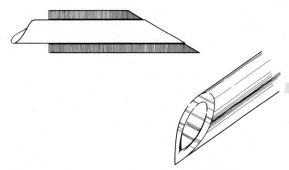

Figure 9–2. Schematic drawing of the tip of the fine caliber cholangiography needle. A 30-degree noncutting bevel minimizes the risk of hemorrhagic complications.

usually begun 24 hours before the procedure but can be initiated on a more abbreviated schedule in emergency cases. Thus, in very ill patients the timing of FNPTC can be adjusted to occur within a 2- to 3-hour time span to coincide with the optimal effects of administered blood products and antibiotics. Antibiotic coverage is continued for a minimum of three to four days if surgery or catheter insertion is not carried out. We have employed a combination of ampicillin (2 gm/24 hr IV) and gentamicin (80 mg/24 hr IM) with good results. It is to be noted that the principal side effect of gentamicin is renal toxicity; therefore, parameters of renal function should be observed carefully.

Table 9–3. PERCUTANEOUS TRANSHEPATIC TECHNIQUES — CHOLANGIOGRAPHY AND DRAINAGE: PATIENT PREPARATION

Preprocedure
1. Bleeding parameters
   Prothrombin time: <3 seconds beyond control (correct with vitamin K, fresh frozen plasma)
   Platelets: >75,000/cc (correct with platelet transfusions)
   Thromboplastin time: normal range (correct with vitamin K, fresh frozen plasma)
   Bleeding time: <10 minutes (usually a platelet defect, hematology consult)
2. Prophylactic antibiotics
   Ampicillin 2.0 gm/24 hr IV (start day before)
   Gentamicin 80 mg IM/24 hr (? substitute tobramycin) (start day of procedure)
3. Premedication
   Demerol and/or Valium

Periprocedure
1. Intravenous fluids running
2. Blood presure monitored continuously
3. Sterile technique (gowns, drapes, etc.)

Medication with narcotics and sedatives is essential before and during the procedure to ensure safety and success. A typical combination is meperidine (Demerol), 25 mg intravenously, and diazepoxide (Valium), 2.5 mg intravenously, repeated at 30- to 40-minute intervals as needed. Continuous intravenous fluid administration and monitoring of blood pressures at timely intervals are also mandatory.

2. Choice of Puncture Site

A lateral (mid axillary line) approach is generally employed, with the puncture site located in the eighth or ninth intercostal space as determined by clinical and fluoroscopic evaluation of hepatic size and configuration. The lateral approach is selected because a long needle tract is created through the liver substance, which promotes tamponade of subsequent bleeding or bile leakage from the interior of the liver. In selecting the puncture site it is essential to avoid transgression of the costophrenic sulcus. The approximate target for termination of the needle thrust can be identified fluoroscopically with the use of a metallic marker on the skin over the subxiphoid region.

3. Needle Path

Following sterile preparation of the puncture site and local administration of 1 per cent Xylocaine anesthesia, the needle and stylet are introduced in a single rapid thrust during a brief period of end-expiratory apnea. The needle is passed toward the opposite axilla in a plane horizontal and parallel to the tabletop, slightly above the confluence of the main intrahepatic ducts. The needle tip is deposited just to the right of the eleventh or twelfth thoracic vertebral body. Generally this represents an approximately 30-degree cephalad angulation of the needle. Subsequent serial passes, if required, are made in small incremental angles in a sequentially more caudad direction (Fig. 9–3). The initial cephalically directed punctures may be inserted more deeply (medially and dorsally) because of the presence of the bulk of the left hepatic lobe. Lacking the protection of the left lobe, caudally directed punctures should be more shallow (to a point short of the midline). To avoid an extrahepatic puncture in a caudal insertion, the needle should rarely progress beyond the

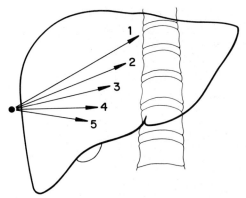

Figure 9–3. Preferred sequence of needle passes into liver parenchyma. Initial punctures should begin cephalad, medial, and dorsal and should proceed caudally, laterally, and more superficial. This sequence minimizes the risk of an extrahepatic puncture. (From Mueller, P. R., et al.: Am. J. Roentgenol. *136*:85, 1981.)

right mid clavicular line. However, judicious use of more caudal punctures has occasionally been the only maneuver to allow successful puncture of the duct system.

4. Puncture Thrust

The actual motion of needle placement is generally done under continuous fluoroscopic

control and is thus "guided" rather than "blind," minimizing the risk of inadvertent puncture of lung, heart, or bowel. Fluoroscopy is also critical during the performance of multiple or successive punctures to create appropriate "searching" alterations in the needle path, especially if re-entry into a partially opacified duct system is being attempted in a complicated case.

5. Contrast Injection

Under fluoroscopic control, the stylet is withdrawn and a syringe containing contrast material (usually 30 per cent methylglucamine diatrizoate) is attached and shallow respirations are resumed. The needle is slowly withdrawn in several millimeter increments with intermittent injections of 1 to 2 ml of contrast material under fluoroscopic monitoring until the ducts are opacified.

6. Fluoroscopic Observations

As the needle is withdrawn through the hepatic parenchyma, a distinct tract is created, which may appear as a persistent, irregular, linear streak of contrast material often reaching several centimeters in length (Fig. 9–4).

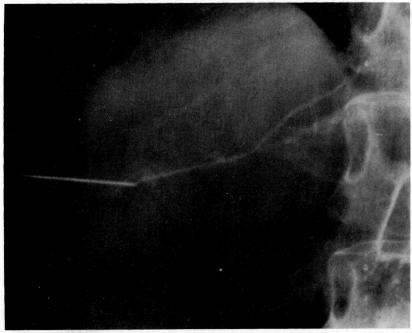

Figure 9–4. Transparenchymal needle tract. Contrast opacifies an irregular linear needle tract created by entry-withdrawal needle motion. In some cases the tract may act as a conduit for the preferential flow of contrast material into coincidentally punctured venous channels. (From Ferrucci, J. T., Jr., and Wittenberg, J.: Am. J. Roentgenol. *129*:11, 1977.)

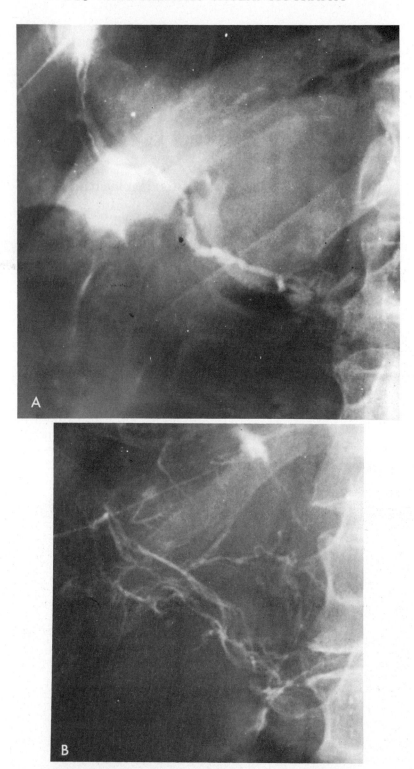

Figure 9–5. Hepatic lymphatics. Beaded, serpiginous lymphatic vessels often fill after intrahepatic contrast deposition and course medially and inferiorly from the porta hepatis. They may appear as a single trunk *(A)*, which could be misinterpreted as an irregular or sclerosed biliary radicle, or as a branching multichannel network *(B)*. Visualization of hepatic lymphatics at FNPTC carries no diagnostic significance relative to the prediction of extrahepatic biliary obstruction.

However, in some cases the tract may act as a conduit for the preferential flow of contrast material into venous structures previously punctured deep within the liver substance, even though the needle has been withdrawn far peripherally. The net effect of this preferential flow of contrast from the needle tip into previously punctured venous branches is that contrast material tends to be diverted from small biliary radicles, which may be entered as the needle is further withdrawn, and negative passes result. Further punctures in another plane will usually be required.

Recognition of the site of contrast material deposition is readily made fluoroscopically. Contrast within the hepatic parenchyma persists in an amorphous accumulation; contrast within venous channels flows rapidly toward the right atrium or porta hepatis; contrast within hepatic lymphatics may appear as a single or branching multi-channel beaded network extending inferiorly and medially from the area of the porta hepatis (Fig. 9–5). Hepatic lymphatics rarely exceed 2 to 3 mm in diameter, but they may be initially confused with small caliber or sclerosed intrahepatic biliary radicles, since, fluoroscopically, the rate of contrast flow in both structures is similar. However, the horizontal anatomic course of the lymph vessels toward the midline permits ready recognition. However, visualization of hepatic lymphatics has not been found to have any diagnostic significance in terms of predicting the presence or absence of mechanical biliary obstruction.[31, 32]

Transient visualization of branches of the hepatic and portal venous systems is also a commonplace event during the injection withdrawal sequence (Fig. 9–6). This too is an incidental observation, causing no clinical discomfort, and is of no diagnostic significance.

Deposition of contrast material under the liver capsule produces a typical elongated, smooth, crescentic or semi-lunar appearance and may account for considerable acute epigastric and substernal distress. A few minutes intentional delay will often allow the patient's discomfort to subside.

7. Ducts Opacified

Normal caliber or sclerosed ducts are frequently opacified during FNPTC, principally as a result of the small caliber of the 22-gauge needle (Fig. 9–7). Occasionally, the needle punctures tiny intrahepatic ducts of insufficient size to be recognized during fluoroscopy yet

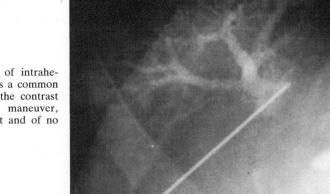

Figure 9–6. Visualization of intrahepatic venous branches. This is a common transient observation during the contrast injection–needle withdrawal maneuver, causing no clinical discomfort and of no diagnostic significance.

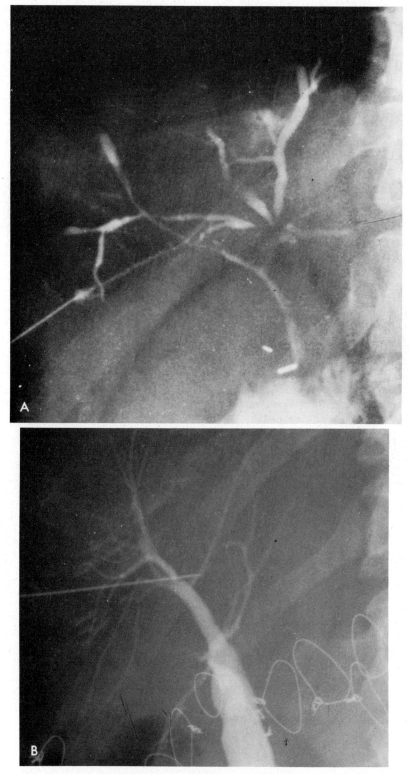

Figure 9–7. Opacification of small caliber sclerosed biliary ducts at FNPTC. *A,* Sclerosing cholangitis. *B,* Biliary cirrhosis. Note the tiny caliber of the biliary radicle in which the tip of the needle is located.

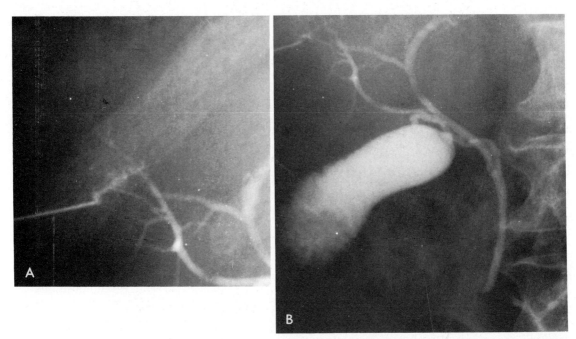

Figure 9–8. Opacification of tiny, nearly invisible intrahepatic biliary radicals with satisfactory filling of the remainder of a normal caliber extrahepatic biliary tree. *A,* Spot view of the intrahepatic ducts during contrast injection. *B,* View of the entire biliary tree, and lymph channels, but the common duct proper is adequately filled. Brief fluoroscopic scanning over the region of the distal common duct is recommended at the conclusion of "negative" needle passes to detect such serendipitious duct opacification from tiny intrahepatic radicles.

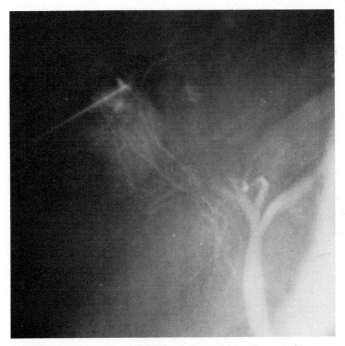

Figure 9–9. Common duct filling from tiny "invisible" biliary radicles. The actual puncture site of the intrahepatic biliary tree is obscured by parenchymal stain. (From Ferrucci, J. T., Jr., and Wittenberg, J.: Am. J. Roentgenol. *129*:11, 1977.)

large enough to carry contrast distally into the common duct itself (Fig. 9–8). In such cases fluoroscopic screening confined to the intra-parenchymal locus of the needle tip will yield a false impression that a negative pass has been made. Hence, brief fluoroscopic scanning over the region of the distal common duct is recommended at the conclusion of each "negative" puncture to detect such serendipitous duct opacification from tiny intrahepatic radicles (Fig. 9–9).

When dilated ducts are opacified, contrast material is judiciously injected and usually flows rapidly in a centrifugal direction. Often the mixing of viscid bile and contrast material in a dilated duct produces a "melting wax" effect fluoroscopically.

A brief attempt to aspirate bile can be made and is occasionally successful despite the small caliber of the needle, but no prolonged attempt to decompress the ducts is made at this stage. Rather, contrast material is injected with meticulous efforts to avoid undue distention of the duct system (Fig. 9–10). This is a crucial precaution to avoid subsequent septic complications. *Indeed, needless overfilling of the duct system is the cardinal sin of percutaneous transhepatic cholangiography* or for that matter of any cholangiographic procedure involving direct injection of the biliary tree.

8. Positioning

The use of gravity positioning maneuvers is essential for accurate interpretation. Because of the high intraluminal pressure in the presence of biliary obstruction, there is frequent initial poor opacification of the extrahepatic ducts, requiring the use of the erect and left lateral decubitus positions to promote gravity opacification of the caudad duct segments. Use of a tilting fluoroscopic table is therefore crucial. Removing the needle and taking prone films is an additional, although less frequently utilized, maneuver.

9. Filming

Radiographic exposures are made in supine, oblique, semi-erect, and prone positions as necessary. All radiographs should be reviewed before withdrawing the needle to assess the need for further filming.

10. Ducts Not Opacified

Failure to opacify the duct system does not warrant any diagnostic conclusions as to the presence or absence of biliary obstruction.[9, 11, 33] In many instances partially ob-

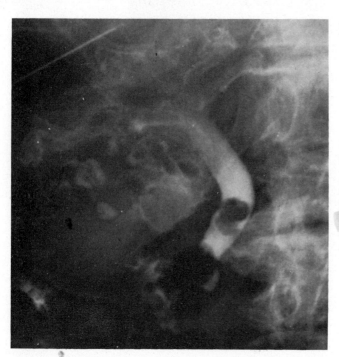

Figure 9–10. Choledocholithiasis. Cholangiographic filling technique adequate or not? Limited contrast filling of the ducts is intentional in this elderly man with suppurative cholangitis. Only enough contrast is injected to establish a definite diagnosis. This is a crucial precaution to minimize the risk of subsequent septic shock. Needless overfilling of the duct system is the cardinal sin of FNPTC.

structed systems have been opacified after more than 15 needle passes, and at least this number of puncture attempts should be made. With lesser degrees of duct obstruction, the frequency of successful opacification has been shown to have an almost linear relationship to the number of passes. The limiting factor in continuing a study is usually patient discomfort owing to subcapsular deposition of contrast material, which may produce deep epigastric distress, nausea, and restlessness. For that reason we and others have recommended a programmed, orderly sequence for locating successive needle passes to optimize results.[12, 33] The puncture sequence should follow the schema given in Figure 9–3, varying the cephalo-caudad and antero-posterior needle planes with each pass.

11. Post-Procedure

If normal or sclerosed ducts have been identified, bile and contrast material are aspirated and the needle withdrawn. If obstructed ducts are disclosed and surgery is intended imminently, bile and contrast material are aspirated and the needle removed. If a catheter drainage procedure is elected, the needle is left in place for further contrast injections during catheter introduction. A STAT hematocrit (or hemoglobin) and chest film (R/O pneumothorax) are obtained. The patient is returned to the ward with instructions for monitoring of vital signs and continuation of intravenous fluids.

Additional approaches to technique for hepatic puncture have been described in the literature. These include a direct anterior or ventral subcostal approach with the needle directed into the region of the confluence of the right and left hepatic ducts and use of ultrasonic real-time aspiration biopsy transducers to directly guide the puncture needle to the site of dilated intrahepatic ducts.[34, 35] Neither of these techniques has won wide acceptance to date.

PRINCIPLES OF FNPTC INTERPRETATION

Diagnostic Pitfalls

Several common fluoroscopic/radiographic appearances may cause diagnostic confusion during the actual performance of FNPTC.

Adventitial Dissection

The small caliber of the needle may permit contrast to be deposited within tightly confined anatomic spaces such as the adventitial planes surrounding the major vascular structures and biliary ducts in the porta hepatis[6] (Fig. 9–11). Dissection of opaque material along the adventitia of these large tubular structures sometimes results in unusual and misleading fluoroscopic/radiographic appearances. Whereas the negative outlines of biliary duct branches can sometimes be identified, occasionally the dissection of contrast material simulates the appearance of intraluminal contrast within the biliary duct system (i.e., a bizarre or distorted ductal system), giving an erroneous impression of an obstructed system (Fig. 9–12). A slower, more resistant flow of contrast material is usually observed fluoroscopically.

Pseudo-Obstruction

In the presence of obstructing lesions of the distal common bile duct, the initial cholangiographic appearance often gives the misleading impression of an obstruction at a higher level, e.g., in the porta hepatis. The combination of several factors is believed to create this pseudo-obstruction effect.[6, 12, 36, 37] First, in the presence of biliary obstruction, intraluminal biliary pressures may be increased two- to three-fold, with subsequent stagnation of the bile column.[6, 12, 36, 37] Second, in such cases, bile viscosity is greatly increased, causing poor mixing of injected contrast material. Third, the gravity gradient disadvantage of contrast material injected into the dependent posteriorly located right hepatic duct system in a supine patient further retards the flow of injected contrast material distally into the extrahepatic ducts. *In combination, these factors almost regularly and universally create a pseudo-obstruction phenomenon during FNPTC and constitute the single most common technical and interpretive error of this procedure.*

Familiarity with the three-dimensional anatomy of the intra- and extrahepatic biliary ducts aids appreciation of the flow dynamics of injected contrast material.[12]

In the sagittal plane, the common hepatic duct occupies a position somewhat dorsal to the common bile duct and follows a gradual ventral course caudally until it is joined by the cystic duct to form the common bile duct (Fig. 9–13). The common bile duct then passes

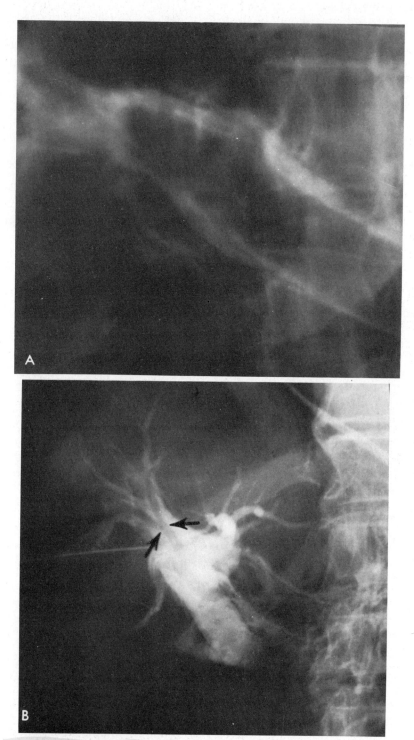

Figure 9–11. Adventitial contrast injection within tissue planes surrounding major ducts and vessels of the porta hepatis. *A,* Splenoportal venous junction. *B,* Periportal dissection disclosing negative outline of hepatic arterial branches (arrows) and opacification of several normal biliary radicles. (From Ferrucci, J. T., Jr., and Wittenberg, J.: Am. J. Roentgenol. *129*:11, 1977.)

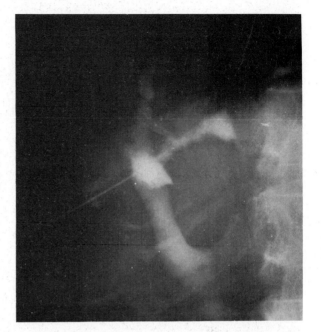

Figure 9–12. Adventitial dissection of contrast material simulating the appearance of intraluminal contrast within a dilated duct system. A slower, more resistant flow of contrast material can be observed fluoroscopically.

ventrally for a short distance to the level of the portal vein, where it turns dorsally to course between the posterior margins of the pancreatic head and the anterior margin of the inferior vena cava, terminating in the second portion of the duodenum. Hence, contrast material injected into an intrahepatic radicle in the supine patient must overcome a 4- to 6-cm ventro-dorsal hydrostatic gradient to flow caudally into the extrahepatic ducts. Awareness of these anatomic space relationships permits the use of gravity maneuvers for greater

precision in delineating the exact location and configuration of the obstructing lesion.

As noted, spurious periportal pseudo-obstruction is almost a rule with high-grade distal common duct obstruction and introduces a false proximal localization of the site of obstruction on initial filming.[6, 12, 36, 37] Because contrast material is deposited in the right hepatic ducts at a level several centimeters dorsal to the plane of the common bile ducts in the supine patient, the elevated biliary pressure and inspissated bile prevent flow beyond the

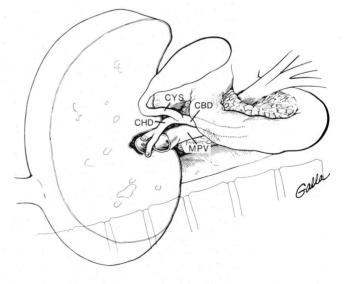

Figure 9–13. Schematic drawing in the supine parasagittal plane of the spatial relationships of the intra- and extrahepatic biliary tree in the supine position. The common hepatic duct (CHD) passes several centimeters ventral to the locus of the needle puncture in the mid right hepatic lobe and courses superficially over the main portal vein (MPV), turning dorsally into the common bile duct (CBD). CYS = cystic duct.

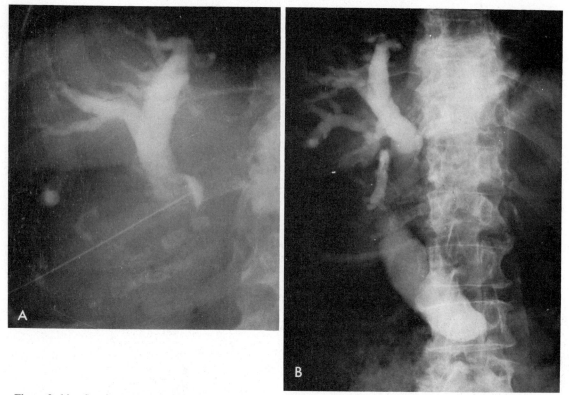

Figure 9–14. Spurious periportal pseudo-obstruction due to high-grade distal common duct block. A falsely proximal localization of the level of obstruction occurs as a result of the combination of high intraluminal biliary pressure, gravity, and inspissation of bile with poor bile and contrast mixing. Gravity maneuvers in the semi-erect and left lateral decubitus positions effectively promote flow of contrast distally. *A,* Initial film showing dilated intrahepatic ducts with no flow beyond the level of the periportal region. Note the indistinct fuzzy termination of the contrast column. (A small amount of extraluminal adventitial contrast deposition is noted.) *B,* Delayed semi-erect film disclosing better mixing with opacification of the entire length of the distal dilated common bile duct. Final diagnosis: carcinoma of the head of the pancreas. The initial appearance might have suggested an unresectable or inoperable lesion, whereas the correct identification of the obstruction in the periampullary region indicates that a surgical resection might still be technically feasible. (From Ferrucci, J. T., Jr., and Wittenberg, J.: Am. J. Roentgenol. *129*:11, 1977.)

porta hepatis (Figs. 9–14 and 9–15). Hence, serious diagnostic errors could result, including undetected distal common duct calculi and a false-positive diagnosis of a high periportal neoplastic infiltration, when only a localized obstructing periampullary tumor is present. The surgical and prognostic implications are radically divergent.

The possibility of spurious periportal obstruction of the contrast column can be suggested by recognition of a hazy, poorly defined interface of the injected contrast with the non-opacified bile column distally.[36] A well-defined sharp configuration of the terminus of the biliary contrast column suggests that a true site of obstruction has been delineated, and if this is not displayed, gravity positional maneuvers should be promptly employed.

The table is first tilted about 45 degrees upright, and the patient is then turned into a left lateral or left posterior oblique position. Most commonly, these maneuvers are carried out concurrently to promote better distal flow of contrast. As a result, the commonly encountered nonspecific fuzzy or blunt termination of the contrast column due to stagnation may be converted to a classic "rat-tail" appearance of pancreatic carcinoma. Usually these maneuvers also obviate the need for injection of additional amounts of contrast, reducing the likelihood of bacterial sepsis and increasing both the volume of contrast injected and the pressure of injection.

Gravity maneuvers frequently also result in opacification of the left hepatic duct, the caliber of which is important preoperative data in patients who may undergo a left hepatic cholangiojejunostomy bypass (Bismuth procedure). Further, since the possibility of percutaneous biliary drainage is now routinely

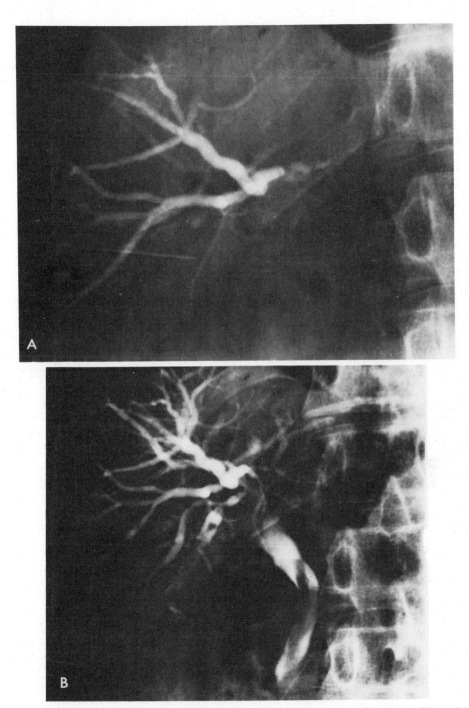

Figure 9–15. Another example of a spurious periportal obstruction. *A*, Initial film shows filling of intrahepatic radicles only. *B*, Film after placing the patient in the semi-erect left lateral decubitus position shows better filling of the distal common bile duct. Areas of incomplete filling at the porta and in the distal duct are due to poor bile contrast mixing and limited volumes of injected contrast material. Final diagnosis: small pancreatic head carcinoma.

considered in nearly all obstructed cases, these maneuvers assure more complete filling of the duct system, which aids selection of the most appropriate duct segment for introduction of a percutaneous biliary drainage catheter. It is worth re-emphasizing that the foregoing discussion represents the critical technical and interpretive aspect of the entire FNPTC procedure.

Admixture Defects

Poor mixture of contrast material with viscid inspissated bile may produce a single, sharply demarcated, elongated filling defect simulating a large oval calculus[6] (Fig. 9–16). This is characteristically located in the ventralmost portion of the mid common bile duct as the duct courses with the portal vein and turns dorsally toward the second portion of the duodenum. Although the appearance varies little from case to case, semi-erect and left decubitus films should be obtained to exclude other causes of intraductal filling defects. Admixture defects are most often seen in association with low-grade distal obstruction and stagnation of bile column and have been encountered during T-tube and intravenous cholangiography as well as FNPTC (Fig. 9–17).

Biliary Obstruction

In the presence of mechanical bile duct obstruction, present-day practices tend to re-

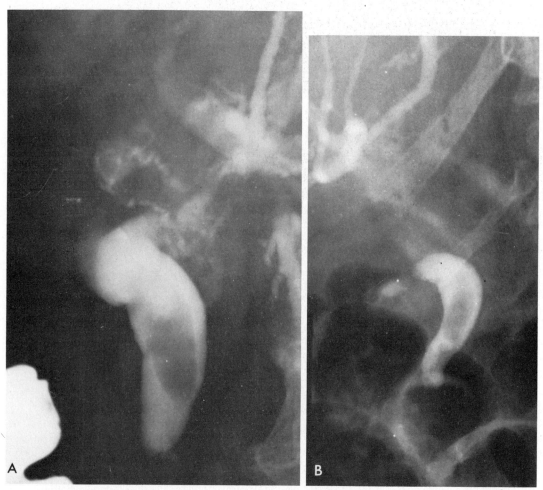

Figure 9–16. *A, B,* Admixture defects. Two different cases. An elongated, sharply demarcated filling defect is visible in the mid common bile duct, simulating a large oval calculus. At surgery both patients were found to have benign periampullary strictures with no stone or other discrete lesion. The defects are considered to arise from poor mixing of viscid bile and injected contrast and are typically found in the mid to distal common bile duct. (From Ferrucci, J. T., Jr., and Wittenberg, J.: Am. J. Roentgenol. *129*:11, 1977.)

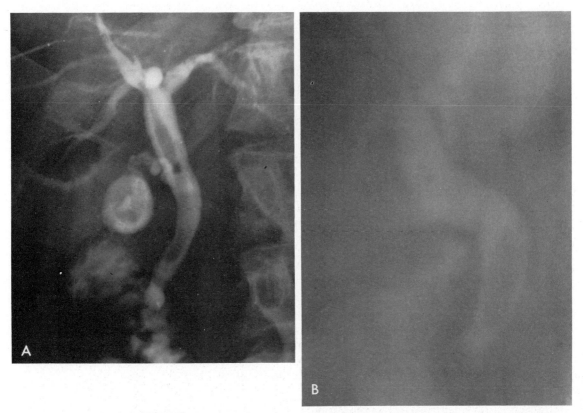

Figure 9–17. Admixture defects in a normal percutaneous cholangiogram *(A)* and an intravenous cholangiogram with mild ampullary stenosis *(B)*. The defect is characteristically located in the ventrally positioned mid portion of the common bile duct where contrast material layers dependently under viscid bile.

quire a more complete delineation of duct anatomy than was previously required. Because surgical approaches have become more highly tailored with regard to the specific type of biliary digestive bypass or anatomic reconstruction attempted, preoperative anatomic delineation of duct anatomy has become critical for planning the operative approach. By the same token, the increasing availability of nonsurgical options for treatment of mechanical lesions of the bile ducts, such as percutaneous catheter techniques and perendoscopic methods, also requires accurate delineation of duct anatomy for selection of the optimal treatment method. This section details some special considerations in the delineation and interpretation of FNPTC in the presence of mechanical obstruction.

Radiographic/Pathologic Correlations

During the initial performance of FNPTC the radiographic appearance of the biliary duct anatomy may reflect a number of variables other than the actual configuration of the mechanical obstruction present, so that correlations with surgical pathologic findings must be made cautiously. As already noted, because injection of contrast is commonly made into a peripheral biliary radicle against considerable pressure and hydrostatic gravity gradients, complete opacification of the bile duct system is often not possible without injection of excessive volumes of contrast at unacceptable levels of pressure with respect to the likelihood of producing septicemia. It is the present authors' view that most of the cholangiograms published in earlier papers on conventional sheathed needle percutaneous transhepatic cholangiography demonstrated dangerously unacceptable degrees of duct distention by present-day standards.

Because of the generally more cautious current approach to injecting contrast into a dilated obstructed system by FNPTC, several interpretive caveats follow. Most "complete" obstructing lesions are in fact not anatomically complete when tested by a probing guide wire or catheter (Fig. 9–18). Rather, the cholangio-

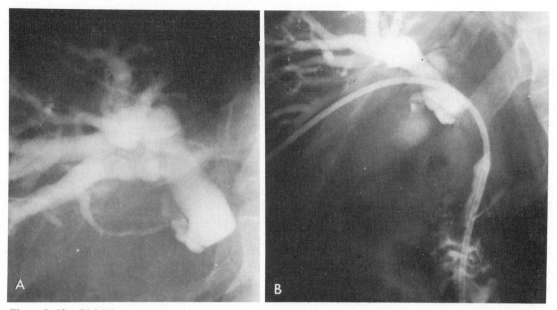

Figure 9–18. Pitfall in cholangiographic appearance of complete obstruction. Initial diagnostic FNPTC *(A)* showing apparent "complete" malignant obstruction in the mid common duct. The obstruction is in fact not anatomically complete, as demonstrated by ready catheterization for internal biliary drainage *(B)*. Diagnosis: carcinoma of the head of the pancreas.

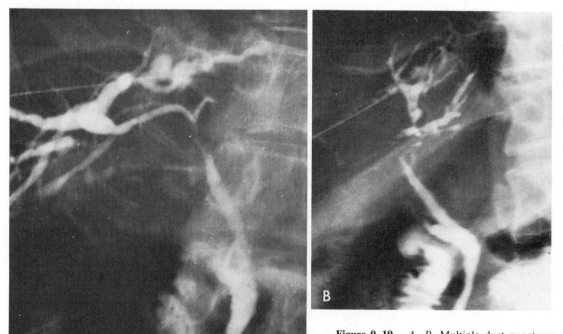

Figure 9–19. *A, B,* Multiple duct punctures. Undifferentiated malignant neoplasm (primary bile duct carcinoma?) causing diffuse multisegmental encasement and distortion of the hepatic bifurcation and multiple intrahepatic ducts. Separate isolated and noncommunicating groups of duct radicles are filled on two separate needle punctures during the same study. In patients with diffuse intrahepatic or periportal disease, several separate duct punctures may be needed for complete delineation of multiple isolated or noncommunicating groups of radicles.

graphic appearance suggesting complete obstruction is in fact due to the spatial and mechanical factors involved. In such cases, percutaneous catheters subsequently advanced closer to the actual site of the obstruction often show a readily discernible trickle of contrast through the stricture distally. By the same token, initial cholangiographic films may show filling of only a subgroup of intrahepatic biliary radicles, which are located in a posterior or dependent portion of the liver in the supine patient. Subsequent cholangiograms made after introduction of a drainage catheter with interval decompression and better anatomic advantage often will show far more complete opacification of the entire duct system including the left hepatic duct. Indeed, in many instances and in some institutions, the initial radiographs obtained during FNPTC are essentially disregarded with respect to their diagnostic content and serve only as a means to guide fluoroscopic introduction of the drainage catheter. After an interval of several days for therapeutic decompression, contrast is then injected through the indwelling catheter for a diagnostic cholangiogram. Such an approach is entirely safe and sensible.

Multiple Duct Punctures

In certain instances adequate delineation of intrahepatic duct anatomy is prevented by multiple isolated areas of duct obstruction so that various divisions of intrahepatic radicles no longer communicate. This is most commonly seen in patients with severe sclerosing cholangitis, diffuse infiltration of the porta hepatis by cholangiocarcinoma, or metastatic disease infiltrating the periportal region. In such instances it may be necessary to puncture several different biliary radicles separately to obtain sufficient anatomic information to plan appropriate therapy (Fig. 9–19).

Selective Left Hepatic Duct Puncture

A specific example of the role of multiple duct puncture is selective cholangiography of the left hepatic duct. This is most often indicated when malignant periportal infiltration selectively isolates and obstructs the left hepatic duct. In such cases specific surgical decompression of the left hepatic duct by a hepaticojejunostomy (Bismuth procedure) or selective percutaneous catheter drainage of the left hepatic duct system may be required.

Analysis of our own material suggests that selective obstruction of the left hepatic duct may be almost universal when malignant periportal infiltration occurs. Unfortunately, in most instances FNPTC is performed from the standard right lateral approach and fails to opacify the obstructed dilated left hepatic duct system. Until the recent popularity of the Bismuth procedure and the availability of ultrasonography to easily demonstrate dilated left hepatic ducts, the frequency of this phenomenon was generally not appreciated.

The technique for selective left duct cholangiography involves the use of preliminary ul-

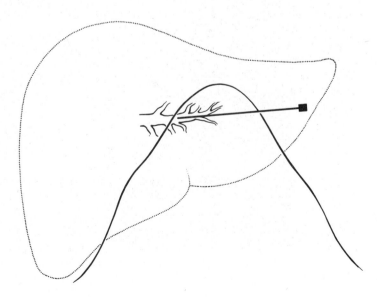

Figure 9–20. Schematic drawing showing technique for selective puncture of the left hepatic duct. The needle is inserted horizontally across the subxiphoid costal arch, with the patient reversed feet first on the fluoroscopic table. Initial ultrasonographic localization of the dilated left hepatic duct segment greatly facilitates selective left duct puncture.

trasonography to demonstrate and localize on the skin the presence and level of the dilated left hepatic duct system. Ordinarily, the left lobe of the liver is located superficially below the anterior abdominal wall in the subxiphoid region rarely more than 3 to 4 cm deep to the skin surface. The patient is placed in a reverse (feet first) position on the fluoroscopic table to bring the left upper quadrant into the operator's working area, and the needle is inserted horizontally across the subxiphoid costal arch (Fig. 9–20). The actual cutaneous needle puncture site is made as close to the margin of the left costal arch as possible, directing the needle tip medially and dorsally into the left hepatic lobe (Fig. 9–21). Over 35 selective left

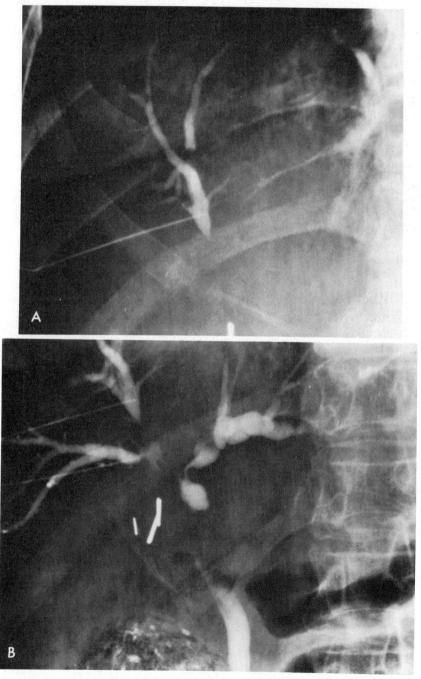

Figure 9–21 *See legend on opposite page*

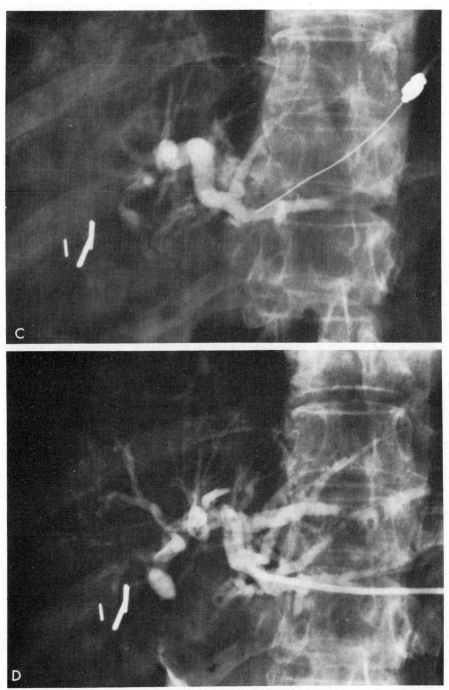

Figure 9–21. Another example of multiple needle punctures including selective puncture of the left hepatic duct. Undifferentiated carcinoma infiltrating the periportal region. Final diagnosis: primary bile duct carcinoma. *A*, Initial needle puncture showing a single isolated intrahepatic biliary radicle. *B*, Second needle puncture opacifying lower branches of the right duct, a portion of a dilated left hepatic duct, and normal caliber distal common duct. *C*, Selective cholangiogram of the left hepatic duct showing obstruction at the confluence with negligible flow into the common duct. *D*, Selective external drainage catheter placed in the left hepatic duct.

duct cholangiograms have now been performed in our department with no specific untoward results.

Periampullary Obstructions

Periampullary obstruction presents a special diagnostic problem in that such lesions are often nonspecific in radiographic appearance, may be either benign or malignant in nature, and may arise from either the distal common bile duct, the duodenum, or the head of the pancreas. Useful ancillary maneuvers in the evaluation of such cases include the use of glucagon for hypotonic cholangiography and barium duodenography, often in combination.

Inflammatory diseases of the choledochoduodenal junction, especially pancreatitis, a recently passed common duct stone, and ampullary stenosis, may be associated with considerable smooth muscle spasm at the time of

FNPTC. Thus, exclusion of a small impacted common duct stone or an ampullary or pancreatic neoplasm is often impossible. Because the distalmost part of the common duct is encircled by smooth muscle fibers originating from the musculature of the duodenal walls, an antispasmodic drug such as glucagon can be effective in aiding the differential diagnosis.[38] The drug is given in a dose of 1.0 mg intravenously, and immediate relaxation of periampullary smooth muscle spasm may be demonstrated, allowing the free flow of common duct contrast into the duodenum (Fig. 9–22). When glucagon is not available, other spasmolytic agents, including propantheline bromide (Pro-Banthine), are also effective.

When response to glucagon or other antispasmodic agents is inconclusive or when the possibility of a duodenal, ampullary, or pancreatic cause for distal common duct obstruction is suggested, a simultaneous barium duodenogram is sometimes of value (Figs. 9–23

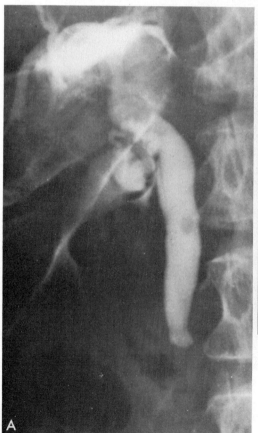
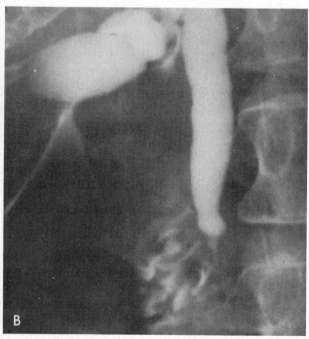

Figure 9–22. Role of antispasmodic drugs (glucagon) in periampullary obstructions. *A,* Initial study disclosing blunt attenuation of the contrast column with no flow into the duodenum. Differential between small impacted ampullary calculus and neoplasm is difficult. *B,* Immediately following the administration of intravenous glucagon, periampullary smooth muscle sphincter spasm relaxes, allowing contrast material to flow into the duodenum. Slight narrowing of the periampullary distal common duct with nodular appearing mucosa is evident. No definite calculi or tumor. Final diagnosis: recently passed common duct stone with ampullary sphincter spasm.

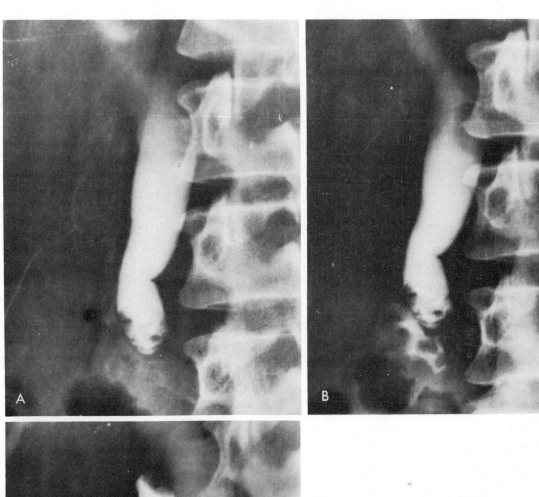

Figure 9–23. Cholangiographic aids for peri-ampullary obstruction. Combined hypotonic cholangiogram and barium duodenogram. *A,* Initial FNPTC showing complete periampullary obstruction with a blunt termination of the contrast column suggesting neoplasm. Several tiny irregular nodular defects are noted in the distal portion of the contrast column. *B,* Film immediately following intravenous administration of glucagon (1.0 mg) shows partial relaxation of the choledochoduodenal sphincter with flow of contrast into the duodenum. Nodular thickened duodenal mucosal folds are apparent. *C,* Simultaneous barium duodenogram confirms diffuse nodular duodenal mucosal fold thickening. Diagnosis: villous adenoma of the duodenum obstructing the distal common bile duct. This diagnosis was correctly made prospectively.

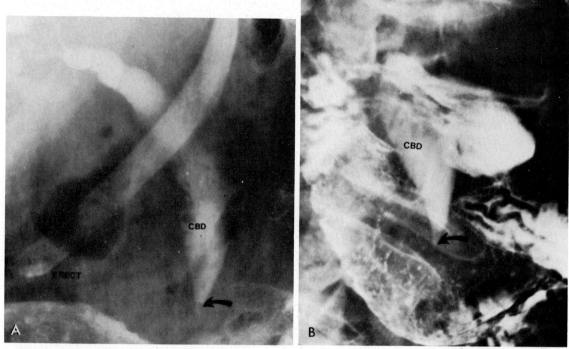

Figure 9–24. Combined cholangiogram barium duodenogram in another patient with villous adenoma of the duodenum obstructing the distal common bile duct. *A*, Erect view following the administration of glucagon showing an elongated, tapered narrowing of the distal common duct but with no flow into the duodenum despite glucagon. *B*, Simultaneous barium duodenogram showing diffuse frond-like thickening of mucosal folds and widening of the duodenal lumen. The correct diagnosis was made prospectively on the basis of the radiographic features.

and 9–24). Glucagon and barium are satisfactorily administered when given in quick succession with the patient in the right lateral decubitus position. This position promotes adequate gastric emptying of barium into the duodenum before the full hypotonic effect of the glucagon occurs. Timing is of some importance during a combined hypotonic cholangiography-duodenography, since delayed administration of the barium will result in poor gastric emptying and impaired duodenal filling.

RESULTS

Success Rate

Because of the wide safety margin of the fine caliber needle and the ability to make an almost unlimited number of needle passes, the success rate for satisfactory duct opacification should approach 100 per cent.[9, 11, 12] In the largest series reported to date, Harbin, Mueller, and Ferrucci reported the results of a multi-institutional survey in the United States and found an overall success rate of 97.8 per cent in 1,293 patients with dilated bile ducts.[11]

They also noted a 70.2 per cent success rate in 476 patients with nondilated bile ducts. The data from that study also indicated that success rates improved slightly when the number of needle passes reached 15. It is noteworthy that neither this study nor a study by Ariyama from Japan was able to demonstrate an increase in clinically significant complications with the increased number of needle passes.[9, 11]

Although the 70 per cent rate of visualization of nondilated ducts is less than that usually quoted for endoscopic retrograde cholangiography (ca 90 per cent), it should be emphasized that FNPTC is an effective means of demonstrating biliary ducts regardless of the degree of dilatation. Thus, when endoscopic retrograde cholangiography is precluded because of previous gastrointestinal surgery, such as a Billroth II gastroenterostomy or biliary enteric anastomosis, FNPTC becomes the preferred method[40] (Fig. 9–25).

Complications

Because transhepatic cholangiography, even if performed with a fine caliber needle, can

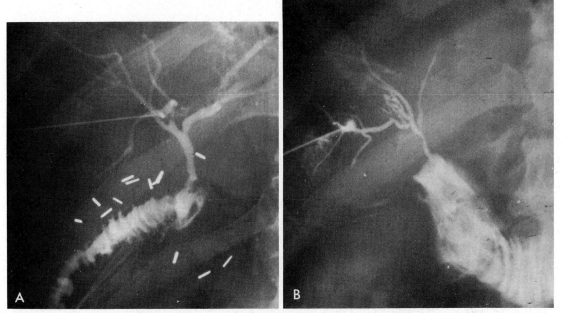

Figure 9–25. FNPTC following previous biliary enteric bypass surgery. Two different cases showing appearance following choledochojejunostomy with normal intrahepatic ducts *(A)* and slightly sclerosed, attenuated intrahepatic ducts *(B)*. In patients in whom prior surgical reconstructions have been performed, endoscopic cholangiography is frequently precluded for anatomic reasons, and FNPTC thus becomes the principal method for direct cholangiography and can be successful regardless of the degree of duct dilatation. (Figure 9–25*B* from Ferrucci, J. T., Jr., et al. Am. J. Roentgenol. *127*:403, 1976.)

lead to lethal complications, including bile peritonitis, hemorrhage, and septic shock, an understanding of the mechanisms of these complications and an awareness of the measures to prevent or minimize their occurrence are essential[9, 11] (Fig. 9–26).

If sporadic reports of high (37 to 80 per cent) complication rates in the hands of non-radiologist cholangiographers are excluded as nonrepresentative, the incidence of major complications remains well below 5 per cent.[41, 42] The survey of complications of FNPTC reported by Harbin, Mueller, and Ferrucci noted a 3.28 per cent major complication rate in 3,596 procedures recorded.[11] The principal complications of FNPTC as derived from the data of Harbin, Mueller, and Ferrucci are presented in Table 9–4.

Sepsis

Septic shock, defined as fever and chills accompanied by hypotension, a positive blood culture, or severe prostration, is the most common serious complication, occurring in approximately 2 per cent of patients. Sepsis following FNPTC is almost invariably limited to patients with biliary obstruction and is believed

to result from infected bile entering the blood stream via direct communication between the biliary canaliculi and the liver sinusoids.[43-47] Septic complications are virtually nonexistent

Table 9–4. FINE-NEEDLE TRANSHEPATIC CHOLANGIOGRAPHY: COMPLICATIONS*

Complication	Percentage of Patients
Septicemia (defined as hypotension, prostration, or positive blood culture)	1.8
Bile Leakage Bile staining/biloma Bile peritonitis	1.0
Hemorrhage Intraperitoneal Intrahepatic hematoma	0.3
Death	0.1
Other Pneumothorax Hepatic A-V fistula/pseudo-aneurysm Hemobilia Perihepatic abscess Bent/broken needle	0.1
Total	3.3

*Data from reference 11.

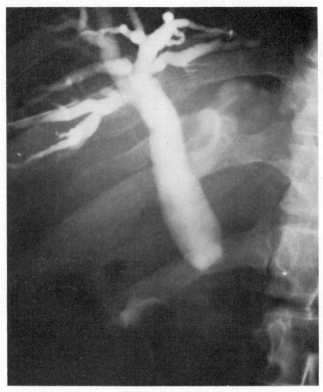

Figure 9–26. A lethal FNPTC. This patient with high-grade periampullary obstruction proven at surgery to be due to an impacted common duct calculus developed septic shock several hours after the procedure and underwent emergency surgery, which was complicated by an intraoperative myocardial infarction. The patient expired on the third postoperative day.

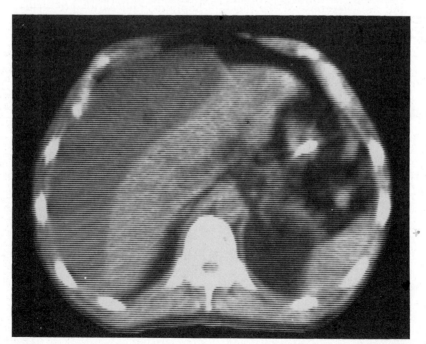

Figure 9–27. Perihepatic bile collection shown by CT 24 hours following FNPTC. The collection was evacuated by CT guided–percutaneous catheter drainage.

when ducts are of normal caliber or are non-obstructed. Infection of the bile is quite common in patients with common duct stones (80 per cent) but occurs less frequently (25 to 30 per cent) in patients with malignant biliary obstruction. The common organisms found on blood culture include *E. coli, Klebsiella,* and *Streptococcus.*

Septic shock following FNPTC may occur as early as 30 minutes to one hour after the procedure. The probable exact mechanism is vasomotor collapse mediated by the release of endotoxins rather than bacterial seeding of the blood *per se.*[43-47] Thus, strictly speaking, antibiotics may not prevent sudden endotoxemia caused by organisms extruded from the biliary ducts into the blood stream during cholangiography. Nevertheless, antibiotic prophylaxis is obviously crucial for preventing septicemia and should be administered 24 hours prior to the study, if possible.

The optimal choice of antibiotics for prophylaxis against biliary sepsis has been studied by Keighley and colleagues.[48, 49] They noted that antibiotic concentration in the bile is almost always inadequate for sterilization when obstruction is present, but a sufficient serum concentration is easily achieved in most patients. In their studies, more than 60 per cent of patients with infected bile had multiple organisms, both gram positive and gram negative. For these reasons, we currently recommend parenteral administration of both ampicillin and gentamicin. A newer aminoglycoside analogue, tobramycin, carries less renal toxicity than gentamicin and may be substituted. The usual doses are ampicillin 2.0 gm/24 hr IV and gentamicin 80 mg/24 hr IM.

Septic shock can usually be effectively managed with intravenous fluids and pressors but can obviously precipitate lethal cardiovascular events, such as stroke and myocardial infarction, especially in elderly or debilitated patients. Prophylactic antibiotics, avoidance of excessive volumes of injected contrast, and increasing use of catheter decompression are the most important measures to reduce septic complications.

Bile Leakage

The incidence of bile leakage reported at surgery is 3 to 4 per cent, although the incidence of clinically occult asymptomatic bile leaks detected by ultrasound or CT is probably somewhat higher (Fig. 9–27).[9, 11, 41, 42, 50] Thus, it is not uncommon to observe a moderate amount of loculated bile or bile-stained peritoneal fluid in the right upper quadrant as an incidental observation at laparotomy with no apparent effect on clinical course or patient management.[50] Frank bile peritonitis with right upper quadrant pain, fever, and signs of guarding and rebound tenderness requiring emergency surgery occurs less frequently. In Harbin, Mueller, and Ferrucci's survey of over 2000 procedures, only four required emergency laparotomy.[11]

Bile leakage most often occurs as a consequence of biliary obstruction when intraductal pressures are markedly elevated and bile decompresses through the needle puncture site. However, the incidence of bile leakage is markedly increased when the puncture site is inadvertently made too caudad at the level of the extrahepatic bile ducts, where there is no protective effect of surrounding hepatic parenchyma to tamponade leaking bile[11] (Fig. 9–28). Thus, of the 13 patients in Harbin, Muel-

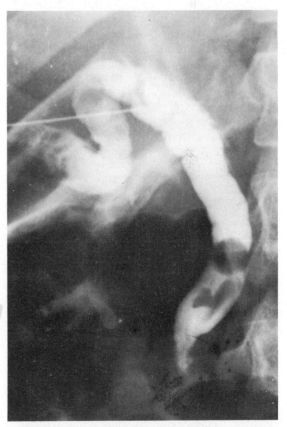

Figure 9–28. Extrahepatic puncture predisposes to bile leakage. This patient with inadvertent caudal puncture of the common hepatic duct below the protection of the hepatic parenchyma developed bile peritonitis, requiring emergency surgery 24 hours after the procedure. Recognition that the extrahepatic ducts have been inadvertently punctured warrants especially close post-procedure monitoring.

ler, and Ferrucci's survey studied with signs and symptoms of bile peritonitis, the extrahepatic ducts were inadvertently punctured in nine. Therefore, recognizing that the extrahepatic ducts have been entered during FNPTC warrants exceptionally close post-procedure monitoring. In general, protection against bile peritonitis is afforded by post-procedure aspiration and drainage of the duct system. With the increasingly widespread use of percutaneous biliary drainage as a means of preoperative decompression or definitive palliative drainage, the incidence of clinically significant bile leakage has remained at the acceptably low level of 1 to 2 per cent.[21-26]

Hemorrhage

Intraperitoneal hemorrhage occurs in 0.5 to 1 per cent of cases on the basis of surgical reports, although small clinically asymptomatic intrahepatic hematoma formation is undoubtedly more common.[9, 11, 50] Experience in our department suggests a 10 to 15 per cent incidence of sonographically detectable intrahepatic hematoma formation immediately following FNPTC (Fig. 9–29). Hemobilia (blood clots in the biliary ducts) is only rarely encountered during FNPTC, although it is much more frequent during percutaneous biliary drainage and will therefore be discussed in Chapter 12.

If a coagulation disorder is present, ERCP is preferable to FNPTC. If ERCP is unavailable, hematologic consultation is necessary to restore bleeding parameters to a point where needle puncture studies can be safely carried out.

Death

Several fatalities have been recorded in which FNPTC-associated sepsis, bile peritonitis, or hemorrhage precipitated sudden death or emergency surgery resulting in postoperative demise (Fig. 9–26). Harbin, Mueller, and Ferrucci's data disclosed five deaths in 3,596 total procedures (0.14 per cent).[11] Undoubtedly many more have occurred.

Miscellaneous

Tension pneumothorax and intrahepatic arteriovenous fistulas may rarely occur but can be expected less frequently than with large sheathed needle techniques. In Okuda's study of 79 patients undergoing FNPTC and follow-up hepatic arteriograms, three instances of intrahepatic A-V fistula (3.8 per cent) were encountered, all of which were clinically silent.[51] Bending of the fine-caliber needle is not an uncommon event, especially when the liver

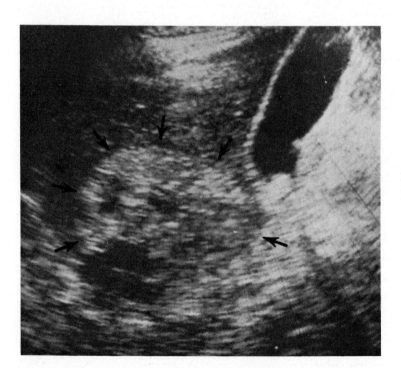

Figure 9–29. Intrahepatic hematoma following FNPTC shown sonographically as a rounded echogenic mass in the right hepatic lobe. Note the gallstone.

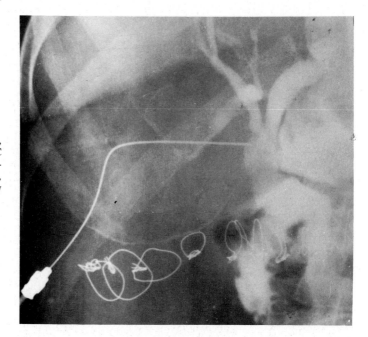

Figure 9–30. Bending of the thin-walled, fine caliber 22-gauge needle during FNPTC is not uncommon when firm fibrotic or neoplastic hepatic tissue is traversed. Usually, bending of the needle produces no clinically evident sequelae.

is replaced by firm fibrotic or neoplastic tissue, but this usually causes no untoward effects (Fig. 9–30). Broken needle shafts have also been reported verbally to the authors.

RADIOGRAPHIC FEATURES

The expectation in performing percutaneous transhepatic cholangiography is that it will demonstrate (1) the presence or absence of biliary obstruction, (2) the level or site of obstruction, and (3) the probable cause.[52-56] With appropriate FNPTC technique, the presence and level of the obstructing lesion are now almost invariably demonstrable. However, prediction of the precise etiologic cause is considerably less exact.

Although the number of diseases affecting the extrahepatic ducts is limited, only a few regularly display entirely typical cholangiographic features. Thus, common duct calculi are usually readily identifiable as are other distinctive morphologic entities such as sclerosing cholangitis and choledochal cyst. However, the differential diagnosis of malignant obstructions, either primary or secondary, and benign stenosing lesions is seldom clear-cut. There are many "look alike" entities, and several conditions may present varied appearances. It is frequently difficult to determine whether an area is stenotic owing to intrinsic or extrinsic constriction, and the termination

of the contrast column often has a nonspecific configuration whether blunt or symmetrically tapered. In short, benign and malignant obstructions of the extrahepatic ducts are often difficult to differentiate.

Notwithstanding these uncertainties, a useful working differential diagnosis can be offered by considering those disorders most commonly presenting at the level where the obstruction is demonstrated (Fig. 9–31). Obstruction at the level of the liver hilus in the periportal region is most often due to cholangiocarcinoma, carcinoma of the gallbladder, metastatic lymph node enlargement from remote primaries, or infiltration from primary hepatocellular carcinoma. Obstruction of the suprapancreatic portion of the mid common duct is commonly due to carcinoma of the pancreas or bile duct but may be due to iatrogenic stricture, metastatic disease, or benign stricture from sclerosing cholangitis, chronic pancreatitis, or an unusual manifestation of common duct calculus disease. Periampullary or infrapancreatic obstruction is most often due to carcinoma of the head of the pancreas or ampulla of Vater but may be due to a variety of benign disorders including common duct stone, ampullary stenosis, choledochal cysts, villous adenoma of the duodenum, choledochocele, and duodenal diverticulum.

It is of considerable importance to note that the practical value of cholangiographic differential diagnosis has recently assumed new di-

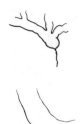

PERI-PORTAL

CHOLANGIOCARCINOMA
CA GALLBLADDER
METASTATIC DISEASE
HEPATOMA INVADING BILE DUCT

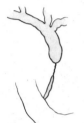

MID-COMMON DUCT

CA PANCREAS
CA BILE DUCT
IATROGENIC STRICTURE
METASTATIC DISEASE
SCLEROSING CHOLANGITIS
CHRONIC PANCREATITIS
COMMON DUCT STONE

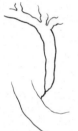

PERI-AMPULLARY

CA PANCREAS
AMPULLARY CA
COMMON DUCT STONE
AMPULLARY STENOSIS
CHOLEDOCHAL CYST
VILLOUS ADENOMA OF DUODENUM
CHOLEDOCHOCOELE
DUODENAL DIVERTICULUM

Figure 9–31. Common sites and causes of bile duct obstruction.

mensions with the current widespread use of new nonsurgical methods for treatment of biliary obstruction such as percutaneous catheter techniques and endoscopic papillotomy. Laborious speculation over the exact patho-anatomic extent and nature of a malignant stricture becomes somewhat academic if transhepatic catheter insertion is chosen for nonsurgical palliative decompression, followed by percutaneous needle biopsy to establish a pathologic diagnosis. By the same token, the identification of common duct stones or an apparently benign disorder of the choledochoduodenal junction such as ampullary stenosis may suggest a need for perendoscopic papillotomy and basket extraction, possibly averting the need for formal laparotomy.[57-60] The opportunity to make such therapeutic choices based on cholangiographic localization of obstruction and prediction of probable cause has become one of the predominant themes in the present-day clinical management of biliary disease.

Neoplasms

Carcinoma of the Pancreas

Complete or nearly complete stricture-obstruction of the mid or distal common duct should be considered a carcinoma of the head of the pancreas until proved otherwise (Fig. 9–32). When the site of obstruction is at the superior margin of the pancreatic head, the suprapancreatic portion of the duct may assume a medially directed, almost horizontal, course as if retracted toward the mid line by a pancreatic mass (Fig. 9–33). Proximal dilatation of the extrahepatic ducts may be moderate to marked, and in post-cholecystectomy patients considerable dilatation of the cystic duct may occur with the spiral valves of Heister in the intramural portion of the cystic duct, sometimes giving a bizarre beaded appearance (Fig. 9–34).

Although the "rat-tail" configuration of the distal common duct has been deemed typical of obstructing pancreatic carcinoma, the terminus of the contrast column may be smoothly and symmetrically tapered in a conical fashion or may show a slightly eccentric and irregular appearance. Equally often, however, the termination of the contrast column shows a completely obstructed blunt or rounded terminus (Fig. 9–35). This configuration simply reflects pooling of contrast material in the dilated prestenotic segment of the distal common duct with little or no opacification of the "rat-tail" beak itself (Fig. 9–36). If a percutaneous drainage catheter is subsequently advanced into this segment, reinjection of contrast will often disclose a more characteristic, irregularly tapered, beak-like "rat tail."

Ampullary Carcinoma

The classic appearance of an ampullary carcinoma obstructing the distal common bile duct is that of an irregular polypoid intraluminal mass growing within the immediate supraduodenal portion of the common duct (Fig. 9–37). In such cases, the lumen of the distal duct is often locally widened at the level of the obturating mass. However, ampullary carcinomas may also produce an irregular tapered stricture or a squared-off, flattened termination of the contrast column at the level of the duodenum, which may be identical to an appearance of a small pancreatic head cancer and may be difficult to distinguish from benign ampullary

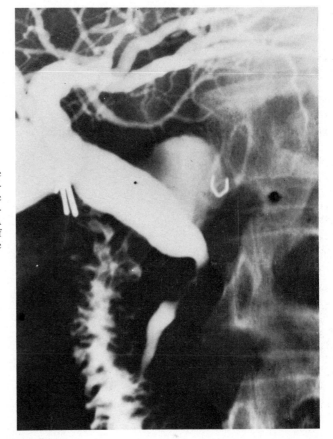

Figure 9–32. Carcinoma of the head of the pancreas with a typical high-grade stricture-obstruction in the mid common duct at the level of the pancreatic head. There is moderate proximal dilatation including dilatation of the cystic duct. A small, normal caliber infrapancreatic segment of the distal common duct is opacified below the tumor.

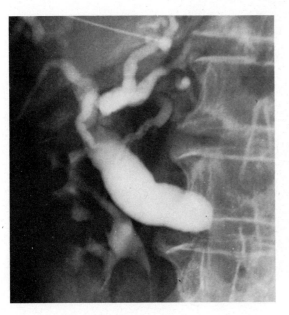

Figure 9–33. Carcinoma of the head of the pancreas showing a high-grade complete obstruction at the superior margin of the pancreatic head, with a medially directed horizontal course of the distal common duct as if retracted toward the midline by the pancreatic tumor. This is a common FNPTC pattern in obstructing carcinoma of the pancreatic head.

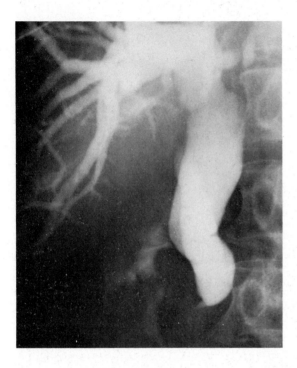

Figure 9–34. Carcinoma of the head of the pancreas with high-grade obstruction and proximal dilatation. A "rat-tail" configuration is apparent. Note the striking dilatation of the cystic duct in this patient.

Figure 9–35. Carcinoma of the pancreatic head with complete obstruction and a blunt or rounded termination of the contrast column. This is an equally common cholangiographic appearance in pancreatic cancer and reflects pooling of contrast material in the dilated prestenotic segment of the distal common duct.

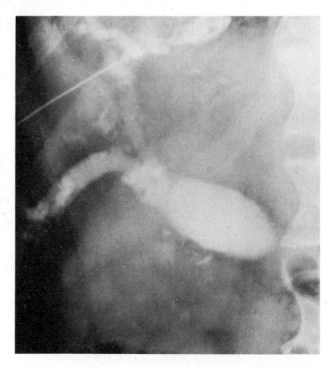

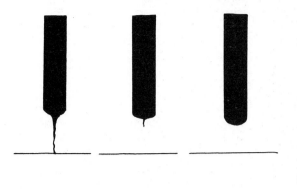

Figure 9–36. Schematic drawing showing the common "rat tail" and blunt terminations of the contrast column in carcinoma of the pancreas.

and growing cephalad into the distal common duct may produce an indistinguishable appearance, especially if histologic malignancy supervenes.

Carcinoma of the Bile Duct

This may occur at any level in the extrahepatic ducts, usually is a glandular adenocarcinoma, and typically presents as a short area of stenosis with varying degrees of proximal dilatation.[61, 62] Some produce considerable fibrotic desmoplastic reaction, giving a long stricture resembling diffuse metastatic periductal infiltration (Fig. 9–39). Less frequently, it presents as a polypoid intraluminal mass.

Bile duct carcinoma may be biologically indolent in its growth pattern, progressing gradually over months to years. Initial biopsies often yield only inflammatory tissue, interpreted pathologically as sclerosing cholangitis. Lesions located high in the porta hepatis have been referred to as Klatskin tumors and have

stenosis (Fig. 9–38). As previously noted, the use of intravenous glucagon and simultaneous barium hypotonic duodenography may be of considerable diagnostic value in such cases. Primary villous adenomas of the duodenum infiltrating the choledochoduodenal junction

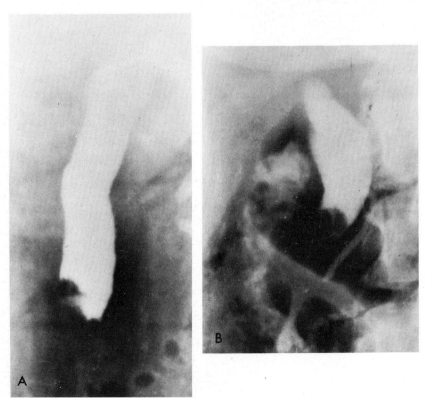

Figure 9–37. *A, B,* Carcinoma of the ampulla of Vater. Two different cases showing obstruction of the distal common bile duct by irregular polypoid intraluminal growth of tumor. This appearance can also be produced by a villous adenoma of the duodenum growing cephalad into the distal bile duct lumen.

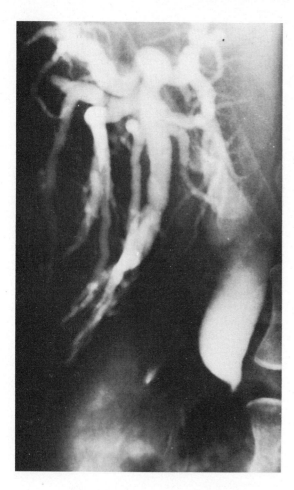

Figure 9–38.   Carcinoma of the ampulla of Vater producing an irregular, eccentric, tapered stricture. This appearance may be impossible to distinguish from small pancreatic head carcinoma or benign ampullary stenosis. The use of glucagon and combined simultaneous barium duodenography may be of considerable diagnostic value in such cases.

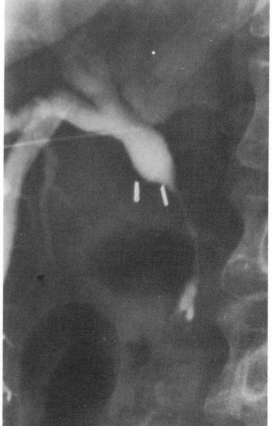

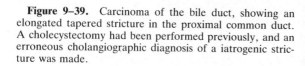

Figure 9–39.   Carcinoma of the bile duct, showing an elongated tapered stricture in the proximal common duct. A cholecystectomy had been performed previously, and an erroneous cholangiographic diagnosis of a iatrogenic stricture was made.

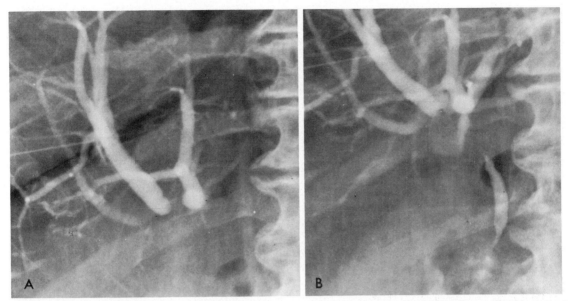

Figure 9–40. *A, B,* High, periportal stenosing bile duct carcinoma. These tumors are referred to as Klatskin tumors and are often misdiagnosed pathologically or overlooked at the time of initial surgical operation.

been somewhat controversial because of the frequency with which they have been misdiagnosed pathologically and overlooked at the time of initial surgical exploration[63] (Figs. 9–40 and 9–41).

Cholangiocarcinoma

Cholangiocarcinoma is a primary bile duct carcinoma arising from intrahepatic biliary radicles. It typically produces an infiltrating mass effect within the hepatic parenchyma and is associated with varying degrees of distortion, stretching, crowding, and dilatation of intrahepatic bile ducts cholangiographically (Fig. 9–42). Separate isolated obstructions of the right and left intrahepatic duct systems are not infrequent when the tumor arises from a centrally located periportal duct segment. Differentiation from hepatocellular carcinoma can be made angiographically by the finding of small thin neoplastic vessels with irregular encased or obstructed arteries, whereas hepatomas generally reveal abundant neovascularity.

Periductal Metastatic Disease

Infiltration, encasement, and obstruction of the extrahepatic biliary tree may occur by direct neoplastic invasion from primary malignancy in adjacent organs such as the gallbladder, stomach, and hepatic flexure of the colon or by metastatic replacement of periportal lymph nodes. The commonest remote primaries to metastasize to periportal lymph nodes are colon, breast, lung, and lymphoma. The importance of this form of neoplastic biliary

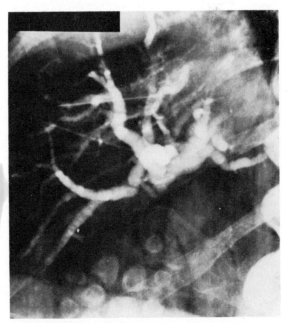

Figure 9–41. Another Klatskin-type primary bile duct carcinoma in the hilus of the liver. Numerous calcified gallstones are evident.

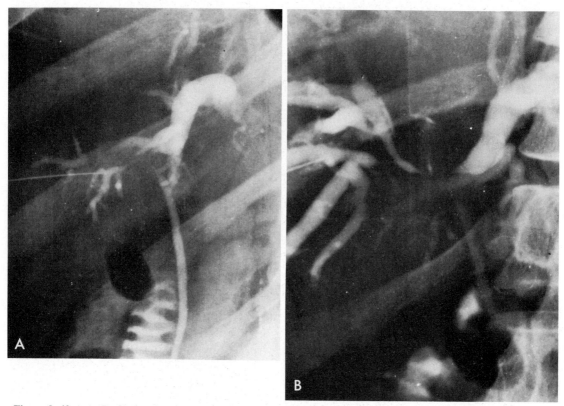

Figure 9–42. *A, B,* Cholangiocarcinoma. Two different cases showing an infiltrating intrahepatic mass effect with varying degrees of encasement, distortion, and dilatation of intrahepatic radicles. Separate isolated obstructions of the right and left duct systems are not infrequent.

obstruction is that considerable beneficial effect may result from radical aggressive therapy using a combination of percutaneous catheter drainage, local irradiation, and adjuvant chemotherapy. In fact, our own experience indicates that, overall, this group of patients with malignant obstruction of the biliary ducts has a much better prognosis than do patients with primary pancreatic carcinoma.

Several cholangiographic patterns are observed. The classic appearance is a long, relatively smooth-appearing stricture, the margins of which may be concentrically tapered or may show an irregular shelf (Fig. 9–43). A second pattern is that of an abrupt, sharply demarcated pseudocalculus-like appearance producing a meniscus-like defect, presumably due to external compression from enlarged periductal lymph nodes (Fig. 9–44). In our material this has occurred in several instances of periportal metastasis from bronchogenic carcinoma. Direct local extension from recurrent or primary malignancies of the gallbladder, colon, or duo-

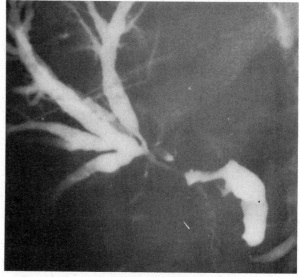

Figure 9–43. Periductal metastatic lymphadenopathy encasing the common hepatic duct in the hilus of the liver. Percutaneous fine needle aspiration biopsy yielded adenocarcinoma, primary site unknown. Note the typical elongated, irregular shelf-like constriction.

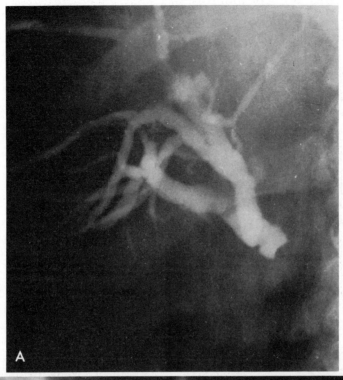

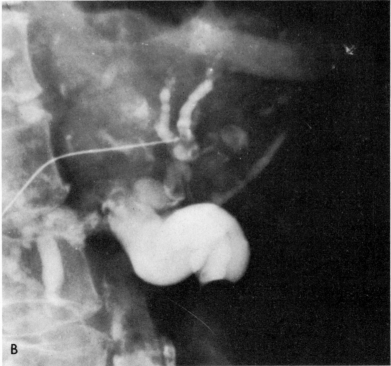

Figure 9–44. *A, B,* Periductal metastatic lymphadenopathy from bronchogenic carcinoma, producing an abrupt, sharply demarcated pseudocalculus appearance, giving a meniscus-like defect due to external compression. Two different cases. This is a typical pattern for periductal metastatic lymphadenopathy.

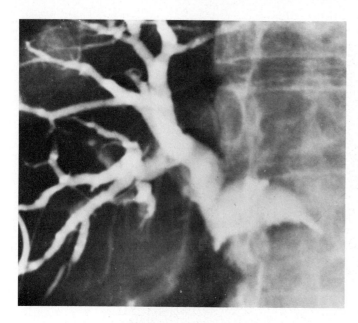

Figure 9–45. Recurrent carcinoma of the hepatic flexure of the colon presenting as a massive obturating irregular intraluminal tumor growth.

denum may also invade, encase, and obstruct the distal common duct (Fig. 9–45).

Hepatoma

It has recently been recognized that hepatocellular carcinoma (hepatoma) may invade the periportal segment of the extrahepatic bile ducts and cause mechanical biliary obstruction with a typical cholangiographic appearance of bulky, lobulated, fleshy intraluminal filling defects obstructing the flow of contrast and expanding the duct lumen[64] (Fig. 9–46). Soft fleshy tumor masses can usually be extracted from the ducts at surgery. Differential diagnosis includes a variety of other rare benign and malignant biliary tumors such as sarcoma botryoides, biliary adenomas, cyst adenomas, and papillomas.

Choledocholithiasis

Common duct lithiasis is usually a straightforward cholangiographic diagnosis and often a most welcome one, given the prognostic implications of most of the alternatives. However, there has been little discussion of the varied manifestations of calculous disease as seen by FNPTC. Some pose interesting diagnostic problems, and some carry important clinical implications. Similarly, the differential

diagnosis of intraluminal filling defects in the extrahepatic ducts is not common knowledge (Table 9–5).

Although the degree of calculous duct obstruction obviously varies greatly, calculi impacted in the periampullary region may produce high-grade obstruction and dense jaundice (Fig. 9–47). Infection of the bile is likely to be present in 80 per cent of these cases, and extreme care must be taken to avoid overinjection and subsequent septicemia. Although it has been long apparent that common duct calculi may be present without biliary

Table 9–5. CHOLEDOCHOLITHIASIS

Cholangiographic Features
Obstructing/nonobstructing
Dilated/normal caliber duct
Impacted (ampullary) obstructing stone
Bile plug/cast
Adherent stone
Recently passed stone

Differential Diagnosis
Blood clot
Bile-contrast admixture defect
Intraluminal tumor
  Ampullary CA, hepatoma, melanoma, sarcoma
   botryoides
Extramural tumor impression — "ductal
  pseudocalculus"
Choledochal sphincter—"ampullary pseudocalculus"

obstruction, it has been increasingly evident in recent years that common duct stones may also exist in the presence of entirely normal caliber extrahepatic ducts (Fig. 9–48). Such cases would likely give a false-negative ultrasound or CT result. False-negative ultrasound results may also occur when a common duct is completely filled with calculi (as with a completely

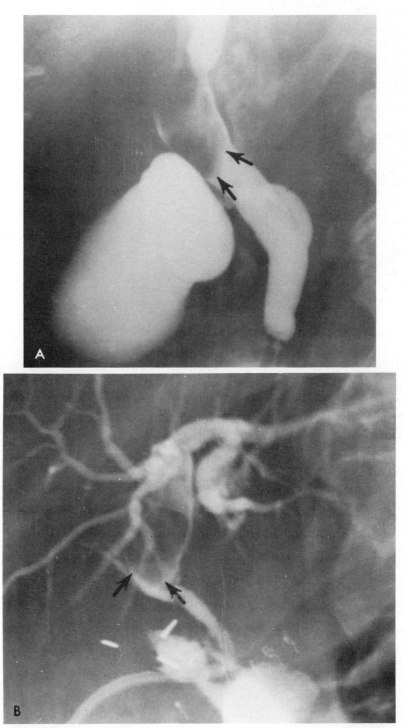

Figure 9–46. *A–C,* Invasion of the bile ducts by hepatocellular carcinoma (hepatoma). Three different cases showing bulky, lobulated, sharply demarcated intraluminal masses obturating and expanding the bile duct lumen at the level of the liver hilus.

Illustration continued on following page

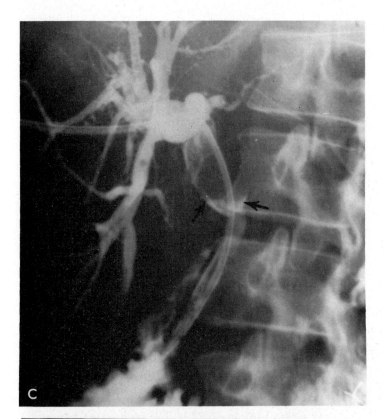

Figure 9–46 *Continued*

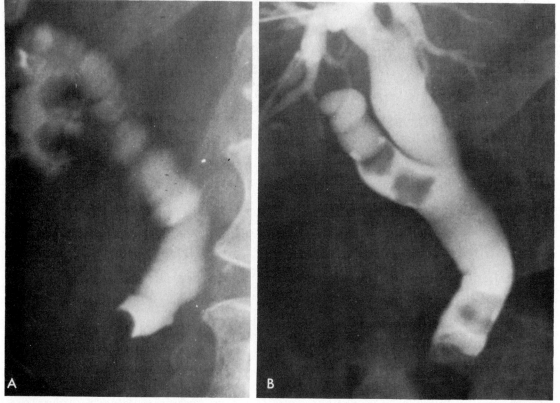

Figure 9–47. *A, B,* Impacted ampullary calculi. Two different cases. High-grade obstruction with dense jaundice and suppurative cholangitis are common clinical presentations.

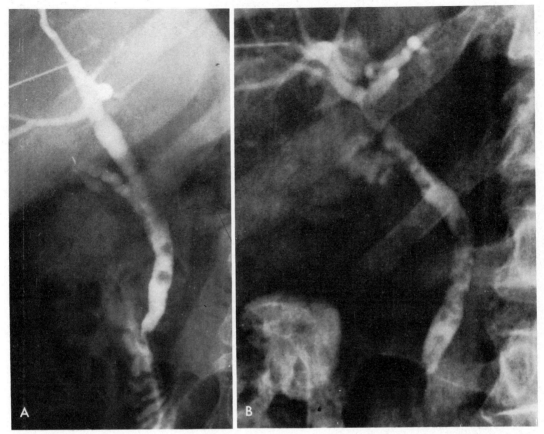

Figure 9–48. *A, B,* Nonobstructing common duct calculi with normal caliber ducts. Such cases could give a false-negative ultrasound or CT result. This fact leads to the premise that all patients suspected of biliary tract complications should be considered for direct cholangiographic duct opacification regardless of the results of ultrasound or CT.

stoned-filled gallbladder), and the inability of these noninvasive studies to reliably exclude the presence of extrahepatic biliary disease is now well known.

Cholangiographic recognition and differentiation of calculi from admixture defects due to distal obstruction and stagnation of the bile column can be a difficult diagnostic problem. Cautious injection of adequate volumes of contrast material (Fig. 9–49) and awareness of the potential for confusing appearances (Fig. 9–50) are most helpful.

Soft, amorphous, mud-like bile plugs or casts may form and fill the entire duct lumen, producing elongated defects in individual radicles or complete mechanical obstruction (Fig. 9–51). Occasionally, mud-like calculi adhere to one or more walls of the duct system, simulating a fixed mural mass (Fig. 9–52).

Recently passed common duct stones are another familiar cholangiographic problem. Such patients are usually admitted with a his-tory of biliary colic and a modest elevation of serum bilirubin level, which promptly subsides after hospitalization. Transhepatic cholangiography in such cases reveals a minimally dilated common bile duct and a short, focal, tapered stenosis at the sphincter of Oddi but no residual calculi in the duct (Fig. 9–53). The mucosa of the distal common duct may be irregular and granular in appearance, and there is often a moderate amount of associated choledochal smooth muscle spasm, which responds to the administration of intravenous glucagon. Clinical management of such patients is sometimes a dilemma and may include the options of cholecystectomy and common duct exploration, endoscopic papillotomy, or expectant observation.

As indicated in Table 9–5, the differential diagnosis of choledocholithiasis includes blood clot (hemobilia), admixture defects due to poor bile-contrast mixing (Fig. 9–16), and intraluminal neoplasms such as ampullary car-

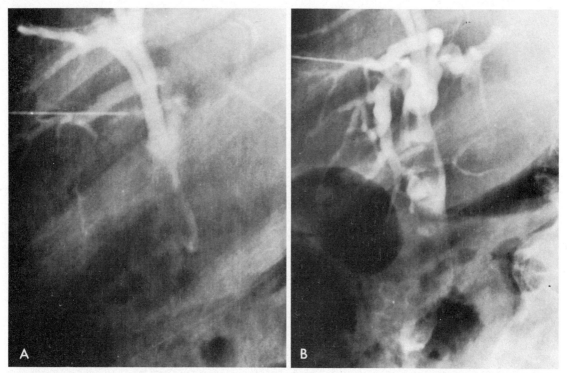

Figure 9–49. Pitfall in the diagnosis of common duct stones due to high-grade distal obstruction and stagnation of the bile column. *A,* Initial film showing apparent stenosis in the proximal common duct but no calculi. *B,* With further cautious filling, a proximal faceted calculus and amorphous distal mud-like debris are demonstrated. The initial appearance presumably reflected poor mixture of injected contrast with calculi and stagnant bile.

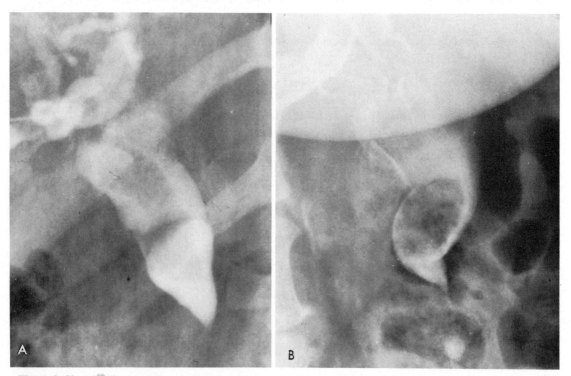

Figure 9–50. Admixture defect simulating a large oval calculus. Frontal *(A)* and left lateral *(B)* views showing a tapered distal obstruction ultimately proved to be due to a pancreatic carcinoma. An elongated oval radiolucent filling defect above the neoplastic stricture was initially misinterpreted as a large common duct calculus.

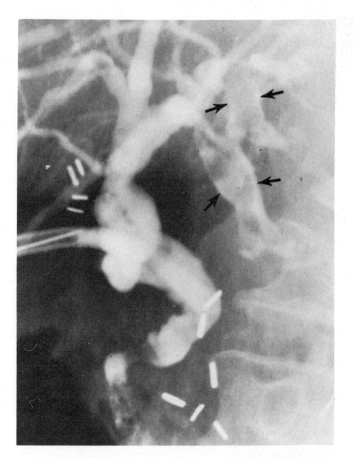

Figure 9–51. Elongated, radiolucent mud-like bile plugs or casts are present within two segmental radicles of the left hepatic duct on this oblique cholangiogram. Focal areas of stricture formation at the origin of these segmental radicles were presumed to account for the appearance.

cinoma (Fig. 9–37), intraluminal growth of primary hepatocellular carcinoma (Fig. 9–46), periductal lymph node metastases (Fig. 9–44), and sarcoma botryoides in children.

Benign Stricture

Iatrogenic

Unfortunately, post-cholecystectomy ligature and inflammatory stricture are not uncommon occurrences. A ligature or traumatic disruption of the duct is often apparent within a few days or weeks following cholecystectomy, and cholangiography may show a complete obstruction, irregular narrowing, or even extravasation of contrast material (Fig. 9–54). Delayed onset of strictures often occurs several months to years after cholecystectomy and may be manifested by an elongated or irregularly annular stenotic lesion in the mid common duct. It is a reasonable working rule that a mid common duct stricture in a patient who has undergone previous cholecystectomy is a

benign iatrogenic stricture, whereas a similar finding in a patient with an intact gallbladder should be considered a malignant stricture until proved otherwise.

Anastomotic strictures occur in 30 per cent of patients undergoing biliary-enteric bypass or reconstructive procedures.[65] Since endoscopic cholangiography is usually precluded for anatomic reasons, FNPTC is the method of choice for direct cholangiography.[40] Varying degrees of circumferential stenosis occur, which are not infrequently associated with formation of intrahepatic duct calculi (Fig. 9–55).

Sclerosing Cholangitis

This idiopathic disorder is a diffuse periductal inflammatory process principally affecting the extrahepatic ducts but often involving the intrahepatic ducts as well.[66, 67] Grossly, the extrahepatic ducts appear thickened, beaded, and nodular with a fibrotic proliferation in the ductal wall. A significant percentage of these patients have associated chronic ulcerative co-

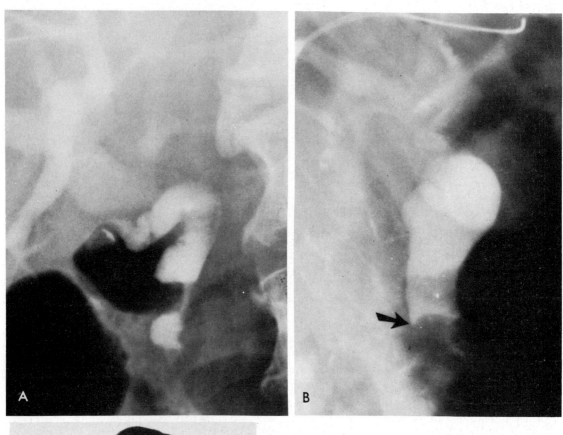

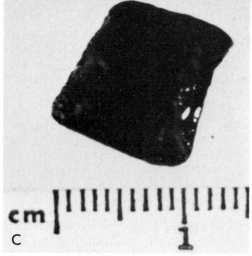

Figure 9–52. Adherent calculus simulating a fixed mural tumor mass. Frontal *(A)* and left lateral *(B)* views showing a unilateral fixed-appearing radiolucent filling defect suggesting a neoplasm. *C,* Square, faceted calculus removed at surgery.

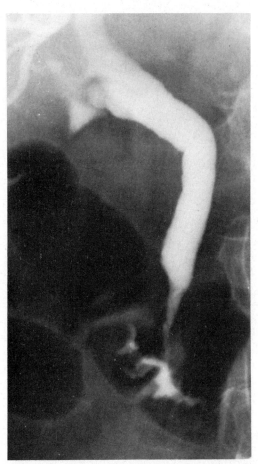

Figure 9–53. Recently passed common duct stone. Short focal tapered stenosis at the sphincter of Oddi with slightly irregular granular-appearing mucosa. Associated smooth muscle spasm often responds to glucagon.

litis, although the exact frequency of this association is difficult to ascertain.[68] A smaller percentage of patients develop a secondary carcinoma of the bile duct engrafted on the sclerosing cholangitis.

Typical cholangiographic features of sclerosing cholangitis include irregular multi-segmental narrowing of both extra- and intrahepatic ducts.[69, 70] A nodular beaded appearance of the duct is characteristic (Fig. 9–56). Intrahepatic ducts may show varying degrees of stretching, attenuation, and distal segmental dilatation (Fig. 9–57). However, discrete or focal areas of stricture formation in the extrahepatic ducts occurring in patients with known sclerosing cholangitis or in patients with chronic ulcerative colitis always require consideration of a superimposed bile duct carcinoma. Usually this diagnosis is impossible to exclude short of exploratory laparotomy.

Chronic Pancreatitis

Severe stricturing of the intrapancreatic portion of the common duct may occur as a result of periductal induration and pancreatic glandular fibrosis in chronic relapsing pancreatitis.[71] Serious sequelae of chronic biliary tract obstruction may occur in such patients including suppurative cholangitis and biliary cirrhosis. Typically, the extrahepatic common duct shows a gently undulating, smooth, elongated stricture but usually not complete obstruction (Fig. 9–58). Calcareous deposits in the pancreatic head and the clinical history usually confirm the differential diagnosis. Similar biliary duct deformity can be produced by an adjacent pseudocyst in the pancreatic head, but a greater degree of curvilinear displacement of the duct is usually apparent. Ultrasonography and CT scanning are ordinarily confirmatory in such cases.

Ampullary Stenosis

Benign stenosis of the ampulla of Vater (papillitis) is undoubtedly a real but difficult

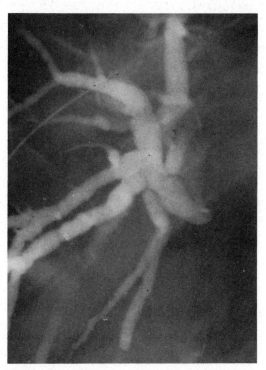

Figure 9–54. Iatrogenic suture ligature obstruction of the common hepatic duct presenting three weeks following cholecystectomy.

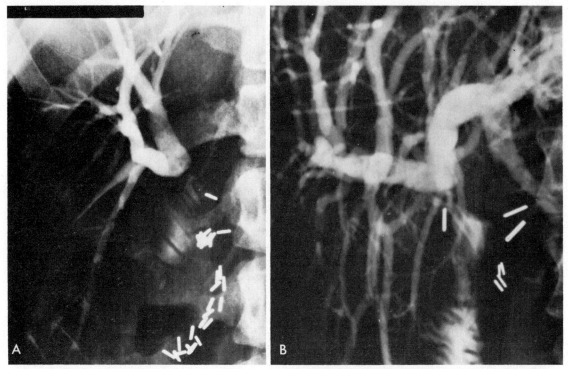

Figure 9–55. *A, B,* Anastomotic stricture following biliary enteric hepaticojejunostomy reconstructive anastomosis. Circumferential annular stenosis and dilatation of intrahepatic ducts are the typical features. Intrahepatic duct calculi are frequently present as well. Two different patients.

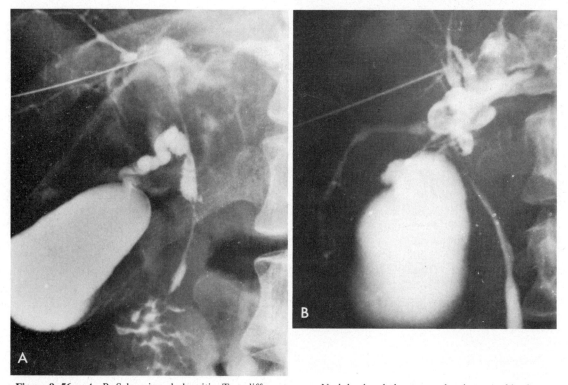

Figure 9–56. *A, B,* Sclerosing cholangitis. Two different cases. Nodular beaded segmental strictures of both extra- and intrahepatic ducts are the typical cholangiographic features. Superimposed bile duct carcinoma are common and frequently are difficult to exclude on radiologic grounds.

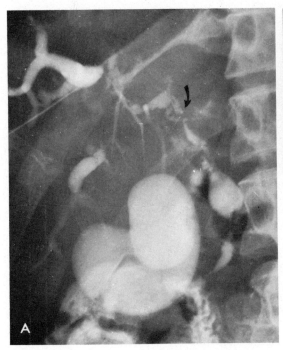

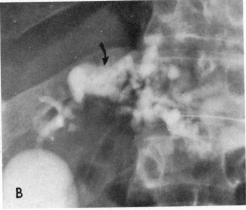

Figure 9–57. Sclerosing cholangitis diffusely involving both intra- and extrahepatic ducts with complete segmental obstruction of the left hepatic duct at the confluence *(A)*, requiring a selective left hepatic duct puncture *(B)* as part of complete preoperative delineation of the anatomy. A left hepatic duct jejunostomy (Bismuth procedure) was subsequently performed.

Figure 9–58. Chronic pancreatitis. Smooth, gently undulating elongated stricture of the intrapancreatic portion of the distal common duct. Typically, the obstruction is incomplete, and calcareous deposits are visible within the head of the pancreas.

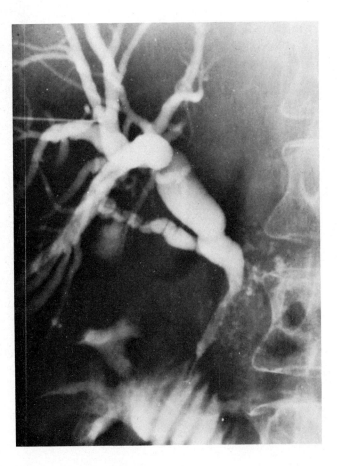

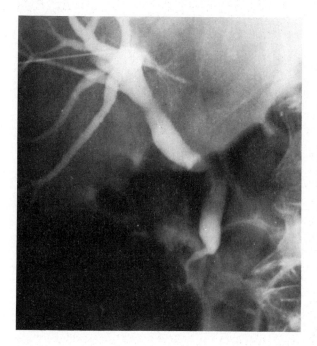

Figure 9–59. Ampullary stenosis. Short, symmetrical, tapered narrowing of the ampullary portion of the distal common duct with varying degrees of proximal dilatation is the usual feature. Differentiation from a recently passed common duct stone and small ampullary or pancreatic head carcinoma is sometimes difficult.

to define entity. With the increasing availability of effective nonsurgical therapy via endoscopic papillotomy, refined diagnostic criteria are emerging.[72, 73] Tapered narrowing of the distal common bile and pancreatic duct with moderate proximal dilatation is the typical radiographic feature (Fig. 9–59). Histologic evidence of fibrosis, manometric findings of a pressure gradient across the ampulla, chronic pain, and chemical abnormalities of liver and pancreatic function have been considered essential to the diagnosis. The principal concern in clinical evaluation is exclusion of a small infiltrating carcinoma of the pancreatic head. In practical terms, the differentiation from a recently passed common duct stone may be impossible. Response to operative or endoscopic sphincteroplasty confirms the diagnosis.

Intrahepatic Ducts

Cholangiographic features of disorders affecting the intrahepatic ducts are thoroughly considered in Chapter 10. However, important intrahepatic duct abnnormalities are often encountered during transhepatic cholangiography. Intrahepatic abscesses communicating with the biliary duct system are frequently encountered in the presence of high-grade distal obstruction (Fig. 9–60). Rounded to oval

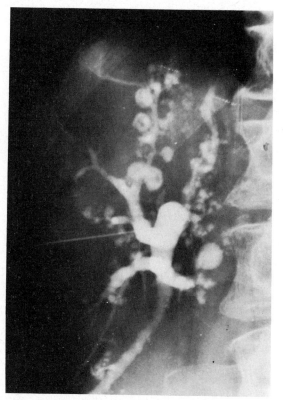

Figure 9–60. Multiple intrahepatic abscesses due to malignant periportal obstruction. Numerous small, rounded intraparenchymal cavities communicate with multiple intrahepatic duct segments. This is often a preterminal event, but the abscess cavities may respond to percutaneous or surgical decompression of the obstructing lesion.

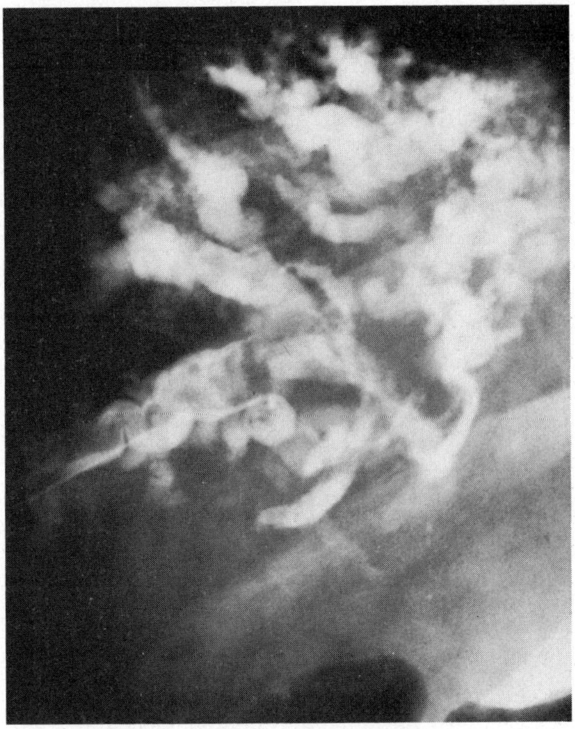

Figure 9–61. Cirrhosis of the liver. Tortuous corkscrew appearance of intrahepatic ducts in advanced hepatic cirrhosis with considerable shrinkage of liver volume. The ducts are markedly dilated because of obstruction at the porta hepatis by superimposed primary hepatocellular carcinoma invading and obstructing the duct confluence.

amorphous collections of intraparenchymal contrast associated with one or more dilated intrahepatic radicles are the typical features. Resolution of the abscesses may occur after transhepatic catheter drainage.

Cirrhosis of the liver may produce a variety of cholangiographic appearances including stretching and attenuation of branches by associated fat and fibrous tissue infiltration or by regenerating nodules. When the liver volume shrinks in the late stages of the disease, a corkscrew tortuous duct configuration may be encountered (Fig. 9–61).

Diffuse neoplastic infiltration of the liver may produce a similar appearance of duct stretching, attenuation, and distal segmental dilatation. It is often difficult to predict the origin of such changes in that metastatic carcinoma, hepatocellular carcinoma, and cholangiocarcinoma may give nearly identical appearances (Fig. 9–62).

RADIOGRAPHIC APPROACH TO THE JAUNDICED PATIENT

Berk and Clemett have urged that "no jaundiced patient should be operated on without preoperative confirmation of the presence of bile duct obstruction and the determination of its location, extent, and probable cause."[56] Our philosophy of biliary duct imaging concurs with this aggressive approach and perhaps extends it even farther. We urge direct cholangiography for all patients with clinically suspected surgical disease of the biliary ducts regardless of whether jaundice is present. Several groups have recently documented early surgical obstruction by sonography and computed tomography in the presence of normal serum bilirubin values,[74, 75] and we now consider sonographic evidence of duct dilatation an indication for fine-needle percutaneous transhepatic cholangiography in symptomatic patients regardless of the serum bilirubin value.[12] As a corollary, we consider the issue to be one of imaging the biliary ducts rather than the "jaundiced patient." Further, since the advent of percutaneous transhepatic biliary drainage, fine-needle transhepatic cholangiography can be considered both the end point for answering the diagnostic questions in terms of documenting the presence, site, and cause of obstruction or providing a "surgical road map" and a starting point for providing definitive nonsurgical therapy by percutaneous catheter techniques.

Nevertheless, because of the small but defi-

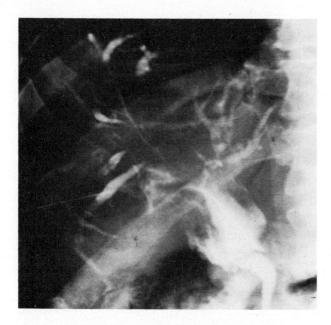

Figure 9–62. Diffuse neoplastic infiltration of the liver producing distortion, attenuation, stretching, and segmental obstructive dilatation of multiple intrahepatic branches. Thus, cholangiographic appearance may be produced by a variety of tumors including metastatic disease, hepatoma, and cholangiocarcinoma.

nite risk of fine-needle transhepatic cholangiography, it is not an ideal screening procedure.[12] Not only is fine-needle transhepatic cholangiography an invasive procedure but further diagnoses, i.e., metastasis, lymphadenopathy, and so on, may be demonstrated by sonography and computed tomography. Moreover, in many cases, specific differentiation between medical and surgical jaundice can be made with these noninvasive modalities. Fine-needle transhepatic cholangiography, therefore, must be integrated with sonography/computed tomography in a contributory and nonrepetitive or competitive way. One must examine both the contributions and limitations of all the various modalities now available for investigation of suspected biliary duct obstruction. With the obvious requirements for a safe, cost-effective approach to diagnosis, a reasonably rapid algorithmic approach to suspected biliary obstruction is appropriate, emphasizing fine-needle transhepatic cholangiography as a focal point of the investigation (Fig. 9–63).

Role of Sonography/Computed Tomography

Sonography and computed tomography remain the accepted initial screening methods

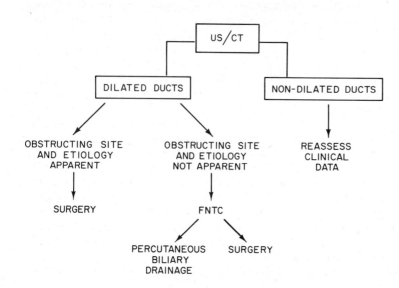

Figure 9–63. Radiographic approach to suspected biliary obstruction.

for evaluation of suspected biliary duct disease. Both have proved to be accurate, noninvasive techniques for determining both intra- and extrahepatic duct dilatation.[76-88] Although computed tomography has also been shown to be highly sensitive in defining dilated biliary systems, owing to its lack of wide availability, high cost, and radiation exposure, ultrasound should be considered the screening method of choice. It is our further, but difficult to substantiate, view that ultrasound by virtue of flexible sagittal and oblique scanning planes and the logistic advantages of real time is in fact substantially more sensitive than computed tomography, especially in detecting minimal dilatation of the extrahepatic ducts. Further, the documentation of dilated ducts by ultrasound or computed tomography does provide reassurance of the necessity to perform and pursue multiple needle punctures during FNPTC if initial passes are unsuccessful. Failure of opacification of the bile ducts after five to six punctures does not exclude either a dilated system or significant biliary duct pathology. Even in the presence of a known dilated ductal system, 15 to 20 punctures can be required; although the rate of serious complication is not thereby increased, the time and attendant minor risks are more readily justified when a dilated system is known to be present. When there is selective obstruction of the right or left hepatic duct system due to stone, inflammation, or tumor, ultrasound may be of special value in localizing ducts for selective puncture of the specific lobar ductal system.

Obviously, both ultrasound and computed tomography may contribute further by providing evidence of associated or additional pathology in a jaundiced patient. Thus, findings of liver or retroperitoneal metastasis, hydronephrosis, and so on, significantly alter the hospital course of a jaundiced patient.

Limitations of Ultrasound/Computed Tomography Vis-à-Vis Fine-Needle Transhepatic Cholangiography

In the specific instance of a patient presenting with a surgical disorder of the biliary ducts, both ultrasound and computed tomography often give incomplete and/or inadequate morphologic data as to the exact site and etiology of biliary obstruction. For example, it has been well documented that significant surgical disease, especially choledocholithiasis, may exist without evidence of biliary duct dilatation.[89]

Common duct stones not infrequently produce a ball-valve effect, causing substantial symptomatology without obstructive dilatation. Similarly, a dilated but completely stone-filled extrahepatic biliary tree may give a misleading negative appearance by ultrasound. Finally, sclerosing cholangitis may cause severe chronic obstruction without accompanying ductal dilatation. In such instances ultrasound and computed tomography may give false-normal results, with the offending process disclosed only after aggressive performance of fine-needle transhepatic cholangiography. Therefore, in patients in whom there is strong clinical suspicion of biliary duct disease, a negative ultrasonogram or computed tomogram does not obviate the need for fine-needle transhepatic cholangiography.

Clinical Correlation

As noted earlier, increasing reliance is now being placed on the use of fine-needle transhepatic cholangiography in patients with nonicteric hyperbilirubinemia or elevation of serum alkaline phosphatase. Clinicians are well aware of the value and sensitivity of an elevated alkaline phosphatase level as an indicator of biliary obstruction, even in a normobilirubinemic patient, and several series have now been reported documenting obstructive duct dilatation with only alkaline phosphatase elevation.[75] Even if bile duct dilatation is not demonstrated by ultrasound, persistent elevation of alkaline phosphatase alone may warrant aggressive evaluation of the biliary tract with fine-needle transhepatic cholangiography. It is precisely in the common subgroup of patients with low-grade obstruction and small caliber ducts, nonobstructing stones, ampullary strictures, and sclerosing cholangitis that a vigorous attempt at fine-needle transhepatic cholangiography must be made for definitive diagnosis.

In our present schema, screening of a patient with suspected biliary duct disease, even if nonjaundiced and nonhyperbilirubinemic, is performed noninvasively by ultrasound[12] (Fig. 9–63). If dilated ducts and the exact etiology of the obstruction are delineated, fine-needle transhepatic cholangiography may proceed primarily as a prelude to percutaneous biliary drainage. If the exact etiology of an obstruction is not defined, fine-needle transhepatic cholangiography will be performed for specific diagnosis.

If ultrasound demonstrates a nondilated duct

system, fine-needle transhepatic cholangiography will only be performed in specific cases in which clinical re-evaluation strongly suggests biliary obstruction or a process unlikely to lead to significant dilatation, i.e., sclerosing cholangitis. In such instances fine-needle transhepatic cholangiography may be clinically necessary to document the presence of an obstructed nondilated system or a normal nonobstructed system. Alternatively, intravenous cholangiography may be employed with some expectation of success, but its role has been increasingly relegated to near obscurity by the effectiveness of the ultrasound/fine-needle transhepatic cholangiography combination.

References

1. Okuda, K., Tanikawa, K., Emura, T., et al.: Nonsurgical percutaneous transhepatic cholangiography. Am. J. Dig. Dis. 19:21, 1974.
2. Redeker, A. G., Karvountzis, G. G., Richman, R. H., et al.: Percutaneous transhepatic cholangiography: improved technique. J.A.M.A. 231:386, 1975.
3. Tabrisky, J., Lindstrom, P. L., Hanelin, L. G., et al.: Chiba percutaneous transhepatic cholangiography. Am. J. Roentgenol. 126:755, 1975.
4. Ferrucci, J. T., Jr., Wittenberg, J., Sarno, R. A., et al.: Fine needle transhepatic cholangiography: a new approach to obstructive jaundice. Am. J. Roentgenol. 217:403, 1976.
5. Pereiras, R., White, P., Dusol, M., et al.: Percutaneous transhepatic cholangiography utilizing the Chiba University needle. Radiology 121:219, 1976.
6. Ferrucci, J. T., Jr., and Wittenberg, J.: Refinements in Chiba needle transhepatic cholangiography. Am. J. Roentgenol. 129:11, 1977.
7. Ayre-Smith, G.: Fine needle cholangiography in post cholecystectomy patients. Am. J. Roentgenol. 130:697, 1976.
8. Fraser, G. M., Cruikshank, J. G., Sumerling, M. D., and Buist, T. A.: Percutaneous transhepatic cholangiography with the Chiba needle. Clin. Radiol. 29:101, 1978.
9. Ariyama, J., Shirakabe, H., Ohashi, K., et al.: Experience with percutaneous transhepatic cholangiography using the Japanese needle. Gastrointest. Radiol. 2:359, 1978.
10. Gold, R. P., Casarella, W. J., Stern, G., et al.: Transhepatic cholangiography: the radiological method of choice in suspected obstructive jaundice. Radiology 133:39, 1979.
11. Harbin, W. P., Mueller, P. R., and Ferrucci, J. T., Jr.: Complications and use patterns of fine needle transhepatic cholangiography: a multi-institutional study. Radiology 135:15, 1980.
12. Mueller, P. R., Harbin, W. P., Ferrucci, J. T., Jr., et al.: Fine needle transhepatic cholangiography: refinements and reflections after 450 cases. Am. J. Roentgenol. 136:85, 1981.
13. Frankel, M., and Gordon, R. L.: Investigation of the nonjaundiced patient by percutaneous transhepatic cholangiography. Clin. Radiol. 28:129, 1977.
14. Elias, E., Hamlyn, A. N., Jain, S., et al.: A randomized trial of percutaneous transhepatic cholangiography with the Chiba needle versus endoscopic retrograde cholangiography for bile duct visualization in jaundice. Gastroenterology 71:439, 1976.
15. Matzen, P., Haubek, A., Holst-Christensen, J., et al.: Accuracy of direct cholangiography by endoscopic or transhepatic route in jaundice—a prospective study. Gastroenterology 81:237, 1981.
16. Kaude, J. V., Weidenmier, C. H., and Agee, O. F.: Decompression of bile ducts with the percutaneous transhepatic technique. Radiology 93:69, 1969.
17. Molnar, W., and Stockum, A. E.: Relief of obstructive jaundice through percutaneous transhepatic catheter—a new therapeutic method. Am. J. Roentgenol. 122:356, 1974.
18. Burcharth, F., and Nielbo, N.: Percutaneous transhepatic cholangiography with selective catheterization of the common bile duct. Am. J. Roentgenol. 127:409, 1976.
19. Mori, K., Misumi, A., Sugiyama, M., et al.: Percutaneous transhepatic bile drainage. Ann. Surg. 185:111, 1977.
20. Tylen, U., Hoevels, J., and Vang, J.: Percutaneous transhepatic cholangiography with external drainage of obstructive biliary lesions. Surg. Gynecol. Obstet. 144:13, 1977.
21. Hoevels, J., Lunderquist, A., and Ihse, I.: Percutaneous transhepatic intubation of the bile ducts for combined internal drainage in preoperative and palliative treatment of obstructive jaundice. Gastrointest. Radiol. 3:23, 1978.
22. Nakayama, T., Ikeda, A., and Okuda, K.: Percutaneous transhepatic drainage of the biliary tract: techniques and results in 104 cases. Gastroenterology 74:554, 1978.
23. Ring, E. J., Oleaga, J. A., Freiman, D. B., et al.: Therapeutic applications of catheter cholangiography. Radiology 128:333, 1978.
24. Pollock, T. W., Ring, E. J., Oleaga, J. A., et al.: Percutaneous decompression of benign and malignant biliary obstruction. Arch. Surg. 114:148, 1979.
25. Hansson, J. A., Hoevels, J., Simert, G., et al.: Clinical aspects of nonsurgical percutaneous transhepatic bile drainage in obstructive lesions of the extrahepatic bile ducts. Ann. Surg. 189:58, 1979.
26. Ferrucci, J. T., Jr., Mueller, P. R., and Harbin, W. P.: Percutaneous transhepatic biliary drainage: techniques, results and applications. Radiology 135:1, 1980.
27. Burcharth, F.: A new endoprosthesis for nonoperative intubation of the biliary tract in malignant obstructive jaundice. Surg. Gynecol. Obstet. 146:76, 1978.
28. Pereiras, R. V., Jr., Rheingold, O. J., Hutson, D., et al.: Relief of malignant obstructive jaundice by percutaneous insertion of a permanent prosthesis in the biliary tree. Ann. Intern. Med. 89:589, 1978.
29. Russell, E., Nunez, D., Jr., and Yrizarry, J.: A 23 gauge sheathed needle: an alternative in transhepatic cholangiography. Radiology 128:822, 1978.
30. Hawkins, I. F.: New fine needle for cholangiography with optimal sheath for decompression. Radiology 131:252, 1979.
31. Okuda, K., Sumikoshi, T., and Kanda, Y.: Hepatic lymphatics as opacified by percutaneous injection of contrast medium. Radiology 120:321, 1976.
32. Goldberg, H. I., Dodds, W. J., Lawson, T. L., et al.: Hepati lymphatics demonstrated by percutaneous trans-hepatic cholangiography. Am. J. Roentgenol. 123:415, 1976.

33. Jaques, P. F., Mauro, M. A., and Scatliff, J. H.: The failed transhepatic cholangiogram. Radiology *134*:33, 1980.
34. Makuuchi, M., Bandai, Y., Ifo, T., et al.: Ultrasonically guided percutaneous transhepatic bile drainage. Radiology *136*:165, 1980.
35. Ohto, M., Karasawa, E., Tsuhiya, Y., et al.: Ultrasonically guided percutaneous contrast medium injection and aspiration biopsy using a real-time puncture transducer. Radiology *136*:171, 1980.
36. Kittredge, R. D., and Baer, J. W.: Percutaneous transhepatic cholangiography: problems in interpretation. Am. J. Roentgenol. *125*:35, 1975.
37. Latshaw, R. F., and Rohrer, G. V.: Semi-erect and erect position in percutaneous transhepatic cholangiography. Am. J. Roentgenol. *131*:171, 1978.
38. Ferrucci, J. T., Jr., Wittenberg, J., Stone, L. B., et al.: Hypotonic cholangiography with glucagon. Radiology *118*:466, 1976.
39. Jaques, P. F., and Bream, C. A.: Barium duodenography as an adjunct to percutaneous transhepatic cholangiography. Am. J. Roentgenol. *130*:693, 1978.
40. Gold, R. P., and Price, J. B.: Thin needle cholangiography as the primary method for the evaluation of the biliary-enteric anastomosis. Radiology *136*:309, 1980.
41. Juler, G. L., Conroy, R. M., and Fullerman, R. W.: Bile leakage following percutaneous transhepatic cholangiography with the Chiba needle. Arch. Surg. *112*:954, 1977.
42. Kreek, M. J., and Balint, J. A.: "Skinny needle" cholangiography—results of a pilot study of a voluntary prospective method for gathering risk data on new procedures. Gastroenterology *78*:598, 1980.
43. Keighley, M. R. B., Wilson, G., and Kelly, J. P.: Fatal endotoxic shock of biliary tract origin complicating transhepatic cholangiography. Br. Med. J. *3*:147, 1973.
44. Holtborn, A., Jacobsson, B., and Rosengren, B.: Cholangiovenous reflux during cholangiography: an experimental and clinical study. Acta Chir. Scand. *123*:111, 1962.
45. Flemma, R. J., Capp, M. P., and Shingleton, W. W.: Percutaneous transhepatic cholangiography. Arch. Surg. *90*:5, 1965.
46. Keighley, M. R. B., Lister, D. M., Jacobs, S. I., et al.: Hazards of surgical treatment due to micro-organisms in the bile. Surgery *75*:578, 1974.
47. Keighley, M. R. B.: Micro-organisms in the bile: a preventable cause of sepsis after biliary surgery. Ann. R. Coll. Surg. Engl. *59*:328, 1977.
48. Keighley, M. R. B., Drysdale, R. B., Quoraish, A. A., et al.: Antibiotics in biliary disease: the relative importance of antibiotic concentrations in the bile and serum. Gut *17*:495, 1976.
49. Keighley, M. R. B., Baddeley, R. M., Burdon, D. W., et al.: A controlled trial of parenteral prophylactic gentamicin therapy in biliary surgery. Br. J. Surg. *62*:275, 1975.
50. Tylen, U. L. F., Hoevels, J., and Nilsson, U. L. F.: Computed tomography iatrogenic hepatic lesions following percutaneous transhepatic cholangiography and portography. J. Comput. Assist. Tomogr. *5*:15, 1981.
51. Okuda, K., Musha, H., Nakajima, Y., et al.: Frequency of transhepatic arteriovenous fistula as a sequela to percutaneous needle puncture of the liver. Gastroenterology *74*:1204, 1978.
52. Isley, J. K., and Schauble, J. F.: Interpretation of the percutaneous transhepatic cholangiogram. Am. J. Roentgenol. *88*:772, 1962.
53. Mujahed, Z., and Evans, J. A.: Percutaneous transhepatic cholangiography. Radiol. Clin. North Am. *4*:535, 1966.
54. Fleming, M. P., Carlson, H., and Adson, M. A.: Percutaneous transhepatic cholangiography: the differential diagnosis of bile duct pathology. Am. J. Roentgenol. *116*:327, 1972.
55. Lang, E. K.: Percutaneous transhepatic cholangiography. Radiology *112*:283, 1974.
56. Berk, R. N., and Clemett, A. R.: Radiology of the Gallbladder and Bile Ducts. Philadelphia: W. B. Saunders Co., 1977.
57. Classen, M., and Sarany, L.: Endoscopic papillotomy and removal of gallstones. Br. Med. J. *4*:371, 1975.
58. Safrany, L.: Duodenoscopic sphincterotomy and gallstone removal. Gastroenterology *72*:338, 1977.
59. Geenen, J. E., Hogan, J., Shaffer, R. D., et al.: Endoscopic electrosurgical papillotomy and manometry in biliary tract disease. J.A.M.A. *237*:2075, 1977.
60. Koch, H., Rosch, W., Shappner, O., et al.: Endoscopic papillotomy. Gastroenterology *73*:1393, 1977.
61. Legge, D. A., and Carlson, H. C.: Cholangiographic appearance of primary carcinoma of the bile ducts. Radiology *102*:259, 1972.
62. Altemeier, W. A., et al.: Sclerosing carcinoma of the major intrahepatic bile ducts. Arch. Surg. *75*:450, 1957.
63. Klatskin, G.: Adenocarcinoma of the hepatic duct at its bifurcation within the porta hepatis. Am. J. Med. *38*:241, 1965.
64. vanSonnenberg, E., and Ferrucci, J. T., Jr.: Bile duct obstruction in hepato-cellular carcinoma—clinical and cholangiographic characteristics. Radiology *130*:7, 1979.
65. Molnar, W., and Stockum, A. E.: Transhepatic dilatation of choledochoenterostomy strictures. Radiology *129*:59, 1978.
66. Warren, K. W., Athanassiades, S., and Monge, J.: Primary sclerosing cholangitis. A study of forty-two cases. Am. J. Surg. *111*:23, 1965.
67. Cutler, B., and Donaldson, G.: Primary sclerosing cholangitis and obliterative cholangitis. Am. J. Surg. *117*:502, 1969.
68. Thorpe, M. E. C., Scheuer, P. J., and Sherlock, S.: Primary sclerosing cholangitis, the biliary tree, and ulcerative colitis. Gut *8*:435, 1967.
69. Krieger, J., Seaman, W. B., and Porter, M. R.: The roentgenologic appearance of sclerosing cholangitis. Radiology *95*:369, 1970.
70. Ruskin, R. B., et al.: Evaluation of sclerosing cholangitis by endoscopic retrograde cholangiopancreatography. Arch. Intern. Med. *136*:232, 1976.
71. Warshaw, A. L., et al.: Persistent obstructive jaundice, cholangitis, and biliary cirrhosis due to common bile duct stenosis in chronic pancreatitis. Gastroenterology *70*:562, 1976.
72. Nardi, G. L., and Acosta, J. M.: Papillitis as a cause of pancreatitis and abdominal pain: role of evocative test, operative pancreatography and histologic evaluation. Ann. Surg. *164*:611, 1966.
73. Zimmon, D. S., Ferrara, T. P., and Clemett, A. R.: Radiology of papilla of Vater stenosis. Gastrointest. Radiol. *3*:343, 1978.
74. Shanser, J. D., Korobkin, M., Goldberg, H. I., et al.: Computed tomographic diagnosis of obstructive

jaundice in the absence of intrahepatic ductal dilatation. Am. J. Roentgenol. *131*:389, 1978.

75. Weinstein, D. P., Weinstein, B. J., and Brodmerkel, G. J.: Ultrasonography of biliary tract dilatation without jaundice. Am. J. Roentgenol. *132*:729, 1979.
76. Taylor, K. J. W., and Rosenfield, A. T.: Gray-scale ultrasonography in the differential diagnosis of jaundice. Arch. Surg. *112*:820, 1977.
77. Goldstein, C. I., Sample, W. F., Kadell, B. M., et al.: Gray-scale ultrasonography. Evaluation in the jaundiced patient. J.A.M.A. *238*:1041, 1977.
78. Neiman, H. L., and Mintzer, R. A.: Accuracy of biliary ultrasound: comparison with cholangiography. Am. J. Roentgenol. *129*:979, 1977.
79. Stanley, R. J., Sagel, S. S., and Levitt, R. G.: Computed tomography of the liver. Radiol. Clin. North Am. *15*:331, 1977.
80. Havrilla, T. R., Haaga, J. R., Alfidi, R. J., et al.: Computed tomography and obstructive biliary disease. Am. J. Roentgenol. *128*:765, 1977.
81. Levitt, R. G., Sagel, S. S., Stanley, R. J., et al.: Accuracy of computed tomography of the liver and biliary tract. Radiology *124*:123, 1977.
82. Sample, W. F., Sarti, D. A., Goldstein, L. I., et al.: Gray scale ultrasonography of the jaundiced patient. Radiology *128*:719, 1978.
83. Cooperberg, P. L.: High resolution real-time ultrasound in the evaluation of the normal and obstructed biliary tract. Radiology *129*:477, 1978.
84. Weill, F., Eisencher, A., and Zeltner, F.: Ultrasonic study of the normal and dilated biliary tree. The "shotgun sign." Radiology *127*:221, 1978.
85. Parulekar, S. G.: Ultrasound evaluation of common bile duct size. Radiology *133*:703, 1979.
86. Shimizu, H., Ida, M., Takayama, S., et al.: The diagnostic accuracy of computed tomography in obstructive biliary disease: a comparative evaluation with direct cholangiography. Radiology *138*:411, 1981.
87. Pedrosa, C. S., Casanova, R., and Rodriguez, R.: Computed tomography in obstructive jaundice. Part I: The level of obstruction. Radiology *139*:627, 1981.
88. Pedrosa, C. S., Casanova, R., Lezana, A. H., et al.: Computed tomography in obstructive jaundice. Part II: The cause of obstruction. Radiology *139*:635, 1981.
89. Greenwald, R. A., Pereiras, R., Jr., Morris, S. J., et al.: Jaundice, choledocholithiasis, and a non-dilated common duct. J.A.M.A. *240*:1983, 1978.

ENDOSCOPIC RETROGRADE CHOLANGIOGRAPHY

by Edward T. Stewart, M.D.
and Joseph E. Geenen, M.D.

10

Endoscopic retrograde cholangiopancreatography (ERCP) is a technique that employs the skills of endoscopists as well as radiologists. Although a few radiologists perform endoscopy, most commonly retrograde cannulations are performed by gastroenterologists and some surgeons. Interpretation of the radiographic results, however, usually falls on the shoulders of an experienced radiologist who works closely with the endoscopist. Under optimal circumstances, the radiologist is in attendance during the procedure. Since the appearance of retrograde cannulation in the early 1970s, there has been a proliferation of expertise so that now retrograde cannulation is available in most communities.[17, 18, 44, 59, 74] Whether or not retrograde cannulation is employed to evaluate the biliary tree as opposed to antegrade studies such as transhepatic cholangiography depends on a variety of factors including availability, expertise, and the clinical problem as well as the possible use of interventional techniques.[94] Retrograde cannulation, therefore, does not stand alone, and there may be considerable overlap in some of the diagnostic information provided by this technique compared with procedures such as transhepatic cholangiography. This chapter will stress the unique advantages of retrograde cannulation as well as its shortcomings as it applies to the biliary tree.

Retrograde cannulation of the biliary tree is rarely employed without attempts to cannulate the pancreatic duct as well. In many instances, ERCP is performed in an effort to determine whether or not the patient's problem arises primarily in the pancreas, in the biliary tree, or in both. Obviously it is therefore difficult to divorce endoscopic retrograde cholangiography (ERC) from endoscopic retrograde pancreatography (ERP). Realizing this fact, an effort will be made in this chapter to separate out those conditions involving the biliary tree primarily. Reference, when appropriate, will be made to pancreatic pathology masquerading as primary biliary tract disease.

INDICATIONS

Indications for endoscopic retrograde cholangiography at this time can be divided into diagnostic as well as therapeutic indications (Table 10–1). Initially, the use of retrograde cannulation was reserved exclusively for diagnostic purposes, centering primarily on the explanation of jaundice of undertermined etiology. As with other forms of direct cholangiography, visualization of the biliary tree allows separation of mechanical causes of obstructive jaundice from hepatocellular disease. The level of obstruction and frequently its etiology are well defined by cholangiographic means. Usually stones as well as benign or malignant strictures are easily identified. Nonjaundiced patients in whom biliary tract disease is suspected, regardless of prior negative evaluations, are now frequent candidates for retrograde cannulation, especially those with sphincter of Oddi dysfunction. Patients in whom the gallbladder is intact as well as patients in whom the gallbladder has been removed are studied. Harvesting malignant cells from brushings, fluid, percutaneous aspiration, or direct endoscopic biopsy is commonly employed.

Therapeutic indications have been rapidly expanded following the introduction of safe electrosurgical catheters. These catheters for endoscopic sphincterotomy are most commonly applied in the management of patients

Table 10–1. INDICATIONS FOR ENDOSCOPIC RETROGRADE CHOLANGIOGRAPHY

I. Diagnostic indications
  A. Jaundice of undetermined etiology
    1. Extrahepatic biliary obstruction
      a. Stones
      b. Tumor
      c. Strictures
      d. Sclerosing cholangitis
      e. Sphincter of Oddi dysfunction (papillary stenosis)
    2. Intrahepatic biliary obstruction
      a. Hepatitis
      b. Drug-induced cholestasis
      c. Cirrhosis
      d. Malignancy
        i. Primary
        ii. Secondary
  B. Endoscopic cytology and biopsy
    1. Brush cytology or biopsy
    2. Fluid collection cytology
    3. Percutaneous cytology
II. Therapeutic indications
  A. Endoscopic papillotomy
    1. Stones
    2. Sphincter of Oddi dysfunction (papillary stenosis)
  B. Placement of nasobiliary catheters
    1. Drainage of partial obstruction
    2. Perfusion of Mono-Octanoin or other solubilizing solutions
  C. Internal transpapillary stents
  D. Balloon catheter dilatation

with retained common duct stones and sphincter of Oddi dysfunction. Long or short catheters can now be placed across areas of partial obstruction for decompression or can be left in place following sphincterotomy for attempted dissolution of gallstones that cannot be successfully removed. The use of balloon catheters for dilation of benign strictures, such as postoperative strictures or sclerosing cholangitis, will soon be attempted.

CONTRAINDICATIONS

Contraindications to ERC are quite limited. Clinically unstable patients in whom endoscopy for any reason cannot be performed are obviously excluded from this type of study. Such patients include those with severe cardiopulmonary disease. The procedure has generally been avoided in patients with acute pancreatitis. However, when pancreatitis is suspected to be the result of passage of common duct stones, ERCP may be employed to document common duct stones in spite of the presence of clinical acute pancreatitis. How-

ever, other means, such as transhepatic cholangiography, may be more suitable in such cases to visualize the biliary tree. Patients with Australian antigen-positive hepatitis can be studied endoscopically, but contamination of scopes and equipment as well as personnel may occur in such cases and precautions are necessary.[53] Contrast hypersensitivity does not appear to be a major problem, as discussed hereafter.

COMPLICATIONS

The complications that are unique to ERCP include pancreatitis, drug reactions, instrumental injury, cholangitis, and pancreatic sepsis (Table 10–2).[10, 40, 58, 79, 96]

Approximately 70 per cent of patients undergoing ERCP develop a significant rise in serum amylase level, which returns to normal in one to four days. Amylase levels as high as several thousand units are frequently seen. These are usually unassociated with clinical symptoms. The cause for the rise in amylase level is not known but is undoubtedly related to manipulation of the pancreatic duct in some way. Occasionally the patient will develop clinical pancreatitis manifested by abdominal pain, fever, and leukocytosis. This is the most common complication associated with the procedure, and the incidence has been reported to be from 0.7 to 7.4 per cent. The cause of pancreatitis is unknown but is very likely influenced to some degree by the technique of the examiner. The pressure applied as well as the rate of injection of contrast material may well have something to do with the incidence of pancreatitis. Overfilling of the pancreas is to be avoided.[48] The incidence of pancreatitis is probably inversely related to the experience of the endoscopist. Because the incidence of asymptomatic hyperamylasemia is so high following the procedure it has been our practice to confirm amylase levels only in those patients in whom clinical symptoms of pancreatitis appear.

Table 10–2. ERCP COMPLICATIONS

Complication	Incidence (%)
Pancreatitis	0.7–7.4
Drug reaction	0.1–0.6
Instrumental injury	0.07–0.3
Cholangitis	0.6–0.8
Pancreatic sepsis	0.5–1.3

There is a low risk of reaction to the drugs used in the examination. As noted previously, contrast media reactions seem to be uncommon. Contrast material is absorbed from the biliary tree as well as the pancreas during the study and is excreted by the kidneys.[46] Although patients with contrast sensitivity are obviously at risk for contrast reactions, the observed number of reactions appears to be quite small. The authors are unaware of any serious complications from contrast media hypersensitivity.[10] In the face of documented prior hypersensitivity reaction, it is our policy to inform the patient of the possible risk and premedicate him with steroids and Benadryl, although any possible benefit from these drugs is not entirely known at this time. Because these patients must be sedated for the procedure, there is a risk of reaction to either the sedatives or the analgesics that are used. These may produce either cardiac or respiratory depression. In addition, occasional patients develop thrombophlebitis at the site of diazepam injection.

Cannulation with the relatively stiff cannula can produce injury to the mucosa of the duodenum or ductal structures. Occasional injection into the wall of the duodenum occurs and is almost always unrelated to subsequent symptoms. Perforation of the common duct as well as the pancreatic duct has been reported, and such patients are at risk for the development of subsequent pancreatitis.

The mortality rate associated with ERCP is reported to vary between .01 and .08 per cent. The majority of these fatalities have been associated with bacterial infections, in either the biliary tree or the pancreas. Cholangitis and pancreatic sepsis or abscess formation are, therefore, the two most serious complications. Sepsis usually occurs above partial obstruction of a duct. Early surveys of ERCP complications suggested that fatal cholangitis was usually superimposed on partial obstruction of the biliary tree.[10, 58] Cholangitis usually occurs within 72 hours after retrograde cannulation, and the onset of chills, fever, and hypotension signifies the significance of the infection. A variety of organisms have been cultured including *E. coli* and *Pseudomonas aeruginosa*.[21, 36, 52] Sepsis above the partially obstructed pancreatic duct also may occur, and when a pancreatic pseudocyst is filled, the risk of abscess formation within the pseudocyst increases.

The incidence of bacteremia following ERCP has been reported to be between 0 and 14 per cent.[61] When bacteremia does occur, the organisms in the blood are often the same as those cultured from endoscopic equipment. Scopes and cannulas, therefore, must be adequately disinfected.[36] Although transient bacteremia may occur because of contaminated equipment, significant pathogenic bacterial infections are rare. In some cases, bacteria may already be present in the biliary tree.[23] Patients with chronic partial obstruction, such as patients with sclerosing cholangitis, very likely already have bacteria in the biliary tree above the obstruction.

The efficacy of prophylactic antibiotics is in question.[56] However, when partial obstruction of the biliary tree or pancreatic duct is encountered, it has been our practice and the practice of others to immediately place the patient on antibiotics. Patients in whom an unsuspected pseudocyst is filled with contrast are also placed on antibiotics. Once a high-grade obstruction of either a duct or a pseudocyst is encountered, further injection of contrast is to be avoided.[83] The use of antibiotics and carefully limiting injection of contrast above an obstruction or into a pseudocyst seem to have diminished the incidence of septic complications significantly.[55] It should be noted that when ascending cholangitis does complicate ERC, decompression is necessary either by endoscopically placing a stent, by percutaneous transhepatic decompression, or by surgery. ERP complicated by pancreatic abscess or sepsis requires immediate surgical decompression of the abscess.

ENDOSCOPIC TECHNIQUE

ERCP is generally performed using fluoroscopic rooms in radiology departments. The examining room must be of sufficient size to accommodate the endoscopist, the gastrointestinal assistant, the radiologist, and the radiology technician. Space is required for endoscopic equipment as well as special monitoring equipment that may be needed. Support equipment, such as oxygen and suction equipment, is always available. This procedure is performed on patients who are sedated; the most common sedative is diazepam or opiates such as meperidine. Sedation of the visceral muscle is accomplished using varying amounts of atropine and glucagon. All of these medications are given intravenously during the procedure. Obviously, close monitoring of the patient being examined in a darkened room is necessary.

ERCP is carried out using flexible fiberoptic endoscopes. The type of endoscope employed is generally a side-viewing duodenoscope (Fig. 10–1) unless the procedure is being performed through a Billroth II anastomosis, in which case a forward-viewing duodenoscope is used. *It is not the intent of this chapter to provide an in-depth discussion of the cannulation technique. The reader is referred to descriptions available in the literature.*[86] ERCP is only attempted after the endoscopist has had considerable experience with upper GI endoscopy, and endoscopic sphincterotomy should only be attempted after the examiner has wide experience performing ERCP. Initial attempts at ERCP are frequently unsuccessful, but a skilled endoscopist generally achieves expertise rapidly.[8, 45] Cannulation is generally not a hit-or-miss proposition, and with experience successful cannulation of the papilla is achieved in well over 90 per cent of patients. Because of the anatomy of the ductal structures at the papilla, cannulation of the common duct is slightly more difficult than cannulation of the pancreatic duct. As alluded to previously, cannulation through the afferent loop of a Billroth II anastomosis can be successful, and in our hands cannulation is accomplished in excess of 50 per cent of patients. Fluoroscopy is seldom necessary to assist in locating the papilla in patients with normal anatomy. When a Billroth II cannulation is contemplated, fluoroscopy is frequently helpful in selecting the appropriate limb of the gastrojejunostomy.

There is no time limit for cannulation procedures. Uncomplicated studies may take as little as 5 to 15 minutes; however, procedures in excess of one hour are not uncommon. Therefore, scheduling of patients must take into account the possible length of the procedure.

RADIOGRAPHIC TECHNIQUE

ERCP is a team effort. The radiologist and endoscopist work together closely to achieve adequate images of the ductal structures. The division of labor is such that the endoscopist is responsible for the cannulation and management of the patient and the radiologist is

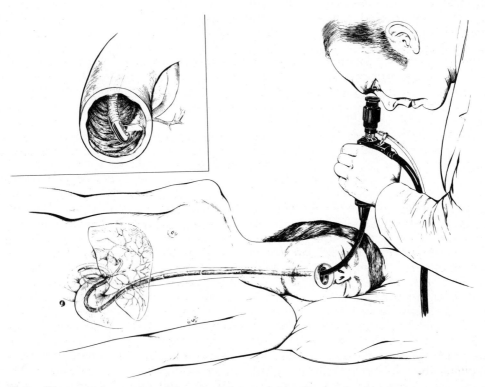

Figure 10–1. Diagrammatic overview of the cannulation procedure showing the side-viewing duodenoscope in the duodenum. Cannulation is taking place using the cannula through the biopsy channel of the scope. The insert depicts the appearance of the papilla as cannulation is performed. (From Stewart, E. T., Vennes, J. A., and Geenen, J. E.: Atlas of Endoscopic Retrograde Cholangiopancreatography. St. Louis: C. V. Mosby Co., 1977.)

responsible for the filming sequence and directing the injection.

Obviously the fluoroscopic details of the procedure are extremely important since the reasons for continuing or stopping injection depend on the fluoroscopic appearance. Inferior monitoring equipment, therefore, leads to errors in judgment and filming, which must be avoided. It goes without saying that if adequate fluoroscopic equipment is not available, the procedure should not be performed. Optimally, the radiographic equipment should have a focal spot of between 0.3 and 0.6 mm and a generator capable of providing short exposures. Although we initially used 105-mm spot films, we quickly discarded them and now favor the use of standard spot film devices. This allows for a larger field of view so that the entire ductal anatomy can be displayed on a single film.

Television monitoring allows the radiologist as well as the endoscopist to visualize the ductal structures as they are being filled and is an indispensable part of the radiographic procedure.

Although ERCP is initially performed with the patient in the prone-oblique or supine position, many films of the biliary tree and frequently the pancreatic duct are taken with the patient in the erect position and, occasionally, in the Trendelenburg position. A tilting fluoroscopic table is therefore necessary. ERCP is only performed as an inpatient procedure, and all of these comments about radiographic equipment apply to hospital-based radiology departments.

The reader is referred to standard texts, which give a very detailed description of the radiographic aspects of the procedure.[86] However, we would like to stress several important points.

As ERCP has developed, it has become standard practice to use certain concentrations of contrast for the study. When the pancreatic duct is studied, 60 per cent diatrizoate is employed. This generally provides sufficient resolution to see both the main pancreatic duct and its lateral branches. In the biliary tree it has been accepted practice to dilute the contrast to a concentration of 30 per cent. We would like to stress that although 30 per cent diatrizoate may be adequate for visualizing the normal biliary tree, there may be some problems owing to the concentration of contrast. A duct measuring 4 or 5 mm in diameter may be quite readily seen using 30 per cent contrast. However, as dilatation occurs in the biliary

tree, even 30 per cent contrast becomes so dense that small and occasionally even large stones are rapidly obscured. We have to take this into account, especially when looking at the intact gallbladder. A gallbladder measuring several centimeters in diameter is so dense when filled with 30 per cent contrast that virtually nothing can be seen within the gallbladder. Gallstones in the common duct or gallbladder may be seen when initially filling with contrast and are subsequently obscured as filling is completed. Early filming is, therefore, quite important.

Because of this frequent problem, we have begun to employ compression much more frequently and now use it routinely. Compression using a balloon paddle produces remarkable results. Compression greatly reduces the amount of scattered radiation and at the same time compresses ductal structures so that intraluminal filling defects can be seen (Fig. 10–2). Compression can be used with the patient in the *recumbent* as well as the *erect* position. Several of the examples shown in this chapter were selected to demonstrate the use of the compression paddle.

The number of films employed in recording ERCP varies from only a few to many. The filming sequence should be kept to a minimum but should be adequate to record all of the necessary ductal abnormalities. It is the radiologist's responsibility to move the patient so that ductal structures are seen from a variety of angles. Also, radiation exposure should be closely monitored and all personnel maximally protected.[16, 62] Prolonged fluoroscopy is reserved for ductal filling only, since radiation causes slow deterioration of the fiberoptic light bundles.[4]

When examining the biliary tree, attempts should be made to fill the entire ductal system so that both the left and right intrahepatic ducts are completely filled. When the gallbladder is intact, filling of the cystic duct and gallbladder should also be accomplished. Because of its oblique position relative to the long axis of the body, the common hepatic duct is anterior to the distal common duct. Also, the left intrahepatic ducts are anterior to the right intrahepatic ducts (Fig. 10–3). Since the procedure is performed in the prone-oblique position, dense contrast runs down the dependent wall of the extrahepatic bile ducts and preferentially fills the left intrahepatic ducts. A "streaming artifact" produced by the contrast running down the dependent wall of the extrahepatic bile ducts may initially give a

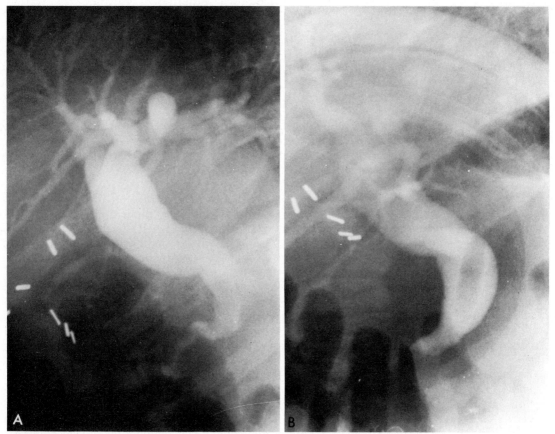

Figure 10–2. Use of compression devices. *A,* This postcholecystectomized patient was being evaluated for recurrent symptoms of biliary obstruction. Initially the dilated biliary tree was seen fluoroscopically. No definite stones could be seen. *B,* When the patient was placed supine and compression applied using a balloon paddle, an ovoid stone was easily seen in the distal common duct. Compression decreases scattered radiation as well as compresses the duct. In a dilated bile duct even very dilute contrast may be so dense as to obscure large stones. We recommend compression of all bile ducts regardless of size.

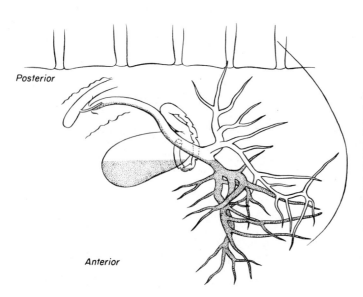

Figure 10–3. Gravity markedly influences the flow of heavy contrast. In the prone position, the left intrahepatic ducts fill preferentially owing to their anterior position in the liver. Note that the extrahepatic ducts are positioned obliquely relative to the long axis of the body. Contrast streams down the bile duct and may give a falsely narrow appearance to the duct. (From Stewart, E. T., Vennes, J. A., and Geenen, J. E.: Atlas of Endoscopic Retrograde Cholangiopancreatography. St. Louis, C. V. Mosby Co., 1977.)

falsely narrowed appearance of the diameter of the common duct. The true diameter of a dilated common duct is appreciated only later when contrast is mixed with the unopacified bile. If only the left intrahepatic ducts can be filled, it may be necessary to visualize those on the right by placing the patient in the supine position and allowing gravity to fill the posteriorly located right-sided ducts.

Underfilling of the ductal structures, especially the intrahepatic ducts, can give a very bizarre appearance to the biliary tree. Interpretation of underfilled ductal structures is hazardous. Therefore, attention to proper filling of the biliary tree and technique is very important for interpreting abnormalities, especially of the intrahepatic bile ducts. Also, preferential flow into the gallbladder can make filling of the intrahepatic ducts suboptimal.

When drainage of the biliary tree is being evaluated, the patient is placed in the supine position. The normal post-cholecystectomy biliary tree should empty within 45 minutes.[9] In the presence of delayed drainage, the source of delayed drainage should be sought, such as sphincter of Oddi dysfunction or benign or malignant strictures. In the presence of an intact gallbladder, drainage times of the biliary tree are invalidated.

One of the unique advantages of ERCP is the information provided by the companion pancreatogram. Abnormalities of the distal common bile duct are much more easily interpreted when the pancreas is shown to be normal or abnormal. Therefore, every effort should be made to obtain a companion pancreatogram when examining the biliary tree.

ABNORMALITIES OF THE BILIARY TREE

When considering pathologic findings in the biliary tree, it is easier to divide the bile ducts into intrahepatic and extrahepatic ducts. Extrahepatic abnormalities will be considered first, since they are the first that are encountered during retrograde filling. Extrahepatic bile duct components include the origin of the left and right intrahepatic ducts, the common hepatic duct, the cystic duct, the gallbladder, the common duct, and sphincter areas (the sphincter of Oddi will be considered separately in the section on endoscopic papillotomy).

EXTRAHEPATIC BILE DUCT ABNORMALITIES

The most common abnormalities seen in the extrahepatic bile ducts are choledocholithiasis and some type of stricture. Filling defects within the common duct, when persistent, are almost always due to calculus material. Occasionally a polypoid tumor within the lumen of the common duct will mimic a stone. Stones rarely completely obstruct the common duct unless impacted at the level of the papilla. Also, stones do not locally expand the common duct. A filling defect that causes local expansion of the diameter of the common duct should be suspected of representing a growing lesion such as some type of tumor. As noted before, compression of the common duct may be necessary to fully evaluate the presence or absence of calculus material.

Strictures of the common bile duct have different possibilities depending on their location.[81, 82] Since the common bile duct passes behind or within the pancreas for a short distance, strictures involving the distal common duct include pathology in the pancreas within the differential diagnosis. If a stricture is encountered, the mucosal details should be examined in the region of the stricture. An infiltrating process may lead to irregularity, which makes the likelihood of malignant stricture much more likely. Unfortunately, malignant strictures may have a very smooth and symmetric appearance (Fig. 10–4). Therefore, any stricture involving the distal common duct includes a malignant stricture in the differential diagnosis. Primary bile duct carcinoma, carcinoma of the pancreas, metastatic carcinoma, and tumors of the papilla can all involve the distal common duct and can produce similar strictures.

Benign strictures of the distal common duct are most commonly seen in chronic pancreatitis. Chronic pancreatitis complicated by pseudocyst may produce significant narrowing of the distal common duct simply because of compression by the adjacent pseudocyst. In the absence of definitive radiographic criteria for malignancy, the companion pancreatogram may be extremely useful in determining the etiology of the stricture (Fig. 10–5). Primary carcinoma of the pancreas almost always is accompanied by ductal abnormalities, which allow differentiation between carcinoma of the pancreas and primary bile duct carcinoma (Fig.

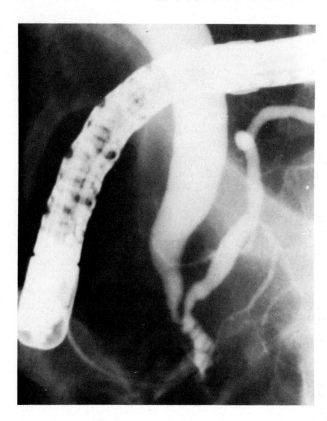

Figure 10–4. This radiograph demonstrates a long common channel, which is frequently seen in normal persons. Notice the irregular mucosal pattern of the common channel. This is normal and represents mucosal pleats or excrescences, which have no pathologic significance.

Figure 10–5. Common bile duct carcinoma. A dilated, partially obstructed biliary tree is seen above an irregular stricture of the distal common bile duct (1). The stricture certainly has malignant characteristics as evidenced by its very irregular margins. The diagnosis of primary bile duct tumor is much more secure when viewing the normal companion pancreatogram (2).

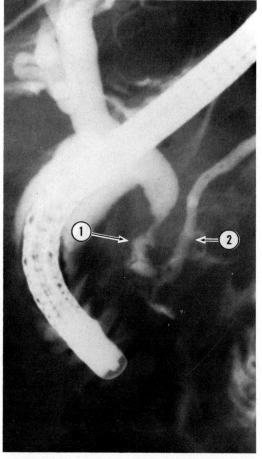

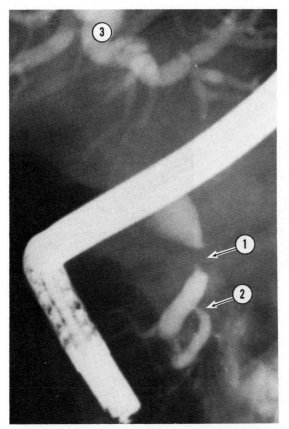

Figure 10–6. Carcinoma of the pancreas. The cannula is simultaneously filling both ducts via a common channel. A smooth, slightly asymmetric stricture of the common duct is present *(1)*. Complete obstruction of the pancreatic duct is present *(2)*. The combination of strictures of both ducts makes the diagnosis of carcinoma of the pancreas a virtual certainty in this nonalcoholic patient. Notice the dilated intrahepatic ducts *(3)*. Further injection above this high-grade stricture of the common duct would increase the risk of cholangitis following the procedure. This patient should be placed on antibiotics prophylactically in any event.

10–6).[24] The companion pancreatogram may confirm the presence or absence of chronic pancreatitis radiologically. The appearance of benign strictures of the pancreatic duct and common duct in the presence of chronic pancreatitis is indistinguishable from the appearance of malignant strictures (Figs. 10–7 and 10–8). Unfortunately, one can never be confident that cancer is not present. Percutaneous aspiration cytology or brush cytology at the stricture is a logical next step. When cytology is negative, it has been our policy simply to follow the patient unless surgery is to be performed to manage a complication of chronic pancreatitis such as pain. ERCP can be repeated to evaluate interval changes, which might increase the confidence level for diagnosing cancer.

There is great value in directly visualizing the papilla of Vater in patients with carcinoma involving this structure. Usually this is an endoscopic diagnosis. Although cannulation through a tumor involving the papilla of Vater is usually successful, the presence of the tumor mass extending into the lumen of the duodenum generally is all that is necessary to suggest the diagnosis. Without direct visualization of the papilla of Vater, the radiographic findings of carcinoma in this area could be indistinguishable from primary carcinoma of the bile duct or pancreas radiologically. Endoscopic biopsy generally confirms the malignant nature of the mass.

Strictures involving the extrahepatic biliary tree in the proximal duct have a different differential diagnosis from those involving the distal common bile duct. Strictures in this area, in the absence of previous surgery, must be considered to represent malignant disease until proved otherwise. There is very little evidence to radiologically distinguish one type of malignancy from another, since findings in primary bile duct carcinoma overlap those of metastatic disease and carcinoma of the gallbladder.

Complete obstruction of the extrahepatic bile ducts is almost invariably due to some malignant lesion, since it is very uncommon for benign strictures to completely obstruct the biliary tree (Fig. 10–9). (Injury to the bile ducts and other postoperative changes secondary to previous surgery will be discussed separately.)

Primary sclerosing cholangitis, an entity frequently accompanying chronic ulcerative colitis, most often has both extrahepatic and intrahepatic manifestations. Although not all cases involve both the intra- and extrahepatic ducts, when the extrahepatic ductal system is involved it makes it much easier to differentiate from cirrhosis, which has similar changes involving the intrahepatic ducts (Fig. 10–10). Primary sclerosing cholangitis is now being found quite often owing to more frequent visualization of the biliary tree by ERC as well as by transhepatic cholangiography.[11] The involvement of the extrahepatic bile ducts is often stark and bizarre in appearance. Multiple areas of stricture, deformity, and frequently small intramural-appearing diverticula can be seen. These patients should be placed on antibiotics following ERC because of the increased risk of cholestasis and sepsis. It should be noted that, radiologically, primary scleros-

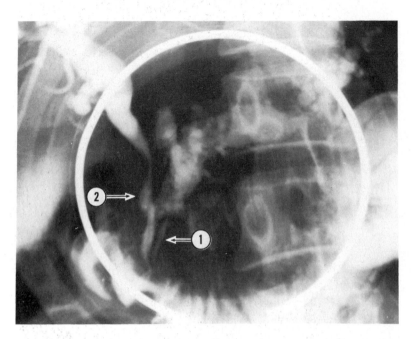

Figure 10–7. Chronic pancreatitis with stricture of common bile duct and pancreatic duct. With compression, the details of both ducts are well seen. The main pancreatic duct is dilated with irregular contours. These findings extend out into the lateral branches. A strictured segment is present near the papilla *(1)*. The common duct is narrowed as it passes through the fibrotic pancreas *(2)*. The common duct in this case is narrowed throughout its entire intrapancreatic portion.

Figure 10–8. Chronic pancreatitis. Dilatation of both ductal systems is present. Ectasia and irregularity of the lateral branches and main pancreatic duct are characteristic of chronic pancreatitis. Strictures of the distal common duct and main pancreatic duct are present and are evident when one knows the location of the papilla of Vater *(1)*. Unfortunately, a carcinoma in the head of the pancreas could cause similar findings. In spite of a history of alcohol abuse, a carcinoma cannot be excluded. In such patients, direct percutaneous aspiration cytology from the suspected area can be done quickly using the ERCP as a guide.

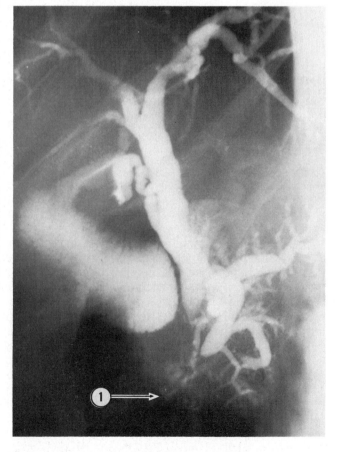

Figure 10–9. Primary bile duct carcinoma. This 46-year-old jaundiced male has a high-grade stricture involving the origin of the right and left intrahepatic ducts. In the absence of previous surgery, as in this case, a stricture located in this area is malignant, with very few exceptions. Although the stricture is due to primary bile duct carcinoma in this case, metastatic disease can produce identical findings. (From Stewart, E. T., Vennes, J. A., and Geenen, J. E.: Atlas of Endoscopic Retrograde Cholangiopancreatography. St. Louis: C. V. Mosby Co., 1977.)

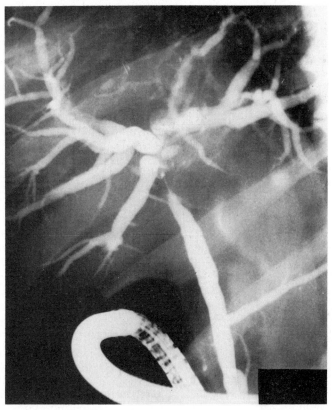

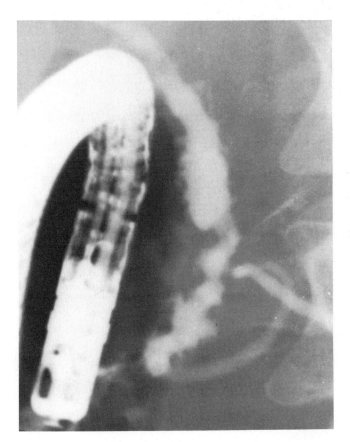

Figure 10–10. This magnified view of the distal common duct demonstrates the stark and bizarre appearance of advanced sclerosing cholangitis. The multiple strictures and numerous "diverticular" outpouchings in the wall are characteristic of this disease. It should be remembered that antibiotics are indicated in these patients following ERC because of the stasis and multiple strictures.

ing cholangitis appears to spare the gallbladder and cystic duct from the bizarre abnormalities seen elsewhere. Occasionally coexistent gallstones are present in patients with primary sclerosing cholangitis, but this has been the exception in our experience.

There are several congenital abnormalities involving the biliary tree that are quite nicely demonstrated by ERC. ERC is particularly well suited for studying choledochoceles[78, 95] as well as choledochal cysts (Fig. 10–11).[1, 38] The anatomy of both these lesions is well displayed, especially the relationship of these congenital abnormalities to the pancreatic duct. Although ERC is not commonly employed to confirm the diagnosis of congenital absence of the gallbladder, failure to fill the cystic duct and gallbladder in conjunction with nonvisualization of the gallbladder by ultrasound might suggest the presumptive diagnosis of congenital absence of the gallbladder (Fig. 10–12). This condition is so uncommon, however, that diagnostic evaluation of such patients is not considered a practical use of ERC.

Occasionally very bizarre congenital abnormalities are seen such as multiple common ducts. The examiner should be prepared to encounter random asymptomatic as well as symptomatic abnormalities, some of which will be congenital in nature (Fig. 10–13). The number of unusual anatomic variations is growing each year.

Nothing has been said up to this point about diameter measurements. Generally, the extrahepatic ducts are measured at their widest point.[50] An estimate of size is made by comparing the diameter of the duct with that of the endoscope (12 mm). There is substantial compliance in the bile ducts, and diameter is greatly affected by injection pressure. One such study demonstrated a 3-mm difference in common bile duct diameter when IVC and ERC were compared.[9] We generally interpret size along with other observations such as drainage, stones, stricture, and so on. Ultrasound or CT measurements of diameter are probably closer to actuality because technique artifacts such as injection pressure are absent.

INTRAHEPATIC BILE DUCT ABNORMALITIES

As noted previously, adequate filling of the intrahepatic bile ducts is necessary before cor-

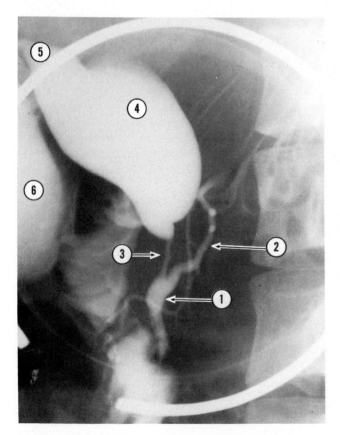

Figure 10–11. ERCP is uniquely suited to showing the usual anatomy of a choledochal cyst. This single film taken using compression shows the detail very well. A long common channel (1) gives rise to the main pancreatic (2) and the common bile duct (3). The narrowed distal common bile duct expands into the hugely dilated choledochal cyst (4). The anatomy of the communication of the ducts was obscured until compression moved the huge redundant cyst superiorly and exposed the anatomy, as seen here. The cystic duct (5) and gallbladder (6) communicate with the cyst.

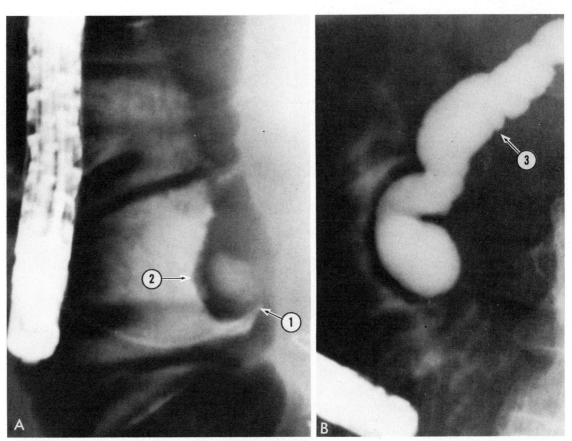

Figure 10–12.   Choledochocele. *A*, Endoscopically, a smoothly bulging papilla was seen. The orifice of the papilla was located inferiorly *(1)*. This magnified view of the duodenum shows the filling defect due to the enlarged papilla *(2)*. *B*, The anatomy of the choledochocele is nicely demonstrated when the common duct is opacified. Notice the caliber irregularities of the common duct *(3)*, which were due to coexistent sclerosing cholangitis in this patient with ulcerative colitis.

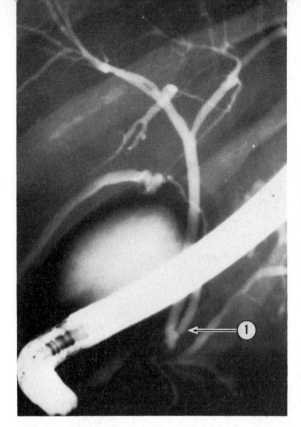

Figure 10–13. Low insertion of the cystic duct. Notice the cystic duct as it joins the common duct just above the sphincter area *(1)*. Such low insertion of the cystic duct is a frequent finding at ERC.

Figure 10–14. An intraluminal obstructing lesion in the left lobe of the liver could be a stone or tumor but in this case was proved to be an intraductal papillary carcinoma.

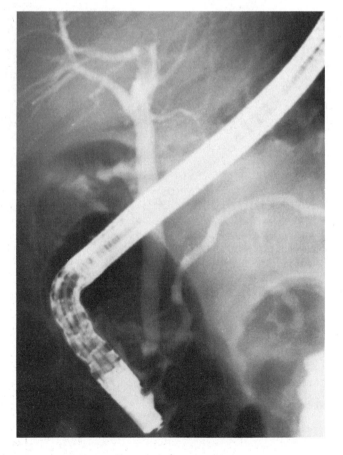

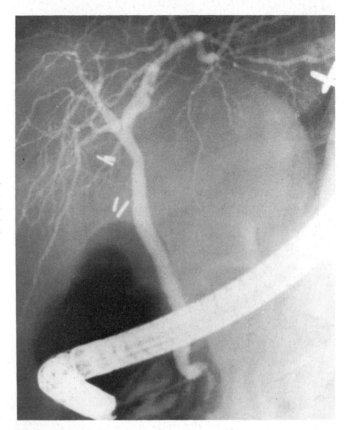

Figure 10–15. The crowded, irregular intrahepatic ducts are consistent with advanced cirrhotic changes in this patient. It is well to note that early cirrhosis may not produce any significant changes on the cholangiogram. Note the normal extrahepatic ducts.

rect interpretation of abnormalities involving these structures is undertaken. The use of ERC has not substantially added to the long list of intrahepatic abnormalities previously seen in the liver by other means such as transhepatic cholangiography. However, the retrograde instillation of contrast in the liver provides another access route to the bile ducts. Observations on bile ducts that need to be made to interpret the cholangiogram correctly include diameter, splaying, separation or crowding, caliber irregularities, strictures, presence or absence of stones (Fig. 10–14) or other foreign material, communication with parenchymal spaces (such as abscess), and obstruction, either partial or complete.[5, 67]

The value in assessing the intrahepatic cholangiogram is in differentiating the normal from the abnormal ducts as well as providing a differential diagnosis in those patients suspected of having diffuse parenchymal or infiltrating disease or some type of space-occupying lesion within the liver.[22]

Cirrhosis is the most common clinical entity encountered and produces very bizarre-appearing ductal structures depending on its severity.[87] Generally, advanced cirrhosis is nec-

essary before significant ductal abnormalities appear on the cholangiogram (Fig. 10–15). Areas of stenosis and ectasia and ductal irregularities due to regenerating nodules and chronic fibrosis are frequently quite marked. Cirrhosis must be distinguished from sclerosing cholangitis, which has similar findings involving the intrahepatic ducts.[70] As noted before, it is the involvement of the extrahepatic bile ducts that allows the easy distinction between cirrhosis and sclerosing cholangitis (Fig. 10–16). Metastatic disease is the most common malignant process encountered in the liver, and this may be unifocal or multifocal. The most commonly seen changes in the ducts include stenosis, obstruction, and mass effect.

Inflammatory diseases in the liver, such as single or multiple abscesses, may produce mass effect or, on occasion, may directly communicate with the biliary tree. Sometimes extravasation of contrast into such structures is dependent upon the injection pressure at the time of the examination.

As in the extrahepatic bile ducts, occasional congenital abnormalities involving the liver are now seen (Fig. 10–17). Polycystic liver disease, as expected, produces a large liver with mul-

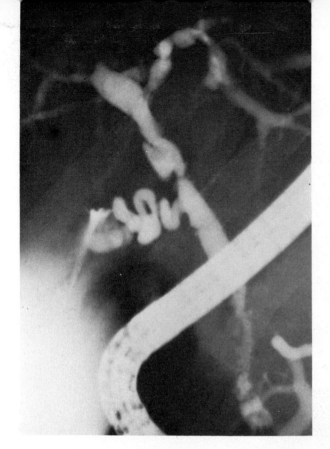

Figure 10–16. The characteristic involvement of the extrahepatic as well as the intrahepatic ducts identifies this patient as having sclerosing cholangitis as opposed to cirrhosis, which can have a similar appearance of the ducts within the liver. Notice the numerous strictures and small diverticular outpouchings in the wall of the common duct. An air bubble is present in the common hepatic duct.

Figure 10–17. Anatomic variant. Here the right lobe of the liver is partially drained by a small duct that joins the common duct at about the same level as the cystic duct. Normal variants are occasionally seen in the biliary tree.

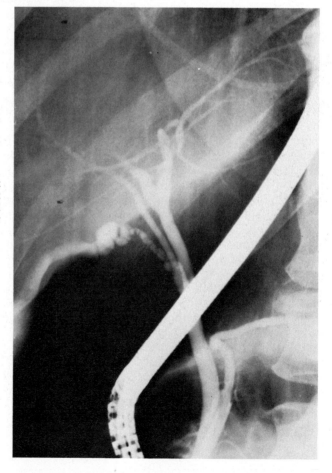

382

tiple space-occupying lesions. Generally the bile ducts are displaced smoothly by the enlarging cysts. Some of these patients may be at risk for developing cholangitis following the procedure due to the multiple stretched and possibly partially obstructed ducts owing to the cysts. Antibiotics are indicated if this diagnosis is established. Caroli's disease, a very uncommon clinical problem, should be easily diagnosed by retrograde study.

Since ERC is a retrograde study, high-grade obstruction of the bile ducts at any level may not yield the definitive answer. Although the diagnosis of malignancy may be well established from the appearance of the obstructed ducts, the important clinical information as to whether the upper level of the obstruction is or is not accessible to the surgeon may be absent. In those cases in which high-grade obstruction does not allow significant contrast above the obstruction to define the upper level, a companion transhepatic cholangiogram is necessary to completely define the anatomy.

One other note of caution should be re-emphasized. The presence of high-grade obstruction in the biliary tree places the patient at risk for sepsis following the procedure. Because of this, injection of contrast above a partial obstruction is generally limited, and the amount of contrast may be insufficient to adequately define the ducts above the level of obstruction. It is wiser to place the patient on antibiotics and restudy the patient with a preoperative transhepatic cholangiogram than to proceed with the study and completely opacify the entire biliary tree.

ENDOSCOPIC CYTOLOGY AND BIOPSY

Strictures of the intra- or extrahepatic bile ducts can be examined histologically by obtaining cells. Brushing of the stricture directly or collection of bile for cytology can confirm the malignant nature of a stricture (Figs. 10–18

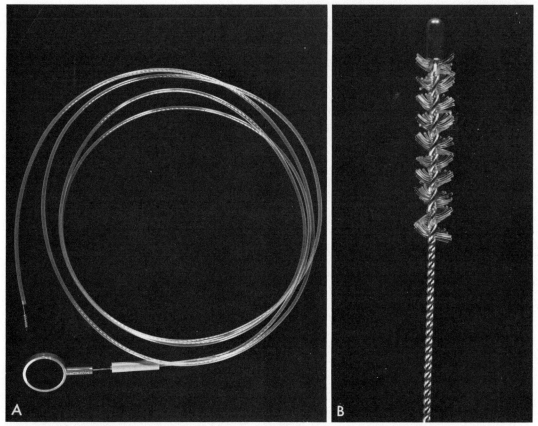

Figure 10–18. Endoscopic brush for cytology. *A,* This 200-cc endoscopic brush can be placed down the biopsy channel and at or through a stricture of the duct by cannulating the papilla. *B,* This magnified view of the brush demonstrates the bristles, which dislodge the malignant cells for cytologic exam. *It should be remembered that cells harvested in this manner must be preserved in 95 per cent alcohol.* (Manufactured by Medi Tech.)

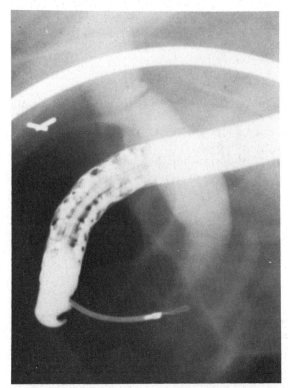

Figure 10–19. A brush may be placed in the common duct or in the pancreatic duct to collect cytologic specimens. As seen here, the brush is in the distal common duct. Note that compression is also being applied to improve resolution.

and 10–19).[60, 66] The closer the tumor is to the scope, the higher the yield of malignant cells. Yields of positive cells are reported to be as high as 50 per cent or greater. If a brush cannot be introduced, the cholangiogram can be used as a guide for percutaneous aspiration.[25, 41] The technique is similar to that described using THC (transhepatic cholangiography) to guide the needle. Samples are taken from the strictured area.

The papilla is directly visualized and ampullary carcinoma is usually obvious. Endoscopic biopsy of the mass generally confirms the diagnosis preoperatively.

POST-CHOLECYSTECTOMY SYNDROME (Table 10–3)

Cholecystectomy is usually performed in patients with acute cholecystitis accompanied by cholelithiasis with or without choledocholithiasis. Cholecystectomy is also performed in patients with asymptomatic gallstones. The third indication for surgery is recurrent right upper quadrant symptoms with an acalculous gallbladder.

When a patient complains of pain or discomfort following cholecystectomy, he is generally evaluated for the possibility of the post-cholecystectomy syndrome. This syndrome is a nonspecific constellation of symptoms that usually includes recurrent pain following gallbladder surgery. The incidence of the post-cholecystectomy syndrome varies between 5 and 50 per cent; however, only about 3 per cent of the patients present with severe, recurrent abdominal pain. Some present with jaundice.

Thus, the post-cholecystectomy syndrome affects a group of patients with continuing or recurrent symptoms following indicated gallbladder surgery, such as cholelithiasis or acute cholecystitis, or those patients in whom a normal gallbladder was found at surgery. Those with normal gallbladders at surgery are the patients who most often have other problems such as a hiatal hernia, irritable colon, and so on.

The role of ERCP in the evaluation of the post-cholecystectomy syndrome is becoming increasingly prominent.[12, 37, 69] Such patients present a particularly vexing clinical problem for the referring clinician. The unique advantage of ERCP is that it allows direct visualization of the biliary tree to detect anatomical abnormalities as well as the presence or absence of stones. At the same time, patients at risk for sphincter of Oddi dysfunction can be studied using manometric means. An entirely normal biliary tree following ERC and manometry generally precludes any further evaluation of the biliary tree as a source of the patient's symptoms.

POSTOPERATIVE BILE DUCTS

ERC is uniquely suited to the evaluation of the postoperative biliary tree. The presence of deformity of the extrahepatic bile ducts secondary to surgical accidents or surgical manip-

Table 10–3. CAUSES OF THE POST-CHOLECYSTECTOMY SYNDROME

Recurrent or residual common duct stones
Postoperative stricture of common bile ducts
Long cystic duct stump with or without cystic duct stones
Sphincter of Oddi dysfunction (papillary stenosis)
Unrelated diseases such as hiatal hernia, peptic ulcer, irritable colon, and possibly liver disease

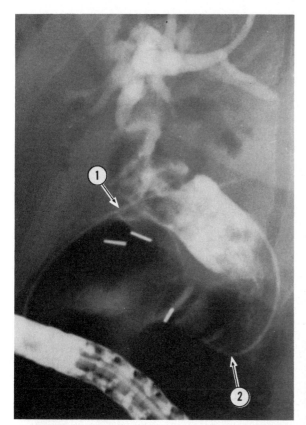

Figure 10–20. Side-to-side choledochoduodenostomy. The cannula enters the biliary tree through the choledochoduodenostomy *(1)*. The tip has re-emerged into the duodenum through the papilla *(2)*. Much food and debris are present in the common duct. Air is seen in the intrahepatic ducts. In this patient with a "sump" syndrome, the study confirmed the anatomy and presence of much foreign material in the extrahepatic ducts.

ulation of the biliary tree is a common problem (Fig. 10–20). This includes patients with and without surgically created biliary enteric anastomoses.[32, 75] ERC is the preferred method for evaluation of biliary enteric anastomoses. Patients who have had end-to-side or side-to-side anastomosis between the common bile duct and the duodenum can be cannulated through the papilla or through the enteric anastomosis.[6] The study assesses whether the anastomosis is patent, the diameter of the anastomosis, the presence or absence of stones or foreign material within the common bile duct as well as some information about the anatomy in patients with questionable previous surgical procedures (Fig. 10–21).

Deformity of the common duct following exploration is frequently seen (Fig. 10–22). Mild narrowing, presumably at the site of T-tube placement, is well documented. Occa-

sional severe stricture occurs, but in our experience this has generally followed transection of the common duct and reanastomosis. We have had no experience with changes that might occur following arterial infusion of chemotherapeutic agents.

TRAUMATIC INJURY TO THE BILIARY TREE

Trauma to the bile ducts is seldom mentioned as an indication for retrograde cannulation; however, ERC is uniquely suited to studying the traumatized biliary tree. Trauma involving the biliary tree can involve intra- or extrahepatic structures.[57] Trauma may be blunt, due to high impact injury, or iatrogenic

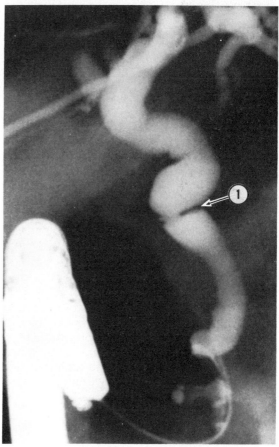

Figure 10–21. Benign postoperative stricture. This patient had prior cholecystectomy and T-tube insertion. The web-like stricture *(1)* in the mid common duct has a benign appearance. In this patient the finding was incidental and no symptoms were present. This location is the most common site of postoperative stricture of the common bile duct.

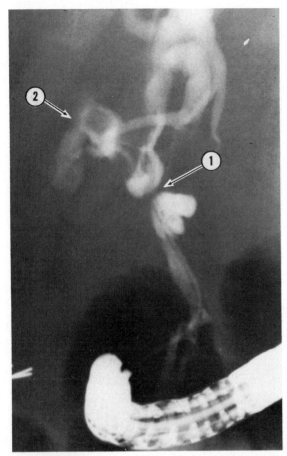

Figure 10–22. This patient had prior cholecystectomy and known common duct injury. A severe stricture is present in the mid portion of the duct *(1)*. The cannula has passed through the stricture. A limited injection of contrast material demonstrates ectasia of the intrahepatic ducts *(2)* and calculus material. A nasobiliary stent might be temporarily placed in such a patient for drainage until surgery could be planned. This patient has done well following a choledochojejunostomy.

at the time of surgery.[2] ERC has been used to demonstrate perforation of the gallbladder as well as laceration of the liver or extrahepatic bile ducts. At the time of endoscopy, hematobilia may be demonstrated, a finding that is not likely to be shown by any other technique short of visceral angiography.

INTERVENTIONAL TECHNIQUES

Endoscopic Sphincterotomy

There are currently several types of patient who might benefit from endoscopic sphincterotomy (Tables 10–4 and 10–5) (Fig. 10–

Table 10–4. INDICATIONS FOR ENDOSCOPIC SPHINCTEROTOMY

Residual or recurrent common bile duct stone following cholecystectomy
Choledocholithiasis in high surgical risk patients with gallbladder *in situ*
Sphincter of Oddi dysfunction (papillary stenosis)
Tumors of papilla
Gallstone pancreatitis

23).[30, 31, 49, 64, 71, 73] The most common indication is a post-cholecystectomy demonstration of common bile duct stones.[19, 84, 85] Retained common duct stones following cholecystectomy is a continuing clinical dilemma. It is said that of the 750,000 patients undergoing cholecystectomy each year, a large number also have common duct exploration. Following exploration, it is believed that between 4.3[33, 39] and 14 per cent of patients will have retained common duct stones. There are variables affecting this number, but these primarily relate to the sur-

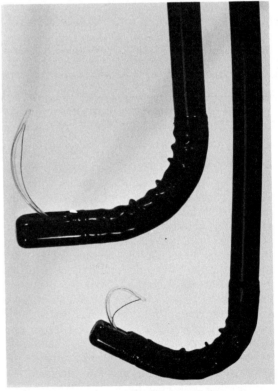

Figure 10–23. The sphincterotome is advanced out of the scope; the open and closed positons of the cutting wire are demonstrated. The cutting current passes through the wire. (Manufactured by Sonderanfertigung Med Gerate, West Germany.)

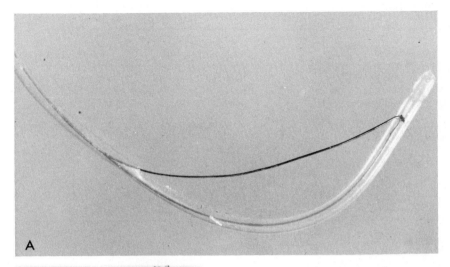

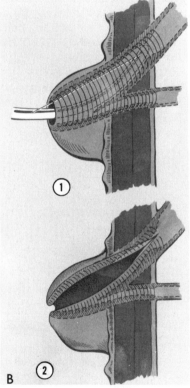

Figure 10–24. *A,* Magnified view of the sphincterotome in the open position. In this position the incision is made by passing current through the wire. (From Stewart, E. T., Jennes, J. A., and Geenen, J. E.: Atlas of Endoscopic Retrograde Cholangiopancreatography. St. Louis: C. V. Mosby Co., 1977.) *B,* Sphincterotome selectively inserted into common bile duct in cutting position *(1).* Following electrosurgery, incision extends through sphincter into distal bile duct *(2).* (From Geenen, J. E., et al.: J.A.M.A. *19*:2075, 1977.)

gical technique and the performance of operative cholangiograms as well as the newer use of choledochoscopes.[91] Endoscopic sphincterotomy is an acceptable alternative to operative sphincteroplasty and stone extraction for the treatment of common duct stones.[14, 15, 47, 68] Most patients who come to endoscopic sphincterotomy have had stones identified months to years following cholecys-

tectomy. Obviously some of these patients have primary bile duct stones rather than undetected common duct stones.

The second indication for sphincterotomy is choledocholithiasis with complications of either jaundice or cholangitis in the high-risk patient who has not had a previous cholecystectomy (Fig. 10–24). If endoscopic sphincterotomy is successful in removing the common

Table 10–5. INDICATIONS FOR ENDOSCOPIC SPHINCTEROTOMY

Indication	Geenen (Unpublished data)	Safrany[72] (Worldwide)
Common duct stones	257 (80.3%)	3070 (84.9%)
Post-cholecystectomy	237	2183
Gallbladder *in situ*	20	887
Sphincter of Oddi dysfunction (papillary stenosis)	51 (16.0%)	471 (13.0%)
Tumor of papilla	3 (0.9%)	57 (1.5%)
Miscellaneous	9 (2.8%)	21 (0.6%)
Total	320	3618

duct stones in this group of patients, subsequent cholecystectomy may be performed on a stabilized patient.

Sphincter of Oddi dysfunction (papillary stenosis) is the third indication (Fig. 10–25). This entity is somewhat poorly defined and is receiving considerable attention.[3, 65] Sphincter of Oddi dysfunction is defined clinically as cholestasis, dilatation of the bile ducts, and radiographic evidence of delayed drainage with or without right upper quadrant pain.[97] This entity is usually superimposed on a prior history of cholecystectomy and, frequently, common duct exploration or passage of stone. The use of endoscopic manometry to examine the sphincter of Oddi indicates that many of the

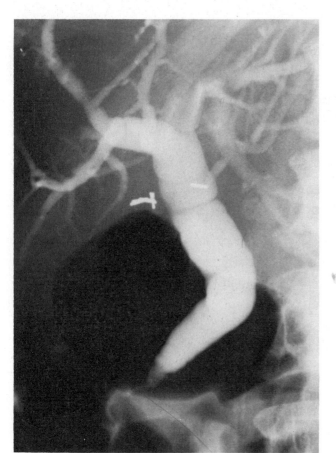

Figure 10–25. Sphincter of Oddi dysfunction. Recurrent symptoms of cholestasis following cholecystectomy prompted evaluation of this patient. There was evidence of clinical jaundice, delayed drainage (> 45 minutes) of the common duct at ERC, and markedly elevated pressures in the sphincter of Oddi. Following endoscopic sphincterotomy, the symptoms disappeared. As noted in the text, the entity of sphincter of Oddi dysfunction is gaining considerable attention and is probably the most frequent indication for manometry in our hands.

Table 10–6. CONTRAINDICATIONS FOR ENDOSCOPIC SPHINCTEROTOMY

Coagulation disorders
Long strictures of distal bile duct
Abnormalities of proximal bile ducts
Large stone >2.5 cm
Acute pancreatitis

patients, if not most, have markedly elevated pressures in the region of the sphincter.[7] Clinically this syndrome is not clear-cut, and it is hoped that identification of these patients will be easier in the future, especially with the more common use of manometric techniques.

The fourth indication for sphincterotomy is a very rare indication. Some patients with tumors involving the papilla of Vater have undergone palliative endoscopic sphincterotomy to relieve the obstructive jaundice caused by the invasive tumor. It is hoped that the patient would then be a better surgical risk for a more radical procedure. Experience with these patients is very limited.

The last indication for endoscopic sphincterotomy is acute pancreatitis related to the passage of common bile duct stones. The stones may have been passed spontaneously or may be impacted in the papilla. Although ERCP is not usually employed in patients with acute pancreatitis, this particular situation warrants such consideration, especially in those patients with pancreatitis severe enough to make them poor operative risks.

Contraindications to endoscopic sphincterotomy include patients with bleeding disorders, since this procedure is associated with occasional hemorrhage (Table 10–6). When strictures of the common duct are so long that they extend beyond the wall of the duodenum, the procedure cannot be done safely and therefore these patients are excluded. Obviously, if the patient has additional strictures above the level of the sphincter, sphincterotomy is of little benefit and should not be performed. Stones that are larger than 2.5 to 3 cm in diameter rarely pass spontaneously following endoscopic sphincterotomy and are difficult to extract with the Fogarty balloon or basket. These patients should be treated with operative management rather than attempts at sphincterotomy.

As mentioned previously, acute pancreatitis

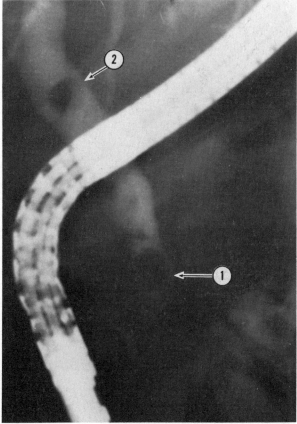

Figure 10–26. Following sphincterotomy, stones are frequently extracted by simply grasping them with the sphincterotome, as in this case *(1)*. A second stone above *(2)* is seen. As noted in the text, most stones of this size will pass spontaneously following sphincterotomy.

is a relative contraindication except in those patients with gallstone pancreatitis who are poor surgical risks.

The last contraindication is the technical inability of the endoscopist to properly align the sphincterotome. The sphincterotome must be precisely positioned so that the incision is extended in the proper direction.[89] Obviously endoscopic sphincterotomy should not be attempted by endoscopists who are not highly skilled in ERCP.

How good is endoscopic sphincterotomy for the removal of stones? If the stones are less than 2.5 cm in diameter it is very likely that they can be removed (Fig. 10–26). Eighty-eight per cent of our patients have had successful removal of the stones by either spontaneous passage or extraction with the balloon, sphincterotome, or Dormia basket (Figs. 10–27 and 10–28). Most stones will spontaneously pass, and repeated attempts to manually extract stones are not warranted until follow-up studies demonstrate failure of spontaneous passage. The sphincterotomy can be extended if necessary at that time.

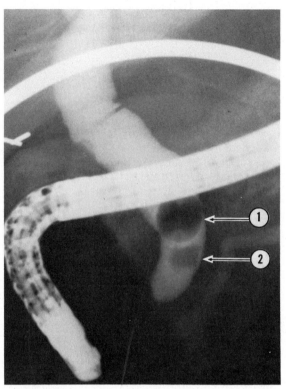

Figure 10–28. Following sphincterotomy, a Fogarty catheter *(1)* is inflated above a stone *(2)* and, by withdrawing the balloon, the stone is removed. The balloon catheter can be pulled through the sphincterotomy to give a good estimate of the size of the incision.

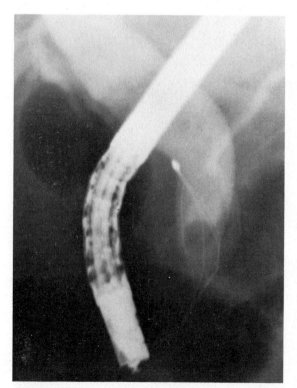

Figure 10–27. Dormia basket retrieval of a stone. A sphincterotomy has been performed. The basket has been inserted into the common duct and is in the process of extracting a stone.

Our experience is similar to that reported in Europe. Safrany reported the results from 15 centers throughout the world[72] (Table 10–5). Endoscopic sphincterotomy was successfully accomplished in 3,618 of 3,853 patients (94 per cent). Of 3,070 patients with common bile duct stones, 1,795 (58.5 per cent) passed their stones spontaneously. In 984 patients (32 per cent) stones were extracted from the common duct, and 291 patients (9.5 per cent) had residual stones and required surgery.

Complications unique to endoscopic sphincterotomy include hemorrhage, cholangitis, pancreatitis, perforation, and stone impaction (Fig. 10–29) (Table 10–7). Our own experience has been similar to the statistics gathered world-wide and reported by Safrany. The mortality for this procedure is reported to be 1.4 per cent. The figure has not changed a great deal. Most of the patients in whom this procedure is performed represent very high-risk patients. Mortality rates at these levels are relatively low when compared with the surgical mortality statistics, which range between 1.1

Table 10–7. COMPLICATIONS OF ENDOSCOPIC SPHINCTEROTOMY

Complication	Geenen (320 pts. Unpublished data)	Geenen[31] (1250 pts. US)	Safrany[72] (3618 pts. Worldwide)
Hemorrhage	8	29	90
Cholangitis	2	25	49
Pancreatitis	7	41	48
Perforation	1	14	40
Stone impaction	3	—	27
Total	21 (6.6%)	109 (8.7%)	254 (7.0%)
Mortality	2 (0.6%)	15 (1.2%)	50 (1.4%)

and 13 per cent in different series.[35, 43, 65] Patients over 50 years of age in whom re-exploration of the common bile duct and operative sphincteroplasty are performed can be expected to have a mortality rate approaching 5 per cent.[34] Thus, the available evidence indicates that endoscopic sphincterotomy is a safe approach when compared with operative removal of common bile duct stones in high-risk and/or elderly patients. The role of sphincterotomy in younger, low-risk patients still needs definition.

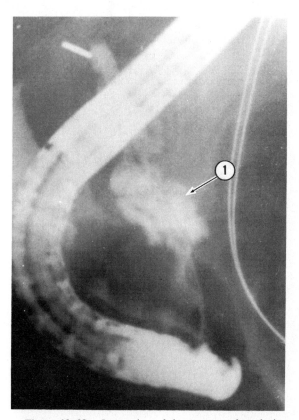

Figure 10–29. Laceration of the common duct during sphincterotomy. Following sphincterotomy for stones, the common duct was cut outside of the intramural portion. Contrast has extravasated from the duct (1). The patient recovered uneventfully. However, as noted in the text, an injury such as this may increase the risk of the procedure for subsequent pancreatitis or other complications. Most patients are treated conservatively with antibiotics and bed rest. In our experience this has rarely led to further difficulty.

Placement of Nasobiliary Catheters

A 300-cm catheter can be placed through the endoscope and into the common bile duct above a stricture, stone, or tumor and left in position for days or weeks.[93, 94] In patients with ascending cholangitis, the bile duct can be perfused with antibiotics or the catheter can be connected to a drainage bag to decompress the biliary tree. This catheter functions like a T-tube or percutaneous transhepatic catheter. If stones are present that are unable to be removed following endoscopic sphincterotomy, the common bile duct can be perfused by means of the transnasobiliary catheter with Mono-Octanoin or bile salts such as cholate in an attempt to reduce the size of stones for subsequent removal (Fig. 10– 0).[42, 88, 90-92] The nasobiliary catheter is then used to perform repeat cholangiography to assess the size of the stones and to see if they have been passed (Fig. 10–31).[20, 77] Transnasobiliary stents can also be positioned in the bile ducts across a benign or malignant obstruction for long-term management in the high surgical risk patient.

Internal Transpapillary Stent

Internal transpapillary stents can be placed endoscopically. This is usually done for benign or malignant strictures in high-risk patients. Pigtail catheters can be fashioned with either a single or a double pigtail placed across bile duct strictures (Fig. 10–32). This is accomplished by first placing a guide wire through

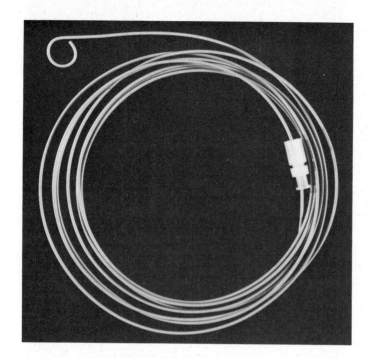

Figure 10–30. Nasobiliary stent. This 300-cm catheter can be placed in the biliary tree with the pigtail left above a stricture for drainage. An alternate use would be for perfusion of stone-solubilizing solution in the case of retained stones following endoscopic sphincterotomy. (Manufactured by Cook Inc.)

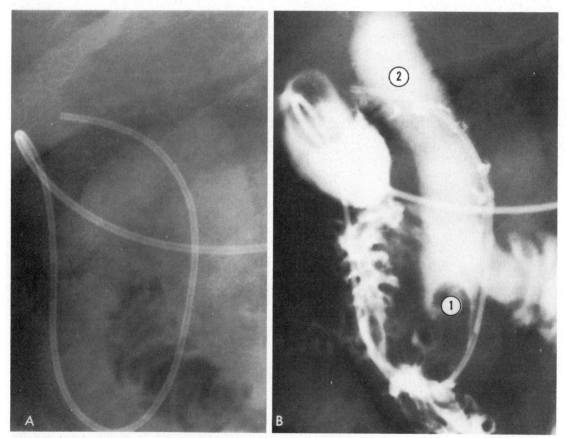

Figure 10–31. Nasobiliary stent. *A,* Following unsuccessful sphincterotomy to remove large stones, a nasobiliary stent was left in place. The stent provides drainage and protects the patient against stone impaction. *B,* A cholangiogram performed through the stent several days later demonstrates that the stone is still present *(1).* At this point the sphincterotomy may be extended, if feasible, or solubilizing solutions can be infused in the common duct *(2)* in an attempt to dissolve the stone.

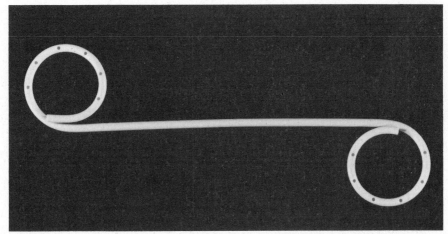

Figure 10–32. Internal stent. This is a double pigtail stent that can be placed internally across a low stricture of the biliary tree. One end remains in the duodenum and can be withdrawn if necessary using the biopsy forceps. (Manufactured by Vance Products.)

the stricture, then subsequently placing the stent across the stricture and leaving it in place (Fig. 10–33). Since the tip of the stent protrudes into the lumen of the duodenum, it can be endoscopically withdrawn and replaced at any time.

Balloon Catheter Dilatation

Although experience with balloon catheters is limited at this time, we expect that their use will rapidly increase. Balloon dilatation of benign strictures from below is logical, since long catheters can be manufactured with balloons of various lengths and diameters. If the catheter can be placed across a stricture, dilation can be performed repeatedly (Fig. 10–34). We are in the process of evaluating balloon catheters, and the preliminary results of feasibility in dilating benign strictures such as sclerosing cholangitis are encouraging.

EXPERIMENTAL USES OF ERC

An exciting and productive application of ERC has been the development of precise manometric measurements of the biliary tree. This procedure combines recent technological refinement in perfused catheter systems with retrograde cannulation to record pressure events as they occur in the biliary tree. Until the present time there has been little infor-

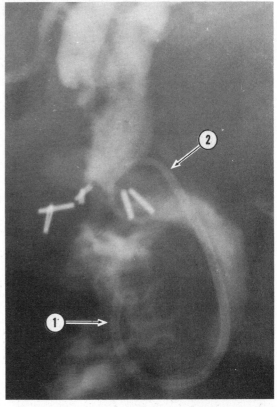

Figure 10–33. Internal stent. This stent has been placed to provide drainage in a patient with common duct stones. The stones are not well seen but recurred following cholecystectomy. The tip of the stent is in the duodenum *(1)*, whereas the proximal portion is in the common bile duct *(2)*. The stent can be removed by pulling it out with the biopsy forceps.

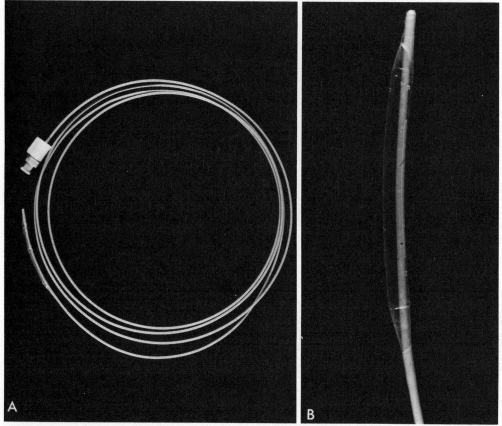

Figure 10–34. Transluminal dilatation balloon. *A,* This 200-cm balloon catheter can be placed across benign strictures for pneumatic dilatation. (Courtesy of Cook Inc.) *B,* Magnified view of the balloon, which is partially inflated.

mation available about the pressure dynamics occurring in the sphincter of Oddi in human subjects.[13, 54]

Over the last several years, we have had the opportunity to study several hundred patients. Pressure recordings were accomplished using two Teflon catheters, each with an internal diameter of 0.8 mm and an outer diameter of 1.6 mm (Fig. 10–35). The length of the catheters was 200 cm. Both catheters were constantly infused with bubble-free water at 0.25 ml/min. Initially, a lateral recording orifice of

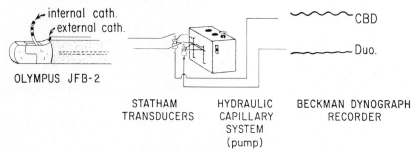

Figure 10–35. Pressure tracings are made in the bile ducts by cannulating with the internal catheter and measuring pressures. Simultaneous pressure events in the duodenal lumen are recorded from the external catheter. Both catheters are constantly perfused with water at 0.25 ml/min. (From Geenen, J. E., and LoGuidice, J. A.: Adv. Surg. *14*:31, 1980.)

SPHINCTER PULL-THROUGH

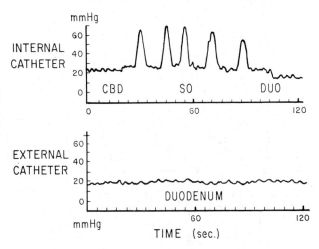

Figure 10–36. In this normal patient, the CBD pressure (internal catheter) is about 22 mm/Hg. As the sphincter is entered, the basal resting pressure of the sphincter is 4 to 5 mm Hg higher. Phasic high pressure contraction waves occur 4 to 6/min. As the catheter is pulled into the duodenum, duodenal pressure is recorded at about 15 mm Hg.

0.8 mm diameter was cut in each catheter. Subsequent refinement in catheters now allows us to incorporate three recording orifices separated by 2 mm. The recording orifices can be arranged in a radial fashion to measure the radial distribution of pressures in the sphincter. To obtain biliary pressure recordings, one catheter is placed in the biopsy channel of the endoscope. This cannula is placed selectively into the biliary tree, and pressures then can be recorded in the common bile duct and the sphincter of Oddi as the catheter is slowly withdrawn through the sphincter. Usually pressure events are measured following slow withdrawal by several millimeter increments (Fig. 10–36). Continuous pressure recordings in the duodenum are compared with the biliary pressure events. The duodenal pressures are recorded using the second catheter, which is taped to the endoscope. Pressure events can also be recorded, using the same technique, in the pancreatic duct.

We as well as others have had an opportunity to examine manometric events occurring in normal and abnormal patients.[26, 29, 76] In our series of 26 normal patients, the sphincter of Oddi segment was found to be between 4 and 6 mm in length. The sphincter had a basal steady-state pressure about 4 mm Hg higher than that of the common bile duct or pancreatic duct. Pronounced phasic contractions were superimposed on the basal sphincter of Oddi pressure (Fig. 10–37). These phasic contractions measured 101 $\pm$ 50 SE mm Hg in amplitude and 4.3 $\pm$ 1.5 sec in duration. They had a frequency of 4.1 $\pm$ .9/min.[27] The phasic contraction seen in the sphincter appears to be unique to this area. No phasic contractions occurred in the main pancreatic duct or common bile duct. These pressure events were independent of other muscle activity occurring in the duodenal wall such as normal peristaltic activity.

A natural extension of this type of investi-

SPHINCTER OF ODDI: PHASIC CONTRACTIONS

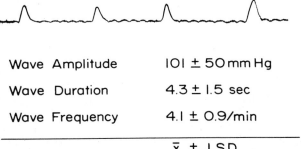

Figure 10–37. Collective data from 26 normal patients. (From Geenen, J. E., and Hogan, W. J.: Endoscopy Suppl.:47, 1980.)

Wave Amplitude	101 $\pm$ 50 mm Hg
Wave Duration	4.3 $\pm$ 1.5 sec
Wave Frequency	4.1 $\pm$ 0.9/min

$$\bar{x} \pm 1\,SD$$

gation is to examine the effect of enteric hormones on the sphincter. Intravenous pulse doses of cholecystokinin-octapeptide and glucagon depressed the sphincter of Oddi muscle activity, whereas pentagastrin increased sphincter of Oddi pressure (Fig. 10–38). Secretin causes a mixed response of excitation followed by inhibition. There are problems in dealing with doses of enteric hormones that may be pharmacologic rather than physiologic. In spite of this, there continues to be significant interest in biliary manometry and evaluation of the normal physiologic events occurring in the sphincter region.

What role, if any, the sphincter of Oddi contractions play in regulating biliary pancreatic duct emptying remains to be determined. It is logical to presume that the sphincter functions as an impedance mechanism. Contraction of the sphincter would cause delay in emptying of the common duct, whereas relaxation would allow the contents of the common duct to empty into the duodenum (Fig. 10–39).[51] Fluoroscopic observations of sphincter activity correspond to the phasic activity seen manometrically. As the four to six/min phasic contractions occur, they are quite easily seen fluoroscopically. Between the phasic contractions, the common duct is seen fluoroscopically to empty some of its contents into the duodenum.

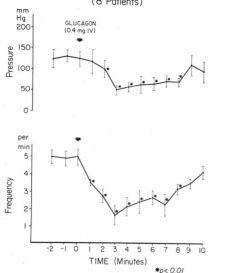

GLUCAGON EFFECT ON PHASIC SO CONTRACTIONS
(8 Patients)

Figure 10–38. Effect of glucagon on the amplitude and frequency of phasic pressure waves recorded from the sphincter of Oddi. An asterisk indicates a significant change from control values (p < 0.01). (From Geenen, J. E., et al.: Gastroenterology 78:317, 1980.)

As alluded to earlier in this chapter, the use of manometry to evaluate patients with sphincter of Oddi dysfunction probably represents one of the more important areas of clinical investigation. This poorly documented entity may be better understood when pressures are investigated. Our preliminary observations as well as those of others suggest that patients with sphincter of Oddi dysfunction have abnormally high resting pressures as well as higher than normal phasic pressures in the sphincter region.[28] The significance of such findings at this time is not entirely clear, and obviously the criteria for establishing the diagnosis of sphincter of Oddi dysfunction are undergoing clarification. It may well be, however, that manometric recordings in the sphincter will be one of the more important objective criteria for making the diagnosis of sphincter of Oddi dysfunction (Fig. 10–40).

There is a considerable difference between operative sphincteroplasty, at which time the incised sphincter is sewn open by the surgeon, and endoscopic sphincterotomy, during which only electrosurgical incision is performed.[35, 43, 80] One of the objections to electrosurgical incisions has been the theoretical problem of restenosis of incision. As noted earlier, restenosis seems to be an infrequent complication of endoscopic sphincterotomy.[63] The use of manometry to restudy the sphincter following endoscopic sphincterotomy suggests that significant restenosis is not very frequent. Long-term follow-up over a period of years, however, still needs to be documented. These studies are currently ongoing.

CONCLUSION

The last ten years have seen the development and rapid proliferation of expertise with fiberoptic endoscopic equipment. The additions of endoscopic retrograde cholangiography and pancreatography have greatly aided in the management of patients with diseases involving the biliary tree as well as pancreas. The innovative use of cannulation has greatly expanded our knowledge of the normal anatomy as well as pathology. There is now a large body of well-documented examples of pathology involving the hepatobiliary tree and pancreas. It is unusual for patients to go to surgery without having a definitive diagnosis. The use of endoscopic cytology and percutaneous aspiration cytology now allows reliable confirmation of malignancy prior to surgery. In many

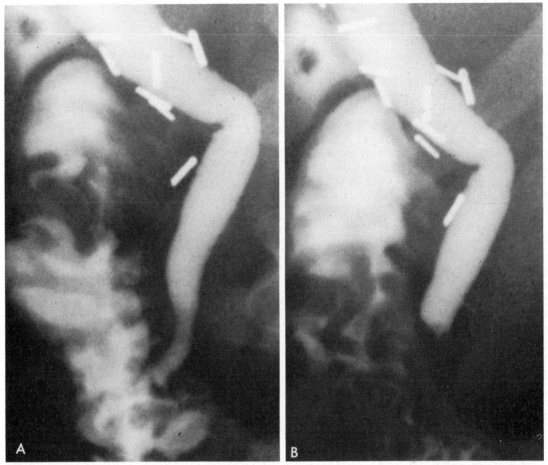

Figure 10–39. Phasic contraction of the sphincter. *A,* This magnified view nicely demonstrates the normal resting sphincter. *B,* A few moments later, the sphincter segment has contracted and obliterated the contrast filled lumen. Manometry shows identical pressure events with phasic contraction occurring four to six times per minute.

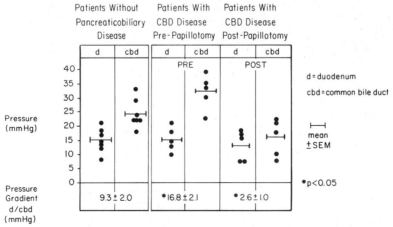

Figure 10–40. From Geenen, J. E., et al.: J.A.M.A. *19:*2075, 1977.

cases surgery is now avoided since the malignant nature of strictures can be confirmed without laparotomy. The availability of endoscopic sphincterotomy has opened a new and exciting alternative for the treatment of common duct stones and sphincter of Oddi dysfunction. The application of endoscopic techniques to manage benign and malignant strictures with stents as well as the dissolving of gallstones is an example of the imaginative uses of endoscopy. There is still much to be learned about the normal and abnormal physiology of the sphincter region, and the future should bring considerable expertise to bear on these areas.

Retrograde cannulation is only one of a number of very sensitive and specific tools now at the disposal of the clinician for diagnosing biliary tract disease. The wise application of such procedures requires that we be informed of the unique strengths and weaknesses of each procedure as well as of overlapping information that might be provided. The preceding has been an attempt to convey the current status of retrograde cannulation at this time, with primary emphasis on the biliary tree.

References

1. Agrawal, R. M., and Brodmerkel, G. J.: Endoscopic retrograde cholangiopancreatography diagnosis of choledochal cyst. Am. J. Gastroenterol. 70:393, 1978.
2. Agrawal, R. M., Mitre, R., Brodmerkel, G. J., and Brooks, D. H.: The diagnosis of post-cholecystectomy cystic duct fistula utilizing endoscopic retrograde cholangiopancreatography. Endoscopy 11:193, 1979.
3. Anacker, H., Weiss, H. D., and Kramann, B.: Endoscopic retrograde pancreaticocholangiography in chronic diseases of the pancreas and in papillary stenosis. Gastrointest. Radiol. 3:325, 1978.
4. Ashby, B. S., and Goodman, D. A.: Effects of x-radiation on fibreoptic endoscopes. Gut 21:717, 1980.
5. Ayoola, E. A., Vennes, J. A., Silvis, S. E., Rohrmann, C. A., and Ansel, H. J.: Endoscopic retrograde. intrahepatic cholangiography in liver disease. Gastrointest. Endosc. 22:156, 1976.
6. Barkin, J. S., and Grunwald, R.: Endoscopic therapy of the "sump" syndrome. Dig. Dis. Sci. 25:597, 1979.
7. Bar-Meir, S., Geenen, J. E., Hogan, W. J., Dodds, W. J., Stewart, E. T., and Arndorfer, R. C.: Biliary and pancreatic duct pressures measured by ERCP and manometry in patients with suspected papillary stenosis. Dig. Dis. Sci. 24:209, 1979.
8. Belholavek, D., Koch, H., Rosche, W., Schaffner, O., Maeder, H. U., Flory, J., Classen, M., and Demling, L.: Five years experience in endoscopic retrograde cholangiopancreatography (ERCP). Endoscopy 8:115, 1976.
9. Blesito, A. A., Marta, J. B., Cramer, G. G., and Dickinson, P. B.: Measurement of biliary tract size and drainage time. Comparison of endoscopic and intravenous cholangiography. Radiology 122:65, 1977.
10. Bilbao, M. K., Dotter, C. T., Lee, T. G., and Katon, R. M.: Complications of endoscopic retrograde cholangiography (ERCP): a study of 10,000 cases. Gastroenterology 70:314, 1976.
11. Blackstone, M. O., and Nemchausky, B. A.: Cholangiographic abnormalities in ulcerative colitis associated with pericholangitis which resemble sclerosing cholangitis. Dig. Dis. 23:579, 1979.
12. Blumgart, L. H., Carachi, R., Imrie, C. W., Benjamin, I. S., and Duncan, J. G.: Diagnosis and management of post-cholecystectomy symptoms: the place of endoscopy and retrograde choledochopancreatography. Br. J. Surg. 64:809, 1977.
13. Boyden, E. A.: The sphincter of Oddi in man and certain representative mammals. Surgery 1:25, 1937.
14. Classen, M., and Demling, L.: Endoskopische Sphincterotomie der Papilla Vateri und Steinextraktion aus dem Ductus choledochus. Dtsch. Med. Wochenschr. 99:496, 1974.
15. Classen, M., and Ossenberg, F. W.: Progress report—non-surgical removal of common bile duct stones. Gut 18:760, 1977.
16. Cohen, G., Brodmerkel, G. J., and Lynn, S.: Absorbed doses to patients and personnel from endoscopic retrograde cholangiopancreatographic (ERCP) examinations. Radiology 130:773, 1979.
17. Cotton, P. B.: Progress report. Cannulation of the papilla of Vater by endoscopy and retrograde cholangiopancreatography (ERCP). Gut 13:1014, 1972.
18. Cotton, P. B.: Progress report—ERCP. Gut 18:316, 1977.
19. Cotton, P. B.: Non-operative removal of bile duct stones by duodenoscopic sphincterotomy. Br. J. Surg. 67:1, 1980.
20. Cotton, P. B., Burney, P. G. J., and Mason, R. R.: Transnasal bile duct catheterisation after endoscopic sphincterotomy—method for biliary drainage, perfusion and sequential cholangiography. Gut 20:285, 1979.
21. Dye, M., MacDonald, A., and Smith, G.: The bacterial flora of the biliary tract and liver in man. Br. J. Surg. 65:285, 1978.
22. Falkenstein, D. B., Riccobono, C., Sidhu, G., Abrams, R. M., Seliger, G., and Zimmon, D. S.: The endoscopic intrahepatic cholangiogram—clinicopathologic correlation with postmortem cholangiograms. Invest. Radiol. 10:358, 1975.
23. Flemma, R. J., Flint, L. M., Osterhout, S., and Shingleton, W. W.: Bacteriologic studies of biliary tract infection. Ann. Surg. 166:563, 1967.
24. Freeny, P. C., Bilbao, M. K., and Katon, R. M.: "Blind" evaluation of endoscopic retrograde cholangiopancreatography (ERCP) in the diagnosis of pancreatic carcinoma: the double duct and other signs. Radiology 119:271, 1976.
25. Freeny, P. C., Kidd, R., and Ball, T. J.: ERCP-guided percutaneous fine-needle pancreatic biopsy. West. J. Med. 132:283, 1980.
26. Funch-Jensen, P., Csendes, A., Kruse, A., Oster, M. J., and Amdrup, E.: Common bile duct and Oddi sphincter pressure before and after endoscopic papillotomy in patients with common bile duct stones. Ann. Surg. 190:176, 1979.
27. Geenen, J. E., Hogan, W. J., Dodds, W. J., Stewart, E. T., and Arndorfer, R. C.: Intraluminal pressure recording from the human sphincter of Oddi. Gastroenterology 78:317, 1980.
28. Geenen, J. E., Hogan, W. J., Shaffer, R. D., Stewart, E. T., Dodds, W. J., and Arndorfer, R. C.: Endoscopic electrosurgical papillotomy and manometry in biliary tract diseases. J.A.M.A. 237:1075, 1977.

29. Geenen, J. E., Hogan, W. J., Stewart, E. T., Dodds, W. J., and Arndorfer, R. C.: ERCP manometry of the sphincter of Oddi. International workshop—the papilla of Vateri and its diseases. Verlag Gerhard Witzstrock. Cologne, Germany, 1979.

30. Geenen, J. E., and LoGuidice, J. A.: Endoscopic sphincterotomy for diseases of the biliary tree. Adv. Surg. 14:31, 1980.

31. Geenen, J. E., Vennes, J. A., and Silvis, S. E.: Resume of a seminar on endoscopic retrograde sphincterotomy (ERS). Gastrointest. Endosc. 27:31, 1981.

32. Ghazi, A.: Enterobiliary fistula and ERCP. Am. J. Gast. 68:81, 1977.

33. Glenn, F.: Retained calculi within the biliary ductal system. Ann. Surg. 179:528, 1974.

34. Glenn, F., and Hays, D. M.: The age factor in the mortality rate of patients undergoing surgery of the biliary tract. Surg. Gynecol. Obstet. 100:11, 1955.

35. Goinard, P., and Pelissier, G.: Total sphincteroplasty without drainage of the common bile duct in the treatment of biliary tract disease. Surg. Gynecol. Obstet. 111:339, 1960.

36. Greene, W. H., Moody, M., Hartley, R., Effman, E., Aisner, J., Young, V. M., and Wiernik, P. H.: Esophagoscopy as a source of Pseudomonas aeruginosa sepsis in patients with acute leukemia: the need for sterilization of endoscopes. Gastroenterology 67:912, 1974.

37. Gregg, J., Clark, G., Barr, C., McCartney, A., Milano, A., and Volcjak, C.: Postcholecystectomy syndrome and its association with ampullary stenosis. Am. J. Surg. 139:374, 1980.

38. Hadad, A. R., Westbrook, K. C., Campbell, G. S., Caldwell, F. T., and Morris, W. D.: Congenital dilatation of the bile ducts. Am. J. Surg. 132:799, 1976.

39. Hall, R. C., Sakiyalak, P., Kim, S. K., Rogers, L. S., and Webb, W. R.: Failure of operative cholangiography to prevent retained common duct stones. Am. J. Surg. 125:51, 1973.

40. Ihre, T., and Heller, G.: Complications and endoscopic retrograde cholangiopancreatography. Acta Chir. Scand. 143:167, 1977.

41. Ihre, T. H., Pyk, E., Raaschou-Nielsen, T., and Seligson, U.: Percutaneous fine-needle aspiration biopsy during endoscopic retrograde cholangio-pancreatography. Scand. J. Gastroenterol. 13:657, 1978.

42. Jarrett, L. N., Balfour, T.W., Bell, G. O., Knapp, D. R., and Rose, D. H.: Intraductal infusion of monooctanoin: experience in 24 patients with retained common duct stones. Lancet 1:68, 1981.

43. Jones, S. A., and Smith, L. L.: A reappraisal of sphincteroplasty (not sphincterotomy). Surgery 71:565, 1972.

44. Kasugai, T., Kuno, N., Aoki, I., Kizu, M., and Kobayashi, S.: Fiberduodenoscopy: analysis of 353 examinations. Gastrointest. Endosc. 18:9, 1971.

45. Katon, R. M., Lee, T. G., Parent, J. A., Bilbao, M. K., and Smith, F. W.: Endoscopic retrograde cholangiopancreatography (ERCP). Experience with 100 cases. Am. J. Dig. Dis. 19:295, 1974.

46. Kaufman, B., Gambescia, R., Maldonado, A., and Raskin, J. B.: Systemic absorption of contrast agent during endoscopic retrograde cholangiopancreatography. Gastrointest. Endosc. 22:175, 1976.

47. Kawai, K., Akaska, Y., Murakami, K., Tada, M., Kohli, Z., and Nakajima, M.: Endoscopic sphincterotomy of the ampulla of Vater. Gastrointest. Endosc. 20:148, 1974.

48. Koch, H., Belholavek, D., Schaffner, O., Tympner, F., Rosch, W., and Demling, L.: Prospective study for the prevention of pancreatitis following endoscopic retrograde cholangiopancreatography (ERCP). Endoscopy 7:221, 1975.

49. Koch, H., Rosch, W., Schaffner, O., and Demling, L.: Endoscopic papillotomy. Gastroenterology 73:1393, 1977.

50. Lasser, R. B., Silvis, S. E., and Vennes, J. A.: The normal cholangiogram. Dig. Dis. 23:586, 1978.

51. LoGiudice, J. A., Hogan, W. J., Geenen, J. E., Dodds, W. J., Arndorfer, R. C., and Stewart, E. T.: Variations in propagation of phasic waves in the human sphincter of Oddi. Gastroenterology 76:1187, 1979 (abstract).

52. Low, D. E., Micflikier, A. B., Kennedy, J. K., and Stiver, H. G.: Infectious complications of endoscopic retrograde cholangiopancreatography. A prospective assessment. Arch. Intern. Med. 140:1076, 1980.

53. McDonald, G. B., and Silverstein, F. E.: Can gastrointestinal endoscopy transmit hepatitis B to patients? Gastrointest. Endosc. 22:168, 1976.

54. Mann, F. C.: A comparative study of the anatomy of the sphincter at the duodenal end of the common bile-duct with special reference to species of animals without a gallbladder. Anat. Rec. 18:355, 1920.

55. Martin, T. R., Geenen, J. E., Raskin, J. B., Vennes, J. A., and Silvis, S. E.: The reduction of septic complications following endoscopic retrograde cholangiopancreatography (ERCP) in obstructed patients. Gastrointest. Endosc. 25:43, 1979 (abstract).

56. Martin, T. R., Silvis, S. E., and Vennes, J. A.: The reduction of septic complications following ERCP in obstructed patients. Clin. Res. 24:566A, 1976.

57. Mitre, R. J., and Brodmerkel, G. J.: Traumatic rupture of the gallbladder: preoperative diagnosis by endoscopic retrograde cholangiopancreatography (ERCP). Gastrointest. Endosc. 25:74, 1979.

58. Nebel, O. T., Silvis, S. E., Rogers, G., Sugawa, C., and Mangelstam, P.: Complications associated with endoscopic retrograde cholangiopancreatography: results of the 1974 A/S/G/E survey. Gastrointest. Endosc. 22:34, 1975.

59. Oi, I.: Fiberduodenoscopy and endoscopic pancreatocholangiography. Gastrointest. Endosc. 17:59, 1970.

60. Osnes, M., Serck-Hanssen, A., and Myren, J.: Endoscopic retrograde brush cytology (ERBC) of the biliary and pancreatic ducts. Scand. J. Gastroenterol. 10:829, 1975.

61. Parker, H. W., Geenen, J. E., Bjork, J. T., and Stewart, E. T.: A prospective analysis of fever and bacteremia following ERCP. Gastrointest. Endosc. 25:102, 1979.

62. Peters, P. E., Kautz, G., Safrany, L., and Weitemeyer, R.: Radiation exposure in patients undergoing retrograde cholangiopancreatography and endoscopic papillotomy. Gastrointest. Radiol. 3:353, 1978.

63. Reidel, D., Geenen, J. E., Hogan, W. J., Dodds, W. J., Stewart, E. T., and Arndorfer, R. C.: Endoscopic sphincterotomy: follow-up evaluation of effects on sphincter of Oddi. Gastrointest. Endosc. 25:47, 1979.

64. Reiter, J. J., Bayer, H. P., Mennecken, C., and Manegold, B. C.: Results of endoscopic papillotomy: a collective experience from nine endoscopic centers in West Germany. World J. Surg. 2:505, 1978.

65. Riddel, D. H., and Kirtley, J. A.: Stenosis of the sphincter of Oddi. Transduodenal sphincterotomy and some other surgical aspects. Ann. Surg. 149:773, 1959.

66. Roberts-Thomson, I. C., and Hobbs, J. B.: Cytodiagnosis of pancreatic biliary cancer by endoscopic duct aspiration. Med. J. Aust. 1:370, 1979.

67. Rohrman, C. A., Ansel, H. J., Ayoola, E. A., Silvis, S. E., and Vennes, J. A.: Endoscopic retrograde intrahepatic cholangiogram: radiographic findings in

intrahepatic disease. Am. J. Roentgenol. *128*:45, 1977.

68. Rosseland, A. R., and Osnes, M.: Endoscopic papillotomy: technique and experience with 204 patients. Curr. Surg. *37*:152, 1980.

69. Ruddell, W. S., et al.: Endoscopic retrograde cholangiography and pancreatography in investigation of post-cholecystectomy patients. Lancet *I*:444, 1980.

70. Ruskin P. B., Katon, R. M., Bilbao, M. K., and Smith, F.: Evaluation of sclerosing cholangitis by endoscopic retrograde cholangiopancreatography. Arch. Intern. Med. *136*:232, 1976.

71. Safrany, L.: Duodenoscopic sphincterotomy and gallstone removal. Gastroenterology *72*:338, 1977.

72. Safrany, L.: Endoscopic treatment of biliary-tract diseases. An international study. Lancet *2*:983, 1978.

73. Safrany, L., and Neuhaus, B.: Intraduodenal manipulations of the common bile duct. Surg. Annu. 301, 1980.

74. Safrany, L., Tari, J., Barna, L., and Torok, I.: Endoscopic retrograde cholangiography. Experience of 168 examinations. Gastrointest. Endosc. *19*:163, 1973.

75. Safrany, L., VanHusen, N., Kautz, G., Wittrin, G., Clemens, M., and Weitemeyer, R.: Endoscopic retrograde cholangiography (ERC) in surgical emergencies. Ann. Surg. *187*:20, 1978.

76. Salik, J. O., Siegel, C. I., and Mendeloff, A. I.: Biliary-duodenal dynamics in man. Radiology *106*:1, 1973.

77. Schenk, J., Schmack, B., Riemann, J. F., and Rosch, W.: Treatment of choledocholithiasis using the transpapillary perfusion technique. Endoscopy *12*:224, 1980.

78. Scholz, F. J., Carrera, G. F., and Larsen, C. R.: The choledochocele: correlation of radiological, clinical and pathological findings. Radiology *118*:25, 1976.

79. Shahmir, M., and Schuman, B. M.: Complications of fiberoptic endoscopy. Gastrointest. Endosc. *26*:86, 1980.

80. Siegel, J. H.: Endoscopic papillotomy: sphincterotomy or sphincteroplasty. Am. J. Gastroenterol. *72*:511, 1979.

81. Silverstein, F. E., Rohrmann, C. A., and Templeton, F. E.: Extrahepatic conditions of the biliary tree. *In* Stewart, E. T., Vennes, J. A., and Geenen, J. E. (eds.): Atlas of Endoscopic Retrograde Cholangiopancreatography. St. Louis: C. V. Mosby Co., 1977, Chapter 11.

82. Silvis, S. E., Rohrmann, C. A., and Vennes, J. A.: Diagnostic accuracy of endoscopic retrograde cholangiopancreatography in hepatic, biliary and pancreatic malignancy. Ann. Intern. Med. *84*:438, 1976.

83. Silvis, S. E., Vennes, J. A., and Rohrmann, C. A.: Endoscopic pancreatography in the evaluation of pa-

tients with suspected pancreatic pseudocysts. Am. J. Gastroenterol. *61*:452, 1974.

84. Sloff, M., Baker, R., Lavelle, M. I., Lendrum, K., and Venables, C. W.: What is involved in endoscopic sphincterotomy for gallstones? Br. J. Surg. *67*:18, 1980.

85. Stewart, E. T., Vennes, J. A., and Geenen, J. E. (eds.): Atlas of Endoscopic Retrograde Cholangiopancreatography. St. Louis; C. V. Mosby Co., 1977.

86. Stout, D. J., Swak, M. V., and Sullivan, B. H.: Endoscopic sphincterotomy and removal of gallstones. Surg. Gynecol. Obstet. *150*:673, 1980.

87. Summerfield, J. A., Elias, E., Hungerford, M. D., Nkoapota, V. L. B., Dick, R., and Sherlock, S.: The biliary system in primary biliary cirrhosis—a study by endoscopic retrograde cholangiopancreatography. Gastroenterology *70*:240, 1976.

88. Thistle, J. L., Carlson, G. L., LaRusso, N. F., and Hofman, A. F.: Effective dissolution of biliary duct stones by intraductal infusion of mono-octanoin. Gastroenterology *74*:1103, 1978.

89. Urakmi, Y., Kishi, S., and Seifert, E.: Endoscopic papillotomy (EPT) in patients with juxtapapillary diverticula. Gastrointest. Endosc. *25*:10, 1979.

90. Venu, R. P., Geenen, J. E., Toouli, J., Hogan, W. J., Kozlov, N., and Stewart, E. T.: Gallstone dissolution using mono-octanoin infusion through an endoscopically placed nasobiliary catheter. Am. J. Gastroenterol. *77*:227, 1982.

91. Way, L. W., Admirand, W. H., and Dunphy, J. E.: Management of choledocholithiasis. Ann. Surg. *176*:347, 1972.

92. Witzel, L., Widerholt, J., and Wolbergs, E.: Dissolution of retained duct stones by perfusion with mono-octanoin via a Teflon catheter introduced endoscopically. Gastrointest. Endosc. *27*:63, 1981.

93. Wurbs, D., Phillip, J., and Classen, M.: Experiences with the long-standing nasobiliary tube in biliary diseases. Endoscopy *12*:219, 1980.

94. Zimmon, D. S., Chang, J., and Clemett, A. R.: Advances in the management of bile duct obstruction—percutaneous transhepatic cholangiography and endoscopic retrograde cholangiopancreatography. Med. Clin. North Am. *63*:593, 1979.

95. Zimmon, D. S., Falkenstein, D. B., Manno, B. V., and Clemett, A. R.: Choledochocele: radiologic diagnosis and endoscopic management. Gastrointest. Radiol. *3*:349, 1978.

96. Zimmon, D. S., Falkenstein, D. B., Riccobono, C., and Aaron, B.: Complications of endoscopic retrograde cholangiopancreatography. Gastroenterology *69*:303, 1975.

97. Zimmon, D. S., Ferrara, T. P., and Clemett, A. R.: Radiology of papilla of Vater stenosis. Gastrointest. Radiol. *3*:343, 1978.

OPERATIVE AND POSTOPERATIVE CHOLANGIOGRAPHY

by George Berci, M.D.,
and J. Andrew Hamlin, M.D.

11

The number of biliary tract operations performed annually in the United States is estimated to range from 500,000 to 750,000.[1] These figures are increasing along with the growth in the general population and the advances in diagnostic modalities for establishing the presence of biliary tract disease. Morbidity and mortality are low (mortality less than 1 per cent) in the uncomplicated case but increase significantly when complications, such as retained stones or iatrogenic injuries, occur.

UNSUSPECTED STONES

Stones are occasionally found within the bile ducts of patients whose clinical and laboratory presentation did not suggest their presence. The reported incidence of these unsuspected stones is 4 to 10 per cent.[2] In our own experience with 500 cholelithiasis patients, 25 (5 per cent) were found by operative cholangiography to harbor unsuspected stones.[3]

COMMON BILE DUCT EXPLORATION

In 10 to 20 per cent of all biliary operations the common bile duct is explored. Indications for common duct exploration include a history of jaundice or pancreatitis, demonstration of choledocholithiasis on intravenous cholangiography, demonstration of multiple small stones within the gallbladder, and surgical discovery of a dilated common bile duct or palpable

stones. Unfortunately, the incidence of negative exploration is high when these clinical criteria are the sole indications for opening the duct.

RETAINED STONES

In 1957, Smith and colleagues reported that, at the time of postoperative T-tube cholangiographic examination, retained stones were discovered in up to 28 per cent of those patients who had undergone common bile duct exploration.[4] A quarter of a century later, the figures were similar.[5] These patients must then face a second procedure for the removal of the residual stones. The additional procedure could be stone extraction through the T-tube tract,[6] infusion of chemicals through the T-tube for stone dissolution, endoscopic sphincterotomy, or a second operation. All of these procedures prolong the recuperative period. Spontaneous passage of these residual stones is unpredictable and cannot be relied upon. In our experience with 55 cases of well-documented retained stones, spontaneous passage was observed in four patients (7 per cent).

BILE DUCT INJURIES

Iatrogenic injuries occur in approximately 0.25 per cent (1/400) of those patients undergoing biliary operations. Although the incidence is low, the consequences of such an injury are tragic. These patients become biliary cripples and often undergo multiple subsequent operations in an attempt to correct the original injury. Recurrence of strictures or narrowing of anastomoses can present after a symptom-free interval of five to ten years.[7, 8]

We are indebted to Mrs. Paz-Partlow for her photographic assistance, to Maureen DeBose for her helpful illustrations, and to Meredith Miller for preparing the manuscript.

Note: Illustrations appear at the end of the chapter.

INCIDENCE OF BILIARY SURGERY

An overview of biliary surgery using mid range figures can be expressed as follows. There will be 625,000 cholecystectomies performed in the United States this year. Of this number, 93,750 patients (15 per cent) will undergo common bile duct exploration. Of this group, approximately 9000 to 10,000 will have a negative exploration. At the time of postoperative T-tube examination, approximately 14,000 patients (15 per cent of 93,750) will be found to have residual stones. Since 31,250 patients (5 per cent of 625,000) with no suggestive clinical history will harbor unsuspected stones within the common duct (which would be undetected without routine operative cholangiography), there will be a potential population in excess of 20,000 to 40,000 patients who will leave the operating table this year with stones remaining in the common duct. It is estimated that 1,500 patients (0.25 per cent of 625,000) will have sustained an injury to their bile ducts that is highly likely to result in biliary strictures requiring further surgical intervention.

The utilization of routine operative cholangiography, carefully performed by interested surgeons and radiologists with the best equipment available, would contribute significantly to improving these statistics.

OPERATIVE CHOLANGIOGRAPHY

Intraoperative cholangiography was introduced by a surgeon, Paolo Mirizzi, a half century ago.[9] His aim was not only to discover overlooked stones before the abdominal wall was closed but to eliminate injuries to the ductal system. The complications following biliary surgery had been extensively studied by biliary fistulography, and Mirizzi noted that "the bile in the peritoneum observed by surgeons, who believe its presence is due to slipping of the ligature, in most cases is a testimony that there is an anatomofunctional lesion of the hepatic and common bile ducts that has not been noted because of the inaccuracy, deceptiveness, and lack of precision in the methods of exploration used." Although intraoperative cholangiography has been available for decades, there has been little effort to refine the techniques and streamline the procedure to encourage its greater use. Surgeons continue to condemn peroperative cholangiography; they claim that it is time consuming, has an unacceptable technical failure rate, has

frequent false-positive or false-negative results, and is too expensive.

Operative cholangiography has been an "unwanted child" trying to find a home with two families, surgeons and radiologists. When it falls short of expectations, surgeons point to the radiologic side of the family, blaming equipment failure, poor exposure techniques, developing time delay, interpretive errors, and so on, while feeling generally frustrated at their lack of understanding and control of radiologic factors. Radiologists, on the other hand, feel that the examination is poor because they lack direct control, blaming the surgeons for not understanding the basic technique of detailed cholangiography, for instance, the importance of patient positioning, and the careful injection of contrast material as well as the removal of clamps, retractors, opaque sponges, and air bubbles from the field of view. If progress is to be made, a genuine cooperative effort must be made by surgeons and radiologists to the ultimate benefit of the patient.

In many hospitals, physical separation of the operating room and x-ray department means that either the technician or the radiologist must travel between the two departments to properly evaluate films and communicate with personnel. If direct discussion with the surgeon regarding the findings is necessary, the radiologist must change into a scrub suit before entering OR, which further prolongs surgery. Installation of an inexpensive audio-intercommunication system between the x-ray department and the OR would help alleviate this delay. Surgeons are not trained in radiologic interpretation, and, although many have developed a skill for reading their own cholangiograms, the difficult or troublesome case requires the trained eye of the radiologist to assist in intraoperative decision making. For this reason, operative cholangiography should be regarded as an *emergency procedure, necessitating the presence or availability of the radiologist.*

The degree of sophistication of x-ray equipment to be used in operative cholangiography is related to the size of the hospital and the volume and type of surgery requiring radiographic assistance. Too often, outdated portable x-ray machines are relegated to surgery and a double standard of film quality is established between surgery and the x-ray department. Although equipment purchase and maintenance is expensive, in institutions where large numbers of biliary (150 to 200) and orthopedic (500 to 1000) operations and pacemaker and catheter insertions are performed each year, the radiologist should insist on obtaining the best x-ray units available to optimize patient care. The outlay for proper equipment must be weighed against the cost to the individual patient and society (i.e., the bill-paying public) when a retained stone or iatrogenic injury results in a prolonged recovery and additional procedures, e.g., percutaneous stone retrieval, endoscopic sphincterotomy, or further surgery.

INITIAL AND/OR COMPLETION CHOLANGIOGRAM

Optimally, both initial and completion cholangiography should be performed in cases of choledocholithiasis; if circumstances permit only one procedure, the initial cystic duct cholangiogram, or in the case of a secondary exploration, the primary choledochocholangiogram is preferred. The reasons for this are many. Much more information is available to the surgeon prior to a potentially difficult dissection if the cholangiogram is performed initially because the anatomy will be displayed, attention will be drawn to important anomalies, and the number and location of stones will be indicated. With a well-performed negative cholangiogram, an unnecessary exploration of the common bile duct with its higher morbidity can be avoided.

The completion cholangiogram is often more difficult to interpret than the initial cholangiogram. Following duct exploration, air bubbles may be incompletely evacuated. After prolonged manipulation or stone extraction attempts, desquamative or cholangitic debris and blood clots may produce radiolucencies obscuring or simulating a calculus, thereby reducing the confidence level in film interpretation. In these instances, operative biliary endoscopy can solve the dilemma. The initial or preliminary cholangiogram is therefore more reliably interpreted because it involves a closed system prior to the introduction of potential artifacts.

Operative cholangiography may be performed by various techniques. In this discussion, we will include the standard technique and fluorocholangiography.

Standard Technique[10, 11]

The orthodox two- and three-film operative cholangiography is usually performed with a portable x-ray machine. In many instances, it is a unit that has been "retired" from service on the floor and given to surgery. Consequently, the performance of the machine may be suboptimal.

The production of an adequate abdominal film with portable equipment is difficult at best, and patients with cholelithiasis are often overweight, adding to the difficulty. Therefore, an x-ray machine with greater capacity is recommended to achieve a satisfactory image with the shortest exposure time possible. An exposure of 300 mA is sufficient for most nonobese patients. Hospitals with four or five active operating rooms for general and orthopedic surgery would do well to obtain such a machine, which would remain in the area and be earmarked for operating room use only. The time delay that frequently occurs when calling for a portable machine to be brought in from another area of the hospital prolongs the anesthesia time unnecessarily.

Various film cassette–holding devices have been designed for use with the standard operating room table. If a film tunnel is made to rest on top of the operating table, care must be taken to adequately pad the holder as well as build up the table at either end of the holder. Operating room tables are now available with radiolucent tops and built-in cassette holders. In either case, access to the film cassette is difficult when sterile drapes hang over the side of the table.

The use of a grid will greatly improve film quality during standard operative cholangiography, but its use requires precise alignment of the tubes and grid by the technician to avoid interfering grid lines. If a standard line grid is used, it should be oriented perpendicular to the table to avoid grid lines if the table (and cassette holder) is tilted to the right during filming. Attention to detail permits the use of a criss-cross grid, which further enhances film quality. These grids must be perpendicular to the beam, however, so the patient but not the table must be tilted with the grid-containing cassette. The use of a grid, of course, increases the required radiation dose.

Patient Positioning

With the patient supine, the common bile duct is often projected over the spine, and the superimposed structures can increase the difficulty in assessing the CBD. To avoid this problem, the patient should be tilted 15 to 20 degrees to the right, thereby casting the CBD to the right of the vertebral column. Various methods have been developed for obtaining this obliquity. Wedges of radiolucent material, sponge, or rolled linen may be placed under the left side of the patient prior to surgery but have the disadvantage of making the surgeon operate at an angle. Some tables are capable of lateral tilting. A tabletop that is hinged along the right side may be elevated during the cholangiographic studies and then lowered to complete the operation. A balloon-like pad placed under the patient's left flank will roll the patient to the right when inflated.

Because of uncertainty in positioning, the film format used for standard cholangiography tends to be larger than that necessary to record the biliary tree. The competent technician may attempt to use a 10 × 12 in. film, but more often an 11 × 14 or 14 × 17 in. film is used in the hope that the bile duct will appear somewhere on the film. The x-ray collimator is, of course, fully opened to expose the entire film, losing the advantage of tighter coning.

Scout Films

Taking a preliminary scout film prior to surgery aids the technician in achieving an appropriate technique. Although this may be regarded as a waste of time by the surgeon or anesthesiologist, the assurance of equipment function as well as the ability of obtaining a properly exposed film will ease anxiety at the time of cholangiography.

Injected Volume

It is virtually impossible to predict the volume of the biliary system. Small ducts may be filled with 5 to 10 ml of contrast material, whereas dilated ducts may require 20 to 50 ml. Schedules for injection volumes have been suggested based on an estimate of the CBD diameter (Table 11–1). These are only esti-

mates, however, because sphincter tone can also influence the degree of duct filling. A relaxed sphincter, for instance, results in good opacification of the duodenum with little visualization of the proximal ducts. When the opposite occurs, the degree of opacity within the ducts may obscure small stones.

Contrast Material

For contrast material, we prefer to use a 25 per cent Hypaque solution, which is diluted slightly further as it enters the bile duct. This concentration penetrates sufficiently to visualize small calculi within the ducts. A range of 70 to 80 kV is used, although some have suggested a higher kilovoltage to achieve greater penetration of the contrast column. This may be useful when larger volumes of contrast material are used.

Great care must be exercised in the cannulation and injection techniques so as not to introduce air, which could be mistaken for calculi. Also critical is having the anesthesiologist produce complete apnea during the exposure. Films we have reviewed reveal that too little attention has been given to this latter aspect. Exposure time required by the portable machines is often long enough to result in unsharpness due to either respiratory motion or duodenal peristalsis.

Fluorocholangiography

Because of the difficulty in producing consistently reliable cholangiographic radiographs of diagnostic quality and because of the number of cholecystectomies performed yearly at the Cedars-Sinai Medical Center (150 to 200 cases/year) requiring this examination, we have developed a fluorocholangiographic technique for operative cholangiography that we believe is superior to the standard method. Since critical decisions are based on the cholangiographic findings, we felt that the examination ought to be of the same high quality as the postoperative T-tube examination performed in the x-ray department. This required the installation of special equipment designed to provide both radiographic and fluoroscopic images.[12-15]

A three-phase generator with a 800 to 1000 mA capacity, a transformer, and a control panel is placed in a clean corridor between two operating rooms. The x-ray tube crane is

Table 11–1. SCHEDULE FOR INJECTION VOLUMES

Duct Size	First Film (ml)	Second Film (ml)	Third Film (ml)
Under 10 mm	3	3	5
Over 10 mm	3	5	8

permanently mounted in the operating room and can be swung to the side and out of the way when not in use.* The x-ray tube and image amplifier (IA) may be joined by a C-arm, or the IA can be wheeled into position under the OR table and fixed in place by floor mounts while the overhead tube is brought to a predetermined position directly above the IA.

Indirect radiography using a 100 × 100 mm film camera provides a permanent record. Fluoroscopy is observed on a mobile floor- or ceiling-mounted television monitor within the operating room as well as on a remote monitor in the x-ray department. A double foot switch allows the surgeon to control both the fluoroscopy and exposure timing.

Two additional pieces of equipment should be mentioned. A surgical table with a radiolucent top that can be moved coordinately is required for such an installation. Commercially produced models are available (Kifa,† Maquet,‡ and Amsco§). In addition, a film processor located within the surgical suite further facilitates the rapid completion of the examination. If films must be taken to the x-ray department for developing and the technician must change again to re-enter the operating room, valuable time is lost.

The advantages of fluorocholangiography over the standard technique include the following:

1. Ease in positioning the patient. The ability to observe the fluoroscopic image permits minor adjustments in the position of the patient using the floating (coordinate) tabletop. These adjustments can even be made during the examination if necessary.

2. Optimal beam collimation. When the technician is certain of the patient's position and assured that the CBD is central to the beam, the shutter can be approximated to improve image quality.

3. Shorter exposure time. The greater capacity of the equipment results in short exposure time (1/20 to 1/30 sec) so that unsharpness due to motion is avoided. (Even in the very obese, it is unnecessary for the anesthesiologist to suspend respiration during the exposure.)

4. Automatic exposure control. Phototiming of the exposures provides uniformity of film quality.

5. Minimal technician activity. Technician movement within the operating room is minimized, since there is no exchange of cassettes between exposures. The film receiver is removed from the head of the table when the examination is completed.

6. Control of exposure sequence. The timing of the exposure is determined by observing the degree of ductal opacification fluoroscopically. The need for repeating the examination because of overfilling or underfilling the duct is avoided.

7. Serial films. The examination is not limited to three exposures, and, in fact, a serial film technique is recommended utilizing 6 to 12 exposures. The acquisition of multiple films taken during the course of the injection is helpful in clarifying the nature of puzzling artifacts or abnormalities encountered on the cholangiograms. *Our average was 10.4 films per patient.*

8. Decreased examination time. Having dispensed with the exchange of film cassettes for each exposure, the total examination time is reduced. The entire cholangiographic process, including slow injection, fluoroscopy, and 6 to 12 exposures, *can be completed within five minutes.* The need for repeat injections and filming because of technical problems is almost completely eliminated.

Objections have been raised to interpreting the images on the small 100 × 100 mm film based on the belief that insufficient detail is obtained. This has not been so in practice, and the small intrahepatic branches are easily seen. We have identified and documented calculi as small as 2 to 3 mm within a normal sized common bile duct.

Image enlargement on the film can be obtained if the IA tube is incorporated with a double input phosphor screen linked to the x-ray camera system. The enlarged image will result in a slight degradation in resolution, but the effect is rarely critical.

The key to successful functioning of this system is close collaboration between radiologist and surgeon. The technician prepares the equipment and takes scout films while the anesthesiologist prepares the patient. He then alerts the radiologist that surgery is starting. When the surgeon asks for the cystic duct cannula, the technician should notify the radiologist through the intercom and be in the room ready for cholangiography. The radiologist observes the fluoroscopy on the remote monitor and gives necessary instructions over the intercom to be sure the cholangiogram is

---

*Manufactured by Siemens X-ray Co., Erlangen, West Germany.

†Kifa, OR table, represented by Siemens Co.

‡Maquet, OR table, represented by Siemens Co.

§Amsco, Special table, American Sterilizing Co.

properly performed. After the films are processed, the radiologist views the developed films and writes his findings on the progress notes in the chart, thus avoiding later confusion over what was said. The surgeon should remove the gallbladder, leaving the cystic duct cannula in place until he receives the radiologist's report. If, for some reason, the examination is not satisfactory or there is uncertainty, additional exposures should be taken. The radiologist should not hesitate to ask for a repeat series.

RADIATION HAZARD

Appropriate precautions should be taken to minimize radiation exposure of all personnel as well as to the patient. During the procedure, the surgeon should wear a gas-sterilized lead apron. If sterilization is not possible, he can double glove and double gown, but an apron must be worn. Extension tubing will allow the surgeon to step back 3 or 4 ft during the injection, thereby further reducing his exposure. The anesthesiologist must also wear a lead apron and should not leave the patient. The scrub nurse and surgical assistants should stand behind a protective screen in one corner of the room. Nonsterile personnel should step out of the room. Film badges are worn by all personnel in the OR to monitor exposure. Fluoroscopic time is reported for each case, and the surgeon is cautioned to keep the time to a minimum (intermittent short exposures) by maintaining a "light" foot. These protective measures require little effort and are very worthwhile. With the increasing number of diagnostic procedures requiring radiographic assistance, the exposure to personnel working within the hospital is ever increasing.[6]

THE CYSTIC DUCT

Our study of the cystic duct has revealed a significant deviation from standard knowledge in regard to its course and relationship to the common duct. In our cases, we found that the cystic duct entered the right or lateral side of the common duct *in only 17 per cent of patients*. In 41 per cent, the duct entered the anterior or posterior aspect of the common duct. Of particular interest was the 35 per cent of patients in whom the cystic duct passed around the choledochus, usually posteriorly, to enter on the medial aspect of the common bile duct. These are referred to as spiral cystic ducts. A long parallel drainage was seen in only 7 per cent of patients. It is clear that *in a high percentage of cases* (83 per cent in our studies) that portion of the cystic duct stump lateral to the common bile duct is only a fraction of its total length. The incidence of a long cystic *duct remnant is higher than previously thought.*[14] During common duct exploration or stone manipulation in the postoperative period, calculi have been found to disappear into a dilated spiral cystic duct.

ANOMALIES

The anomalies of greatest surgical interest are those of the cystic duct and its relation to the common duct as well as aberrant hepatic ducts. Surgeons should become aware of their presence as soon as possible during surgery. This information may prevent an iatrogenic injury. Aberrant ducts often course through the triangle of Calot and are particularly vulnerable to the unwary surgeon. The cystic duct may either enter the hepatic ducts or be joined by an aberrant duct before entering the common duct.[18] In either case, ductal division or ligation may result in irreversible complications. In these situations, the potential for injury is compounded if the dissection is difficult because of acute inflammation, bleeding, or obesity. In our series, anomalies of interest to the surgeon occurred in 8 per cent of cases and were discovered in time by routine cystic duct cholangiography.

CONCLUSIONS

Questions regarding the usefulness of operative cholangiography contribute to the dilemma of whether or not to perform it routinely. Some surgeons question its cost effectiveness by stating that the diagnostic accuracy is low. Others report an accuracy factor of over 95 per cent. What is usually overlooked is *the total cost for the care of the patient who has a retained stone. To the cost of the initial surgery must be added the expense of corrective measures.*

Percutaneous stone extraction through the T-tube tract extends the recovery time from six to eight weeks. Although performed as an outpatient procedure, multiple sessions may be necessary and the overall success rate is only 90 per cent.

If the retained stone is discovered at a later

stage, endoscopic sphincterotomy may be performed. This method requires a few days of hospitalization and is attended by a success rate of 80 per cent and a mortality of 1 per cent.

With cholecystectomy one of the most common operations performed, the complication rate is higher than it should be for what is basically a curable, benign disease. Our goal is that the optimal curative procedure be performed *at the first surgical intervention*. High quality routine operative cholangiography in biliary surgery contributes significantly to reducing the present incidence of complications, i.e., retained stones and iatrogenic injuries with secondary strictures.

Surgeons and radiologists alike must shoulder the responsibility of providing the optimal examination for the patient. If a better way is available, *the status quo should not be accepted.* In an age of technological revolution, the continued performance of an examination in essentially the same manner as that originally described seems out of step. Fluoroscopy utilizing a portable C-arm and image storage devices has been used in the operating room for many years. It has been applied to orthopedic cases as well as pacemaker and catheter insertions and has been used as a guide in performing lung biopsies through the flexible bronchoscope. The same concept, operative fluoroscopy, can also be helpful in biliary cases to monitor and, combined with indirect cholangiography, to observe anatomic detail and sphincter function. The technique demands more than portable equipment, however.

A cooperative venture by surgeons and radiologists should begin with a review of every operative and postoperative cholangiogram performed within a hospital over a period of several years. With continued communication and exchange of ideas, a realistic picture will develop with respect to the status of operative biliary radiology and a plan drawn for implementing improvements.

These comments are based on more than 20 years of research and clinical activities in the field of surgical radiology.[3] In a period of five years we have studied more than 1,200 biliary surgical cases in which modern operative cholangiography was performed as a routine. It was difficult in the beginning to train surgeons, radiologists, nurses, and technicians to use more complex equipment; however, today the system is not only strongly supported, but the surgeons are demanding its availability in other institutions. The gratifying result is the ultimate benefit to the patient.

POSTOPERATIVE T-TUBE CHOLANGIOGRAPHY

Postoperative examination of the biliary tree through the indwelling T-tube usually follows surgery by 7 to 14 days, and, if no contraindication is discovered, the T-tube is pulled within two to three days after the cholangiogram. The examination requires little time and is highly reliable if, as is true with all studies, attention is paid to detail.

For contrast material we use either Hypaque sodium 50 per cent or Renografin 60 per cent, both of which contain similar amounts of iodine, 300 and 288 mg/ml, respectively. Because the degree of opacity produced by a duct filled with straight contrast material can obscure small calculi, we dilute the contrast material with sterile saline in the ratio of two parts saline to one part contrast material. This is done in a 30-cc syringe, which provides a volume that is more than sufficient to examine most ducts. Venous extension tubing and a 21-gauge needle are attached to the prepared syringe and filled with the solution, taking care to flush all bubbles from the system.

The patient is then placed on the fluoroscopic table in a shallow right posterior oblique position, and a scout film of the right upper quadrant is taken. After clamping the T-tube, the rubber tube is cleaned with an alcohol sponge, and the needle, with extension tubing and syringe attached, is inserted. Gentle aspiration with the syringe should reveal a bubble-free interface between the yellow bile and the colorless contrast solution. If a bubble is present, it is coaxed into the syringe by flicking the tubing with the finger while holding the syringe and tubing vertically. Once in the syringe, it is prevented from re-entering the tubing by the orientation of the syringe.

Some surgeons attach the bile drainage bag directly to the rubber T-tube. In this situation, air from the bag rises into the T-tube and bile ducts and is impossible to clear at the time of examination. This problem can be eliminated by having the surgeon add a 2- or 3-ft length of extension tubing between the T-tube and drainage bag and coiling it at the patient's side. This does not interfere with bile drainage and prevents reflux of air from the bag.

A fractionated injection technique is used for the introduction of contrast material. The injection proceeds slowly and intermittently and is monitored fluoroscopically, during which time spot films are taken. Exposures are made during the sequence of filling to record the gradual increase in opacity of the ducts.

By paying close attention to the early filling stage, small calculi can be discovered, which might be obscured if films were taken only after dense duct opacification. The injection continues until second- and third-order intrahepatic ducts are visualized and duodenal drainage is achieved.

The patient is instructed to report any discomfort experienced during the examination and should have little or none. Sphincter spasm is uncommon with this technique, but if it occurs it can be relieved by the intravenous injection of glucagon, 1 mg. Opacification of the tiny tertiary peripheral ducts is unnecessary and may require a volume and pressure sufficient to place the patient at risk of developing bacteremia. Excessive pressure and pancreatic duct reflux can also precipitate pancreatitis. Those concerned with these complications have advocated a gravity filling technique, condemning the "thumb on the plunger" method. Bacteremia and cholangitis or pancreatitis as complications of T-tube cholangiography have not been clinically evident in our experience, and, as with most methods, attention to detail is the key.

When duct opacification is complete, spot films are taken with the patient in various positions: i.e., right oblique, supine, and left oblique. Because of the course of the left hepatic duct, it often is not adequately opacified with the patient supine or in a right oblique position unless excessive injection pressure is used. It is best displayed with the patient turned to the left, which places the left hepatic duct in a relatively dependent position, thus favoring opacification.

If a question arises as to whether a particular filling defect represents a retained stone or an air bubble, raising the head of the examining table, thereby placing the patient in an erect position, and observing the effect on the lu-cency in question can often resolve the problem. If uncertainty persists, it is recommended that the examination be repeated on the following day. Precautions must be taken to prevent the entry of air from the bag and external tubing in the interval.

References

1. Wood, M.: Eponyms in biliary tract surgery (Presidential address). Am. J. Surg. *138*:746, 1979.
2. Farha, G. L., and Pearson, R. N.: Trans-cystic duct operative cholangiography. Am. J. Surg. *131*:228, 1976.
3. Berci, G., and Hamlin, J. A.: Unsuspected stones. *In* Berci, G., and Hamlin, J. A. (eds.): Operative Biliary Radiology. Baltimore: Williams & Wilkins, 1981, Chapter 9.
4. Smith, S. W., Engel, C., Averbook, B., and Longmire, W. P.: Problems of retained and recurrent common bile duct stones. J.A.M.A. *164*:231, 1957.
5. Corlette, M. B., Schatzky, S., and Ackroyd, S.: Operative cholangiography and overlooked stones. Arch. Surg. *131*:729, 1978.
6. Berci, G., and Hamlin, J. A.: A combined fluoroscopic and endoscopic approach for retained and overlooked stones removed through the T-tube tract. Surg. Gynecol. Obstet. *273*:153, 1981.
7. Seror, J., Schmitt, J. C., Pateras, C., and Sava, G.: Operative injuries to the bile duct. Intern. Surg. *63*:108, 1978.
8. Warren, K. W., and Jefferson, M. J.: Prevention and repair of strictures of the extra-hepatic bile ducts. Surg. Clin. North Am. *53*:1169, 1973.
9. Mirizzi, P. L.: La colangiografia durante las operaciones de las vias biliaries. Bol. Soc. Cir. Buenas Aires *16*:1133, 1932.
10. Hicken, N. F., MacAllister, A. J., Franz, B., and Crowder, F.: Techniques in indications and value of operative cholangiography. Arch. Surg. *60*:110, 1950.
11. Schulenberg, C.: Operative Cholangiography. London: Butterworth, 1966.
12. Berci, G., and Seyler, A.: An x-ray television image storage apparatus. Arch. Surg. *197*:577, 1973.
13. Berci, G., and Zheutlin, N.: Improving radiology in surgery. Med. Instrum. *10*:1110, 1976.
14. Berci, G., Hamlin, J. A., Morgenstern, L., and Fisher, D. L.: Modern operative fluorocholangiography. Gastro. Intest. Radiol. *3*:401, 1978.

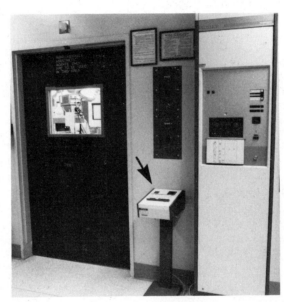

Figure 11–1. The generator (three phase, 1000 mAs) can be installed on the clean corridor in the OR area without interfering with the traffic pattern. Two adjacent ORs can be operated with one generator (time-sharing concept). Modern generators are required to achieve short and traumatic exposures with uniform performance. Mode selector control (arrow).

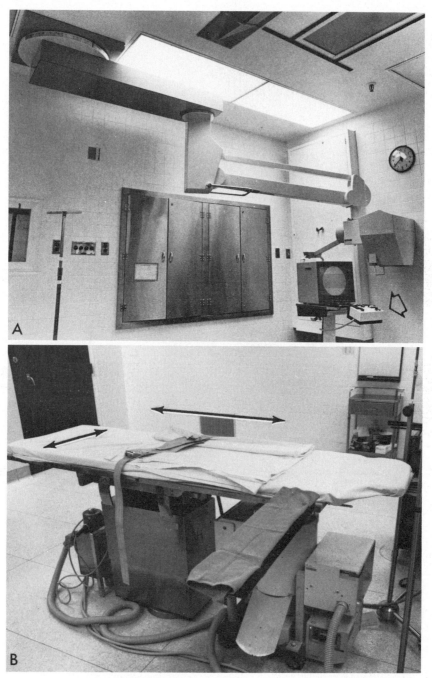

Figure 11–2. *A,* The overhead tube crane is in the parked position. The remote slave control box with TV monitor on wheels is alongside (arrow). *B,* Coordinate tabletop (arrows). Image amplifier is in position underneath.

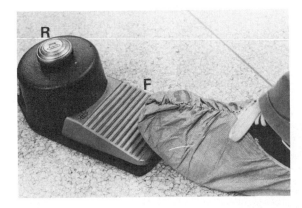

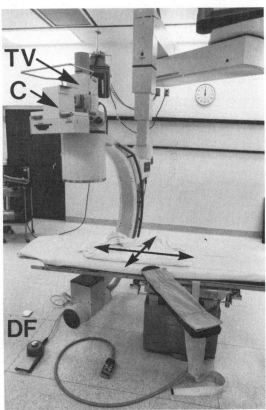

Figure 11–3. The dual control footswitch allows fluoroscopy (*F*) and radiography (*R*). The entire cholangiographic process is expedited by the ability to rapidly change from fluoroscopy to radiography.

Figure 11–4. Similar equipment utilizing a C-arm apparatus suspended from the ceiling. TV = television; C = x-ray camera; DF = double footswitch. Tabletop with coordinate movements (arrows). This equipment permits oblique views.

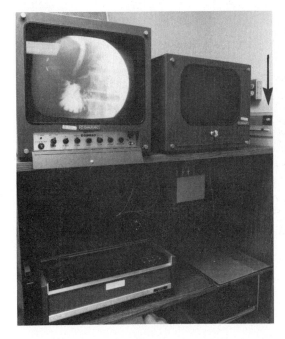

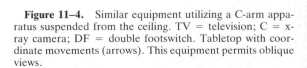

Figure 11–5. Audiovisual intercom system between the OR and diagnostic x-ray department. Wall-mounted audio intercom (arrow) and video tape recorder.

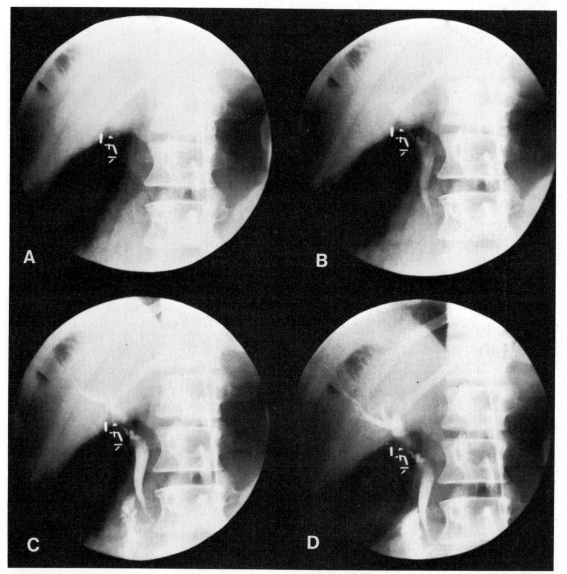

Figure 11–6. *A–H*, Normal cystic duct cholangiogram utilizing the serial film technique. Note the early filling stage (*B, C*). All anatomical areas, the sphincter (*D*), and intrahepatic ducts (*H*) are well seen.

Illustration continued on opposite page

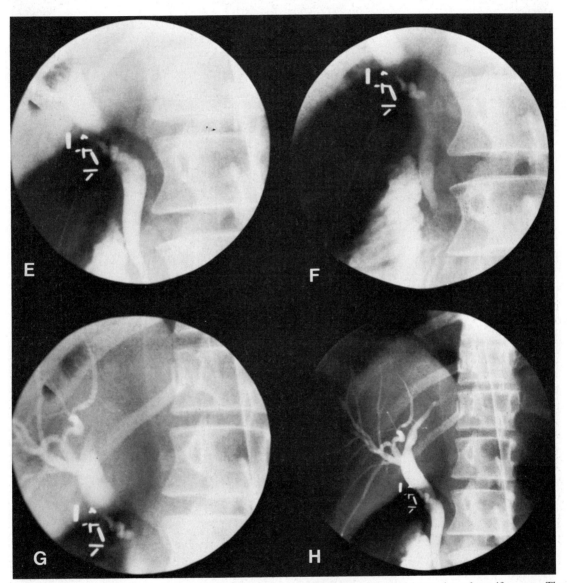

Figure 11–6 *Continued* Electronic enlargement (*E, F, G*) allows more detailed inspection of specific areas. The entire examination, including fluoroscopy and film exposure as well as shifting of the patient's position, did not exceed five minutes.

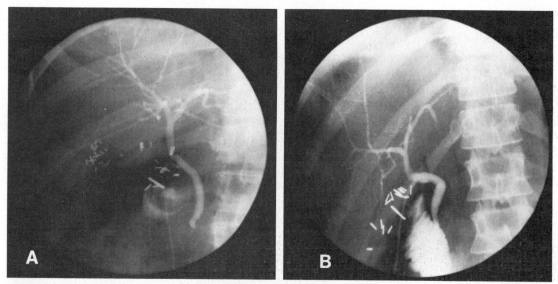

Figure 11–7. Normal cystic duct cholangiogram, selected film. *A,* Good detail of intra- and extra-hepatic ducts prior to duodenal filling. *B,* Note fine detail of intra- and extra-hepatic ducts during the late filling stage.

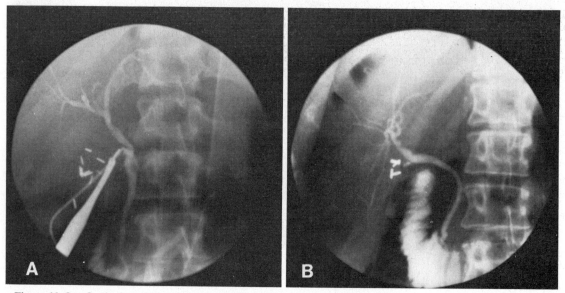

Figure 11–8. Cystic duct cholangiogram. *A,* Biliary ductal tree well displayed, with spiral cystic duct and common bile duct entering the third portion of the duodenum (low entry). *B,* The common bile duct is shown to enter at the junction of second and third portions of the duodenum (low entry).

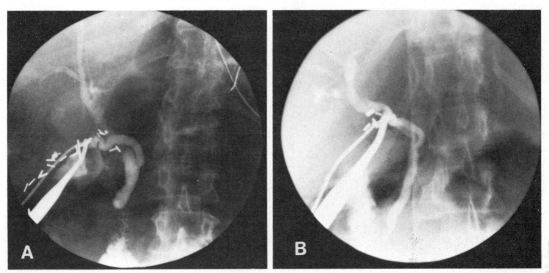

Figure 11–9. Cystic duct cholangiogram. *A,* The slightly dilated common duct demonstrates a spiral-type entry of the cystic duct, which is also slightly dilated. *B,* Spiral-type entry of the cystic duct into a normal caliber common duct.

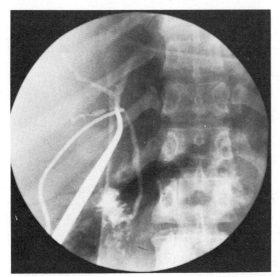

Figure 11–10. Cystic duct cholangiogram, anomaly. The cystic duct enters the common duct high in the subhepatic region near a right hepatic branch, which drains anomalously into the common duct. The potential for iatrogenic injury in this situation is high.

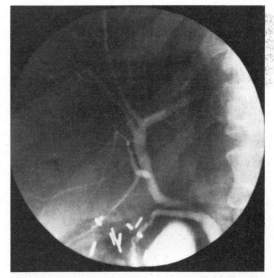

Figure 11–11. Cystic duct cholangiogram, anomaly. Anomalous insertion of the postero-caudal branch from the right lobe of the liver into the common hepatic duct.

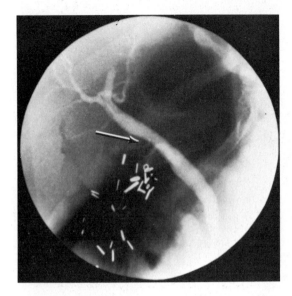

Figure 11–12. Cystic duct cholangiogram, anomaly. A small aberrant right hepatic duct (arrow) enters the common hepatic duct just proximal to the cystic duct entry.

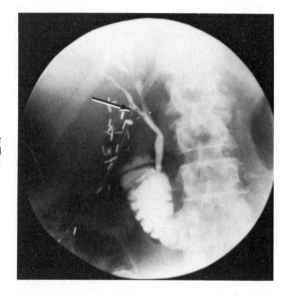

Figure 11–13. Cystic duct cholangiogram, anomaly. The cystic duct enters an aberrant right hepatic duct (arrow), and they drain together into the mid portion of the common duct.

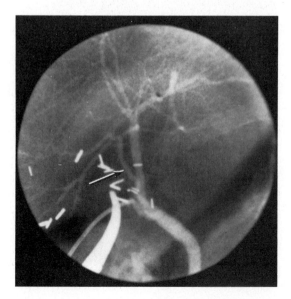

Figure 11–14. Cystic duct cholangiogram, anomaly. Aberrant right hepatic duct (arrow) draining into the common hepatic duct just above the cystic duct entry.

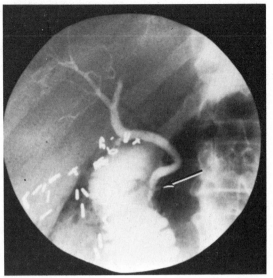

Figure 11–15. Cystic duct cholangiogram, anomaly. Tortuous distal common bile duct with small diverticulum (arrow) arising from the medial aspect. It is important to know the course of the common duct as well as the existence of the diverticulum if biliary endoscopy is contemplated.

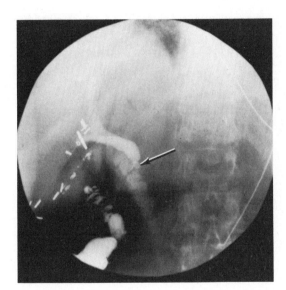

Figure 11–16. Cystic duct cholangiogram, anomaly. A small diverticulum (arrow) arises from the distal common bile duct.

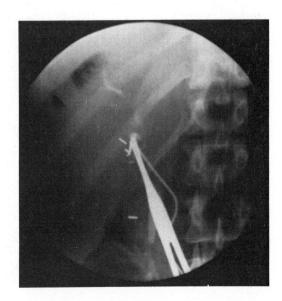

Figure 11–17. Cystic duct cholangiogram, early injection phase. Instruments may obscure the common bile duct. With fluoroscopy, this problem is quickly identified and corrected.

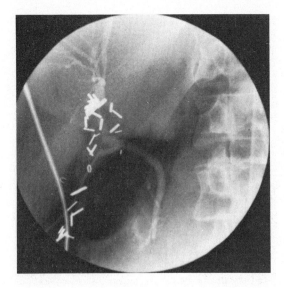

Figure 11–18. Cystic duct cholangiogram. Excessive use of hemoclips can obscure important anatomical areas.

Figure 11–19. Cystic duct cholangiogram. Excessive use of hemoclips here almost obscures a distal common bile duct calculus.

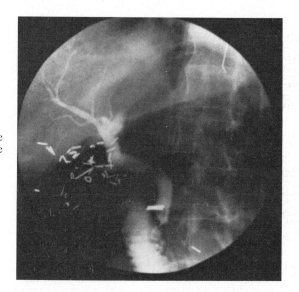

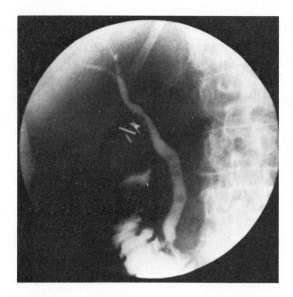

Figure 11–20. Cystic duct cholangiogram. Air bubbles are shown as rounded radiolucencies within the common bile duct. Fluoroscopy aids in distinguishing them from calculi by observing their movement with alternating negative and positive pressure applied to the syringe plunger.

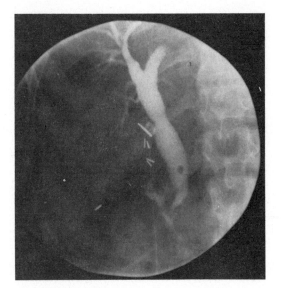

Figure 11–21. Cystic duct cholangiogram. Small, faceted calculus floating within the dilated common bile duct.

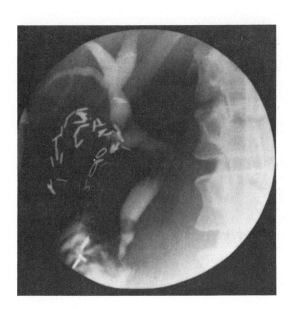

Figure 11–22. Cystic duct cholangiogram. Faceted calculus displayed within the distal common bile duct.

Figure 11–23. Cystic duct cholangiogram. Multiple calculi both proximally and distally within a slightly dilated common bile duct.

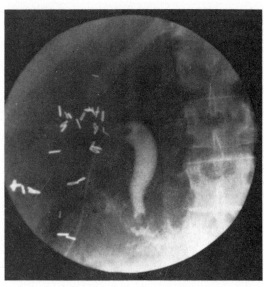

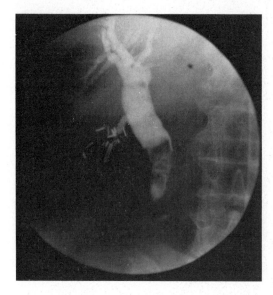

Figure 11–24. Cystic duct cholangiogram. Multiple calculi partially obstructing a dilated common bile duct.

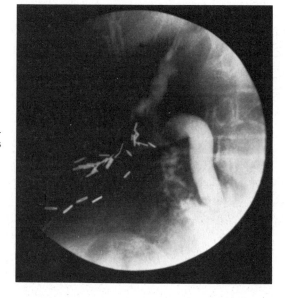

Figure 11–25. Cystic duct cholangiogram. Dilated common bile duct containing multiple calculi plus a single calculus seen in the left hepatic duct.

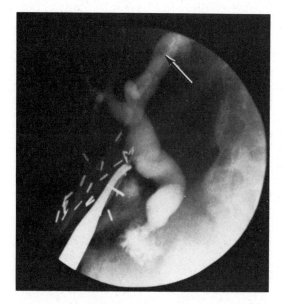

Figure 11–26. Cystic duct cholangiogram. Dilated common duct with calculus present in left hepatic duct (arrow).

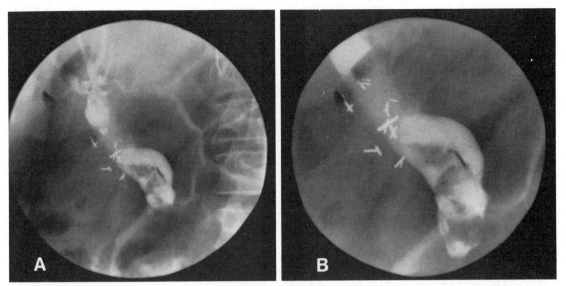

Figure 11–27. Cystic duct cholangiogram. Standard (*A*) and enlarged (*B*) views showing multiple calculi within and obstructing a dilated common bile duct. The spiral cystic duct is also dilated, and care must be exercised to prevent entry of a calculus into the cystic duct remnant where it might be overlooked.

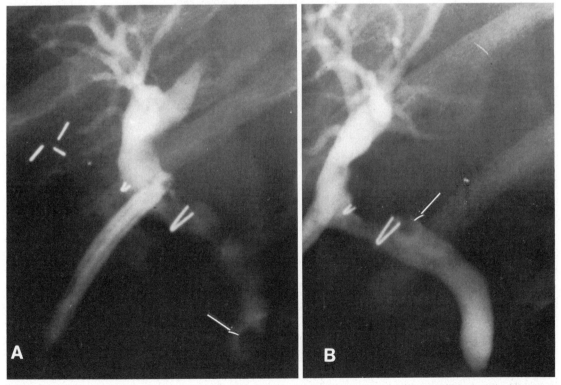

Figure 11–28. In dilated common bile ducts that contain calculi, stones may escape into a dilated cystic duct stump during extraction attempts. Postoperative tube cholangiogram. *A*, Stone shown in the distal common duct (arrow). This stone escaped operative biliary endoscopy. *B*, Same calculus in the cystic stump (arrow). During attempted removal through the T-tube tract in the postoperative period, the stone migrated into the stump and escaped endoscopic discovery. It was subsequently retrieved from the distal common duct.

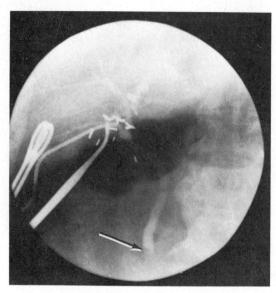
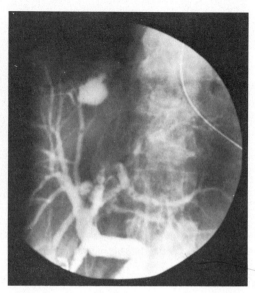

Figure 11–29

Figure 11–30

Figure 11–29. Cystic duct cholangiogram. Normal caliber common bile duct with partially obstructing and unsuspected distal calculus (arrow).

Figure 11–30. Cystic duct cholangiogram. Ruptured intrahepatic duct owing to excessive injection pressure or manipulation with extravasation into liver parenchyma. Multiple small calculi are shown in the left hepatic duct.

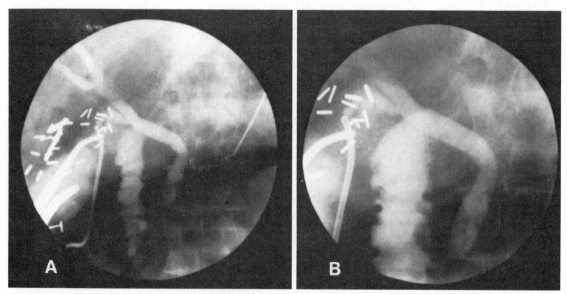

Figure 11–31. Cystic duct cholangiogram. *A*, Nonrotation of patient results in superimposition of the distal common bile duct on the spine with suspicious radiolucencies. *B*, Enlarged view shows "defect" to be due to overlapping of osseous structures.

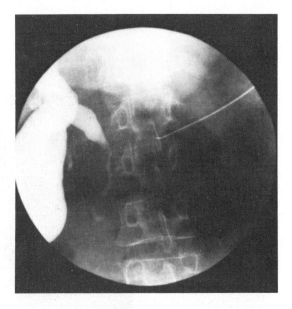

Figure 11–32. Cholecystocholangiogram. The dilated common duct is shown to taper into a long narrowed pancreatic segment. At surgery, chronic pancreatitis was found.

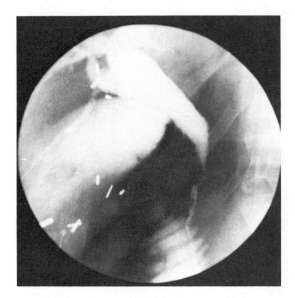

Figure 11–33. Cholecystocholangiogram. Similar appearance to that of Figure 11–32, showing tapering of the dilated common duct into a narrowed and irregular pancreatic segment. At surgery, pancreatic carcinoma was confirmed.

Figure 11–34. Cystic duct cholangiogram. Dilated common bile duct with abrupt narrowing to a long stenotic segment owing to pancreatic carcinoma.

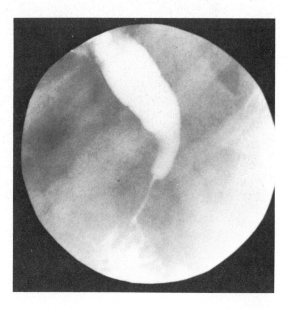

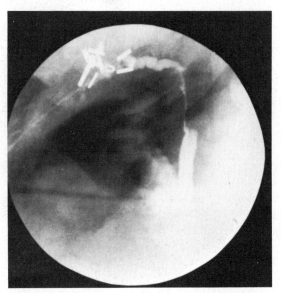

Figure 11–35. Cystic duct cholangiogram. A long stenotic segment of the cystic duct is shown as it courses within the common duct sheath. At surgery this proved to be due to advanced cholangiocarcinoma.

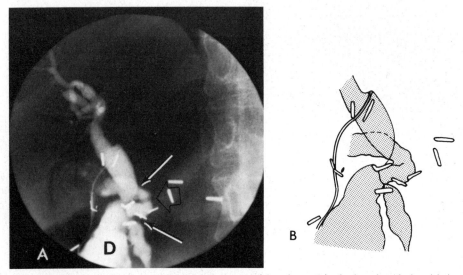

Figure 11–36. Choledochocholangiogram. Multiple strictures (closed arrows) of sclerosing cholangitis in this patient with inflammatory bowel disease. Spiral cystic duct (open arrow) and duodenum (D). *A,* X-ray. *B,* Schematic drawing.

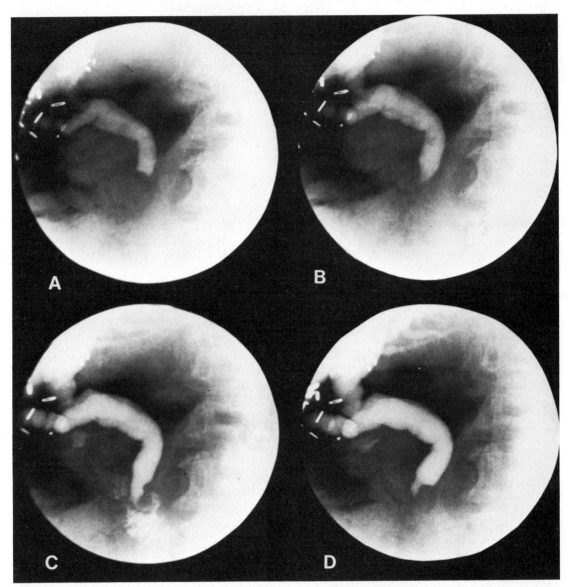

Figure 11–37. *A–D,* Cystic duct cholangiogram. Sphincter spasm will occasionally produce an apparent defect at the lower end of the common bile duct simulating an obstructing stone (pseudocalculous sign), as shown in *A*. Serial films *A* through *D* (selected from a series of eight) as well as fluoroscopy clearly demonstrate the functional changes in sphincteric contraction.

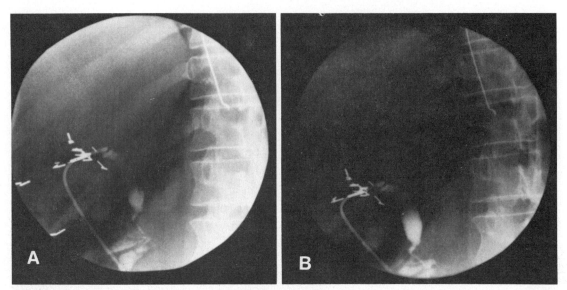

Figure 11–38. *A, B,* Cystic duct cholangiogram. The long, narrowed sphincter segment, unchanging on multiple exposures, as well as a slightly dilated common bile duct suggest sphincteric stenosis.

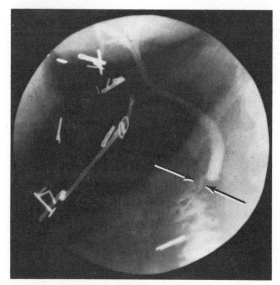

Figure 11–39. Cystic duct cholangiogram. Sphincteric segment appears to drain from the lateral aspect of the distal common bile duct (arrows).

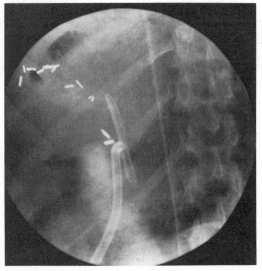

Figure 11–40. The course of the vertical limb of the T-tube is curved with angulation at the entry into the common bile duct. To facilitate potential postoperative stone extraction through the T-tube tract, the tube should be as straight as possible and perpendicular to the horizontal portion.

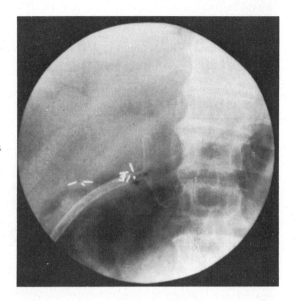

Figure 11–41. Kinking of the tip of the T-tube results from allowing too much length in the horizontal limbs.

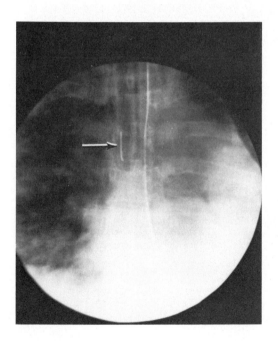

Figure 11–42. When fluoroscopy is available, it is useful to check the position of the endotracheal tube if the anesthesiologist is having difficulty with ventilation. Here, the endotracheal tube tip was in the right mainstem bronchus (arrow).

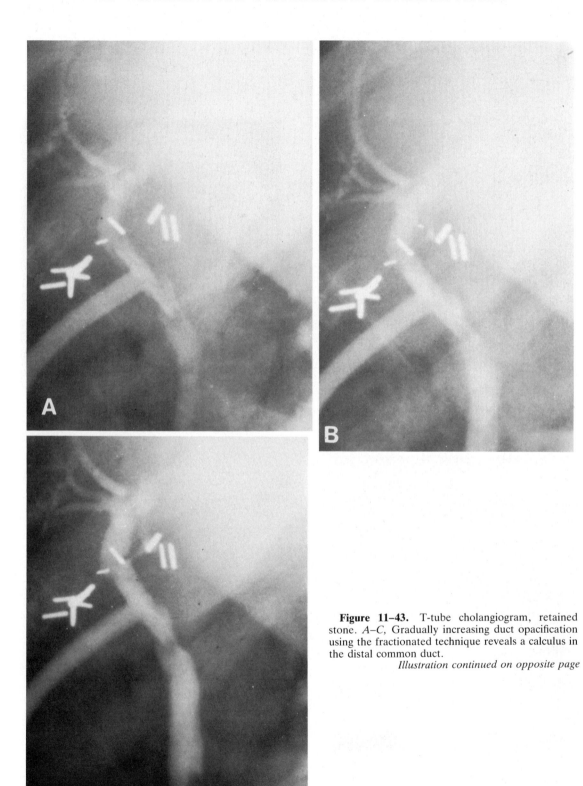

Figure 11–43. T-tube cholangiogram, retained stone. *A–C*, Gradually increasing duct opacification using the fractionated technique reveals a calculus in the distal common duct.

Illustration continued on opposite page

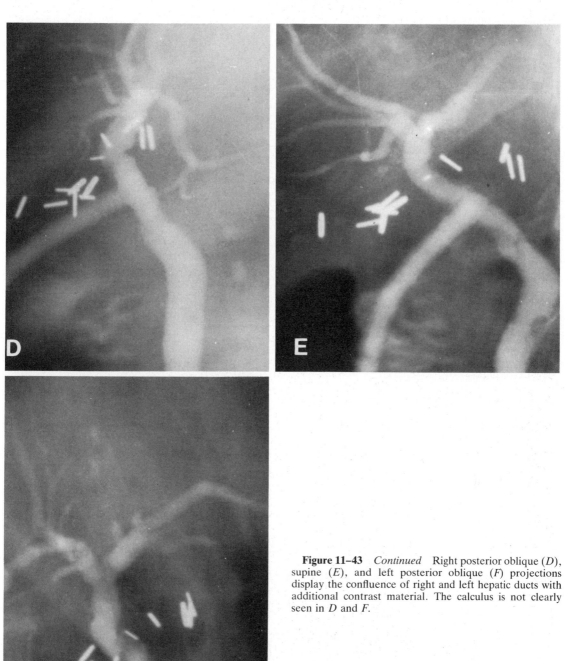

Figure 11–43 *Continued* Right posterior oblique (*D*), supine (*E*), and left posterior oblique (*F*) projections display the confluence of right and left hepatic ducts with additional contrast material. The calculus is not clearly seen in *D* and *F*.

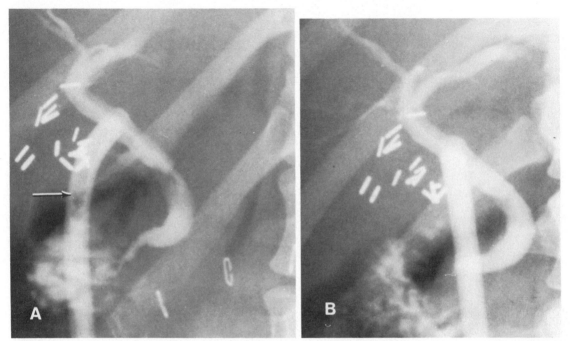

Figure 11–44. Normal T-tube cholangiogram. *A,* Right posterior oblique view with air bubbles (arrow) seen in the vertical limb of the T-tube. Introduction of bubbles into the bile ducts was avoided by elevating the tube and allowing them to rise as additional contrast material was slowly introduced to displace the air. *B,* Supine view showing further duct filling with no air bubbles present.

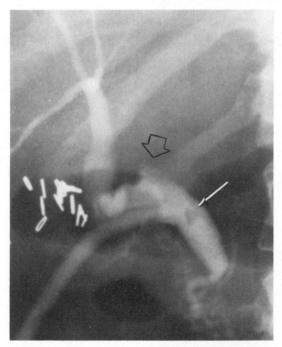

Figure 11–45. T-tube cholangiogram, retained stone (closed arrow). The T-tube has slipped distally so that the upper limb tents the medial wall of the common duct (open arrow). There is pancreatic duct reflux although the intrahepatic ducts are incompletely opacified.

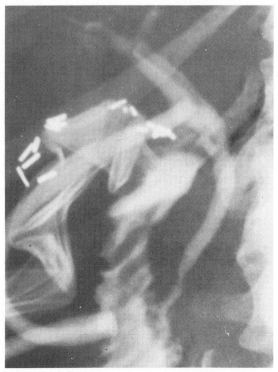

Figure 11–46. T-tube cholangiogram, pancreatitis. Normal biliary ducts drain freely into the duodenum, which features effacement of its medial aspect by an inflamed and enlarged pancreatic head. Opaque drains are present.

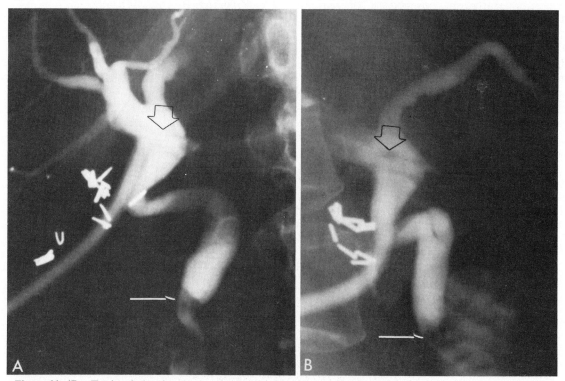

Figure 11–47. T-tube cholangiogram, retained stone (closed arrows). The T-tube has migrated proximally with the upper limb in the right hepatic duct, whereas the lower limb tents the common hepatic duct (open arrows) and appears to protrude from it. *A*, Supine view. *B*, The left posterior oblique position places the left hepatic duct in a dependent position, which favors its opacification.

431

TRANSHEPATIC INTERVENTIONS

12

by Joseph T. Ferrucci, Jr., M.D.,
Peter R. Mueller, M.D., and
Eric vanSonnenberg, M.D.

In recent years, percutaneous transhepatic interventional techniques have begun to assume a major role in the clinical management of biliary tract obstruction. The prototype, percutaneous biliary drainage (PBD) for combined external/internal catheter decompression, provides an effective method for rapid nonoperative biliary decompression and has become an established alternative to standard surgical biliary bypass. It is most commonly employed for palliative drainage of advanced malignant obstruction, but it may also be used for preoperative decompression in patients with dense jaundice or acute suppurative cholangitis.

The basic technique for PBD involves transhepatic insertion of a drainage catheter into the biliary ducts and through areas of bile duct stricture into the duodenum. The catheter is fashioned so that multiple sideholes can be placed above and below the stricture to allow drainage of bile in an antegrade fashion into the duodenal lumen for internal drainage.

In addition to the successful combined external/internal catheter decompression provided by PBD, it also affords a secure initial catheter access to the biliary ducts through which a variety of secondary therapeutic inter-

ventional procedures can be performed (Table 12–1). Using a variety of techniques and instrumentation, various groups have performed indwelling stent endoprosthesis insertion, dilatation of biliary strictures with a Gruntzig angioplasty balloon catheter, tumor biopsy techniques, and basket extraction or solvent dissolution of intrahepatic and common duct calculi. These techniques will be detailed hereafter.

HISTORICAL BACKGROUND

Transhepatic cholangiography performed via a large caliber (18 gauge) sheathed needle during the 1960s was often concluded by leaving the cannula sheath *in situ* for protective decompression while the patient was transported to the operating suite. This reduced the risk of bile leakage during the few hours that might elapse before operation. In the early 1970s, several groups reported attempts to fix the cannula sheath in a more secure position by advancing it over an angiographic guide wire. Thus, Kaude, Weidenmier, and Agee[1]; Molnar and Stockum[2]; Burcharth and Nielbo[3]; and Tylen, Hoevels, and Vang[4] reported small series of patients in whom successful short-term external drainage had been established. Although the wide acceptance of the fine caliber "Chiba" needle cholangiography technique in the late 1970s largely replaced the large caliber sheathed needle technique, Scandinavian and Japanese workers continued to exploit angiographic techniques and reported successful guide wire and angiographic catheter negotiation of areas of bile duct stricture for longer-term positioning of biliary catheters for internal drainage. Hoevels, Lunderquist, and Ihse from Lund reported 15 cases of successful combined external/internal drainage

Table 12–1. TRANSHEPATIC BILIARY INTERVENTIONS

Initial Access	Secondary Procedures
Percutaneous biliary drainage (combined external/internal catheter decompression)	Endoprosthesis Stricture dilatation (Gruntzig balloon) Biopsy techniques (cytology needle brush) Stone removal (basket extraction, solvent dissolution)

for antegrade flow of bile into the alimentary tract in 1978[5] and extended their experience in a subsequent report.[6] Nakayama, Ikeda, and Okuda from Japan also reported a large early series of over 100 patients successfully drained.[7] Subsequently, in the United States, Ring and colleagues[8, 9]; Ferrucci, Mueller, and Harbin[10, 11]; Clark and coworkers[13]; Berquist and associates[12]; and Mueller and coworkers[14, 15] confirmed the efficacy and refined the instrumentation and technical principles involved.

PERCUTANEOUS BILIARY DRAINAGE

Indications

The general and specific indications for PBD are given in Table 12–2.

Palliation—Advanced Malignant Obstruction. The most common indication is palliative biliary decompression for advanced or unresectable malignant obstructions. These are most often carcinomas of the head of the pancreas, primary carcinomas of the extrahepatic bile ducts and/or gallbladder, cholangiocarcinoma, and metastatic periportal lymphadenopathy from other primary sites including lung, breast, and colon.[10-13] Eighty per cent of such patients are unresectable at the time of diagnosis, and the mortality for operative biliary bypass approaches 20 per cent.[16-22] Because carcinoma of the head of the pancreas carries a mean survival of no more than six months, regardless of the mode of therapy,[16-22] these patients comprise the most common indication for PBD in most series.[12, 13] The presence of intrahepatic metastases does not

Table 12–2. INDICATIONS FOR PERCUTANEOUS BILIARY DRAINAGE

General
    Extrahepatic obstruction with:
        Sepsis
        Pruritus
        Hepatic decompensation

Specific
    Palliation—advanced malignant obstruction
    Preoperative decompression
    Sepsis-cholangitis, liver abscess
    Failed biliary-enteric anastomosis
    Secondary therapeutic maneuvers
        Stricture dilatation
        Endoprosthesis
        Stone dissolution/extraction
    Post-THC prophylactic decompression

contraindicate a percutaneous drainage procedure, since intra- and extrahepatic obstruction may coexist and considerable improvement in the patient's clinical status may occur following drainage.[10, 11] For a large group of patients, especially those with obvious liver metastases, high periportal obstruction precluding effective surgical decompression, advanced age, sepsis, or inanition, the availability of a safe, effective alternative to formal surgical exploration with its attendant morbidity, mortality, and cost has been welcomed.

Preoperative Biliary Decompression. Disordered hepatic metabolism following prolonged biliary obstruction produces an operative mortality of up to 25 per cent when laparotomy is performed without prior biliary decompression.[7, 16-22] However, surgical data indicate that the risk of operative death can be reduced by half when bilirubin levels are decreased to less than 10 mg per cent by preliminary decompression by either operative cholecystostomy or radiologic catheter drainage.[7, 12, 13, 16-19, 23] Denning, Molnar, and Carey were unable to demonstrate a reduction in operative mortality but were able to show a significant reduction in postoperative complications from 56 per cent in patients without decompression to 28 per cent in patients undergoing PBD.[24] Pitt and associates have attempted to identify risk factors in jaundiced patients associated with a poor surgical outcome to define those who might benefit most from preoperative PBD.[25] They noted postoperative renal failure, bacteremia, and upper gastrointestinal hemorrhage to be the most common causes of postoperative mortality in high risk patients. Reasons for improved surgical morbidity after preliminary biliary decompression include improvement of liver function (especially bleeding parameters), reversal of secondary portal hypertension, improvement in wound healing, and a decreased incidence of postoperative acute tubular necrosis.[18, 19, 23, 26]

Decline in serum bilirubin levels of 10 to 15 mg per cent can be accomplished in as short a period as four to five days while leaving the extrahepatic common bile duct sufficiently dilated so that surgical anastomosis can still be done without inordinate technical difficulty. By the same token, during the interval, more complete preoperative staging of tumor extent by computed tomography, angiography, and fine-needle aspiration biopsy can be carried out. In many cases, evidence of unresectability (e.g., local extension, liver metastases) will be detected and will preclude attempts at curative resection.

Failed Biliary-Enteric Anastomosis. Biliary-enteric reconstructions for benign strictures carry a 30 per cent recurrence rate, whereas biliary-enteric bypass for malignant obstruction fails in 15 per cent of cases as a result of local disease progression. Cholecystojejunostomy is especially susceptible to failure since the origin of the cystic duct becomes occluded at an early stage by cephalad tumor growth. Thus, many surgeons avoid this procedure if possible. In both circumstances, reoperation on the biliary tract may be precluded by dense adhesions and/or local tumor extension, leaving radiologic catheter drainage as a useful alternative.

Sepsis-Cholangitis, Liver Abscess. Acute biliary tract sepsis is more often due to benign obstruction from common duct stone or stricture than to tumor. It can be associated with profound septic shock and is a *bona fide* surgical emergency that responds dramatically to percutaneous catheter decompression.[7, 10, 11] In such patients therapeutic decompression can be performed as an urgent preoperative resuscitative maneuver while the patient's condition is stabilized for an elective surgical procedure. In our institution, PBD is frequently performed in such cases as an emergency night or weekend procedure. However, in dealing with such gravely ill patients, excessive manipulation of the catheter should be carefully avoided, and PBD in such circumstances is generally restricted to external drainage only.

Secondary Therapeutic Maneuvers. As noted in Table 12–1, successful catheter access to the biliary ducts is often employed as an essential preliminary to further therapeutic manipulations. Following several days of catheter drainage, formation of a discrete tract through the hepatic parenchyma occurs, and subsequent instrumentations are carried out with greater ease. Indeed, the initial step of percutaneous catheter insertion often proves technically far more difficult than the various secondary maneuvers that may be employed.

Post-THC Prophylactic Decompression. Because septicemia is the most common serious complication of diagnostic fine-needle cholangiography, some institutions employ routine post-cholangiography catheter decompression when high grade obstruction is demonstrated. Thus, there is a growing trend for the majority of patients with transhepatic cholangiograms showing noncalculus obstruction to undergo PBD. In our institution approximately 60 per cent of all diagnostic fine-needle cholangiograms are followed by PBD.

Contraindications

Because PBD is often employed in patients who are too ill to undergo formal surgical exploration, there are few absolute contraindications. Thus, once the appropriate medical supportive measures are under way, the procedure may be carried out in patients who are actively septic or are somnolent from hepatic coma or those with ascites or intrahepatic metastases. Marked ascites displacing the liver from the abdominal wall increases the technical problems of bridging this gap with the drainage catheters but is not a contraindication *per se*. Use of stiff guide wires frequently provides success. Routine contraindications to PBD include an uncorrectable bleeding diathesis, massive replacement of the liver by metastatic disease, hepatic cirrhosis with marked distortion and narrowing of intrahepatic bile ducts, and periportal obstruction producing isolated noncommunicating obstructions of two or more separate intrahepatic duct radicles (Fig. 12–1). In the last-named instance, the technical difficulty of catheter placement and the frequent necessity for insertion of multiple simultaneous catheters to obtain satisfactory decompression, combined with a low likelihood of prolonged palliation, are discouraging factors.

Nevertheless, it should be re-emphasized that mere demonstration of intrahepatic metastases should not preclude an effort at decompression of a concurrent extrahepatic block. By the same token, extrahepatic ducts may show only minimal dilatation despite the presence of severe extrahepatic obstruction when there is diffuse neoplastic infiltration or widespread fibrosis in hepatic cirrhosis. Thus, the decision to attempt drainage in any given case must always be individualized. Factors to consider include age, overall medical condition, and prognosis of the underlying process.

CAUTION: Once PBD is initiated, it must be completed. The necessary puncture techniques carry a risk of bile leakage unless a catheter can be successfully inserted. Thus, the anatomic findings, available equipment, and radiologist's experience also enter into the decision to proceed.

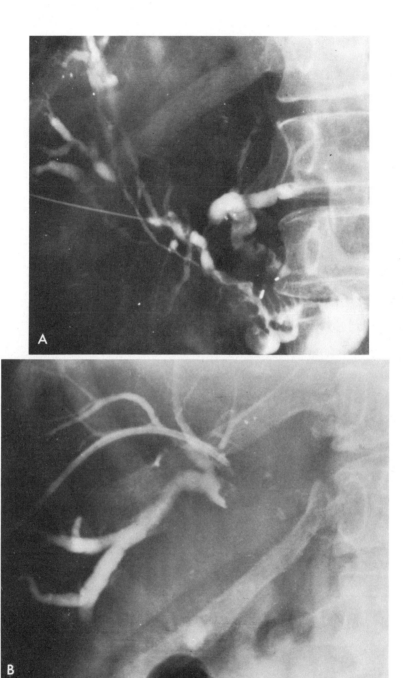

Figure 12–1. Worth draining or not? Absolute contraindications to PBD are few. Relative discouraging factors include multiple areas of distortion and narrowing and obstruction of intrahepatic ducts by tumor or fibrous tissue in hepatic cirrhosis. *A,* Typical malignant periportal infiltration with elongated narrowing of multiple radicles of the right duct, stricture of the left main duct, and poor filling of the common hepatic duct. *B,* In this patient with metastatic disease to the intrahepatic ducts, an external drainage catheter has been placed in a ventral branch of the right hepatic duct. However, gross intraluminal tumor occludes all the other duct radicles. In both cases multiple catheters would be required for any hope of successful palliation, whereas outlook for survival would be poor. Both of these patients died within four weeks.

Instrumentation

Commercially prepared biliary drainage assembly kits are now available.* Nevertheless, the greatest degree of success will be achieved only in well-equipped procedure rooms with an assortment of guide wires, catheter systems, vessel dilators, adaptors, skin fixation devices, and collection bags. Imagination and adaptability remain useful tools as well.

Initial diagnostic cholangiography is performed with a standard 22-gauge, thin-walled Chiba needle, followed by a cannula puncture

---

*Cook Catheter Co., Bloomington, IN.

of an appropriate biliary radicle using a conventional 18-gauge sheathed needle assembly.

Guide Wires

Angiographic guide wires of 0.38-in. size are generally required to provide the degree of rigidity needed to support subsequent catheter insertions. In addition to standard tight J (3 mm) and floppy J (15 mm) tipped configurations and moveable core straight wires, two special wires have been designed specifically for biliary catheter work, the Ring-Lunderquist torque wire and the Lunderquist "coat

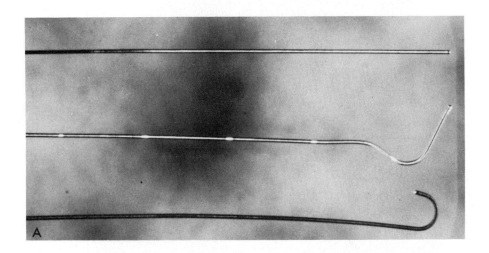

LUND GUIDE   0.38" STAINLESS STEEL — STIFF SHAFT, 10 cm. FLOPPY TIP

RING GUIDE   0.38" STAINLESS STEEL — TORQUE CONTROL

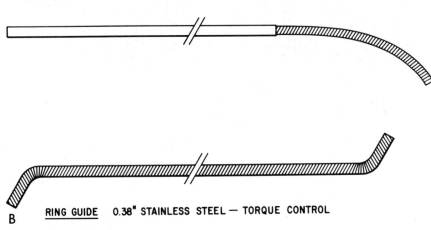

Figure 12–2. Biliary guide wires. *A,* Photograph of Lunderquist wire[28] (top), Ring-Lunderquist memory torque wire[8] (center), and sharp 3.0 mm J 0.38″ angiographic wire (bottom). *B,* Schematic representation. The Lunderquist rigid wire has a straight, long, malleable tip and is used for catheter advancement through densely fibrotic or neoplastic liver tissue. The Ring-Lunderquist memory torque control wire is used for searching maneuvers during initial catheterization.

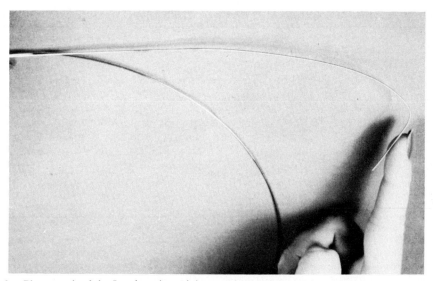

Figure 12–3. Photograph of the Lunderquist stainless steel "coat-hanger" wire showing the long malleable tip.

hanger" wire (Fig. 12–2). The advantages and disadvantages of various guide wires are summarized in Table 12–3. Smaller caliber (0.35- and 0.28-in.) wires are occasionally useful when only smaller caliber catheters can be inserted in difficult problem cases.

The 0.38-in. Ring-Lunderquist torque control guide wire is sufficiently rigid to retain a memory tip and is useful for negotiating sharp turns or areas of tight stricture, especially when proximal dilatation is severe.[8] A rotary motion on the external hub of this wire allows an effective tip-searching motion within the lumen of a dilated duct. Although occasional instances of breaking or uncoiling of the torque control tip of this wire have occurred, the wire readily supports initial catheter insertions and remains the workhorse wire for biliary interventional procedures. High torque J tip wires have also been described by Harrington that combine the advantages of torque control and a conventional sharp J design.[27]

The extremely stiff stainless steel shaft guide wire described by Lunderquist[28] is occasionally used to support catheterization through liver parenchyma that has been replaced by malignant tumor or dense fibrosis. This wire consists of an 80-cm long rigid steel shaft with a 5-cm straight malleable tip welded to its distal portion (Fig. 12–3). The firmness of the shaft has evoked the "coat-hanger" designation, and the soft tip provides a margin of safety.

In routine work the 0.38-in. tight J (3 mm) and 0.38-in. Ring-Lunderquist torque wires prove sufficient in 90 per cent of cases.

Catheters

Various radiopaque multi-sidehole drainage catheters have been employed in different centers. Early workers tailored conventional angiographic catheters of 5 to 7 French size with sideholes specifically made for the configura-

Table 12–3. BILIARY GUIDE WIRES: CLINICAL CHARACTERISTICS

Guide Wires (0.38 in.)	Advantages	Disadvantages
Tight J (3 mm)	Leads with curve Good for tight turns	May not go through tight obstruction May not support catheter in all cases
Floppy J (15 mm)	Leads with curve Good for turns	May not support catheter in all cases
Ring-Lunderquist (torque)	Torque control Supports catheters well	May pierce duct wall Difficult negotiating tight turns
Lunderquist	"Coat-hanger" wire Supports catheters extremely well	Not good for searching

Table 12–4.   BILIARY DRAINAGE CATHETERS: CLINICAL CHARACTERISTICS

Catheter	Advantages	Disadvantages
Ring (8.3/10 F)	Angle/pigtail tip Anchor in duodenum	Not good for external drainage
Mueller (8.3/9.0 F)	External drainage catheter with various curves Fewer sideholes	Too few sideholes for internal drainage
Argyle feeding tubes (10, 12, 14 F)	Soft, large caliber Easier on patient Can tailor sideholes	Too pliable to use initially
Self-retaining (Cope loop)	Soft, large caliber (polyvinyl or Silastic) Anchor effect with inner suture	Too pliable to use initially Long-term patency unclear
Foley type	Standard balloon anchor rubber	Wall necrosis from balloon

tion of the obstructing lesion. At present, numerous catheters of larger caliber size are available commercially.* Important clinical characteristics of biliary drainage catheters are detailed in Table 12–4.

Ring popularized an 8.3 French (OD 2.7 mm, ID 1.8 mm) Teflon catheter with a pigtail configuration to provide an anchoring effect within the duodenal lumen (Fig. 12–4).[8, 29] A right-angle bend in the catheter approximately 3 cm proximal to the tip conforms to the angle between the distal common bile duct and the duodenal lumen. Forty-one sideholes are arranged over the distal 12 cm, with several sideholes located on the intraduodenal portion to aid egress of bile into the alimentary canal lumen. Later modifications include a 10 French size and a model with fewer sideholes (32) for shorter, more distal strictures. The Ring catheter has been proved to be an effective general purpose catheter system for combined external/internal biliary drainage.

Because catheter purchase within the duct and the location of sideholes are important considerations in many different situations, a straight, tapered-tip catheter with multiple sideholes (Mueller series) is often of value (Fig. 12–5).*[10, 11] This is most often a 9 French catheter with sideholes closely spaced over a shorter length near the catheter tip. The tapered tip and stiff polyethylene material add a distinct dilator effect. Variations with a gentle curve are available.

Polyvinyl stomach tubes of 10 to 14 French caliber are effective catheter systems for longer-term drainage (Fig. 12–6).† These radiopaque tubes have a softer wall material and are usually more comfortable for ambulatory patients. Multiple large sideholes can be cut

to conform to the obstructing anatomy. In general, however, the soft wall material requires that these tubes be inserted as a replacement for an initial stiffer, smaller caliber drain-

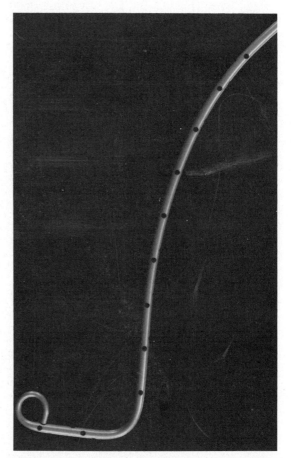

Figure 12–4.   Ring pigtail 8.3 French multi-sidehole biliary catheter for internal drainage.[8] Forty side holes are placed over the distal 12 cm. The pigtail tip provides an anchoring effect within the duodenum, and the right angle bend 3 cm from the tapered tip conforms to the orientation of the choledochoduodenal junction.

---

*Cook Catheter Co., Bloomington, IN.

†Argyl, St. Louis, Missouri

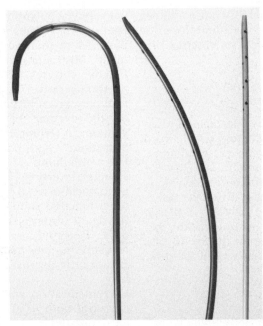

Figure 12–5. Mueller straight, tapered-tip, multi-side hole, 9 French biliary catheters for external drainage.[10, 11] These tapered-tip catheters are fashioned with sideholes over a short distance (6 to 8 cm) and are principally used when there is a short "purchase," as in a high periportal obstruction. Variations with gentle and J curves are shown.

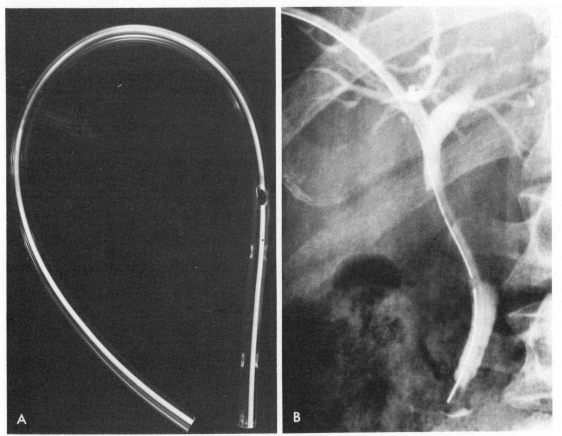

Figure 12–6. Polyvinyl catheter (Argyl stomach tube) for long-term drainage. The soft wall material and large lumen size (10 to 14 F) of these catheters are well suited for chronic external/internal catheter drainage. *A*, Photograph. *B*, Clinical case.

age catheter. Their pliability also allows formation of a terminal crossed limb loop for a self-retaining anchor effect as described by Cope.[30]

Other Materials

Additional materials of value include a variety of smaller caliber catheters with curved and pigtail tips, angiographic vessel dilators, adaptors, stopcocks, and plastic leg bags for bile collection. Catheter fixation to the skin is achieved with a commercially available adhesive Corya material (Stomahesive).* A plastic adhesive disk (Molnar) is less satisfactory because the slippery, lubricating quality of bile weakens long-term skin adherence of the disk.

Patient Preparation

Preparatory measures for percutaneous biliary drainage are identical to those used for ordinary diagnostic fine-needle transhepatic cholangiography (see Table 10–3). Thus, no additional specific modifications are required if a catheter is to be inserted following a diagnostic transhepatic cholangiogram. Nevertheless, attention to preparatory details is crucial for a safe, comfortable, and successful procedure.

Prior to the procedure, a review of the patient's chart is made for a survey of the bleeding parameters and the need for any corrective measures. The prothrombin time should be within two minutes of the control value, and platelets should be above 75,000/cu mm. Initial thromboplastin time values should also be within normal range. Most patients with long-standing biliary obstruction are routinely given vitamin K on admission to the hospital in anticipation of an interventional therapeutic maneuver. Should the bleeding parameters be found abnormal, administration of appropriate corrective agents including fresh frozen plasma, vitamin K, or platelets can be carried out until bleeding functions return to a normal range. The study is then carried out. In very ill patients with severe liver failure or underlying bleeding disorders, the timing of the percutaneous transhepatic manipulation can be adjusted to occur within a two- to three-hour time span to coincide with the optimum effects of specific therapy for the bleeding defect.

---

*E. R. Squibb & Sons, Inc., Princeton, NJ.

Prophylactic antibiotic coverage is instituted routinely beginning the day before the procedure. More than 50 per cent of patients with biliary obstruction will be found to have positive bile cultures, often gram negative, as well as gram-positive organisms. Therefore, drugs routinely given are ampicillin (4 gm/24 hr IV on the evening before the procedure) and gentamicin (80 mg IM early on the day of the procedure). Antibiotic coverage is continued for a minimum of three to four days after catheter insertion. The primary side effect of gentamicin is renal toxicity, and parameters of renal function should be observed carefully if this agent is administered for more than several days. Recently, a derivative of gentamicin, tobramycin, has been introduced that has a significantly decreased incidence of renal toxicity.

Premedication with narcotics and sedatives is crucial both to allay anxiety and to control local discomfort at the puncture site during catheter introduction. Combinations of barbiturates, meperidine (Demerol), and diazepoxide (Valium) are given intramuscularly and/or intravenously and are liberally employed. However, the potential side effect of respiratory depression should be borne in mind, and naloxone (Narcan) should be available for reversal. Atropine is not used routinely but only as necessary for vagal brachycardia.

Preoperative preparations also include completely sterile skin preparation and sterile surgical draping of the fluoroscopic table and the fluoroscopic spot film device. A large sterile equipment table is also invaluable. The procedure is carried out with intravenous fluids running and blood pressure monitored at timely intervals.

Technique

The procedural steps for combined external/internal biliary drainage have been detailed by Hoevels and associates[6, 7]; Nakayama, Ikeda, and Okuda[7]; Ring and colleagues[8, 9]; Ferrucci, Mueller, and Harbin[10, 11]; Berquist and coworkers[12]; Clark and associates[13]; and Mueller, vanSonnenberg, and Ferrucci.[14, 15] A schematic diagram and illustrative cases are presented in Figures 12–7 through 12–11. The procedural sequence detailed hereafter is derived from the authors' series of over 250 cases.

1. Fine-needle transhepatic cholangiography is the requisite first step in all cases. Although some patients are referred specifi-

Text continued on page 446

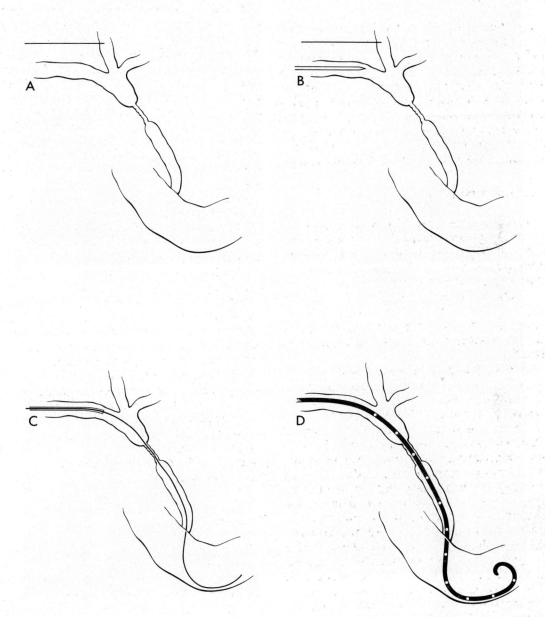

Figure 12–7. Schematic representation of procedure for internal biliary drainage. *A,* Initial diagnostic fine-needle cholangiogram showing stricture. *B,* Selective 18-gauge cannula sheath puncture of horizontal segment of right hepatic duct. *C,* Guide wire advanced through sheath across stricture and into duodenum. *D,* Multi-side hole 8.3 pigtail catheter inserted over guide into duodenum for internal drainage.

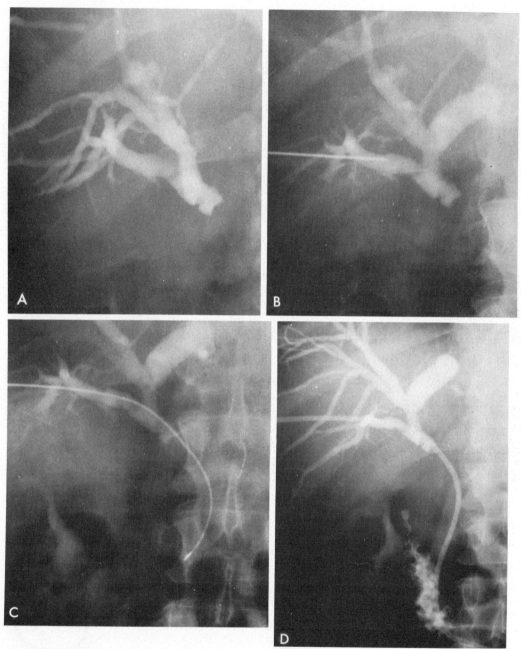

Figure 12–8. Illustrative case of internal drainage. Diagnosis: metastatic periportal adenopathy secondary to oat cell carcinoma of the lung. *A,* Diagnostic cholangiogram showing complete obstruction of common hepatic duct. Abrupt terminus of contrast column is consistent with extrinsic tumor compression. *B,* Separate selective puncture with 18-gauge sheathed needle. A favorable horizontal segment of the right main duct is cannulated with a long length of duct to permit secure purchase for guide wire-catheter exchange. A visible movement of the opacified duct and "pop" will be seen as the large needle punctures the duct walls. If this does not occur, successful puncture is unlikely. *C,* Guide wire advanced through cannula sheath beyond obstruction and into distal common bile duct. Note that the complete obstruction apparent on the initial cholangiogram is readily traversed by guide wire. *D,* Final placement of 8.3 F pigtail biliary drainage catheter into descending duodenum for internal drainage. (From Ferrucci, J. T., Jr., Mueller, P. R., and Harbin, W. P.: Radiology *135*:1, 1980.)

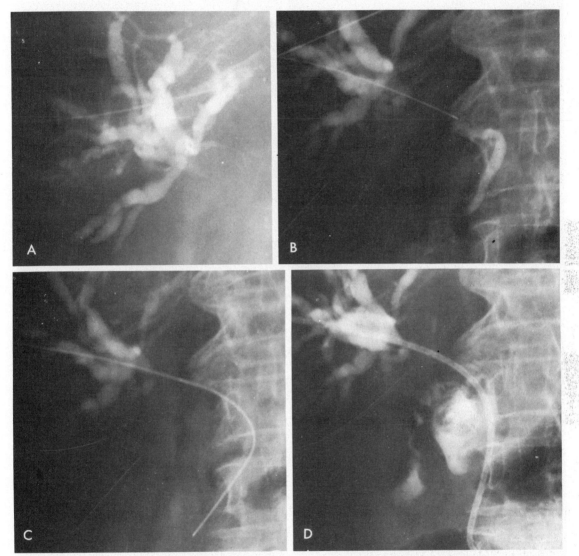

Figure 12–9. Illustrative case of internal drainage sequence. Diagnosis: metastatic periportal lymphadenopathy secondary to carcinoma of the stomach. *A,* Initial cholangiogram showing complete periportal obstruction. The ill-defined blunt terminus of the contrast column is consistent with metastatic disease. *B,* Following successful separate puncture of a dilated right hepatic radicle with an 18-gauge cannula sheath, a guide is passed through the obstruction into a normal caliber distal common bile duct. Additional contrast medium is injected during advancement of the 18-gauge sheath and guide wire, revealing the exact length of the stricture. Note again that "complete" obstruction on an initial cholangiogram can often be negotiated by the guide wire. *C,* Guide wire advanced to level of ampulla. *D,* Internal biliary drainage catheter inserted. (Collection of contrast medium is in duodenal cap.)

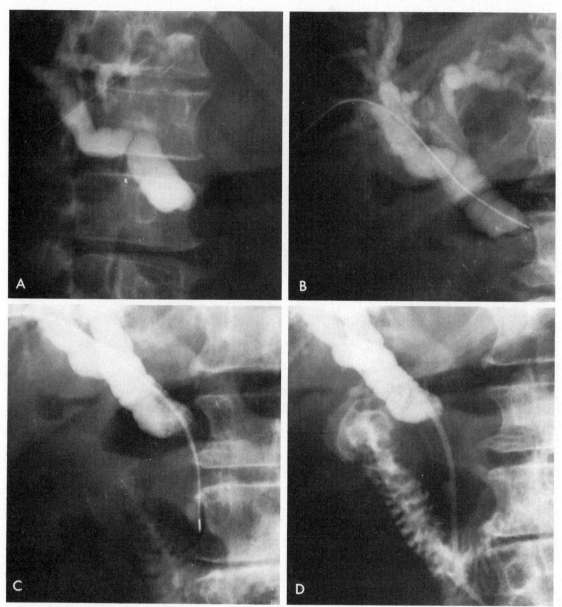

Figure 12–10. Illustrative case of internal drainage. Diagnosis: carcinoma of the head of the pancreas. *A*, Initial cholangiogram showing complete blunt obstruction of the mid common bile duct consistent with a pancreatic carcinoma. No contrast passes distally. *B*, Guide wire advanced to point of obstruction. *C*, Wire and small catheter negotiated through "complete" obstruction into distal common bile duct. *D*, Catheter placed into duodenum for internal drainage. Note: Despite complete obstruction on the initial cholangiogram, wires and catheters can often be successfully negotiated caudally through the obstruction into the distal duct.

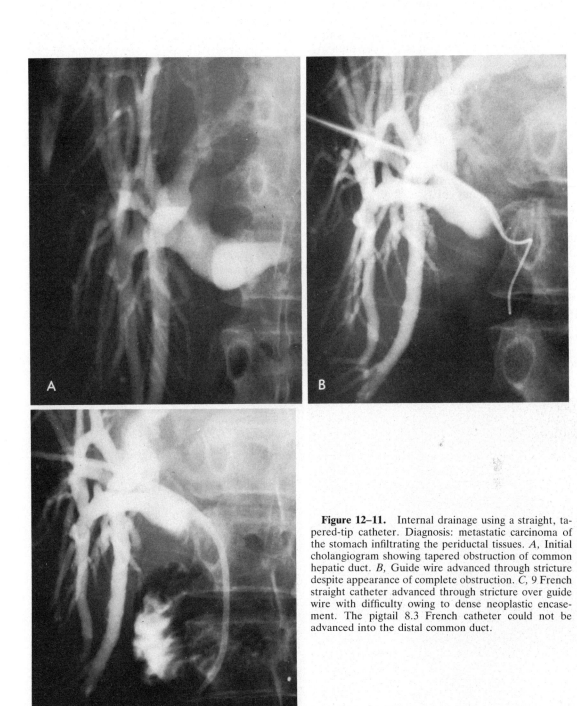

Figure 12–11. Internal drainage using a straight, tapered-tip catheter. Diagnosis: metastatic carcinoma of the stomach infiltrating the periductal tissues. *A,* Initial cholangiogram showing tapered obstruction of common hepatic duct. *B,* Guide wire advanced through stricture despite appearance of complete obstruction. *C,* 9 French straight catheter advanced through stricture over guide wire with difficulty owing to dense neoplastic encasement. The pigtail 8.3 French catheter could not be advanced into the distal common duct.

cally for biliary catheter drainage, more often the procedure derives from a standard diagnostic transhepatic cholangiogram. Following initial demonstration of an obstructing lesion and immediate consultation with the referring physician, a decision is made to proceed with the catheter insertion during the same session. It should be noted that PBD can be carried out despite relatively normal or small caliber intrahepatic ducts (Fig. 12–12). Obviously, such cases do pose a greater technical challenge.

2. Following successful opacification of the biliary ducts by the fine-needle cholangiogram, an optimal segment of the duct system is selected for catheter insertion. Usually this is the horizontal portion of the main right hepatic duct immediately above the confluence. This segment of the duct system is intrahepatic, easily accessible by a direct right lateral intercostal approach, and affords a relatively straight path for advancement of guide wires and catheters.

3. A separate skin puncture site is selected for puncture with the 18-gauge cannula sheath. This is located as cephalad as possible (avoid-ing the pleural space) to minimize the angle of entry into the biliary ducts, thus facilitating subsequent guide wire/catheter insertions. Actual puncture site selection is based on fluoroscopic observations of the position of the opacified bile ducts. It should be noted that the fine-needle cholangiogram needle should be left *in situ* as long as it remains in communication with the bile duct system, since continued opacification of the ducts is essential for guided selective puncture with the cannula sheath.

4. Localization of the anterior-posterior position of the target duct is the next and crucial step. Biplane fluoroscopy is invaluable if available but not essential, and we have not employed it. Methods for anterior-posterior localization of the duct include the use of lead markers with horizontal beam lateral radiographs and fluoroscopic localization of the contrast-filled ducts in the left lateral decubitus position. After experience with only a few cases, however, it is generally possible to directly enter the ducts from a simple mid right coronal puncture site, guiding the advancing cannula sheath tip under continuous fluoro-

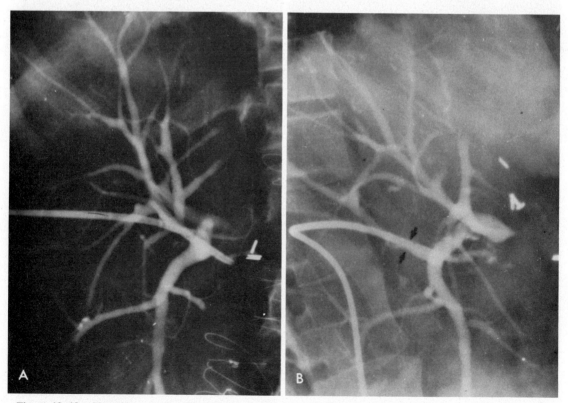

Figure 12–12. Normal or small caliber ducts can be drained. Frontal (*A*) and left posterior oblique (*B*) views. External drainage only. Note small caliber of duct containing the catheter in *B* (arrows).

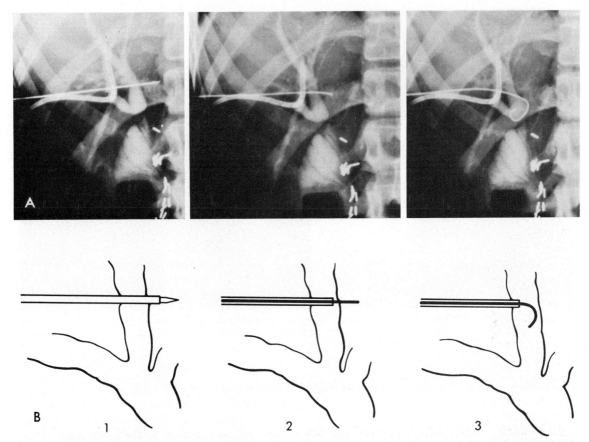

Figure 12–13. Use of the tight (3 mm) safety J wire to avoid perforation of duct wall and false passage. Clinical case *A* and schematic representation *B*. Diagnosis: anastomotic stricture postcholedochojejunostomy for iatrogenic injury. *1,* Cannula sheath inadvertently punctures back wall of vertically oriented intrahepatic radicle. *2,* Straight wire protrudes through hole in back wall, creating false passage. *3,* Sharp J wire misses back wall puncture site and passes caudally to area of stricture. Note: A catheter has been previously placed in the intra-hepatic ducts.

scopic control. Because the right hepatic duct courses posteriorly. the puncture site chosen for catheter insertion is usually 1 cm or more posterior to that used for the fine-needle cholangiogram.

5. The cannula sheath is advanced into the intended duct under continuous fluoroscopic guidance and suspended respiration. Puncture of the duct wall occurs with a visible forward snap and a simultaneous tactile pop. If these are not observed, successful cannulation is unlikely. If possible, a long intraluminal length of cannula is inserted to provide adequate purchase to facilitate subsequent catheter exchanges (Fig. 12–8).

6. Successful entry into the biliary duct system is confirmed by prompt flow of bile. Bile is readily distinguished from blood, even if blood tinged, by its sticky, filmy, or greasy consistency. If blood is returned from the cannula, contrast medium should not be introduced, at least initially, because extraductal deposition of contrast may obscure anatomic detail should repeat punctures be required.

7. When bile flow is observed, a 0.38-in. safety guide wire with a sharp J tip or a 0.38-in. Lunderquist-Ring memory torque guide wire is inserted through the cannula and advanced caudally. The cannula is then advanced over the guide wire as far as possible. If the back wall of the duct has been inadvertently punctured, use of a straight wire will create a false passage; thus it is usually preferable to initially use a tight (3 mm) safety J wire (Fig. 12–13).

In some cases, the guide wire will initially pass readily through areas of stricture and thence into the duodenum. In others, hold-up of the guide wire will be encountered at an area of obstruction. In such cases, withdrawal

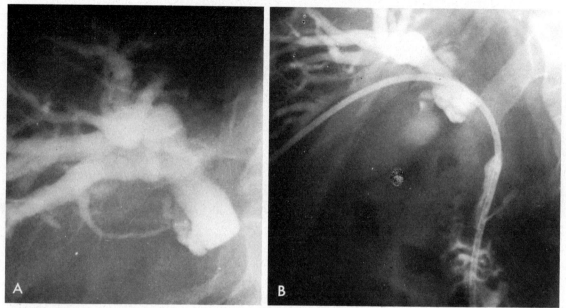

Figure 12–14. *A, B,* "Complete" obstruction on the initial cholangiogram successfully negotiated for internal biliary drainage. Such complete obstruction often represents cholangiographic phenomena rather than actual total occlusions (see also Chapter 9). Diagnosis: carcinoma of the bile duct.

of the guide wire and injection of contrast will provide more complete delineation of the stricture anatomy.

Negotiation of an area of stricture or obstruction by the guide wire is almost invariably successful if the initial cholangiogram shows any passage of contrast into the distal common duct. However, even when a complete obstruction is displayed on the initial cholangiogram, it is not uncommon for the stricture to be successfully negotiated by the guide wire (Figs. 12–14 and 12–15) (see also Chapter 9).

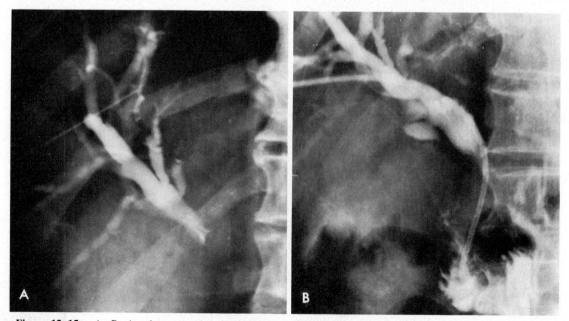

Figure 12–15. *A, B,* Another example of "complete" cholangiographic obstruction in which successful internal drainage was carried out.

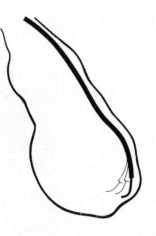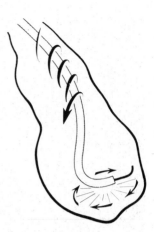

Figure 12–16. Diagnosis: carcinoma of the head of the pancreas. Use of the Ring-Lunderquist wire to search for the lumen when duct dilatation is marked. A rotary motion applied to the external protruding tip of the wire produces a circular searching movement of the wire tip.

At this stage, use of the Ring-Lunderquist memory torque wire with a rotary motion applied to the external protruding end of the wire creates a searching motion, which may be of aid in finding the residual lumen in a dilated duct (Fig. 12–16).

8. When the guide wire has been advanced as far as possible, an appropriate biliary drainage catheter is selected. If the guide wire has passed beyond the stricture, through the ampulla, and into the duodenum, a Ring pigtail catheter is selected. When the guide wire cannot be advanced beyond the stricture, a straight biliary catheter of the Mueller variety is preferred, as its sidehole pattern is more suitable for external drainage. In a few days, attempts can be made to achieve internal drainage and replace the Mueller catheter with a Ring catheter.

9. Catheter insertion can be made over either a Lunderquist-Ring torque wire or a Lunderquist stainless steel guide wire, both of which provide sufficient rigidity and stiffness to support the insertion of the catheter across the liver parenchyma. Conventional 0.38-in. angiographic guide wires are often not firm enough to support biliary catheter insertion.

10. The catheter insertion maneuver requires successive penetration of the abdominal wall, liver capsule, liver parenchyma, and duct wall. Intrinsic resistance of these tissues is overcome by preliminary skin and soft tissue spreading and angiographic vessel dilators, especially if the puncture site on the body wall is thick, fatty, or muscular. Continuous gentle retractile tension on the guide wire as the catheter is advanced, use of a rotary or screw-like motion on the catheter as it is advanced through the liver substance, and use of a tapered-tip catheter as provided by the Ring

and Mueller catheters are also essential. Throughout the catheter insertion maneuver, it is useful to perform continuous fluoroscopic monitoring with an alternate screening of the abdominal wall/liver capsule area and the distal tip of the guide wire to avoid wire/catheter looping and/or loss of distal wire position (Fig. 12–17). These are more likely to occur when there is dense fibrosis or tumor infiltration within the hepatic parenchyma. Use of the stiffest guide wire available will aid in overcoming catheter looping (Fig. 12–18).

Considerable local pain may be experienced

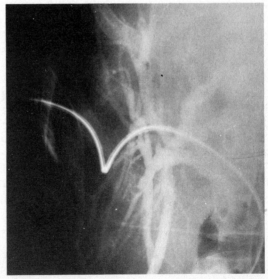

Figure 12–17. Looping of the catheter-guide wire assembly at the liver capsule during catheterization. Increased soft-tissue resistance due to liver parenchymal infiltration and/or duct wall thickening as well as poor catheter purchase may impede further catheter insertion. Use of a Lunderquist stiff steel guide wire will help overcome this problem. (From Ferrucci, J. T., Jr., Mueller, P. R., and Harbin, W. P.: Radiology *135*:1, 1980.)

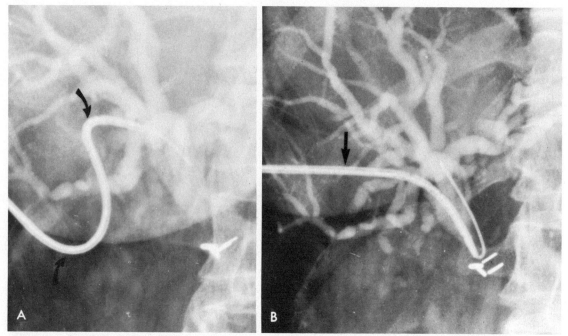

Figure 12–18. Catheter looping corrected by use of a Lunderquist "coat-hanger" wire. *A,* Marked looping. Catheter could not be advanced into duct lumen when using a standard Ring memory torque wire. *B,* Following exchange for the "coat-hanger" wire, sufficient stiffening occurred so that catheter insertion was possible. Note coiled back, long malleable tip of the Lunderquist wire.

during catheter insertion, and booster doses of intravenous analgesics and local lidocaine (Xylocaine) should be administered beforehand. Care should be taken to avoid making more than a single puncture in the liver capsule, with additional passes made without completely retracting the needle. It has been suggested that this maneuver minimizes the likelihood of subsequent bile leak or bleeding.

11. For internal drainage, the 8.3 F Ring biliary catheter is positioned with its tip through the ampulla of Vater in the descending duodenum. The pigtail terminus should be directed toward the third portion of the duodenum to achieve the optimal anchoring effect and minimize subsequent catheter backout due to expiratory excursions. Smaller caliber catheters (4 to 6 F) are not recommended because of their tendency to kink, occlude, or migrate out of position.

12. Catheter position is adjusted so that at least several sideholes are located above the obstruction, as reflected by initial filling of intrahepatic radicles following contrast material injection. If drainage catheters are prepared individually from standard catheter materials, sideholes should be placed through one wall only, spaced according to the anatomic

features of the obstruction and oriented in a spiral. These maneuvers aid drainage and minimize risks of accidental catheter breakage.

13. Acceptable catheter position is confirmed fluoroscopically by complete syringe aspiration of bile and contrast material with resultant decompression of the proximal system. Despite apparently acceptable anatomic placement of the internal catheter, it is not always possible to immediately demonstrate flow of contrast material into the duodenum as a result of ampullary sphincter spasm.

14. When only external drainage can be achieved, it is preferable to use a straight tapered-tip catheter with sideholes located over a shorter catheter length (Mueller catheter). This configuration accommodates the shorter length of drainable duct usually available with complete duct obstructions while still providing adequate decompression of the intrahepatic ducts (Fig. 12–19). In some cases, after several days of external drainage, resolution of inflammatory reaction may permit successful catheterization of the strictured area for conversion to internal drainage. Indeed, in debilitated, elderly, or acutely unstable patients a conservative two-stage procedure may be preferred. External drainage with a straight

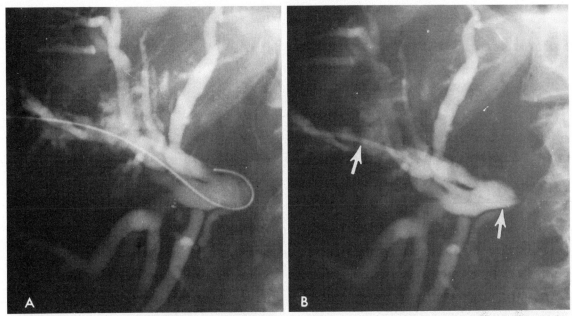

Figure 12–19. External biliary drainage only in complete periportal obstruction due to metastatic lymphadenopathy (presumed and subsequently unproved; patient expired). *A*, The guide wire could not be advanced beyond the obstruction. *B*, A straight multi-side hole catheter specially designed for patients drained externally. (Mueller biliary catheter) is inserted (arrows). Sideholes over a short length of catheter more precisely address the length of drainable duct available. (From Ferrucci, J. T., Jr., Mueller, P. R., and Harbin, W. P.: Radiology *135*:1, 1980.)

catheter is performed on the first day, and on a subsequent sitting the stricture is more readily and more safely negotiated with a guide wire and Ring catheter for internal drainage.

15. The biliary drainage catheter is then fixed to the skin. We prefer to use two pieces of a commercially available Corya adhesive material (Stomahesive) (Fig. 12–20). Alternatively, skin catheter fixation can be accomplished by silk sutures fixed to either an adhesive disk (Molnar) or two strips of surgical adhesive tape pinched against the catheter

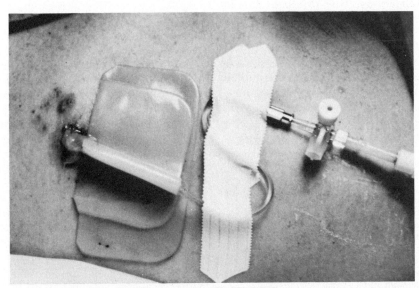

Figure 12–20. Method for catheter skin fixation using Corya (Stomahesive, E. R. Squibb & Co.) strips. An initial strip of Corya is placed on the skin directly. The catheter is then butterfly taped on by a second Corya strip.

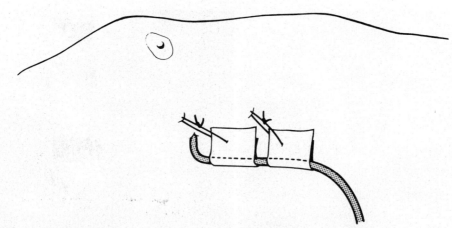

Figure 12–21. Schematic drawing of suture-tape system for fixation of drainage catheter to skin. Two strips of surgical adhesive tape are separately butterfly fastened to catheter and individually sutured to skin. This system prevents catheter back-out by securely fixing catheter at two different sites.

itself and then sutured to the skin (Fig. 12–21). Neither of these techniques is satisfactory, however, as the silk sutures lead to painful skin infections and the disk loses its adhesiveness owing to the lubricating effect of small quantities of leaking bile.

16. A three-way stopcock is connected to standard drainage tubing for easy access during subsequent catheter irrigations. Initial bile samples are collected for culture and cytologic analysis; in 40 per cent of patients with malignant obstruction bile cytology after biliary catheter insertion will yield positive results.

17. The catheter is allowed to drain externally by gravity for three days while the patient is monitored for catheter patency and periprocedural complications. Bile drainage can be collected in a standard T-tube bottle or a urine strap leg plastic bag, which permits more mobility for ambulatory patients.

18. The catheter is clamped on the third or fourth post-procedure day, causing bile to flow in an antegrade manner into the duodenum.

19. Post-procedural care orders are listed in Table 12–5. Most important are 10-ml saline irrigations twice daily. These should be administered gently, especially if the catheter is on external drainage only, since a closed system is involved and the theoretical risk of sepsis following irrigation is higher. Monitoring of bile volume drained and determination of bilirubin, alkaline phosphatase, and electrolytes are also crucial, since external drainage of bile and duodenal contents can result in substantial depletion of both serum sodium and bicarbonate levels, resulting in dehydration and clinical syndromes of electrolyte imbalance. Catheter position can be checked by periodic abdominal radiographs.

Other Techniques

Although the method of percutaneous biliary drainage previously described is the most widely employed, other techniques have been successfully applied by individual groups. Tsuchiya, Ohto, and Ebara from Chiba University, Japan[31] and Makuuchi and coworkers from the University of Tokyo[32] reported real-time ultrasonic guidance for duct localization and cannulation with a single puncture technique. Hawkins also employed a single puncture technique with a specially designed 45-cm long sheathed Chiba needle assembly to introduce a 4 French catheter into the ducts.[33] If the caliber and orientation of the initial duct opacified were favorable, exchange for a larger caliber drainage catheter could be carried out. However, despite their conceptual appeal, sin-

Table 12–5. PERCUTANEOUS BILIARY DRAINAGE—POST-PROCEDURE ORDERS

1. Check vital signs
2. Take chest film
3. Obtain HCT stat
4. Place tube to gravity drainage
5. Determine daily bilirubin and alkaline phosphatase levels
6. Administer antibiotics for three days
7. Measure 24-hour bile drainage
8. Send 24-hour bile sample for cytology/cell block
9. Assess daily electrolytes (hyponatremia)
10. Take KUB every other day
11. Irrigate catheter with 10 ml normal saline b.i.d.

gle puncture techniques suffer from inconsistency of initial duct localization and are not widely employed.

Special Considerations

Conversion to Antegrade Flow

After successful placement of an internal drainage catheter, rerouting of bile from external gravity drainage to antegrade flow into the duodenum finishes the procedure. This maneuver is done by simply closing a three-way stopcock or capping the external protruding hub of the catheter. However, a series of vexing management problems may arise at this stage. An understanding of the physiology of bile production and the dynamics of bile flow are therefore of value.

Physiology of Bile. Normal bile production averages 600 to 800 ml/24 hr and has high electrolyte concentrations, especially sodium and bicarbonates, and a strongly alkaline pH ranging from 7.5 to 9.0.[34, 35] Crucial organic components include bile acids (cholic acid), which solubilize ingested lipids for transmucosal intestinal absorption. The bile acid pool is strictly conserved by the enterohepatic circulation and is nearly completely extracted from portal blood in a single pass through the hepatic parenchyma for re-excretion into the bile. Inavailability of bile acids results in malabsorption and malnutrition.

Although a short period of external biliary drainage (several days) is usually well tolerated, prolonged external biliary diversion produces severe metabolic consequences. Electrolyte depletion, especially hyponatremia, may appear with clinical symptoms of lethargy and altered mental status. Prompt parenteral electrolyte replacement is required. Replacement of wasted bile salts is a more difficult problem, as liquid bile is generally not palatable orally and refeeding of bile requires the creation of either a feeding jejunostomy or gastrostomy. Desiccation or freezing of bile with refeeding offers an acceptable solution. Frozen bile ice cubes crushed and consumed with fruit juice have proved the most acceptable solution in our experience. Unfortunately, only rare patients referred for biliary drainage have a prolonged life expectancy when only external drainage is possible because of a complete bile duct obstruction.

Function of the External/Internal Catheter. Theoretically, the measured daily bile volume collected from an external/internal drainage catheter system placed to gravity represents the overflow residual, with the remainder of bile output assumed to be flowing in a normal antegrade fashion into the bowel. However, evaluation of catheter function at this stage is often complicated by two factors. First, there is often a rather copious postdecompression choleresis with larger volumes of bile produced than under normal conditions. Second, retrograde reflux of duodenal contents frequently occurs with daily volumes of "bile" output often exceeding 1,500 ml. The presence of duodenal contents can be recognized by a more watery appearance and the presence of semisolid particulate matter. Thus, assessment of "successful" internal drainage based on measured bile volumes is difficult. Therefore, despite the theoretical risk of ascending cholangitis due to duodenal reflux, if the patient

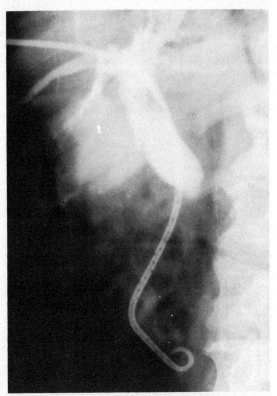

Figure 12–22. Sidehole run-off of injected contrast material allows common duct to fill with no opacification of duodenum. It is impossible to predict whether true obstruction of the catheter is present or not.

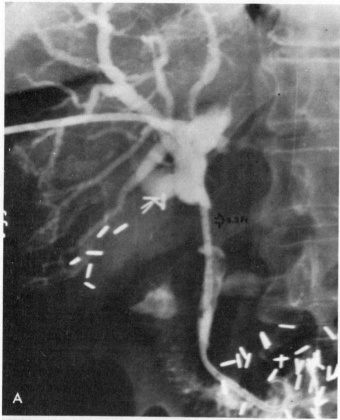

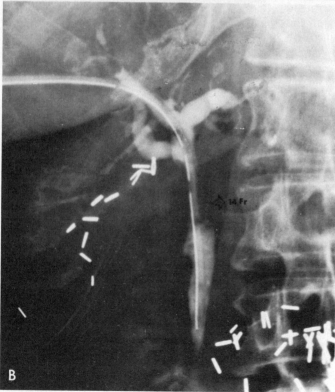

Figure 12–23. *A,* Problem: cholangitis after clamping ideally positioned internal 8.3 F Ring catheter. Diagnosis: periductal lymph node metastases from primary carcinoma of the jejunum. *B,* Solution: exchange for 14 F polyvinyl stomach tube (Argyl) and leave catheter tip in distal common duct rather than across ampulla in duodenum. Larger caliber of tube, larger size of sideholes, and restoration of sphincter of Oddi integrity contribute to improved drainage. Patient tolerated clamping well after exchange. Note diminished caliber of intrahepatic ducts.

with an internal drainage catheter in good position is otherwise doing well, a trial of catheter clamping is routinely carried out on the third or fourth post-procedure day. Should chills, fever, or hypotension occur, prompt unclamping is mandatory.

Post-clamping Cholangitis. Unfortunately, 50 per cent or more of patients with an appropriately positioned internal drainage catheter develop cholangitis after initial clamping, as we have detailed in prior reports.[14]

Contrast injection after unclamping does not usually reveal the cause. Initial low pressure injection of the catheter may show "sidehole run off" with contrast visualized only above the strictured area (Fig. 12–22). Injection with greater pressure carries a greater risk of bacteremic sepsis but occasionally demonstrates contrast material within the duodenum. Removal of the catheter at this stage will not necessarily reveal an obstructing sediment, plug, or debris. We believe that the internal drainage catheter placed through the strictured area accentuates the degree of biliary obstruction, possibly because of the relatively small internal diameter of the commonly used 8.3 French Ring catheter and its rather small caliber sideholes. Further, an externally protruding biliary catheter allows prompt bacterial colonization of the bile. Positive bile cultures can be obtained within 24 hours after PBD. The potential of this combination has been clearly shown in canine studies in which bacteria placed in unobstructed biliary systems have no ill effects, whereas cholangitis and death ensue when even partial obstruction is superimposed.

It is also apparent clinically that patients who drain a large quantity of duodenal contents in the first days after PBD are more susceptible to post-clamping cholangitis. Perhaps duodenal reflux is an indication of sphincter spasm and relative increased intraluminal duodenal pressure with further obstruction of the egress of bile. Patients with distal common duct obstruction from pancreatic head carcinoma tend to have the greatest difficulty with post-clamping cholangitis.

Long-Term Catheter Drainage. In most instances, replacement of the initial 8.3 French drainage catheter with a larger caliber (10 to 14 F) polyvinyl stomach tube (Argyl) provides an effective solution to post-clamping cholangitis (Fig. 12–23). Polyvinyl catheters are well suited for long-term drainage because of their relatively thin walls and soft pliable wall material. Large sideholes may be cut manually and positioned under fluoroscopy to contribute to better drainage. Straight Argyl catheters may be left in the distal common bile duct provided there is sufficient length of normal duct below the stricture. This further decreases duodenal irritation and sphincter spasm and diminishes the likelihood of duodenal reflux. More recently, Silastic biliary drainage tubing has become available commercially.*

Placement of soft long-term drainage catheters is unfortunately not possible at the time of the initial drainage because of intrinsic resistance of liver tissues. However, after initial drainage catheters have been in place for five to seven days, a sufficiently well-formed transparenchymal tract is present, allowing introduction of the softer catheter by a coaxial technique over a 6 or 7 F polyethylene angiographic catheter (Fig. 12–24).

*USCI, Inc., Billerica, MA.

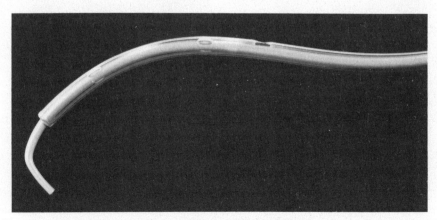

Figure 12–24. Coaxial system for introduction of 10 to 14 F polyvinyl soft wall tube for long-term drainage. The inner, stiffer 7 to 8 F catheter carries the larger catheter in a piggyback fashion.

Both polyvinyl and Silastic catheters may be fashioned as a self-retaining catheter system by forming a crossed limb loop over a suture ligature according to the technique described by Cope (Fig. 12–25).[30] The Cope loop may be formed within the duodenum or within the distal bile ducts (if sufficiently large in caliber) to provide a greater anchor effect than is otherwise available with a straight catheter system.

External Drainage

External drainage is often (and mistakenly) viewed as a "failure" of an attempt at internal drainage and occurs in 20 to 25 per cent of cases, depending on operator expertise and clinical material (Fig. 12–26).[10, 11, 14] Frequently in such cases, dense periportal malignant infiltration causes complete biliary obstruction, and unduly vigorous manipulations result in false passage and bleeding. Further, often only a brief period of palliative drainage can be anticipated. The principal technical concern with external drainage is the lack of stability

of catheter position. Unfortunately, the length of catheter purchase within the biliary ducts in such situations may be minimal (2 to 3 cm or less) and may dispose to dislodgement by simple body movement and respiratory excursions. An effective measure to improve the stability of catheter purchase is to divert the catheter tip from the immediate vicinity of the obstruction and direct it into a more peripheral radicle of either the left or right hepatic duct, significantly lengthening purchase within the lumen of the biliary tree (Fig. 12–27).

Two-Stage Delayed Internal Drainage

It is a sound general rule to refrain from prolonged instrumentation of an obstructed duct system at the initial sitting. In the presence of undecompressed dilated ducts and untreated infected bile, the risks of sepsis, duct perforation, and bile leakage are excessive. Instead, placement of an initial external drainage catheter only should be carried out and followed by a delayed second-stage attempt to catheterize the stricture for internal drainage

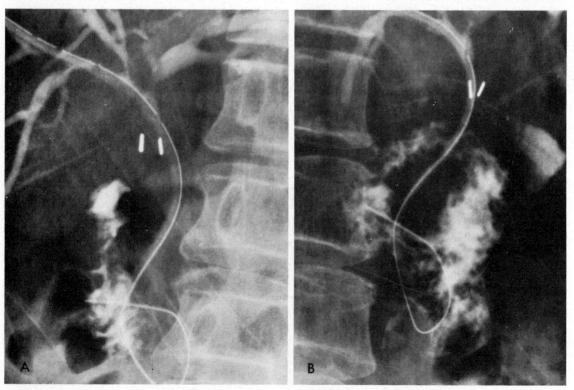

Figure 12–25. *A, B,* Self-retaining crossed limb Cope loop terminus formed with a polyvinyl stomach tube using an inner silk ligature.[30]

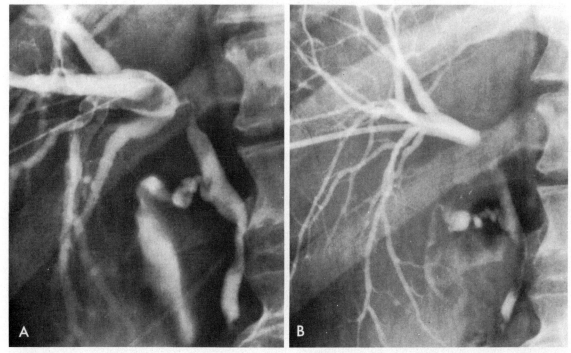

Figure 12–26. External drainage in high periportal obstruction. Diagnosis: cholangiocarcinoma. *A,* Diagnostic cholangiogram. *B,* Drainage catheter placed. Catheter position is relatively unstable owing to a short, 2- to 3-cm length of purchase within the duct lumen. Thus, inadvertent dislodgement is a major concern. Note also the intraluminal clot in the intrahepatic ducts, which is completely lysed on the later study.

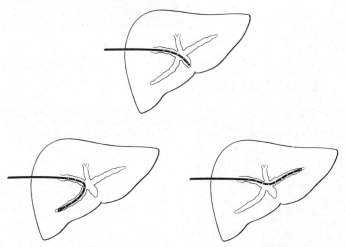

Figure 12–27. Maneuvers to improve catheter stability in high obstruction with external drainage. Direct catheter away from obstruction to left or right duct radicles, lengthening catheter purchase. Risk of inadvertent dislodgement is thereby minimized.

after two to three days of external gravity decompression (Fig. 12–28). This delayed approach minimizes acute morbidity without sacrificing subsequent options. In our institution one-third of cases are now managed in such a fashion. In a few institutions nearly all cases are managed in this fashion, with filming for diagnostic cholangiography postponed until the second sitting. A two-stage approach is especially satisfactory in the presence of marked duct dilatation when the exact position of the residual lumen is unknown and in patients with acute suppurative cholangitis or those who otherwise are medically unstable.

Several factors may account for easier catheterization of the stricture at a delayed second sitting. These include decrease in duct caliber above the obstruction, which straightens the course of the guide wire, directing it into the strictured lumen; resolution of the reactive

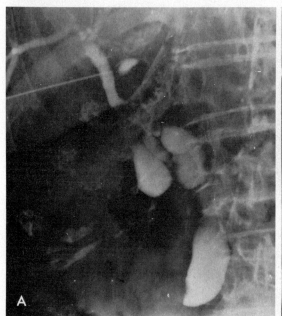

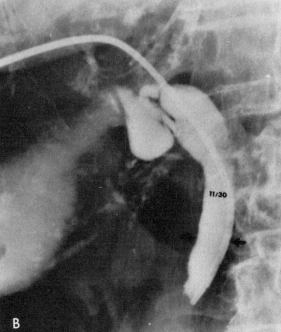

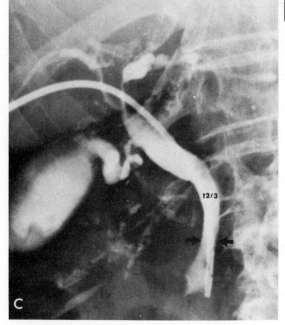

Figure 12–28. Elective two-stage delayed internal drainage is a more conservative, safer approach for elderly or debilitated patients. Diagnosis: carcinoma of the head of the pancreas in a 92-year-old woman. *A,* Diagnostic cholangiogram revealing a tapered complete obstruction of distal common bile duct. *B,* External drainage only with straight (Mueller) biliary drainage catheter on same day. Brief attempts to negotiate guide wire into duodenum were unsuccessful, and further attempts were discontinued in favor of an external catheter. *C,* Repeat cholangiogram four days later showed considerable reduction in bile duct caliber.

Illustration continued on opposite page

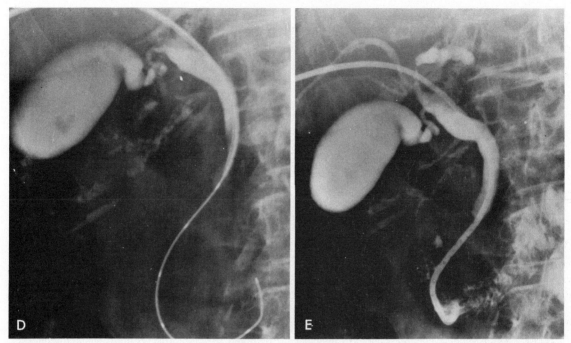

Figure 12–28 *Continued* Guide wire now easily passed through strictured area into duodenum. *E,* Pigtail catheter properly placed for internal drainage. Successful catheterization on the delayed attempt probably represents a combination of resolved edema and more favorable orientation of the guide wire in a small caliber duct lumen.

edema at the site of obstruction; and formation of a transparenchymal tract around the initial drainage catheter, which may facilitate subsequent manipulations.

Periportal Obstruction

Obstructions in the hilus of the liver at the periportal region are often due to malignant disease (cholangiocarcinoma, Klatskin bile duct carcinoma, metastatic lymphadenopathy). Such cases are increasingly being referred for radiologic catheter therapy as a result of the technical difficulty and extreme hazard associated with surgical bypass of intrahepatic duct radicles. The two most common technical issues are the requirement for multiple drainage catheters and the remarkable utility of selective drainage of the left hepatic duct system.

Multiple Drainage Catheters

Periportal obstruction from infiltrating cholangiocarcinoma and metatastic replacement of the liver parenchyma often produce isolated noncommunicating obstructions of multiple separate duct segments. In such cases, effective palliative decompression cannot be achieved unless all major duct segments are drained.

Failing this, cholangitis is highly likely to occur. Although early biliary drainage enthusiasts often placed several separate drainage catheters, subsequent experience suggests that the risks, the difficulty of catheter placement in the face of complicated anatomy, and the low likelihood of prolonged effective palliation should temper enthusiasm when multiple intrahepatic radicles are segmentally obstructed. Indeed, few centers now attempt to place more than two simultaneous drainage catheters (Fig. 12–29).

It is worth noting that when multiple intrahepatic sites of obstruction are present, initial diagnostic cholangiograms often incompletely demonstrate the anatomy, and multiple separate needle punctures are often required to completely delineate the duct anatomy (Fig. 12–30).

Selective Drainage of the Left Duct

Selective obstruction of the left hepatic duct system is a near universal accompaniment to obstructions in the periportal region. The authors recently reviewed this subject, reporting their own experience with selective left-sided catheter decompression in 23 cases.[15]

Data from the surgical literature indicate that the metabolic and clinical sequelae of

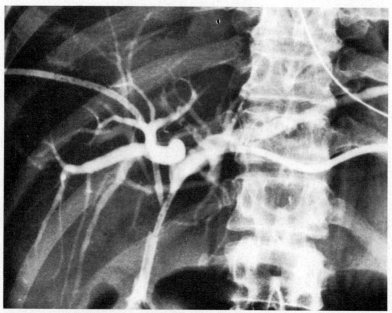

Figure 12–29. Multiple drainage catheters. Simultaneous right and left duct catheters are commonly required to drain separately obstructed noncommunicating duct segments. Diagnosis: cholangiocarcinoma producing periportal obstruction.

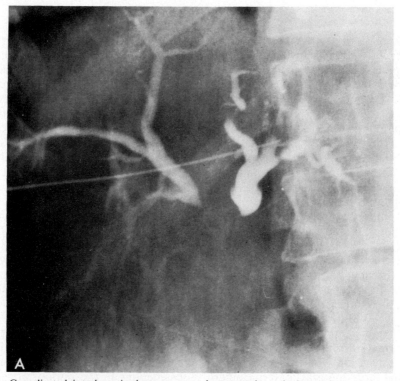

Figure 12–30. Complicated intrahepatic duct anatomy due to periportal obstruction requiring separate selective left-sided fine needle cholangiogram and left duct drainage. Diagnosis: metastatic carcinoma of the ovary to the porta hepatis. *A*, Initial cholangiogram showing opacification of dilated right and left ducts by an infiltrating lesion, producing separate isolated obstruction at the porta hepatis.

Illustration continued on opposite page.

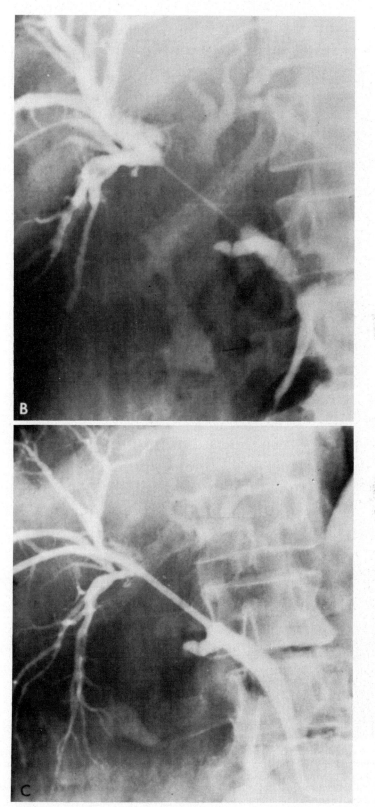

Figure 12–30 *Continued B,* Percutaneous biliary drainage of the right side showing a guide wire placed through the obstruction into a normal-appearing distal common bile duct. *C,* Successful internal drainage of the right hepatic duct with a catheter placed in the distal common bile duct. Notice that there is no filling of the left hepatic duct from the right side, indicating complete, separate, isolated obstruction.
duct from the left side.

Illustration continued on following page.

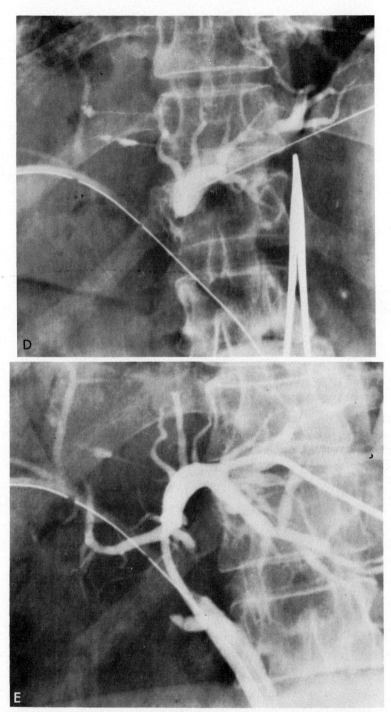

Figure 12–30 *Continued* *D,* Selective wire inserted for left-sided PBD. *E,* Selective left-sided fine needle transhepatic cholangiography performed several days after percutaneous drainage of the right side. Notice the dilated tortuous left hepatic duct with a high grade obstruction at the porta hepatis and no filling of the right system. *E,* Selective internal catheter drainage of the left side carried out with two separate internal drainage catheters well positioned for complete palliative decompression. (Reproduced with permission from Mueller, P. R., and Ferrucci, J. T., Jr.: Radiology, in press 1982.)

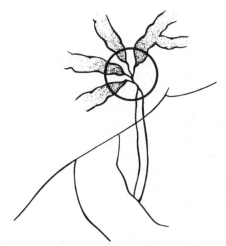

Figure 12–31. Critical locus of tumor infiltration at the porta hepatis separately obstructs multiple successive subdivisions of the right duct, whereas the entire left duct system is obstructed at a single point. Separate catheters will be required for each subdivision of the right duct, whereas a single catheter will drain the entire left duct.(Reproduced with permission from Mueller, P. R., Ferrucci, J. T., Jr., and vanSonnenberg, E.: Radiology, in press. 1982.)

ious surgical procedures have been employed for a bypass of either the right or left hepatic ducts in the presence of high periportal obstruction. At present, use of the left hepatic duct for cholangiojejunostomy (Bismuth procedure) is generally considered safer and more effective than drainage of the right ducts by surgical authorities.[36] Similarly, clinical and anatomic considerations suggest that selective catheter drainage of the left hepatic duct is equally valuable.

Fundamental anatomic differences between the left and right hepatic ductal systems exist. In particular, the left duct gives off fewer major segmental radicles than the right and thus enters the confluence at the porta as a single large lumen biliary duct. Consequently, infiltrating portal neoplasms invariably cause obstruction of the entire left duct system by occlusion at a single point near the hilus (Fig. 12–31). On the other hand, because several segmental ramifications of the right hepatic system arise simultaneously at the confluence, an infiltrating periportal tumor often separately obstructs and isolates several successive segments. This precludes successful catheter decompression unless each obstructed radicle is separately drained. Further, the left duct follows a long extrahepatic course, which al-

biliary obstruction can be effectively palliated even if only one-third of the hepatic parenchyma is adequately decompressed. Thus, var-

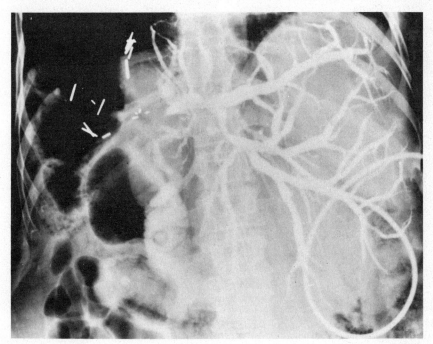

Figure 12–32. Selective left-sided catheter drainage in a patient with obstruction of a markedly hypertrophied left duct, which developed following a right hepatectomy for metastatic renal cell carcinoma. This case illustrates the capability of the liver to undergo regenerative hypertrophy after resection or destruction of liver tissue. Metastatic replacement of the right lobe may result in marked enlargement of the left duct system, facilitating palliative drainage procedures.

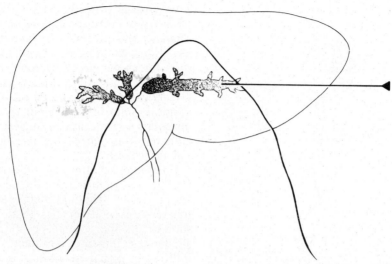

Figure 12–33. Technique for selective left hepatic cholangiogram. Needle puncture is performed from left subcostal area horizontally across epigastrium. Drainage catheter insertion is performed in similar fashion. (Reproduced with permission from Mueller, P. R., Ferrucci, J. T., Jr., and vanSonnenberg, E.: Radiology, in press. 1982.)

lows it to dilate to a greater degree than the right duct since it is rarely compressed or encased by infiltrating tumor. The resulting elongation and tortuosity that occur make the left duct an ideal candidate for catheter insertion or surgical anastomosis. Finally, with complete destruction of the right lobe, marked chronic compensatory hypertrophy of the left lobe occurs and can produce an enormously enlarged left duct should secondary obstruction supervene (Fig. 12–32). It is this contrasting potential for greater early selective obstruc-

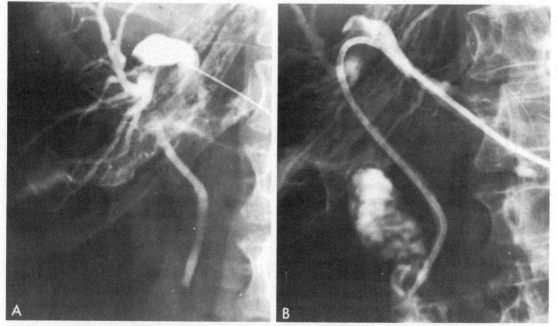

Figure 12–34. Selective internal drainage of the left hepatic duct system. Approach made from the left side. *A*, Initial diagnostic cholangiogram via selective puncture of the left hepatic duct showing a lobulated mass obstructing the lumen at the origin of the left main duct. Biliary radicles draining the right lobe are of normal caliber. *B*, Left duct cholangiogram following selective internal drainage showing the catheter through the lesion into the duodenum. Diagnosis: metastatic carcinoma of the colon. Pathologic confirmation obtained by cytologic analysis of bile aspirated after completion of the drainage procedure.

tion and dilatation of the left duct that allows for its preferential use as a surgical or radiologic drainage route in high periportal obstructions.

Technical steps for performing selective cholangiography and left-sided catheter drainage are analogous to those procedures performed on the right duct system.[15] The principal modifications in technique include the use of an anterior horizontal subxiphoid approach for diagnostic needle puncture and catheter inser-

tion (Fig. 12–33). Reversing the patient's position on the fluoroscopic table usually simplifies the logistics by more readily exposing the left upper chest to the operator's view. Preliminary ultrasonographic or CT localization of the dilated left duct with placement of a skin ink marker greatly facilitates selection of the site for skin puncture entry. Several illustrative cases are demonstrated in Figures 12–34 through 12–36.

On occasion, selective drainage of the left

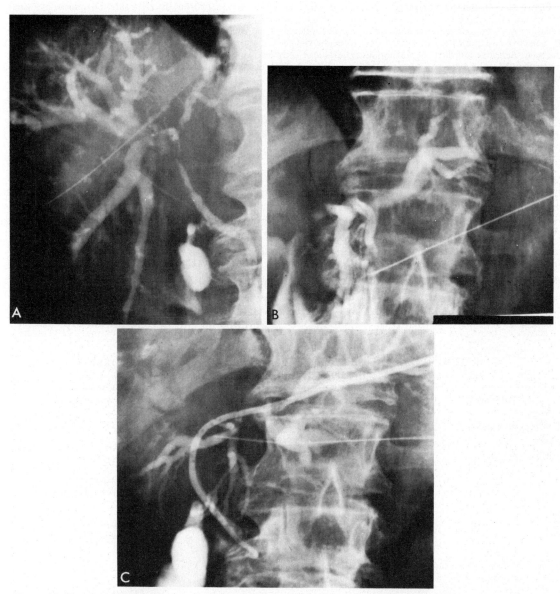

Figure 12–35. Selective left duct drainage for infiltrating hilar cholangiocarcinoma with isolated obstruction of left duct. *A*, Diagnostic fine-needle cholangiogram performed from the right. Notice that the left duct system is not filled. *B*, Selective left duct cholangiogram performed from the left side revealing marked obstructive dilatation of the left duct with no filling of the right side. *C*, Selective catheter drainage of the left duct performed from the left.

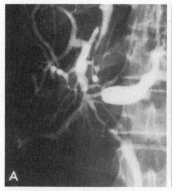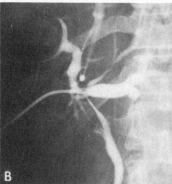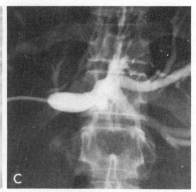

Figure 12–36. Selective drainage of the left hepatic duct. Approach made from the right side. Diagnosis: metastatic carcinoma of the breast. *A,* Initial diagnostic cholangiogram showing diffuse metastatic replacement of the right lobe, encasement of the common hepatic duct in the porta hepatis, and isolated obstructive dilatation of the left main duct. *B,* Selective catheterization of the left duct from the right side. Approach made across the confluence of right and left ducts. *C,* Selective left duct cholangiogram via drainage catheter. Note marked enlargement of the left lobe consequent to metastatic replacement of the right lobe (see Fig. 12–32). (From Ferrucci, J. T., Jr., Mueller, P. R., and Harbin, W. P.: Radiology *135*:1, 1980.)

system may be accomplished from a right-sided approach by advancing catheters across the hilus into the left duct (Fig. 12–36).[15] The principal disadvantage of this approach is that successful internal drainage is often more difficult because of the acute right angle bend as wires and catheters pass caudally into the extrahepatic ducts.

The principal disadvantage of left-sided biliary drainage is the considerable radiation dose to the operator's hand, since catheter and wire manipulations are done over the anterior epigastrium. Meticulous measures for reducing radiation dose are therefore of critical importance.

Catheter Malfunction: Detection/Management

There are many manifestations of biliary catheter malfunction, and their onset may be sudden or gradual. Radiologists performing diagnostic procedures must accept full responsibility for their diagnosis and treatment. Table 12–6 presents the most common problems, causes, and corrective measures.

Catheter Occlusion. The most common cause of catheter occlusion is blockage of the catheter lumen, usually by detritus/encrustations, tumor ingrowth, or clot. Clinical manifestations include sepsis, unrelieved jaundice,

Table 12–6. POST-PROCEDURE CATHETER CARE: COMMON PROBLEMS AND THEIR MANAGEMENT

Problem	Cause	Correction
Bleeding per catheter	Sideholes extraductal → open to liver vascular system → backbleeding	Reposition
Catheter dislodged		Direct reinsertion
Sepsis	1. Catheter occluded* 2. Transampullary catheter placement not tolerated → ascending cholangitis	1. Exchange catheter 2. Withdraw to distal CBD
Unrelieved jaundice	1. Catheter occluded 2. Sideholes too distal 3. Progressive liver failure	1. Exchange catheter 2. Withdraw as required
Drainage of duodenal contents → electrolyte loss	Excessive number of sideholes in duodenum → retrograde reflux	Withdraw to ampulla
Injected contrast does not flow into duodenum	Contrast run-off via proximal sideholes (differential diagnosis: catheter occluded)	Exchange only if clinically malfunctioning

*Signs of catheter occlusion—sepsis, persistent jaundice, leakage of bile around catheter.

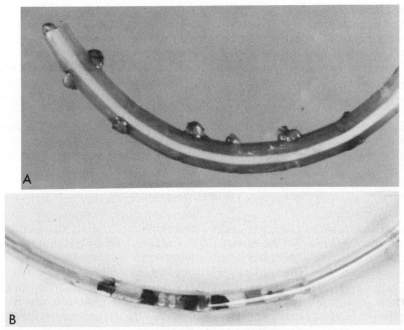

Figure 12–37. Drainage catheters removed because of signs of obstruction. Two different patients, both with 12 French polyvinyl feeding tubes. *A,* Tumor ingrowth protrudes from multiple side holes. *B,* Multiple concretion-encrustations occlude lumen three weeks after insertion. (From Ferrucci, J. T., Jr., Mueller, P. R., and Harbin, W. P.: Radiology *135*:1, 1980.)

or leakage of bile into the skin dressings. Injection of contrast material under fluoroscopic guidance is generally necessary to delineate the problem. If injected contrast does not flow distally, suction on the catheter may deliver a blood clot or passage of a guide wire may dislodge the obstructing material. Usually, however, prompt catheter exchange over a guide wire is a more definitive measure for dealing with catheter occlusion. Examples of detritus and tumor occlusion are illustrated in Figure 12–37.

Figure 12–38. Back bleeding through the catheter. Gross blood emerging during or after catheter placement indicates inappropriate positioning of a side hole within a major hepatic or portal venous channel. *A,* Initial spot radiograph taken when gross blood appeared during catheter insertion. *B,* Injection of contrast material demonstrates venous opacification (arrows). Prompt advancement of the catheter, placing sideholes within the duct lumen, terminates bleeding. (From Ferrucci, J. T., Jr., Mueller, P. R., and Harbin, W. P.: Radiology *135*:1, 1980.)

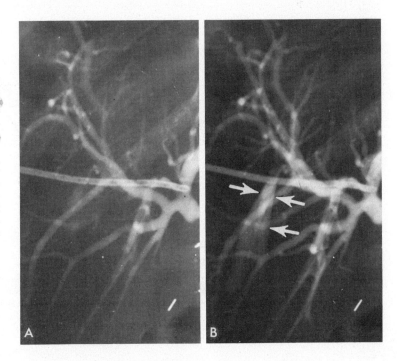

Bleeding per Catheter. The appearance of gross blood via the catheter usually reflects inadvertent positioning of a proximal sidehole within a major hepatic or portal venous channel. The venous communication can be confirmed by injection of contrast material and corrected by advancing the catheter under fluoroscopic control (Fig. 12–38). Backbleeding is most likely to occur during initial catheter insertion but may develop in the postprocedure period if the catheter backs out of position as a result of respiratory excursions or patient movement. Fatal exsanguination has occurred when the cause of such backbleeding has not been recognized.

Catheter backbleeding is most likely to occur in a duct system where purchase of the catheter is rather short, leaving only a minimal intraluminal length of sideholes. Thus, a patient with a vertical orientation of intrahepatic ducts is more vulnerable to this type of complication (Fig. 12–39). Obviously, if advancement of the catheter is required several days after the initial insertion, the external portion of the catheter is no longer sterile and a fresh catheter will have to be employed, with the insertion carried out with complete sterile technique.

Unrelieved Jaundice. Persistent or recurrent hyperbilirubinemia may reflect catheter occlusion, inappropriate distal position of the proximal sideholes preventing drainage of the intrahepatic ducts, or progressive liver failure due to tumor replacement or severe postobstructive parenchymal damage. Failure of injected contrast material to provide initial opacification of the intrahepatic radicles indicates inappropriately distal sideholes (Figs. 12–40 and 12–41). A frequent associated observation is the large volume of duodenal contents refluxing into the drainage receptacle. This is presumed to result from too many sideholes in communication with the duodenal lumen, allowing retrograde reflux of intestinal secretions during periods of active duodenal peristalsis. During these periods, intraluminal duodenal pressures are presumed to transiently rise above the secretory pressure of bile flow in the common duct. Fluoroscopic withdrawal for repositioning is usually straightforward.

Catheter Dislodgement. Inadvertent dislodgement of the indwelling catheter is an uncommon, albeit discouraging, occurrence. However, direct reinsertion through the original cutaneous puncture site is often feasible. After seven to ten days of catheter drainage, a granulating transparenchymal tract forms, usually 2 F larger in caliber than the outer diameter of the catheter itself (Fig. 12–42).[8, 10, 11] The tract will not seal over for 48 to 72 hours and can usually be re-entered primarily, provided the cutaneous entry site can be lined up with the entry point through the liver capsule (Fig. 12–43).

Gordon and coworkers recommend a fluoroscopically guided contrast sinogram via a conical adaptor placed in the cutaneous entry

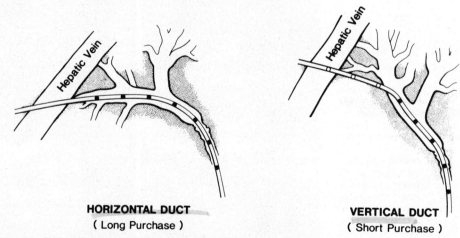

HORIZONTAL DUCT
(Long Purchase)

VERTICAL DUCT
(Short Purchase)

Figure 12–39. Horizontal versus vertical biliary duct configuration. The horizontal configuration is far more favorable for initial duct cannulation, as a longer length of drainage duct is available, assuring adequate purchase for subsequent guide wire–catheter exchanges. The horizontal right duct also provides a safety margin *vis a vis* position of side holes within the bile duct lumen as opposed to hepatic parenchyma. Minimal catheter back-out of a vertical duct places sideholes in potential communication with hepatic venous channels, which could lead to massive back bleeding. Awareness of this anatomic variation helps anticipate complications.

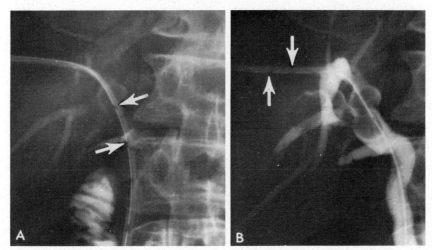

Figure 12–40. Unrelieved jaundice due to catheter malposition. Inappropriate distal location of proximal side holes prevents drainage of intrahepatic ducts. *A,* Initial cholangiogram via a polyvinyl feeding tube. Hyperbilirubinemia persisted on the eleventh postoperative day. Note caudal position of sideholes (arrows) and no filling of intrahepatic ducts. *B,* Cholangiogram after several centimeter withdrawal of the catheter, showing sideholes positioned in the area of the intrahepatic ducts (arrows) and better filling of the proximal system above a lobulated tumor obstructing the common hepatic duct. (From Ferrucci, J. T., Jr., Mueller, P. R., and Harbin, W. P.: Radiology *135*:1, 1980.)

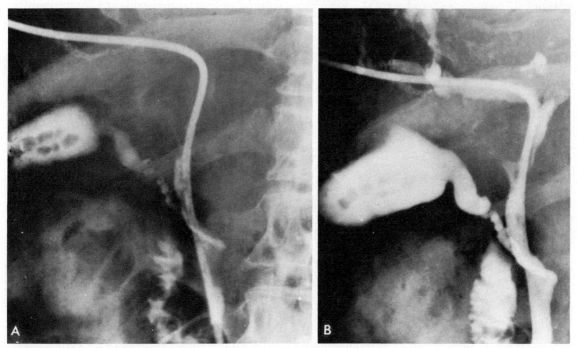

Figure 12–41. Unrelieved jaundice due to inappropriate caudal positioning of sideholes. *A,* Initial catheter injection showing no filling of intrahepatic ducts. *B,* Repeat cholangiogram after catheter is withdrawn several centimeters. Better filling of intrahepatic ducts denotes improved sidehole position for decompression.

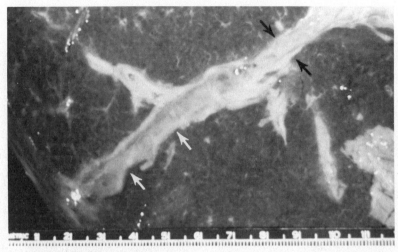

Figure 12–42. Transparenchymal catheter tract (white arrows) extending from a biliary radicle (black arrows) to the liver capsule. Necropsy dissection of the liver was made after six weeks of indwelling biliary catheter drainage. Pericatheter hepatic necrosis and inflammatory response create a tract at least 2 F larger than the caliber of the indwelling catheter. This tract allows direct catheter reinsertion should dislodgement occur. (From Ferrucci, J. T., Jr., Mueller, P. R., and Harbin, W. P.: Radiology *135*:1, 1980.)

site to aid in locating and opacifying the transhepatic tract.[37] Guide wire/catheter systems are then inserted under direct fluoroscopic control. Cope used a small 4 F caliber endoscope to replace drain catheters.[38] We prefer to insert a sheath from an 18-gauge needle directly through the skin entry and into the liver for easy insertion of a guide wire (Fig. 12–44).

Catheter Exchanges. Secondary catheter

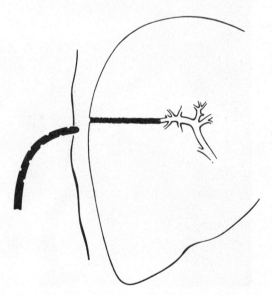

Figure 12–43. Replacement of fallen out biliary catheter can be accomplished by lining up skin opening with liver capsule opening. Direct fluoroscopic contrast opacification of the tract can be carried out via any soft catheter inserted into the skin opening, followed by introduction of a guide wire into the tract.

manipulations or catheter exchanges are required in nearly all cases, especially during prolonged periods of catheter drainage. Ring and associates[8] carried out routine prophylactic exchanges at three-month intervals; we prefer to await indications of catheter dysfunction. In a study of our own results, we found that 27/67 or 40 per cent of patients discharged after PBD required a subsequent tube change.[14] In most cases, these manipulations can be performed on an outpatient basis in less than one hour. A short course of oral broad spectrum antibiotic therapy is given routinely. Patients who present with active sepsis are admitted to the hospital, and catheter exchange is carried out under parenteral antibiotic coverage.

It is assumed that long-term catheter patency is related to the caliber of the catheter and size of the sideholes; therefore, catheter exchanges are generally made to a larger size (10 to 12 F) Argyl polyvinyl catheter (Figs. 12–6 and 12–23). This softer, more flexible material has proved more comfortable in terms of drawing and pulling at the skin level for patients who remain moderately active. Alternatively, some institutions prefer an indwelling stent endoprosthesis for long-term drainage. The merits and drawbacks of this approach are discussed in more detail hereafter.

The Biliary Catheter: Nursing Care

Careful attention to details of catheter care, including instructions to the patient, family,

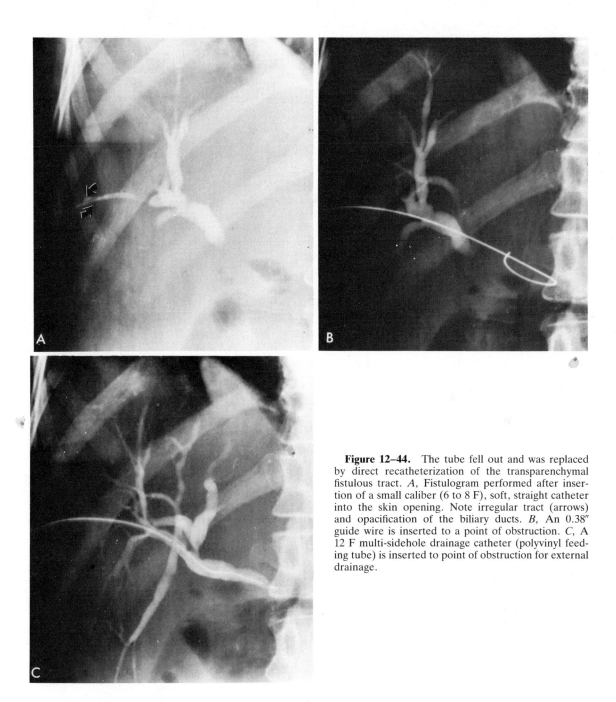

Figure 12–44. The tube fell out and was replaced by direct recatheterization of the transparenchymal fistulous tract. *A,* Fistulogram performed after insertion of a small caliber (6 to 8 F), soft, straight catheter into the skin opening. Note irregular tract (arrows) and opacification of the biliary ducts. *B,* An 0.38″ guide wire is inserted to a point of obstruction. *C,* A 12 F multi-sidehole drainage catheter (polyvinyl feeding tube) is inserted to point of obstruction for external drainage.

and/or visiting nurses, is a vital element for successful long-term catheter drainage after discharge.[11]

Most patients are discharged with the catheter fixed to the skin by Corya (Stomahesive) or a plastic disk, fitted with a three-way stopcock for saline irrigation and covered with dry sterile dressing. Dressings should be changed every two to three days as required by leakage and soiling. Each patient has different skin reactions to bile and sensitivity to tape, but biliary patients are no different from other patients with ostomy bags and many types of skin care products, tapes, and bags are available.

Several specific points of care should be stressed.

1. Patients should bathe by shower, not tub.

2. Skin cleansing of the catheter area can be performed with hydrogen peroxide and bacitracin ointment.

3. Patients should be reminded to protect their catheter from inadvertently catching on clothing, leading to dislodgement.

4. Patients should be taught to irrigate their catheter with saline.

A list of do's and don'ts for the routine care of the catheter should be given to the patient. This is simply a reminder of the procedures to be followed for routine care and also provides instructions for emergency situations including visits to the department for catheter changes.

Care of Your Bile Duct Catheter

You have been instructed by our nursing staff regarding care of your bile duct catheter. This check list will help to remind you of the measures necessary to keep it draining freely with the least discomfort to you.

1. Dressing change: This should be done whenever the dressing appears wet, stained, or crusted. Otherwise, change it every third day. Topper sponge pads and adhesive paper tape can be obtained at your drug store.

2. Irrigate the catheter with sterile saline solution 10 ml once a day or every other day as you were instructed. A new supply of sterile saline and syringes may be obtained from your drugstore or our nurse. We will provide the prescription needed to purchase syringes.

3. Protect your tube! It was inserted at some discomfort, risk, and effort. Keep it well taped and covered with the dressing so that it is not accidentally caught or pulled out on your clothes.

4. Showering is permissible, but do not tub bathe. You should attempt to protect the dressing area by covering it with waterproof material such as a plastic bag or Saran wrap.

---

5. From time to time your tube may need to be changed owing to plugging, blockage, or infection. Therefore, if you develop chills, fever, sweats, jaundice, or leakage around the catheter or into the dressing, contact us without delay. The tube change can be done on an outpatient basis in less than 30 minutes.

Biliary catheter patients tend to become strongly attached to their radiology physician/nurse team, and repeated social visits, telephone calls, and regular outpatient visits are common. In a busy biliary interventional service a special treatment room for ambulatory care may be required for the personal attention necessary. The gratitude of these patients is often freely expressed.

Results

Results of PBD can be assessed at several levels.

Clinical/Metabolic Response to PBD

The initial response to biliary decompression is predictable and often dramatic (Table 12–7). Gravely ill patients with cholangitis and liver abscess may defervesce within 12 to 18 hours, with a diminished requirement for fluids and pressors.[7, 10, 11] Documented liver abscesses proximal to obstructions may show cholangiographic evidence of healing within days (Fig. 12–45).[7, 10] Serum bilirubin levels may drop precipitously, often by as much as 2 to 3 mg per cent/24 hr in the immediate post-drainage period. Net bilirubin declines of 10 to 20 points are not uncommon over a longer period, although the final level of serum bilirubin may remain above normal owing to underlying parenchymal damage or coexistent neoplastic infiltration. Ferrucci, Mueller, and Harbin found that post-procedure bilirubin levels returned to normal in almost 25 per cent of cases.[10] Coinciding with these objective parameters is often a striking subjective response in terms

Table 12–7. RESPONSE TO PERCUTANEOUS DRAINAGE

Bilirubin ↓ —often by 2 mg per cent/24 hr
Fever ↓ —often within 12 hr
Liver shrinks
Function tests improve
Subjective—relief of pruritus and anorexia

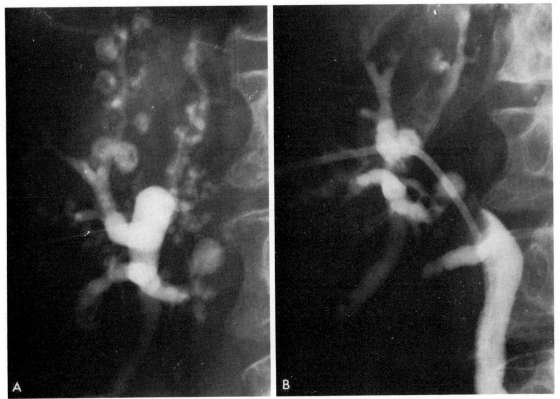

Figure 12–45. Resolution of multiple hepatic abscesses following internal biliary drainage. The patient was a 73-year-old man presenting with signs of acute suppurative cholangitis. *A,* Initial FNTC, revealing multiple, rounded collections of contrast material filling from dilated intrahepatic radicles. There was no flow beyond the confluence. Internal biliary catheter stent drainage was carried out (not shown). Antibiotics were administered. *B,* Follow-up cholangiogram via the catheter on the fourth post-procedural day, showing nearly complete resolution of the intrahepatic abscesses. An obstructing intraluminal mass defect is evident in the common hepatic duct. Defervescence occurred within 18 hours after catheter drainage. The diagnosis of hepatoma was subsequently established by percutaneous fine-needle aspiration biopsy. (From Ferrucci, J. T., Jr., Mueller, P. R., and Harbin, W. P.: Radiology *135*:1, 1980.)

of relief of pruritus and anorexia and an improved sense of well-being. It is noteworthy that reocclusion of a previously placed catheter is often heralded by clinical recurrence of malaise followed by chills and fever.

Rate of Successful Catheterization

Technical success rates for catheter placement obviously vary with operator experience, case selection, instrumentation, and technique. We reviewed the experience in 200 cases treated in our hospital, currently the largest reported series to date; successful catheterization was achieved in 94 per cent of cases, with internal drainage established in 72 per cent (Table 12–8).[14] These results reflect a large general hospital experience with procedures performed by radiologists at varying levels of training. Similar success rates have been recorded by Berquist and associates from the Mayo Clinic[12] and Clark and colleagues from Cincinnati.[13]

Long-Term Results

Long-term results are more difficult to quantitate. It is generally apparent that patients

Table 12–8. PERCUTANEOUS BILIARY DRAINAGE RESULTS*

Successful	188	= 94%
Internal	144	= 72%
External	44	= 22%
Failure	12	= 6%

*200 cases (188 patients) at Massachusetts General Hospital.
Note: 67 of 188 patients left hospital.

Table 12–9. PERCUTANEOUS BILIARY DRAINAGE—CLINICAL OUTCOME*

Discharged from hospital (without surgery)	67
Operation performed	66
Endoprosthesis inserted	15
In-hospital death (any cause)	40

*200 cases (188 patients) at Massachusetts General Hospital.

with advanced malignancy experience effective palliation in the majority of instances. At the Mayo Clinic, Berquist and coworkers found successful palliation in 88 per cent of patients with malignant obstruction.[12] Many patients who have been deemed medically or technically unsuitable for surgical bypass have undergone catheter drainage, which has then been supplemented by adjuvant irradiation and chemotherapy, and have been able to return to an active life, returning only for outpatient treatment. As noted in Table 12–9, of 188 patients completing PBD in our series, 67 or 36 per cent were discharged from the hospital without surgery.[14] Undoubtedly, a significant percentage of these patients would have promptly succumbed to their illness without radiologic catheter decompression. Nevertheless, overall operative mortality (death within 30 days from any cause) for this gravely ill group of patients is substantial, ranging from 11.9 to 31.5 per cent.[16-22] As noted in Table 12–9, 40 of our 188 patients completing PBD succumbed in the hospital.

Data on net survival comparing radiology and surgery are not yet available, as no controlled studies of similar groups of patients have ever been performed. At present, cases referred for radiologic drainage tend to be those declined by surgical consultants. Nevertheless, regardless of mode of therapy, it appears that the initial disease process remains the principal determinant of long-term prognosis. Thus, the six-month life expectancy of patients with pancreatic carcinoma is unlikely to be affected. Indeed, Berquist and colleagues found an average survival of only 39 days in 20 patients with pancreatic carcinoma, whereas patients with carcinoma of the bile ducts and gallbladder had average survival times of 272 and 324 days, respectively.[12] In our series, a number of patients with carcinoma of the bile ducts or gallbladder and several with metastatic lesions sensitive to irradiation or chemotherapy have survived one to two years.

Complications

Acute and chronic complications are listed in Table 12–10.

Acute Complications

Major acute complications occur in 5 to 10 per cent of patients[10–14] and include intra-abdominal hemorrhage, sepsis, and bile leakage with peritonitis. Hemobilia, pancreatitis, pneumothorax, and hepatic traumatic AV fistula and pseudo-aneurysm occur less often. Fatal complications have been reported in several series,[14] and in Mueller's series of 200 cases from our institution there were three postprocedure deaths. Measures to reduce acute major complications are given in Table 12–11.

Bile leakage and bile peritonitis are greatly reduced in frequency if successful catheter insertion has been accomplished. Thus, many centers routinely employ prophylactic PBD following diagnostic cholangiography when obstruction has been demonstrated. Bile peritonitis is usually a major clinical event, commonly occurring within a few hours after duct puncture and characterized by severe upper right quadrant abdominal pain, fever, and prostration. Principal measures to avoid bile leakage include creation of only a single puncture site in the liver capsule and avoidance of puncturing the extrahepatic portion of the bile

Table 12–10. COMPLICATIONS OF CATHETERIZATION

Acute
Bile leakage
Hemorrhage
Sepsis
Death
Hemobilia

Chronic
Cholangitis
Catheter occlusion
  Leakage around catheter
  Recurrent jaundice
  Fever
Catheter dislodgement
Skin infection
Subphrenic abscess
Hepatic AV fistula, pseudo-aneurysm
Empyema
Tumor growth along catheter tract
Antibiotic toxicity

Table 12–11. MEANS TO REDUCE SERIOUS COMPLICATIONS OF CATHETERIZATION

Bile Leak
  Make single puncture site in capsule
  Avoid puncture of extrahepatic ducts

Bleeding
  Carefully position sideholes
  Avoid buckling of catheter
  Occlude tract if catheter removed

Sepsis
  Restrict volume of contrast injection
  Restrict manipulation of catheter in suppurative
    cholangitis
  Start antibiotic prophylaxis

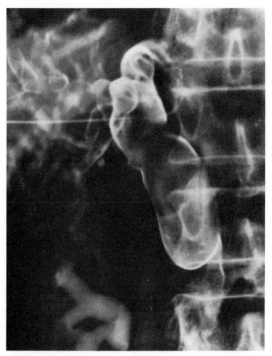

Figure 12–46. Massive blood cast filling entire duct system (hemobilia). Moderate distention of system is also evident. This film was taken after several unsuccessful attempts at insertion of the drainage catheter, which were accompanied by bloody bile returns via catheter. Successful drainage was subsequently established. Following saline irrigation for 24 hours, clear flow of bile began. Diagnosis: pancreatic carcinoma.

duct, where there is no surrounding protective effect of hepatic parenchyma to tamponade bile leakage.

Free intraperitoneal bleeding can occur from needle laceration of an extrahepatic vessel or from an intrahepatic vessel bleeding via the needle tract. Routine deposition of Gelfoam particles has been advocated to reduce the risk of late bleeding; we have not employed this maneuver. External hemorrhage via the catheter may occur if sideholes are inadvertently positioned outside the bile duct lumen in communication with major venous channels. Careful fluoroscopic monitoring of sidehole position at the conclusion of a catheter placement will minimize the risk of inadvertent catheter back-bleeding.

Septicemia (demonstrated by positive blood cultures and hypotension) most commonly occurs in patients who have infected bile or who are febrile prior to the procedure. Careful restriction of the volume of injected contrast material and the amount of catheter manipulation, combined with preprocedure antibiotic prophylaxis, is an effective means of reducing septic complications.

Hemobilia is perhaps more of a technical observation than a frank complication, but it can be a dramatic episode. Acute bleeding into the lumen of the bile duct may occur during the trauma of initial catheterization or as a result of sidehole communication with a major hepatic venous channel (Figs. 12–26 and 12–38). Often, large blood casts are visible within the ducts, greatly distending and obturating the duct lumen (Fig. 12–46).[11, 14, 39] In such cases, the flow of bile through the catheter ceases, and if catheter placement has not yet been completed it may be difficult to determine whether a catheter position within the duct

lumen is satisfactory. Injection of contrast or insertion of guide wires in a testing fashion will usually be necessary. Because the blood casts may obstruct the bile duct and/or the drainage catheter, regular irrigations with 10 ml of normal saline are performed on a one- to 2-hour basis for 12 to 24 hours (Fig. 12–47). Despite a significant amount of thrombus within the ducts, lysis can be anticipated within 24 hours, and a flow of clear bile will usually resume. Should thrombus occlusion persist, a catheter exchange will obviously be required.

Delayed Complications

Delayed complications are unfortunately common, occurring in 40 to 50 per cent of patients and usually related to catheter malfunction[14] (see Catheter Malfunction). Cholangitis has been the most common problem, occurring in 20 to 40 per cent of patients; frank catheter occlusion, catheter dislodgement, and local skin irritation are also frequent

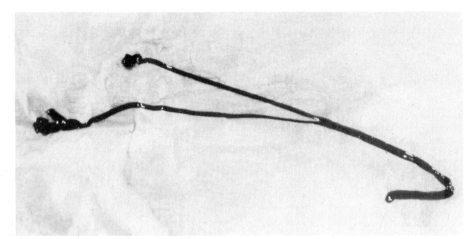

Figure 12–47. Elongated clot recovered from drainage catheter during saline irrigations for hemobilia.

occurrences. Late subphrenic abscess, hepatic AV fistula or pseudo-aneurysm (Fig. 12–48), empyema, and tumor growth along the catheter tract onto the skin surface have also been reported.[40]

SECONDARY PROCEDURES

Endoprosthesis

Disadvantages of a permanently protruding biliary drainage catheter have prompted several groups to employ an indwelling stent endoprosthesis.[41-47] Cited drawbacks of the drainage catheter include frequent malfunction due to occlusion or migration, bacterial colonization and subsequent secondary suppurative cholangitis, local pain at the skin entry point, catheter dislodgement, and the disturbing psychological impact of a permanent externally protruding device.

The indwelling endoprosthesis does not have these negative aspects; the patient is discharged from the hospital with no residual protruding device; typical appearances are shown in Figure 12–49.

Insertion of the endoprosthesis is carried out

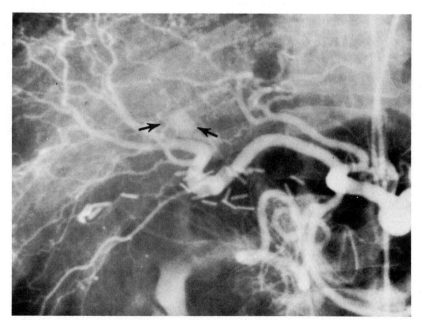

Figure 12–48. Hepatic pseudo-aneurysms following biliary drainage. Angiogram was performed for staging prior to pancreatic resection six days following a moderately difficult catheter insertion. Patient was clinically well.

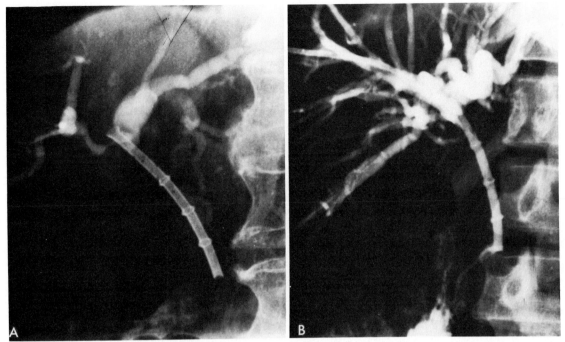

Figure 12–49. *A, B,* Typical appearance of endoprosthesis in two different cases. Note the ridges to prevent irrigation, sideholes to assure effective bile flow, and a proximal flange to facilitate insertion.

as a secondary derivative procedure after initial successful internal PBD. However, insertion of the endoprosthesis is a technically more complex procedure, and the long-term patency rate is yet to be established. Furthermore, if occlusion or migration of the endoprosthesis occurs there is no ready access to the biliary ducts for correction of the problem. Thus, failure of an endoprosthesis becomes *de facto* a preterminal event unless a new drainage catheter is introduced and decompression reestablished.

Technique

The technique for insertion is represented schematically in Figure 12–50 and illustrative cases shown in Figures 12–51 and 12–52. After an internal drainage catheter is placed in the fashion previously described, the endoprosthesis is advanced coaxially over the drainage catheter. The endoprosthesis can be inserted immediately on the initial sitting or after a delayed interval of several days. Pereiras and associates have preferred to proceed with immediate insertion of the endoprosthesis.[42, 43] We have elected to defer for several days. Reasons for delay include the following: (1)

The preliminary interval decompression reduces the potential for sepsis following the forceful dilatation of the stricture prior to insertion of the endoprosthesis. (2) Several days' delay allows formation of a transparenchymal tract, facilitating introduction of a larger dilator and prosthesis catheters. (3) The complete procedure may be excessively long and painful, requiring as much as two to three hours, and Scandinavian workers have employed general anesthesia to carry out this technique. We, therefore, prefer two sessions.

Endoprosthesis devices are now available commercially* or can be fashioned at the time of the procedure from a longer piece of 12 or 14 French Teflon catheter material. Various designs have been employed including curved or angled configurations to conform to duct anatomy. The only commercially available device presently available in the US is fashioned with a series of ridges to prevent migration (Fig. 12–53). Sideholes are also placed near the proximal and distal ends of this prosthesis to ensure adequate bile drainage, whereas the proximal end is flanged to allow it to be pushed into position. The proximal flange also aids in preventing delayed caudal migration.

---

*Surgimed Co. Inc., NC.

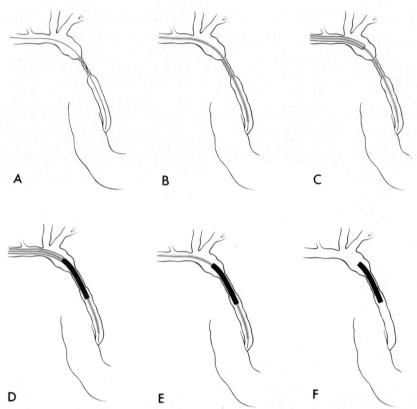

Figure 12–50. Schematic representation of steps for insertion of permanent endoprosthesis. *A*, Guide wire through stricture. *B*, 8 French internal drainage catheter placed. *C*, 12 French dilator catheter coaxially inserted over 8 French drainage catheter and pushed through stricture for forceful dilatation. Dilator catheter then removed. *D*, Preshaped endoprosthesis (solid dark area) pushed coaxially over 8 French drainage catheter by same 12 French dilator catheter. *E*, 12 French dilator catheter withdrawn, leaving endoprosthesis in place over protecting 8 French drainage catheter. Three to four days of gravity drainage is allowed and drainage catheter then removed. *F*, Endoprosthesis alone in place.

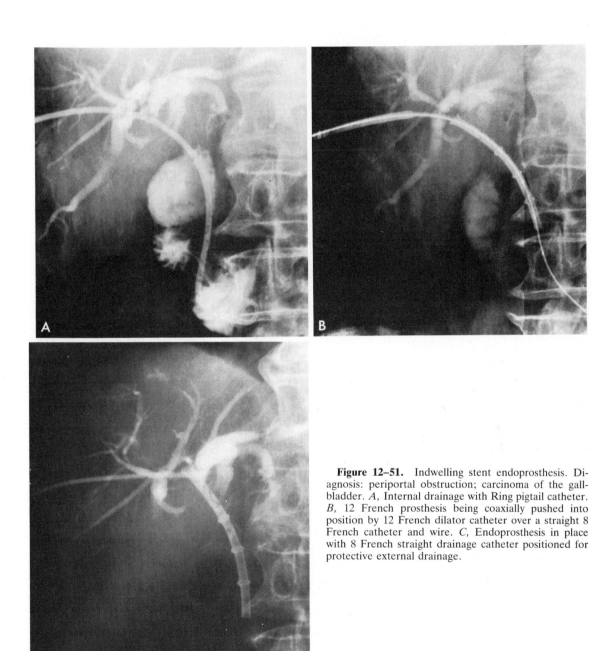

Figure 12–51. Indwelling stent endoprosthesis. Diagnosis: periportal obstruction; carcinoma of the gallbladder. *A*, Internal drainage with Ring pigtail catheter. *B*, 12 French prosthesis being coaxially pushed into position by 12 French dilator catheter over a straight 8 French catheter and wire. *C*, Endoprosthesis in place with 8 French straight drainage catheter positioned for protective external drainage.

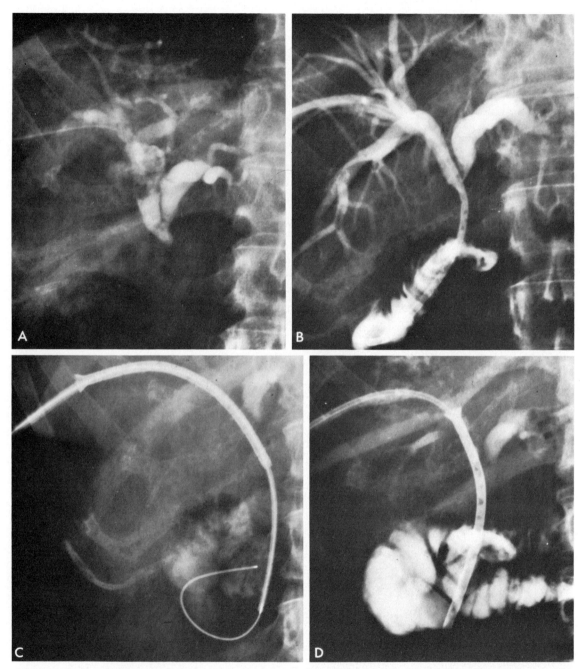

Figure 12–52. Endoprosthesis inserted through choledochojejunostomy for locally recurrent carcinoma of the pancreas following Whipple procedure. *A*, Diagnostic cholangiogram showing complete obstruction at anastomosis. *B*, Internal drainage with Ring catheter. *C*, Endoprosthesis being inserted by pusher catheter over 7 F straight catheter and wire. *D*, Final position of endoprosthesis in jejunum with 7 F drainage catheter still in place.

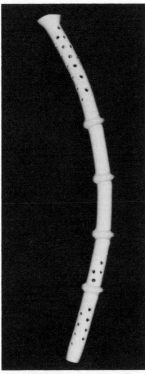

Figure 12–53. Endoprosthesis device (12 to 14 F size) and Teflon material provide a sturdy stent. Ridges prevent migration, proximal flange facilitates insertion, and sideholes increase efficiency of drainage.

The length of the prosthesis to be employed is determined by the length of the stricture evident on diagnostic cholangiography as described by Hellekant, Jonsson, and Genell.[45] A guide wire is passed through the drainage catheter to the distal end of the stricture, and a bend is placed in the wire at the skin surface. The guide wire tip is then withdrawn to the proximal end of the stenotic area and a second bend is made in the guide wire. The difference between the bends gives the necessary length of the prosthetic device.

Precise positioning of the prosthesis can be obtained after insertion by preliminary placement of two silk sutures within separate sideholes at the proximal end of the prosthesis before advancing the device into position (Fig. 12–54). These sutures should be long enough so that they extend out to the skin surface. Once the prosthesis has been inserted these sutures can then be used to withdraw the prosthesis if it has been too deeply advanced.

Prior to insertion of the endoprosthesis the stricture is coaxially dilated by insertion of a large "dilating" 14 French Teflon catheter over the 7 to 8 French drainage catheter through the strictured area. This is then completely withdrawn, and the specially constructed endoprosthesis is placed over the 7 to 8 French catheter and inserted through the skin surface. Next, the large "dilating" catheter is coaxially placed over the original catheter and is used to push the prosthetic device into the bile duct, depositing it in the area of the stricture. The larger catheter is then removed, leaving the prosthesis in place over the smaller drainage catheter.

The drainage catheter is then withdrawn to the proximal end of the prosthesis, and contrast material is injected to confirm patency. The drainage catheter should be left in place for several days to ensure adequate orthograde drainage. If cholangitis or recurrent jaundice

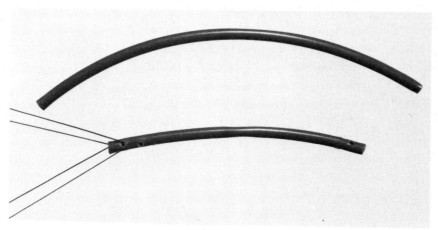

Figure 12–54. End-suture method for adjusting final position of endoprosthesis. Top, prosthesis catheter. Bottom, preplaced sutures through wall of prosthesis brought out to skin allow indwelling prosthesis to be withdrawn for optimal positioning.

does not occur, the drainage catheter is removed, leaving only the prosthesis. Should the distal tip of the prosthesis be placed through the ampulla there is an increased risk of pancreatitis from occlusion of the orifice of the main pancreatic duct; however, in carcinomas of the pancreatic head this may be an unavoidable requirement.

Results and Complications

Although reported experience in the literature numbers fewer than several hundred cases, effective palliation has been reported. Pereiras and coworkers reported a success rate of 47/53 or 88 per cent, with relief of jaundice or pruritus in approximately 80 per cent.[43] Mendez and colleagues reported success in 15 patients.[46] Our own experience with some 20 cases has been comparable.

Major acute complications have been surprisingly infrequent, although cholangitis, proximal and distal migration of the prosthesis (Fig. 12–55), and recurrent obstruction by tumor growth and bile encrustations occur (Fig. 12–56). However, long-term follow-up, particularly relative to patency rates, has not been established, and, despite its technical

appeal, many centers still prefer the catheter approach for decompression, since it preserves access to the bile ducts for delayed corrective manipulations. The decision to insert an endoprosthesis involves a judgment of considerable clinical finality, and we reserve it for patients with far advanced malignancy; the very elderly; and those in whom mental, psychologic, or nursing care reasons preclude care of a standard drainage catheter.

Stricture Dilatation

Benign, iatrogenic, and biliary enteric anastomotic strictures can be effectively managed by percutaneous transhepatic dilatation.[48-52] Benign strictures tend to recur (with a frequency of approximately 30 per cent) following surgical bypass, and such patients often undergo repeated attempts at operative correction, leading to a gradual downhill course. A nonoperative transhepatic approach provides a useful alternative. Following internal catheter drainage, gradual progressive dilatation with catheters of increasing caliber can be employed, leaving an indwelling drainage catheter in place during intervals.

More recently, however, use of a Gruntzig

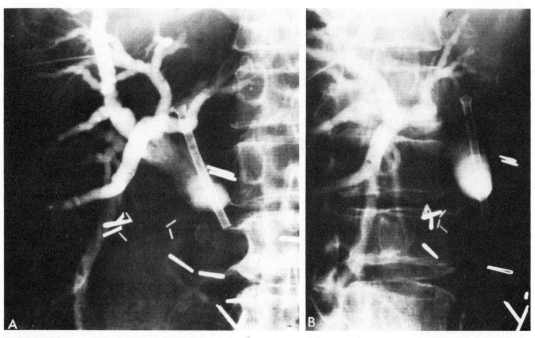

Figure 12–55. *A, B,* Prosthesis failure due to migration proximally. Note the aberrant position above the occluded segment of the common duct. Patient presented with recurrent jaundice and sepsis three weeks after endoprosthesis insertion. Diagnosis: carcinoma of the pancreas.

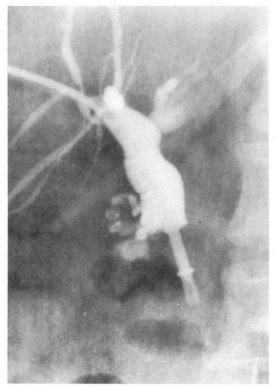

Figure 12–56. Endoprosthesis failure due to tumor occlusion. *De novo* insertion of an external drainage catheter was required for palliation of obstructive symptoms. Diagnosis: metastatic carcinoma of the colon to the common bile duct.

and no waist or indentation remains visible on the balloon walls (Figs. 12–57 and 12–58). We have found 4 to 6 atm pressure (60 to 90 psi) necessary when monitoring with a pressure gauge but generally use only manual inflation. The balloon is inflated five to six times per sitting, although moderate epigastric pain may occur. Repeat cholangiography after successful dilatation discloses a typical widened granular appearance of the abnormal segment, reflecting the traumatization (Fig. 12–59). A protective drainage catheter is left in place, which also allows repeat dilatation if initial response is inconclusive. How long the protective catheter should be left across the stricture to promote re-epithelialization of the traumatized duct lumen without restricturing is presently unclear. We have removed all catheters within a few days; others have left them for up to six months. At present, only a few centers have any real experience with balloon dilatation of benign bile duct strictures, and the long-term success rate for radiologic dilatation is uncertain. Judgment therefore should be reserved. The technique is not recommended for malignant strictures.

Transhepatic Biliary Calculus Removal

Nonoperative transcatheter manipulation of biliary duct calculi through the transhepatic tract can be an alternative technique to the more conventional transfistula or transendoscopic techniques for calculus extraction[10,11,53-55] (see also Chapters 10 and 11). The transhepatic route is particularly well suited for calculi within the intrahepatic ducts, which may be difficult to mobilize by the transfistula or endoscopic route.

Following gradual maturation of the transhepatic tract to an adequate caliber relative to the observed size of calculi, a steerable remote-control catheter can be introduced over a guide wire into the tract.* A conventional biliary stone basket (Dormia) can then be introduced through the steerable catheter. Most calculi can be directly withdrawn through the transhepatic parenchymal tract (Figs. 12–60 and 12–61). Larger calculi may be fragmented and the fragments engaged in the basket and directed caudally through the ampulla into the duodenum where the basket is then opened, releasing the stone. Forceful instrumentation of the ampulla should be assiduously avoided.

angioplasty balloon catheter has been reported.[49-52] Balloon catheter dilatation has two distinct advantages. First, dilatation can be carried out to a 16 to 20 French caliber via only an 8 French catheter placed across the liver. Second, following an interval of protective catheter drainage, all catheters can be withdrawn.

Technique

Balloon catheter dilatation is performed several days after placement of an internal drainage catheter. With opaque contrast material injected into the balloon, the degree of stenosis can be determined visually by inflating the balloon across the site of the stricture, gradually increasing the pressure in the attached syringe. As dilatation progresses the pressure needed to keep the balloon inflated to its initial configuration across the narrowing diminishes. Dilatation is complete when the fully inflated balloon passes smoothly across the stricture

---

*Medi-Tech Inc., Watertown, MA.

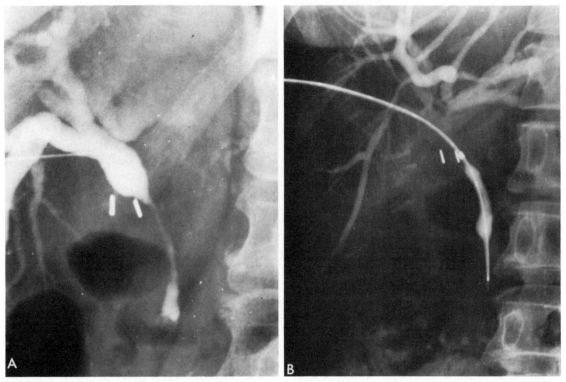

Figure 12–57. Gruntzig balloon catheter dilatation of iatrogenic biliary stricture following cholecystectomy. *A*, Diagnostic cholangiogram revealing long tapered stricture of mid common duct. *B*, Contrast-filled Gruntzig balloon catheter positioned and inflated across stricture.

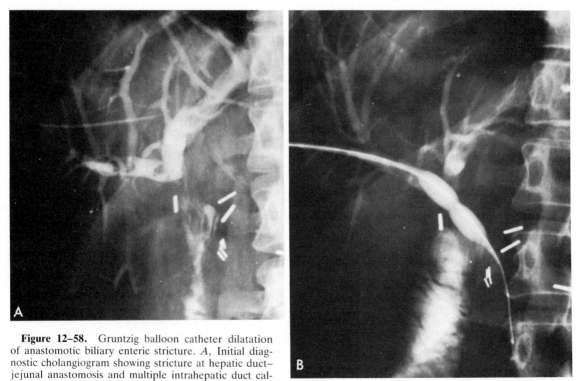

Figure 12–58. Gruntzig balloon catheter dilatation of anastomotic biliary enteric stricture. *A*, Initial diagnostic cholangiogram showing stricture at hepatic duct–jejunal anastomosis and multiple intrahepatic duct calculi. *B*, Contrast-filled Gruntzig balloon catheter positioned and inflated across strictured anastomosis (note impression of stricture on balloon walls). Balloon was dilated to 6 mm in diameter by 6 ATM. A Ring catheter was left across stricture for protecting internal drainage. Stones were subsequently cleared by basket extraction across liver substance.

484

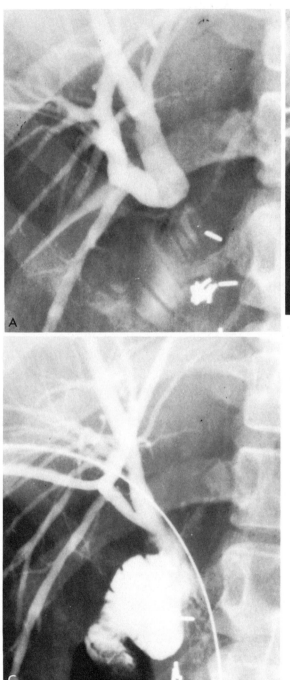

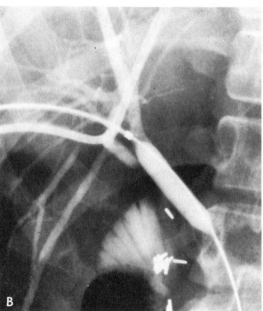

Figure 12–59. Gruntzig balloon dilatation of anastomotic biliary stricture, showing postdilatation appearance. *A,* Diagnostic cholangiogram showing high-grade stricture at choledochojejunostomy performed for iatrogenic stricture. *B,* Balloon in place. No residual waist is evident across stricture. *C,* Postdilatation appearance. Note widened granular area at anastomosis, reflecting traumatization. The jejunal loop is now readily opacified.

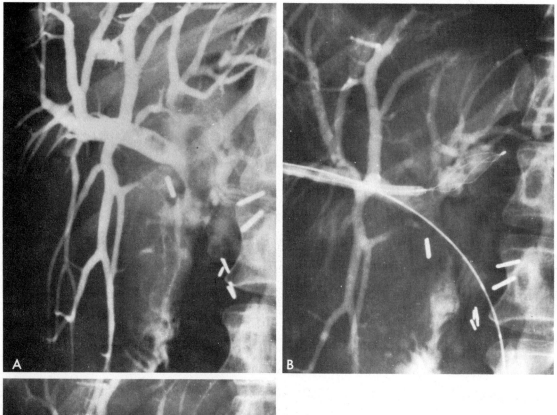

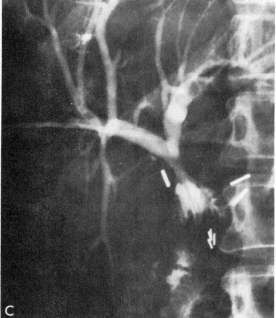

Figure 12–60. Percutaneous transhepatic basket stone extraction via the steerable catheter. *A,* Multiple intrahepatic calculi complicating a strictured biliary enteric anastomosis are shown on an initial diagnostic cholangiogram. Internal drainage was performed and the catheter left in place for two weeks to allow a tract to develop. *B,* Dormia stone basketing of calculi situated within the left hepatic duct. A second wire has been previously placed through the stricture to assure reentry. Eight calculi were extracted through the transhepatic tract. *C,* Post-procedure cholangiogram showing clear ducts and open anastomosis. An air bubble is seen in the left hepatic duct.

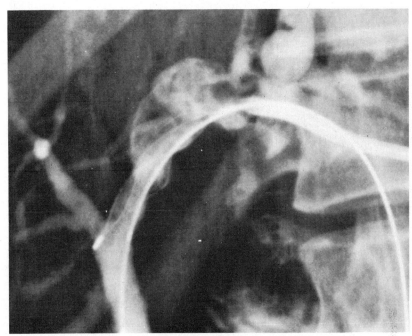

Figure 12–61. Transhepatic Dormia basket extraction of left hepatic duct calculi. Initial catheter access to the left duct was established by selective cholangiography and drainage of the left duct, allowing a tract to mature for four weeks.

However, if a prior papillotomy can be performed via the fiberoptic duodenoscope, calculi might be more easily pushed through the ampulla with the catheter tip. After the procedure, an indwelling drainage catheter should be left for decompression should acute swelling of the ampulla occur. Transcatheter balloon dilatation of the sphincter of Oddi and the use of glucagon to relieve spasm at the sphincter of Oddi have also been employed in an effort to aid stone passage.[56, 57]

Direct transcatheter instillation of stone solvents, especially the cholesterol solvent monooctanoin, has also been reported in a few cases with good results.[58, 59] Continuous infusion at 4 to 10 ml/hr may be required for up to two to three weeks, depending on the number, size, and location of the calculi.

Tissue Biopsy Techniques

Pathologic confirmation of the presence of biliary tract malignancy may be necessary for further management following percutaneous catheter decompression. Available methods for pathologic diagnosis include bile cytology,[10, 11, 60] percutaneous needle aspiration biopsy,[61-63] transcatheter brush biopsy,[64] and transcatheter forceps biopsy.[64]

Cytologic examination of bile obtained following percutaneous catheter insertion yields positive results in approximately 40 per cent of cases, and 10- to 20-ml bile samples are routinely sent for cytologic analysis after initial catheter placement. A 24-hour volume of bile is also sent for centrifugation and cell block. Theoretically, the rate of positive yield is higher after manipulation of a malignant stricture for internal drainage, but positive results have also been obtained following placement of an external drainage catheter only.

Fine-needle aspiration biopsy can be performed in the area of bile duct stricture under fluoroscopic control (Fig. 12–62)[61-63] or of a discrete mass lesion in the liver or elsewhere in the abdomen. The yield of positive cytologic material with fine-needle aspiration techniques approaches 90 per cent in published series.[61-63]

Brush biopsy through the percutaneous catheter can be carried out with to-and-fro and rotary brushing motions. Despite the intrinsic nature of the malignant stricture, positive material can occasionally be obtained.[64]

Transcatheter forceps biopsy techniques have been infrequently reported[64] but would

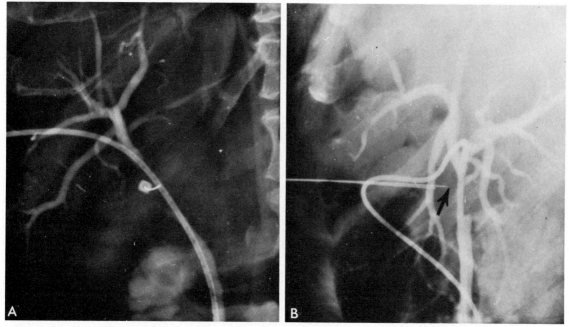

Figure 12–62. Percutaneous fine-needle aspiration biopsy performed via catheter cholangiogram. Samples taken from strictured area after internal drainage established. Frontal (*A*) and cross-table (*B*) lateral radiographs. Three-dimensional localization confirmed by position of needle tip *vis a vis* catheter (arrow) on lateral view.

appear entirely feasible should an obturating intraluminal mass be demonstrated.

Transcatheter Irradiation

Local high dose irradiation of obstructing malignant tumors using a radioactive source (iridium 192) placed in an indwelling catheter has been reported in ten patients by Herskovic and coworkers.[65] Supplemental external beam therapy completed the treatment plan. Further trials appear warranted.

CLINICAL OVERVIEW

The availability of nonoperative access to the biliary ducts via transhepatic catheterization clearly affords new options for clinical management of surgical disorders of the biliary tract. Thus, complete nonoperative management of patients with malignant biliary obstruction can now be provided by radiologic means. Using a combination of percutaneous catheter drainage, bile cytology, needle or brush biopsy techniques, and irradiation or chemotherapy, patients with advanced malignant biliary obstruction can be offered a non-

surgical alternative for palliation. A proposed radiologic approach for management of such cases is given in Figure 12–63.

By the same token, in some cases conventional surgical therapy of biliary obstruction can be modified by a brief preoperative trial of percutaneous catheter drainage. In patients with acute suppurative cholangitis a period of percutaneous catheter decompression contributes to resuscitation prior to elective surgical exploration. In other patients percutaneous drainage may be substituted for surgery when combined with medical measures including antibiotics, instillation of agents for solvent dissolution, transhepatic basket extraction, or endoscopic papillotomy. Thus, a completely new nonoperative approach to common duct stone disease is also possible.

Similarly, patients with dense obstructive jaundice due to presumed operable pancreatic or duodenal carcinoma may experience considerable improvement in liver function, bleeding parameters, and overall metabolic condition following a brief interval of preoperative drainage.[7] In our institution patients are believed to benefit from a brief period of preoperative catheter drainage if bilirubin levels exceed 10 to 15 mg per cent; with lesser degrees of jaundice, surgery is carried out directly.

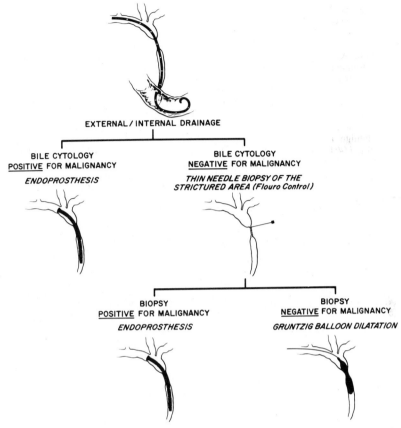

Figure 12–63. Complete nonoperative radiologic management of biliary obstruction.

Questions remain relative to the optimal long-term choice of the nonoperative drainage system, i.e., catheter with protruding hub versus indwelling endoprosthesis. Certainly a combination of biliary obstruction and an indwelling foreign body predisposes to attacks of recurrent cholangitis. The protruding biliary catheter may well provide a source for bacterial contamination as well as cause discomfort and mental annoyance for the patient. On the other hand, the long-term results of an indwelling endoprosthesis are presently unestablished despite the initial successes with this technically dramatic feat.

It is also presently unsettled as to when, if ever, a successfully placed biliary drainage catheter should be removed. Patients and physicians are understandably reluctant to relinquish the security of a functioning catheter system despite the completion of radiation and chemotherapy programs. It might be reasonable to remove the catheter three months after completion of adjunctive therapy provided follow-up cholangiography is normal. However, in our experience only a few patients ever reach this fortunate stage.

In view of the foregoing, it is not inappropriate to suggest that the conventional medical versus surgical categorization of the dilemma of patients with obstructive jaundice can now be expanded to include a third category, namely, radiologic jaundice.

References

1. Kaude, J. V., Weidenmier, C. H., and Agee, O. F.: Decompression of the bile ducts with the percutaneous technique. Radiology 93:69, 1969.
2. Molnar, W., and Stockum, A. E.: Relief of obstructive jaundice through percutaneous transhepatic catheter—a new therapeutic method. Am. J. Roentgenol. 122:356, 1974.
3. Burcharth, F., and Nielbo, N.: Percutaneous cholangiography with selective catheterization of the common bile duct. Am. J. Roentgenol. 127:409, 1976.
4. Tylen, U., Hoevels, J., and Vang, J.: Percutaneous transhepatic cholangiography with external drainage of obstructive biliary lesions. Surg. Gynecol. Obstet. 144:13, 1977.

5. Hoevels, J., Lunderquist, A., and Ihse, I.: Percutaneous transhepatic intubation of bile ducts for combined internal-external drainage in preoperative and palliative treatment of obstructive jaundice. Gastrointest. Radiol. 3:23, 1978.

6. Hansson, J. A., Hoevels, J., Simert, G., Tylen, U., and Vang, J.: Clinical aspects of nonsurgical percutaneous transhepatic bile drainage in obstructive lesions of the extrahepatic bile ducts. Ann. Surg. 189:58, 1979.

7. Nakayama, T., Ikeda, A., and Okuda, K.: Percutaneous transhepatic drainage of the biliary tract. Gastroenterology 74:554, 1978.

8. Ring, E. J., Oleaga, J. A., Freiman, D. B., Husted, J. W., and Lunderquist, A.: Therapeutic applications of catheter cholangiography. Radiology 128:333, 1978.

9. Pollock, T. W., Ring, E. J., Oleaga, J. A., Freiman, D. B., Mullen , J. L., and Rosato, E. F.: Percutaneous decompression of benign and malignant biliary obstruction. Arch. Surg. 114:148, 1979.

10. Ferrucci, J. T., Jr., Mueller, P. R., and Harbin, W. P.: Percutaneous transhepatic biliary drainage. Technique, results and applications. Radiology 135:1, 1980.

11. Ferrucci, J. T., Jr., Mueller, P. R., and Harbin, W. P.: Percutaneous biliary drainage. In Ferrucci, J. T., Jr., and Wittenberg, J. (eds.): Interventional Radiology of the Abdomen. Baltimore: Williams & Wilkins, 1981.

12. Berquist, T. H., May, G. R., Johnson, C. M., Adson, M. A., and Thistle, J. L.: Percutaneous biliary decompression: Internal and external drainage in 50 patients. Am. J. Roentgenol. 136:901, 1981.

13. Clark, R. A., Mitchell, S. E., Colley, D. P., and Alexander, E.: Percutaneous catheter biliary decompression. Am. J. Roentgenol. 137:503, 1981.

14. Mueller, P. R., vanSonnenberg, E., and Ferrucci, J. T., Jr.: Percutaneous biliary drainage. Technical and catheter related problems. Experience with 200 cases. Am. J. Roentgenol. (In press.)

15. Mueller, P. R., Ferrucci, J. T., Jr., and vanSonnenberg, E.: Obstruction of the left hepatic duct: Diagnosis and treatment by selective fine needle transhepatic cholangiography and biliary drainage. Radiology. (In press.)

16. Feduska, N. J., Dent, T. L., and Lindenauer, S. M.: Results of palliative operations for carcinoma of the pancreas. Arch. Surg. 103:330, 1971.

17. Gudjonsson, B., Livstone, E. M., and Spiro, H. M.: Cancer of the pancreas: Diagnostic accuracy and survival statistics. Cancer 42:2494, 1978.

18. Maki, T., Sata, T., Kakizki, G., et al.: Pancreaticoduodenectomy for periampullary carcinomas. Appraisal of two-stage procedure. Arch. Surg. 92:825, 1966.

19. Braasch, J. W., and Gray, B. N.: Considerations that lower pancreaticoduodenectomy mortality. Am. J. Surg. 129:480, 1977.

20. Buckwalter, J. A., Lawton, R. L., and Tidrick, R. T.: Bypass operations for neoplastic biliary tract obstruction. Am. J. Surg. 109:100, 1965.

21. Shapiro, T. M.: Adenocarcinoma of the pancreas. A statistical analysis of biliary bypass vs Whipple resection in good risk patients. Ann. Surg. 182:751, 1975.

22. Brooks, J. R., and Culebras, J. M.: Cancer of the pancreas: palliative operation, Whipple procedure or total pancreatectomy. Am. J. Surg. 131:516, 1976.

23. Wardle, E. N.: Renal failure in obstructive jaundice. Pathogenic factors. Postgrad. Med. J. 51:512, 1975.

24. Denning, D. A., Molnar, W., and Carey, L. C.: Preoperative percutaneous transhepatic biliary decompression lowers operative morbidity in patients with obstructive jaundice. Am. J. Surg. 141:61, 1981.

25. Pitt, H. A., Cameron, J. L., Postier, R. G., and Gadacz, T. R.: Factors affecting mortality in biliary tract surgery. Am. J. Surg. 141:66, 1981.

26. Dawson, J. L.: The incidence of postoperative renal failure in obstructive jaundice. Br. J. Surg. 52:663, 1965.

27. Harrington, D. P.: Teflon-sheath placement in the biliary tree using high-torque J guide wires. Radiology 134:248, 1980.

28. Lunderquist, A., Lunderquist, M., and Owman, T.: Guide wire for percutaneous transhepatic cholangiography. Radiology 132:228, 1979.

29. Ring, E. J., Husted, J. W., Oleaga, J. A., and Freiman, D. B.: A multiside hole catheter for maintaining long term percutaneous antegrade biliary drainage. Radiology 132:752, 1979.

30. Cope, C.: Improved anchoring of nephrostomy catheters: loop technique. Am. J. Roentgenol. 135:402, 1980.

31. Tsuchiya, Y., Ohto, M., and Ebara, M.: PTC and percutaneous transhepatic bile drainage (PTBD) with linear electronic puncture transducer of ultrasound. Jpn. J. Med. Ultrasound 34:315, 1978.

32. Makuuchi, M., Brandai, Y., Ifo, T., Watanbe, G., Wada, T., Abe, H., and Muroi, T.: Ultrasonically guided percutaneous transhepatic bile drainage. Radiology 136:165, 1980.

33. Hawkins, I. F.: New fine needle for cholangiography with optional sheath for decompression. Radiology 131:252, 1981.

34. Bockus, H. L. (ed.): Gastroenterology, 3rd ed. Philadelphia: W. B. Saunders, 1973.

35. Sleisenger, M. H., and Fordtran, J. S.: Gastrointestinal Disease. Philadelphia: W. B. Saunders, 1973.

36. Malt, R. A., Warshaw, A. L., Jameson, C. G., and Hawk, J. C.: Left intrahepatic cholangiojejunostomy for proximal obstruction of the biliary tract. Surg. Gynecol. Obstet. 150:193, 1980.

37. Gordon, R. L., Oleaga, J. A., Ring, E. J., Freiman, D. B., and Funaro, A. H.: Replacing the "fallen out" catheter. Radiology 134:537, 1980.

38. Cope, C.: Endoscopic replacement of drain catheters. Am. J. Roentgenol. 137:426, 1981.

39. Monden, M., Okamura, J., Kobayashi, N., Shibata, N., Horikawa, S., Fujimoto, T., Kosaki, G., Kuroda, E., and Uchida, H.: Hemobilia after percutaneous transhepatic biliary drainage. Arch. Surg. 115:161, 1980.

40. Oleaga, J. A., Ring, E. J., Freiman, D. B., McLean, G. K., and Rosen, R. J.: Extension of neoplasm along the tract of a transhepatic tube. Am. J. Roentgenol. 135:841, 1980.

41. Burcharth, F.: A new endoprosthesis for nonoperative intubation of the biliary tract in malignant obstructive jaundice. Surg. Gynecol. Obstet. 146:76, 1978.

42. Pereiras, R. V., Rheingold, O. J., Hutson, D., Mejia, J., Viamonte, M., Chiprut, R. O., and Schiff, E. R.: Relief of malignant obstructive jaundice by percutaneous insertion of a permanent prosthesis in the biliary tree. Ann. Intern. Med. 89:589, 1978.

43. Pereiras, R., Schiff, E., Barbin, J., and Hutson, D.: Role of interventional radiology in diseases of the hepatobiliary system and pancreas. Radiol. Clin. North Am. 17:555, 1979.

44. Hoevels, J., and Ihse, I.: Percutaneous transhepatic insertion of a permanent endoprosthesis in obstructive

lesions of the extrahepatic bile ducts. Gastrointest. Radiol. *4*:367, 1979.

45. Hellekant, C., Jonsson, K., and Genell, S.: Percutaneous internal drainage in obstructive jaundice. Am. J. Roentgenol. *134*:661, 1980.

46. Mendez, G., Russell, E., Levi, J. U., Koolpe, H., and Cohen, M.: Percutaneous brush biopsy and internal drainage of biliary tree through endoprosthesis. Am. J. Roentgenol. *134*:653, 1980.

47. Jonsson, K., and Hellekant, C.: Percutaneous insertion of an endoprosthesis in obstructive jaundice. Radiology *139*:749, 1981.

48. Molnar, W., and Stockum, A. E.: Transhepatic dilatation of choledochoenterostomy strictures. Radiology *129*:59, 1978.

49. Teplick, S. K., Goldstein, R. C., Richardson, P. A., et al.: Percutaneous transhepatic choledochoplasty and dilatation of choledochoenterostomy strictures. J.A.M.A. *244*:1240, 1980.

50. Martin, E. C., Karlson, K. B., Fankuchen, E. I., Mattern, R. F., and Casarella, W. J.: Percutaneous transhepatic dilatation of intrahepatic biliary strictures. Am. J. Roentgenol. *135*:837, 1980.

51. Burhenne, H. J., and Morris, D. W.: Biliary stricture dilatation. Use of Gruntzig balloon catheter. J. Can. Assoc. Radiol. *31*:196, 1980.

52. Martin, E. C., Fankuchen, E. I., Schultz, R. W., and Casarella, W. J.: Percutaneous dilatation in primary sclerosing cholangitis: two experiences. Am. J. Roentgenol. *137*:604, 1981.

53. Perez, M. R., Oleaga, J. A., Freiman, D. B., McClean, G. L., and Ring, E. J.: Removal of a distal common bile duct stone through percutaneous transhepatic catheterization. Arch. Surg. *114*:107, 1979.

54. Ellman, B. A., and Berman, H. L.: Treatment of common duct stones via transhepatic approach. Gastrointest. Radiol. *6*:357, 1981.

55. Dotter, C. T., Bilbao, M. K., and Katon, R. M.: Percutaneous transhepatic gallstone removal by needle tract. Radiology *133*:242, 1979.

56. Centola, C. A. P., Stauffer, J. A., and Russinovich, N. A. E.: Balloon dilatation of the Papilla of Vater to allow biliary stone passage. Am. J. Roentgenol. *136*:613, 1981.

57. Latshaw, R. F., Kadir, S., Witt, W. S., Kaufman, S. L., and White, R. I., Jr.: Glucagon-induced choledochal sphincter relaxation: aid for expulsion of impacted calculi into the duodenum. Am. J. Roentgenol. *137*:614, 1981.

58. Mack, E., Crummy, A. B., and Babayan, V. K.: Percutaneous transhepatic dissolution of common bile duct stones. Surgery *90*:584, 1981.

59. Hoffman, A. F., Schmack, B., Thistle, J. L., and Babayan, V. K.: Clinical experience with mono-octanoin for dissolution of bile duct stones. An uncontrolled multicenter trial. Letter to the Editor. Dig. Dis. Sci. *26*:954, 1981.

60. Harell, G. S., Anderson, M. F., and Berry, P. F.: Cytologic bile examination in the diagnosis of biliary duct malignant strictures. Am. J. Roentgenol. *137*:1123, 1981.

61. Pereiras, R. V., Meiers, W., Kunhardt, B., et al.: Fluoroscopically guided thin needle aspiration biopsy of the abdomen and retroperitoneum. Am. J. Roentgenol. *131*:197, 1978.

62. Ferrucci, J. T., Jr., Wittenberg, J., Mueller, P. R., et al.: Diagnosis of abdominal malignancy by radiologic fine needle aspiration biopsy. Am. J. Roentgenol. *134*:323, 1980.

63. Harbin, W. P., and Ferrucci, J. T., Jr.: Nonoperative management of malignant biliary obstruction. A radiologic alternative. Am. J. Roentgenol. *135*:103, 1980.

64. Elyaderani, M. K., and Gabriele, O. F.: Brush and forceps biopsy of biliary ducts via percutaneous transhepatic catheterization. Radiology *135*:777, 1980.

65. Herskovic, A., Heaston, D., Engler, M. J., Fishburn, R. I., Jones, R. S., and Noell, K. T.: Irradiation of biliary carcinoma. Radiology *139*:219, 1981.

POSTOPERATIVE INTERVENTION

13

by H. Joachim Burhenne, M.D.

The availability of a steerable catheter[*3] in 1972 made instrumentation of the biliary tract practical as a radiologic procedure under fluoroscopic control (Fig. 13–1). It is applicable to patients with indwelling tubes after surgery on the biliary tract, and it is of significant diagnostic and therapeutic advantage in many postoperative complications. The sinus tract of the indwelling tube is used postoperatively for access to the biliary tract for the following procedures:

1. Selective cholangiography,
2. Relief of obstruction of indwelling tubes,[26]
3. Reinsertion of drainage tubes,[17]
4. Expulsion of retained material,[20]
5. Nonoperative extraction of retained stones from intrahepatic or extrahepatic ducts,[29]
6. Cholecystostomy instrumentation,
7. Transcholecystic intervention,[28]
8. Stricture dilatation,[5]
9. Biopsy,[7]
10. Foreign body removal, and
11. Internal biliary drainage.[5]

GENERAL CONSIDERATIONS

Access to the biliary tract for interventional procedures follows three routes: retrograde via gastrointestinal endoscopy, antegrade through the liver, or through the postoperative drain tract. The latter, or subhepatic, approach is less time consuming and less technically demanding than the transhepatic procedures.

Postoperative subhepatic interventional procedures through the surgical drainage tract are done without anesthesia and are usually performed in the ambulatory patient. About four to five weeks is required for the drain tract to

mature with a good fibrous reaction surrounding the surgical tube. The tract is easily negotiated with a steerable catheter at that time. Earlier postoperative procedures usually require placement of a guide wire through the drainage tube as the initial procedure.

The possibility of excessive radiation to the radiologist's fingers exists during prolonged interventional procedures.[15] Proper technique for radiation protection requires the following precautions:

1. The radiologist's fingers should stay outside the primary beam;
2. Collimation to the smallest possible field, preferably 3×5 cm;
3. An under-the-table x-ray tube;
4. A lead apron drape with a cutout over the patient;
5. Instruments moved as much as possible between fluoroscopic exposures.

A thermoluminescent monitor may be placed in the rubber glove of the operator to record radiation exposure to the fingers. Monitoring of this type should remind the radiologist to pay close attention to his technique.

The biliary tract is also accessible to radiologic intervention in patients with previous cholecystoduodenostomy by transintestinal manipulation with a steerable catheter. It is advanced through the stomach and cholecystoduodenostomy stoma to the cystic duct.[2]

SELECTIVE CHOLANGIOGRAPHY

Use of the steerable catheter permits selective injection of all parts of the intrahepatic and extrahepatic bile ducts. Because of this, better diagnostic spot films of the area of interest are obtained. Selective cholangiography is applicable in the differential diagnosis of retained stones and bile duct tumors and

*Medi-Tech Co., Watertown, MA.

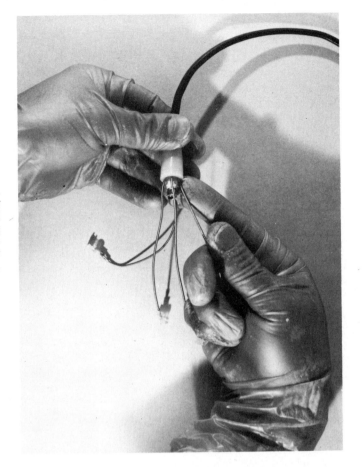

Figure 13–1. The steerable biliary catheter. Four wires are imbedded in the wall of the catheter, permitting multi-directional steering of the catheter tip when applying traction through the wires. This is accomplished by attaching either a control plate or a control handle to the four wires.

spasm and stricture and for better visualization of the junction of the common duct and duodenum. Anatomic variations with anomalous biliary or cystic duct insertion and ampullary entrance into duodenal diverticula with single- and double-channel junction of common and pancreatic ducts are better identified. Selective cholangiography is indicated if conventional T-tube cholangiography is inconclusive concerning the presence of retained stones, air in the biliary ducts, blood clots or sludge, or iatrogenic injuries to the duct (Fig. 13–2).

The T-tube is extracted before selective cholangiography, and the steerable catheter is inserted through the sinus tract. The tip of the catheter is maneuvered to the area of interest for contrast injection, and multiple collimated spot films are obtained in different projections. Forced injection and overdistention films are readily obtained, although care must be taken in patients with partial obstruction. If contrast and bile are forced from the biliary ducts into the vascular bed, septicemia may result.

RELIEF OF OBSTRUCTION OF INDWELLING TUBES

Long-term indwelling tubes in the biliary ducts may become obstructed owing to bile encrustation. If this occurs, a guide wire is introduced through the T-tube to re-establish drainage.[26]

The T-tube is negotiated with a guide wire using a J tip or a steerable tip. Negotiation of the 90-degree angle at the point of T-junction is facilitated by slight traction on the T-tube, rendering the tube angle more obtuse at its junction. The tip of the guide wire also tends to protrude through the wedge-shaped cut at the T-junction. Care must be taken not to direct the guide wire tip into the wall of the duct.

It may be impossible in some obstructed T-tubes to advance the guide wire for this purpose. In these patients, the T-tube is extracted and is replaced by a straight tube for continued drainage, as described hereafter.

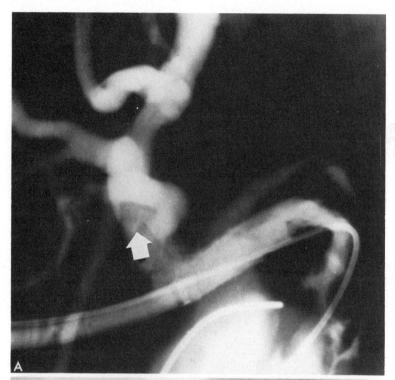

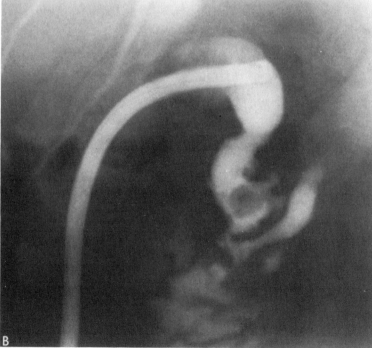

Figure 13–2. *A*, Variation of anatomy of intrahepatic and extrahepatic duct system. One right hepatic radicle enters low into the common hepatic duct (arrow). The long retained cystic duct travels parallel to the common duct on the medial side with low entrance. The anatomy at the junction of common duct and duodenum is not well seen. *B*, Selective cholangiogram in the same patient now outlines the anatomy of distal common duct and pancreatic duct with entrance into the neck of a duodenal diverticulum. The retained stone is now clearly visible.

REINSERTION OF DRAINAGE TUBES

Indwelling tubes may require replacement because of dislodgement, inadvertent extraction, or obstruction by encrustation of bile sediments (Fig. 13–3). Insertion of a torque guide wire under fluoroscopic control can successfully disimpact occlusion as described previously.[22] Obstruction of draining tubes by sediment and bile encrustation, however, is a recurring problem, and we prefer to exchange obstructed tubes by placing a new catheter into the bile ducts. This can readily be accomplished even for T-tubes. Nonoperative replacement of T-tubes in the common duct after inadvertent removal was first described in 1971 with the use of the Seldinger technique.[17] Replacement has also been described with a steerable catheter.[21] T-tubes have been modified for this purpose. Reinsertion over a guide wire[16] or over a stiffer Teflon dilator[33] has been described (Fig. 13–4).

We have found insertion of T-tubes easier with the use of two guide wires. Separate guide wires are placed through the T-tube tract into the proximal and distal bile ducts, and the two short arms of the T-tube are then inserted over the guide wires separately; both guide wires are then fed through the long arm of the T-tube. T-tubes with smaller short arms than long arms have been described[41] and are available for this purpose.* Dilatation of the sinus tract with Grüntzig balloons may be required before T-tube insertion.[12]

T-tubes may be converted into transhepatic U-tubes by a percutaneous approach.[13] This is useful in patients with multiple intrahepatic stones requiring multiple sessions for removal or for long-term stenting in patients with bile duct strictures. The steerable catheter is used for replacement of U-tubes following inadvertent removal.[21]

EXPULSION OF RETAINED MATERIAL

If small amounts of retained stone material are seen on T-tube cholangiography, the T-tube should be clamped for at least four weeks to permit spontaneous passage. If this is unsuccessful, the patient should return five weeks after surgery for roentgenologic instrumentation.

If the selective cholangiogram reveals re-

---

*Whelan-Moss T-tube, Davol Inc., Cranston, RI.

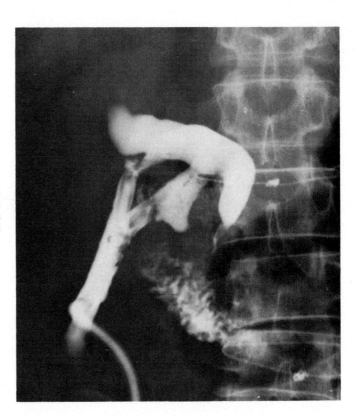

Figure 13–3. Inadvertent partial T-tube extraction with both short arms of the tube lying outside the common duct. The T-tube is withdrawn and the common duct is re-rentered with the use of a steerable catheter.

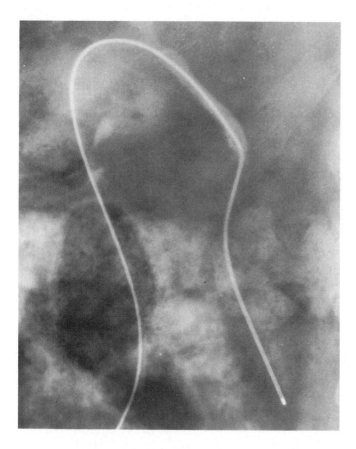

Figure 13–4. A guide wire has been manipulated through the T-tube for tube replacement. The distal end of the guide wire has been introduced into the duodenum. The T-tube is then extracted over the guide wire, and a new straight retention catheter is introduced.

tained material in the bile ducts 4 mm in size or smaller, extraction with the wire basket is usually time consuming and difficult. We prefer to expel the material with the use of the steerable catheter, pushing it through the ampulla into the gut. The technique of radiologic expulsion of retained material was already described in 1970 (Fig. 13–5).[20]

The T-tube is extracted, and selective cholangiography is used to identify the exact location of retained material. This may be quite difficult if the common duct is distended. If the common duct size is larger than 14 mm, we use further contrast dilution for better visualization. One part of 50 or 60 per cent contrast material is diluted with three parts of saline.

A normal diameter ampulla will permit passage of the 10 French steerable catheter in all cases. Approximately every other patient will accept passage of a 13 French steerable catheter. We obtain selective cholangiograms of the ampullary portion and attempt passage of the catheter before we expel the retained material. This may have to be done with the patient in a semi-erect or erect position.

NONOPERATIVE EXTRACTION OF RETAINED STONES FROM INTRAHEPATIC AND EXTRAHEPATIC DUCTS

Retained gallstones following cholecystectomy may be located in any part of the intrahepatic or extrahepatic bile duct system. Nonoperative extraction under roentgenologic control is the procedure of choice for removal. Surgical re-exploration carries twice the operative mortality and morbidity of the initial surgical intervention.

The technique of nonoperative extraction through the sinus tract was first described by Mondet.[29] Mazzariello[27] used a semipliable extraction forceps successfully, even with larger stones, after bougienage of the sinus tract. The ureteral stone basket was first applied to gallstone extraction by Lagrave and colleagues[23] and also has been used by Magarey.[24, 25] The steerable catheter became available in 1972[3] and has greatly simplified nonoperative stone extraction (Fig. 13–6).

If retained stones are detected on the postoperative T-tube cholangiogram, the patient is

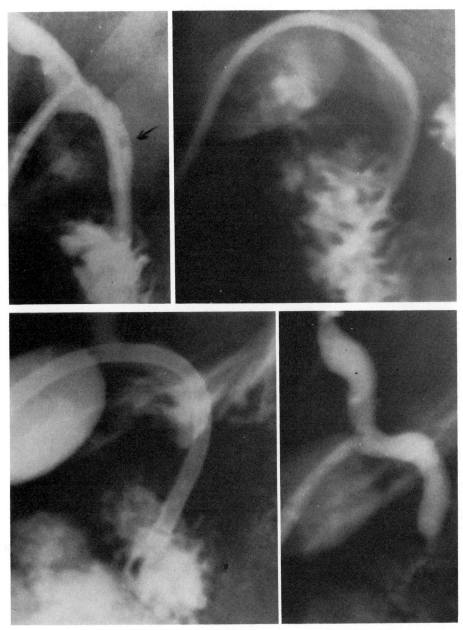

Figure 13–5. There is a small (2-mm) retained common duct stone (arrow). First a #8 and then a #10 French steerable catheter is introduced, and the stone is pushed through the ampulla into the duodenum. Final film shows the duct system clear.

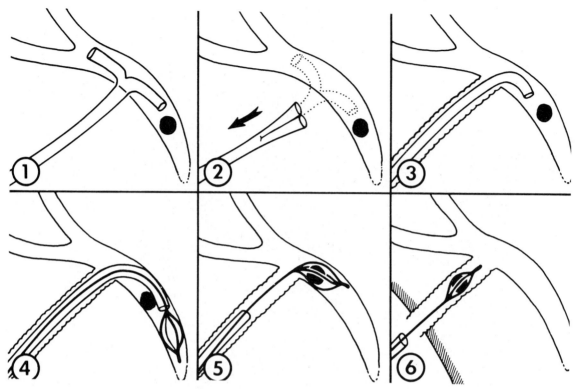

Figure 13–6. Technical steps for retained common duct stone extraction.
1. Repeat T-tube cholangiogram is obtained on the day of stone extraction four to five weeks after choledochotomy.
2. After the location of the retained stone has been ascertained, a T-tube is withdrawn.
3. Using the sinus tract of the T-tube, the steerable catheter is guided into the bile duct, and its movable tip is advanced beyond the retained stone.
4. The basket is inserted through the steerable catheter, the catheter is withdrawn, and the basket is opened.
5. The open basket is withdrawn to engage the stone. The basket is only retracted, never advanced, outside the enclosure of the steerable catheter.
6. The stone is extracted through the drain duct. (From Burhenne: Am. J. Roentgenol. *117*:388, 1973).

asked to return four weeks later for stone extraction, reporting to the radiology department without premedication. No fasting is necessary. Valium may be required for an occasional apprehensive patient.

The T-tube is extracted as the initial step. After introduction of the steerable catheter into the sinus tract, cholangiograms are obtained to ascertain the exact number and location of retained stones.

We have recommended that surgeons routinely use at least a 14 French T-tube after common duct exploration.[11] This permits insertion of the 13 French steerable catheter. Smaller catheters and smaller sinus tracts will often make the extraction procedure unsuccessful. Our 5 per cent failure rate occurred primarily in patients who had small indwelling T-tubes. If the surgeon has used a T-tube of 12 French or less, we prefer to wait several more weeks beyond the usual five-week postoperative period. We also try to manipulate a guide wire through the indwelling T-tube be-

fore its removal. The catheterization of a small sinus tract is more difficult, and injury to the sinus tract is more common during stone extraction. The indwelling guide wire will then permit re-entry of the bile ducts by feeding the steerable catheter over it.

After insertion of the steerable catheter through the sinus tract, its tip is manipulated just beyond the location of the retained stone. The stone retrieval basket is then introduced through the catheter and opened distally to the stone. The open basket ideally should touch the walls of the duct to engage stones readily on withdrawal. Baskets are now available in three different sizes (Fig. 13–7).*

After engagement of the stone by the basket, the entire assembly is slowly but continuously withdrawn through the sinus tract. Initially, we tried to close the basket over the stone after it was engaged. This resulted in

*Medi-Tech Co., Watertown, MA; Cook Inc., Bloomington, IN; V. Mueller, Chicago, IL.

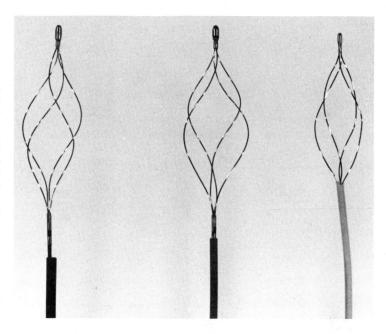

Figure 13–7. Stone extraction baskets are available in different sizes and from different manufacturers. The basket on the left, from the Cook Company, has a black sheath and a medium sized tip. It comes in three sizes. The Dormia basket in the middle comes with a green sheath but in only one size. The stainless steel wire maintains its torque and shape best. The Medi-Tech basket on the right comes with a white sheath and has a smaller tip and less torque to the wire. It is also available in three sizes.

fragmentation in many cases, and we no longer close the basket during withdrawal. If stone fragmentation occurs, the major fragments are extracted, and the patient is asked to return in one week in the hope that the small fragments will have passed spontaneously.

Several passes with the basket may be required before the stone is engaged. Stones smaller than 5 mm often are difficult to see on the television screen, sometimes making blind passes necessary. However, aimed radiographic spot films with close collimation between passes will help to ascertain the exact stone location.

Stones up to 8 or 9 mm in size can be extracted through the sinus tract of a 14 French T-tube. This requires some traction on the wire basket, and only hard stones will be extracted intact. Bilirubin stones usually fragment if they are much larger than the sinus tract.

Large stones (1 cm or larger) almost always require fragmentation, unless a very large T-tube has been inserted. The stone is engaged with a large wire basket or a wire sling and is extracted to the junction of bile duct and sinus tract. Strong traction on the wire stem of the basket is then needed to fragment these large stones. The wires of the basket are sufficiently sharp to accomplish fragmentation. One hand of the operator is held firmly against the abdominal wall, and the wire of the basket is guided between the fingers while strong traction is applied with the other hand. A hemostat

can be clamped to the end of the wire basket to gain sufficient traction. This process may be momentarily painful to the patient. Some bleeding or perforation of the sinus tract has occurred during extraction of large stones, but all signs and symptoms subsided within 48 hours (Fig. 13–8).

Initially, we made a prolonged attempt to extract all fragments on the first sitting. Visualization of fragments, however, becomes difficult if blood clots and air enter the duct system. Therefore, we now extract only the major fragments that are readily visible on the first attempt and then insert a straight catheter; the patient returns for a second session a few days later. We find that about one-third of all patients require multiple sessions (Fig. 13–9).[11]

Dilatation of the sinus tract may be required to extract large stones. If the surgeon has used a 10 or 12 French T-tube, we will usually try to dilate the sinus tract to a 14 or 16 French size before extraction on the first session. This is best accomplished with the use of arterial dilatation balloons.[12]

The routine surgical use of at least a 14 French T-tube is recommended after common duct exploration, even if no retained stones are suspected. If the common duct is small, the short branches of the T-tube are bivalved to permit their insertion into the duct. It also is possible to feed a larger straight catheter over the long arm of the T-tube to form a large sinus tract for subsequent stone extraction.[4]

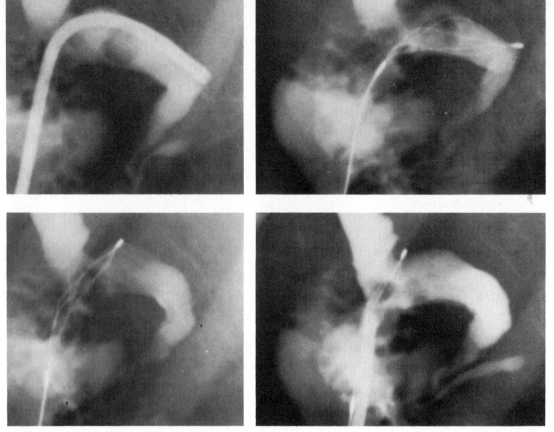

Figure 13–8. A single large retained common duct stone was engaged with the wire basket and moved to the junction of duct and sinus tract. Strong traction resulted in fragmentation of the stone. The fragments were then extracted.

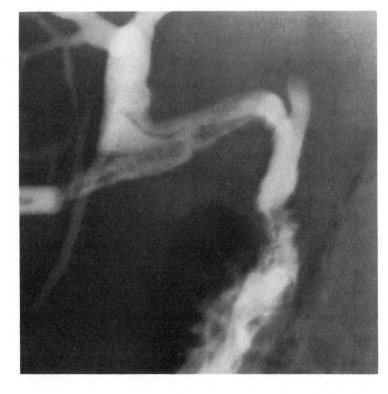

Figure 13–9. Air and blood clots are present following successful stone extraction. A straight catheter was inserted and the completion cholangiogram was obtained one week later. Note also the low medial insertion of the cystic duct.

The T-tube should be brought out through a stab wound in the right flank. If the T-tube is extracted through a midline incision, healing appears to be delayed and instrumentation is much more difficult because the radiologist's fingers will usually be in the fluoroscopic field.

If Penrose drains are present five weeks after surgery, we prefer to extract them and have the patient return two weeks later for extraction of retained stones. This is particularly necessary if the Penrose drain has been placed close to the T-tube. An isolated sinus tract with firm walls will facilitate uncomplicated stone extraction. Penrose drains usually create pockets between the bile ducts and the abdominal wall, complicating the extraction procedure.

Impacted stones located at the distal end of the common duct rarely cause complete obstruction. Surprisingly, most patients tolerate clamping of the T-tube in the presence of distal common duct stones.

Partially impacted distal common duct stones in most instances will not permit passage of the steerable catheter. The tip of the catheter is maneuvered to the stone, and the closed basket is then advanced between the wall of the duct and the stone. Snaring of the stone requires opening of the basket distal to the stone (Fig. 13–10). This is often impossible with stones in a distal common duct location, for which special maneuvers are required. First, attempts are made to move the stone more proximally in the duct system. Suction through a 13 French steerable catheter is applied, and the stone may be moved slightly more proximally. If this does not work, the small 8 French steerable catheter may be maneuvered with its tip alongside the stone, and contrast injection is attempted distal to the stone to flush the stone proximally.

The tip of the steerable catheter also may be maneuvered behind the stone to scoop the stone and move it up. If the basket can be opened alongside the stone, rotation of the basket may cause the stone to enter the basket. In some cases, the basket has to be opened in the duodenum and then carefully retracted to move or ensnare the stone. This requires that contrast be present in the distal common duct and duodenum to observe on the fluoroscopic screen whether the open stone basket is moving back through the ampullary portion of the duct or whether it is engaging the papilla or mucosa. Only gentle traction is permitted. If the basket is seen to be retracting the ampul-

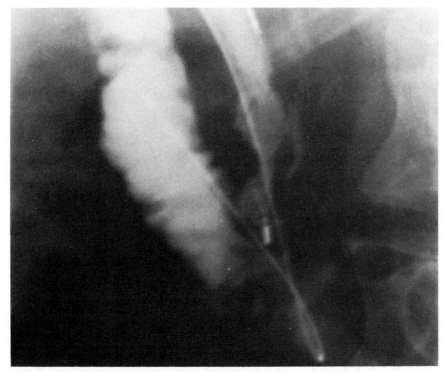

Figure 13–10. The retained distal common duct stone has been engaged with the open basket. A guide wire had been placed into the duodenum preceding extraction.

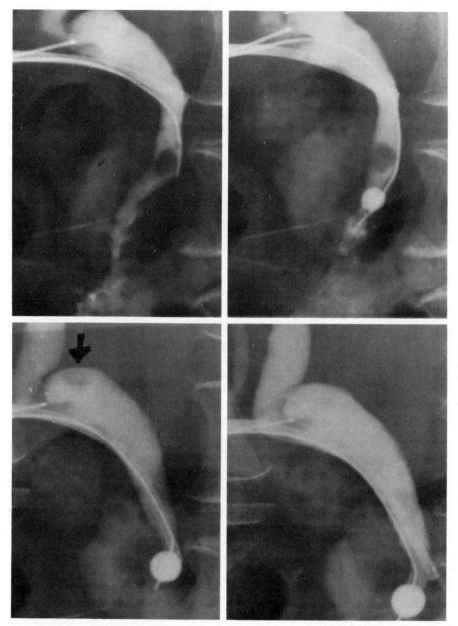

Figure 13–11. Retained common duct stone and dilated cystic duct remnant. The contrast-filled balloon of a Fogarty catheter was placed distal to the stone to avoid impaction. The stone moves freely from the common duct into the cystic duct remnant, requiring erect patient positioning to keep the stone in the common duct. Final film after extraction shows the duct system clear of retained material.

lary portion, it should be moved back into the duodenal loop and closed with the basket sheath before it is extracted.

Another maneuver to mobilize and engage distal common duct stones employs the Fogarty balloon catheter. The balloon is inflated with contrast for fluoroscopic visualization just distal to the location of the stone. Gentle traction is then applied to see whether the stone will move more proximally. We never inflate the Fogarty balloon to a larger caliber than the surrounding duct structure, since iatrogenic injury has been reported from intraoperative instrumentation (Fig. 13–11).[18]

Stones also may be impacted in an intrahepatic location. If stones are seen in hepatic radicles on postoperative T-tube cholangiography, we usually wait to see whether the stones will move into an extrahepatic position for easier extraction. This may require cholangiograms every two or three weeks and a waiting period of as long as three months. If stones do not move and if they are located in major hepatic radicles, extraction may be successful, although this is more difficult than extraction from an extrahepatic duct position (Fig. 13–12). The use of Fogarty balloons is the last resort if intrahepatic stones cannot be otherwise mobilized. Selective cholangiograms must be obtained to ensure that the intrahepatic stone is not situated above an intrahepatic duct stricture. Narrowing of hepatic radicles is then first treated with Grüntzig balloon catheters.

Early in 1975, we conducted a national survey to analyze the complication rate of nonoperative extraction of retained common duct stones. Four hundred and eight patients underwent this procedure in 38 hospitals in different parts of the US and Canada. With the addition of our 223 patients, a total of 631 patients was available for review.[8]

No mortality was reported in the 631 cases of nonoperative roentgenologic extraction of retained stones from the postoperative biliary tract. This is significant compared with the mortality of the alternative of surgical repeat choledochotomy for removal of retained stones.

The morbidity amounted to 5 per cent of patients, with postextraction fever in 12 patients, sepsis in two, pancreatitis in two, vasovagal reaction in two, subhepatic bile collection in two, and perforation of the sinus tract in seven. Extravasation from the sinus tract occurred after extraction of large stones through a small sinus tract. The contrast remained contained, except in two cases with

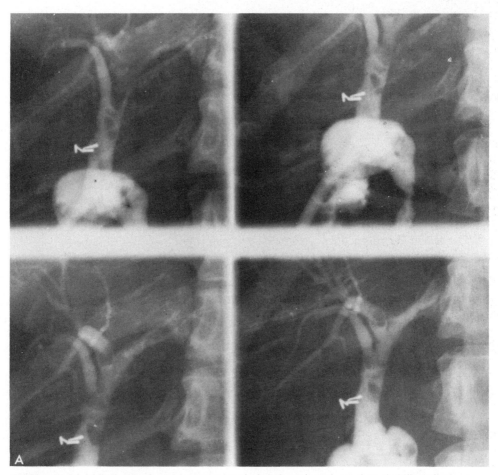

Figure 13–12. *A,* Multiple retained stones are present in intrahepatic and extrahepatic biliary ducts.

Illustration continued on following page

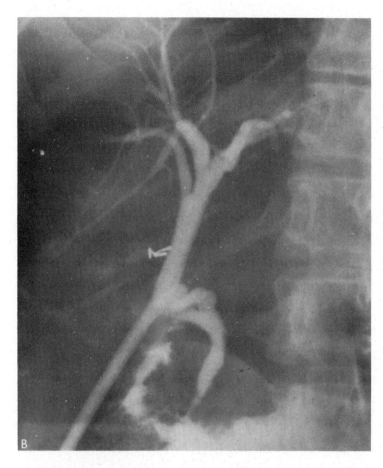

Figure 13–12. *Continued B,* The completion cholangiogram in the same patient shows that all retained stones have been removed. Note again the low and medial insertion of the cystic duct remnant.

free intra-abdominal contrast extravasation. All patients were placed on antibiotics, and no clinical symptoms or signs developed after sinus tract extravasation.

No bile duct perforations have been reported in this survey.

Papillomas of the common duct were mistaken for stones in three patients. The stone extraction basket engaged the papilloma in one case, and operation was required for stone basket removal. One additional patient required operation because of a large subhepatic bile collection that was drained.

Because of the small number of complications, we do not place patients routinely on antibiotics before the extraction procedure. In patients in whom postextraction fever, sepsis, or pancreatitis occurred, all signs and symptoms disappeared within 48 hours of antibiotic therapy.

The results of nonoperative extraction under roentgenologic control are excellent. Our personal experience in nonoperative biliary stone removal through the T-tube sinus tract in 661 patients was reported in 1980.[10] The overall success rate of nonoperative stone extraction was 95 per cent.

Failures occurred primarily in patients with small indwelling T-tubes of 12 French or smaller caliber. Two failures also involved cases in which the T-tube had been placed through a midline incision. Failure occurred in four patients with cystic duct remnant stones. Fifteen of the 33 patients with unsuccessful extractions had intrahepatic stones. The total failure rate was 5 per cent of 661 patients.

It must be remembered that re-exploration for retained stones, the previous method of choice for stone removal, carries a mortality of about 3 per cent.[34] No mortality occurred in a more recent analysis of 661 patients undergoing stone extraction in our institution.[10] Other techniques, such as stone dissolution or endoscopic removal, carry a significantly lower success rate. Also, the complication rate of these techniques is higher

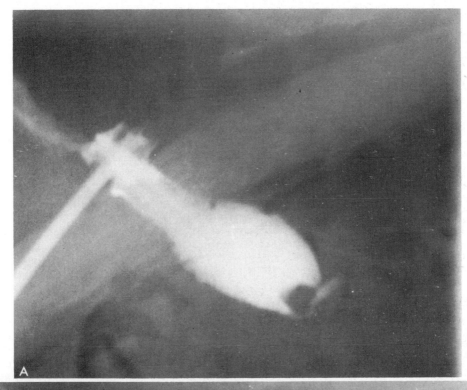

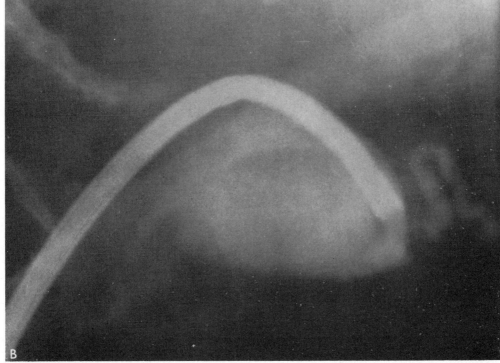

Figure 13–13. *A,* Cholecystostomy tube was placed in the presence of acute cholecystitis. Note partially impacted stone in the neck of the gallbladder. *B,* After removal of the cholecystostomy tube, a #13 French steerable catheter was advanced to the stone, and the stone was successfully extracted using suction.

than that of nonoperative removal under fluoroscopic control.[9] Experienced reviewers agree that our technique of nonoperative postoperative stone removal is the procedure of choice if the T-tube is still in place.[14, 36]

CHOLECYSTOSTOMY INSTRUMENTATION

Nonoperative instrumentation of the gallbladder under fluoroscopic control is feasible if a cholecystostomy tube is present. Stones from the gallbladder can be removed, particularly if the patient presents a poor surgical risk. Partially impacted gallstones in the neck of the gallbladder can be extracted in this fashion (Fig. 13–13). It is usually more difficult to engage free-floating stones in the gallbladder fundus with a stone extraction basket. It is then necessary to dilate the cholecystostomy tract with balloon catheters and use extraction forceps under fluoroscopic control. Large stones have to be fragmented, and the fragments are extracted.

TRANSCHOLECYSTIC INTERVENTION

The same subhepatic interventional approach through the cholecystostomy tract is used to gain access to the bile ducts. Removal of common bile duct stones through the cholecystostomy opening and cystic duct was first described in 1974.[28] This technique was successful in 9 out of 13 patients in the original report.

After cholecystocholangiography, the 8 French steerable catheter over a J guide wire is introduced through the cystic duct. The tip of the guide wire is rotated to negotiate the turns in the cystic duct. After the catheter has entered the bile duct, cystic duct dilatation is performed with Grüntzig balloon catheters.

Other reports of transcholecystic intervention describe both the intraoperative use of the Dormia basket and the postoperative radiologic technique for successful treatment of choledocholithiasis following cholecystostomy.[1, 19]

STRICTURE DILATATION

Interventional dilatation of benign bile duct strictures is indicated if biliary stones are retained proximal to benign narrowing resulting from cholangitis or previous surgery. We have used coaxial arterial catheters, ureteral dilators, or specially designed balloon catheters but now believe that the Grüntzig arterial balloon catheter[12] is best suited for this purpose. The first case was reported in 1974[5] (Fig. 13–14), and experience with seven patients was reported in 1975.[6] Even malignant strictures are readily dilated in one sitting to accommodate a 14 French catheter for internal bile drainage. Also, dilatation of a narrow sinus tract is readily accomplished with the Grüntzig balloon catheter.

It has been suggested that indwelling splint catheters remain within previous strictures for a period of 8 to 24 months to allow the scar to mature and stabilize.[35] We have applied indwelling splinting catheters for periods of up to two and one-half years. Patients tolerate indwelling catheters well; they return to work and are able to take showers without fear of losing the catheter. Should the catheter become obstructed, it is readily exchanged over a guide wire.

Maturing of the previous stricture or possible recurrence can be checked by withdrawing the catheter to a point just outside the previous narrowing. The catheter remains in place to keep the sinus tract open. Should the stricture recur, the splint is again placed through it.

BIOPSY

Biopsy of lesions in the biliary tract can be obtained with the subhepatic approach using the postoperative T-tube tract. This approach was first reported in 1975 (Fig. 13–15).[7] The biopsy forceps employed with the bronchial or duodenal fiberscope has been successfully used for this purpose.[31]

After cholangiographic identification of the filling defect in the bile ducts, the steerable catheter is moved with its tip directly on the lesion. The endoscopic biopsy forceps is then moved through the steerable catheter, and biopsy is obtained under fluoroscopic control. The technique is applicable for biliary masses in hepatic and extrahepatic ducts including carcinoma of the pancreas involving the distal common duct. Our biopsy experience through the subhepatic approach now involves 13 patients. No bleeding and no perforation have resulted. The T-tube tract is kept open with a catheter for several days after biopsy for drainage and to regain access if indicated.

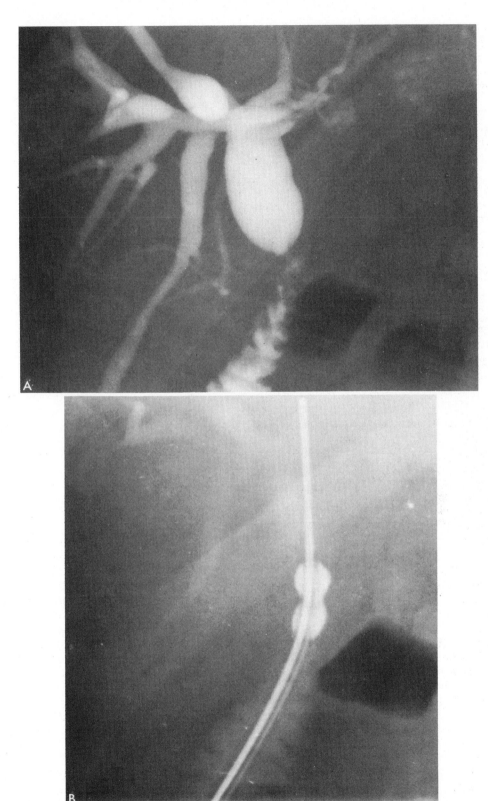

Figure 13–14. *A,* Stricture at the hepatojejunostomy in a jaundiced patient six weeks after anastomosis. *B,* A guide wire was advanced through the stricture, followed by a dilatation balloon. The waist of the contrast-filled balloon indicates the site of the partially dilated stricture.

Illustration continued on following page

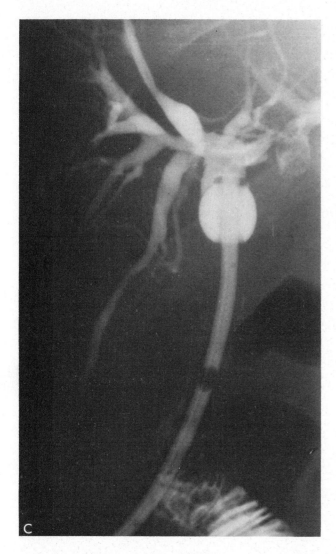

Figure 13–14. *Continued C,* Following dilatation of the stricture, a retention balloon catheter was placed above the anastomosis and left in place for a prolonged period to maintain the diameter of the anastomosis. Note the sidehole in the clamped catheter for intestinal bile drainage. Note also some retained stones in the left hepatic radicle.

FOREIGN BODY REMOVAL

Foreign bodies left behind in the biliary tract after radiologic instrumentation require removal. Like interventional procedures in the vascular system, particular maneuvers have been designed for foreign body removal.

Surgical metallic clips may be disengaged during interventional procedures. They may present as loose bodies in the duct system or the sinus tract. Metallic clips in the sinus tract are best pushed with the steerable catheter into the duct system. This foreign body can then be expelled either spontaneously or by instrumentation with the patient in the erect position through the distal common duct into the duodenum.

Plastic introducer sleeves for guide wires may be deposited in the biliary tract during guide wire and catheter manipulation. These retained foreign bodies can readily be removed with use of the biopsy wire or the wire basket.

We also have had experience with a completely detached stone basket. It separated from the basket wire during instrumentation of a common duct stone. The entire basket was retrieved successfully with the use of the steerable catheter and a guide wire sling, which was manipulated over the tip of the detached basket (Fig. 13–16).[30]

INTERNAL BILIARY DRAINAGE

Internal biliary drainage accomplishes interventional relief of biliary obstruction and normal passage of bile from the liver through the ducts into the gut. It involves placement of a

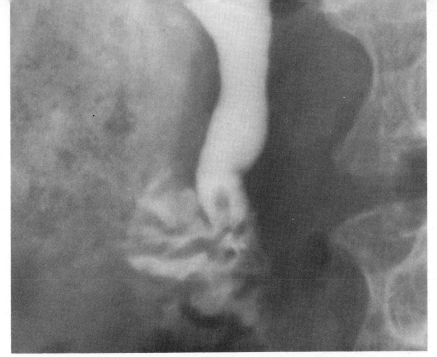

Figure 13–15. The filling defect in the distal common duct was biopsied, closing the wire basket over the lesion. Histology showed normal common duct mucosa, and this lesion apparently represented a mucosal flap elevated with dilatation instruments passed through the ampulla at the time of surgery.

Figure 13–16. The Dormia stone extraction basket detached from the stem during stone removal intervention. The basket was retrieved successfully from the common duct with the use of the steerable guide wire and a wire sling.

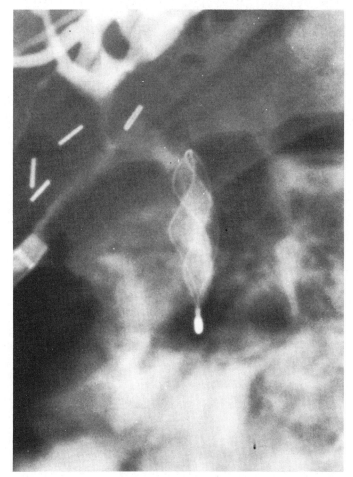

509

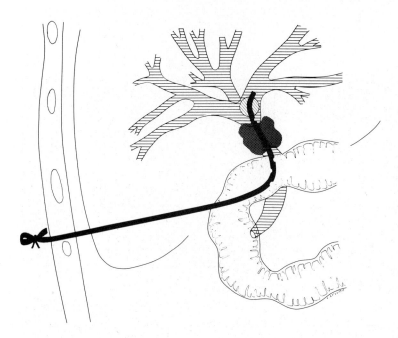

Figure 13–17. The postoperative sinus tract is used for internal drainage of a carcinoma of the common hepatic duct. Sideholes are placed in the common duct and the catheter is closed at the skin. The Silastic-coated balloon catheter is kept in position by inflating the distal catheter balloon with saline.

catheter through a benign or malignant stricture with side- or endholes above and below the lesion. Our first case, reported in 1974, was a stricture at a hepatojejunostomy.[5] The obstructing benign stricture at the anastomosis was entered with a guide wire through a jejunostomy tract, the stricture was dilated with a balloon catheter, and a Silastic-coated balloon catheter was placed to splint the previous stricture. An endhole above and sideholes below the lesion provided for internal drainage. The catheter was clamped at the skin. The balloon above the previous stricture was inflated in the common duct for better retention. The same technique may be applied through the T-tube tract for malignant lesions close to the porta hepatis from duct carcinoma or metastasis or in obstructing carcinoma in the distal common duct. The retention balloon is then placed into the duodenum. No skin fixation of the closed catheter is necessary (Figs. 13–17 and 13–18).

Internal biliary drainage with the subhepatic

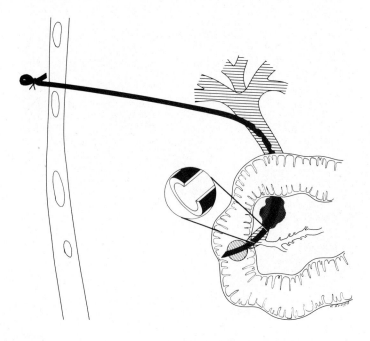

Figure 13–18. A postoperative T-tube tract is used for instrumentation of common duct stricture due to carcinoma of the pancreas. The stricture is dilated and the catheter is placed through it over a guide wire with sideholes in the duct proximally to the lesion. The cut-out demonstrates a lateral groove placed in the drainage catheter to avoid pancreatic duct obstruction. The catheter is closed at the skin and anchored in the duodenum by inflating the balloon.

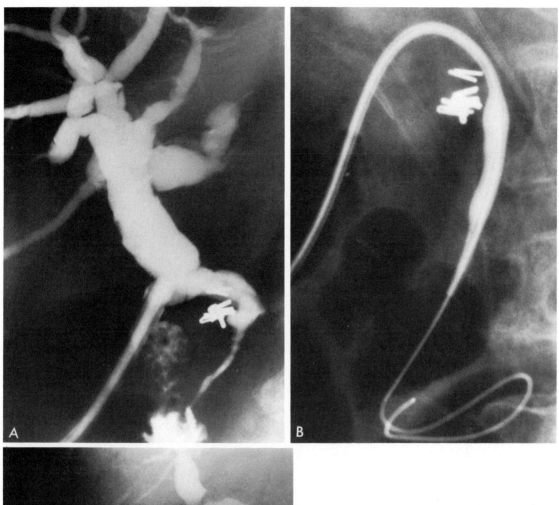

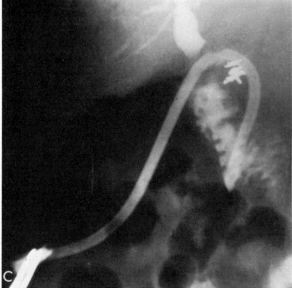

Figure 13–19. *A,* Malignant stricture of the distal common duct due to carcinoma of the pancreas with a postoperative T-tube tract in place. *B,* The malignant stricture is dilated with use of a Grüntzig balloon over a guide wire. *C,* Internal drainage catheter in place and closed at the skin.

postoperative approach is technically easier than with the nonoperative percutaneous transhepatic technique. It requires previous surgical access to the bile ducts but has several advantages. A larger drainage catheter can be placed through the lesion into the duodenum when compared with the transhepatic approach. It provides for long-term drainage. The subhepatic internal drainage technique also requires less technical skill and is less time consuming. It provides for easier dilatation of malignant strictures with Grüntzig balloons. Inadvertent tube removal is less likely, and the complications of the transhepatic approach, such as fluid leak at the capsule, hemorrhage, or parenchymal damage, are avoided. Soft rubber catheters up to a 14 French caliber may be used for patient comfort and long-term internal biliary drainage with the postoperative approach (Fig. 13–19).

References

1. Amberg, J. R., and Chun, G.: Transcystic duct treatment of common bile duct stones. Gastrointest. Radiol. 6:361, 1981.
2. Bastidas, J., and DeIguercio, L. M.: Cholecystocholangiography after cholecystoduodenostomy, Am. J. Roentgenol. 129:534, 1977.
3. Burhenne, H. J.: Extraktion von Residualsteinen der Gallenwege ohne Reoperation. Fortschr. Roentgenstr. 117:425, 1972.
4. Burhenne, H. J.: Nonoperative retained biliary tract stone extraction: A new roentgenologic technique. Am. J. Roentgenol. 117:388, 1973.
5. Burhenne, H. J.: Nonoperative roentgenologic instrumentation technics of the postoperative biliary tract. Am. J. Surg. 128:111, 1974.
6. Burhenne, H. J.: Dilatation of biliary tract strictures. Radiol. Clin. 44:153, 1975.
7. Burhenne, H. J.: Bile duct biopsy with the stone extraction basket. Radiol. Clin. 44:178, 1975.
8. Burhenne, H. J.: Complications of nonoperative extraction of retained common duct stones. Am. J. Surg. 131:260, 1976.
9. Burhenne, H. J.: Nonoperative instrument extraction of retained bile duct stones. World J. Surg. 2:439, 1978.
10. Burhenne, H. J.: Percutaneous extraction of retained biliary tract stones: 661 patients. Am. J. Roentgenol. 134:888, 1980.
11. Burhenne, H. J., et al.: Nonoperative extraction of retained biliary tract stones requiring multiple sessions. Am. J. Surg. 128:288, 1974.
12. Burhenne, H. J., and Morris, D. C.: Biliary stricture dilatation: use of the Gruntzig balloon catheter. J. Can. Assoc. Radiol. 31:196, 1980.
13. Burhenne, H. J., and Peters, H. E.: Retained intrahepatic stones: use of the U tube during repeated nonoperative stone extractions. Arch. Surg. 113:837, 1978.
14. Classen, M., and Ossenberg, F. W.: Nonsurgical removal of common bile duct stones. Gut 18:760, 1977.
15. Cruikshank, J. G., Fraser, G. M., and Law, J.: Finger doses received by radiologists during Chiba needle percutaneous cholangiography. Br. J. Radiol. 53:584, 1980.
16. Crummy, A. B., and Turnipseed, W. D.: Percutaneous replacement of a biliary T tube. Am. J. Roentgenol. 128:869, 1977.
17. Dorsey, T. J., Rowen, M., and Hepps, S. A.: Nonoperative replacement of T tube in common duct after inadvertent removal. Surgery 71:97, 1972.
18. Eaton, S. B., Jr., et al.: Iatrogenic liver injury resulting from ductal instrumentation with Fogarty biliary balloon catheter. Radiology 100:581, 1971.
19. Farinon, A. M., Sianesi, M., and Battistim, C.: Intraoperative transcystic extraction of common bile duct stones by a Dormia-Pironneau catheter. Intern. Surg. 64:31, 1979.
20. Fennessy, J. J., and You, K.-D: A method for the expulsion of stones retained in the common bile duct. Am. J. Roentgenol. 110:256, 1970.
21. Janes, J. O., and McClelland, R.: Fluoroscopic replacement of a choledochal U-tube using a steerable catheter. Radiology 128:828, 1978.
22. Jelaso, D. V., and Hirschfield, J. S.: Jaundice from impacted sediment in a T tube: recognition and treatment. Am. J. Roentgenol. 127:413, 1976.
23. Lagrave, G., et al.: Lithiase biliaire résiduelle: extraction à la sonde de Dormia par de drain de Kehr. Mem. Acad. Chir. 95:530, 1969.
24. Magarey, C. J.: Removal of retained bile-duct calculus without operation: case report. Br. J. Surg. 56:312, 1969.
25. Magarey, C. J.: Non-surgical removal of retained biliary calculi. Lancet 1:1044, 1971.
26. Margulis, A. R., Newton, T. H., and Najarian, J. S.: Removal of plug from T-tube by fluoroscopically controlled catheter. Am. J. Roentgenol. 93:975, 1965.
27. Mazzariello, R.: Removal of residual biliary tract calculi without reoperation. Surgery 67:566, 1970.
28. Mazzariello, R. M.: Transcholecystic extraction of residual calculi in common bile duct. Surgery 75:338, 1974.
29. Mondet, A.: Tecnica de la extraccion incruenta de los calculos en las litiasis residual del coledoco. Bol. Soc. Cir. B. Air. 46:278, 1962.
30. Nichols, D. M., and Burhenne, H. J.: Retrieval of broken Dormia basket. Am. J. Roentgenol. 138:970, 1982.
31. Palayew, M. J., and Stein, L.: Postoperative biopsy of the common bile duct via the T-tube tract. Am. J. Roentgenol. 130:287, 1978.
32. Russell, E., and Koolpe, H. A.: A modified T-tube for use after nonoperative biliary stone removal. Radiology 129:237, 1978.
33. Sniderman, K. W., Baxi, R. K., Rumburg, K. N., and Sos, T. A.: A modified technique for percutaneous insertion of a biliary T-tube. Radiology 131:539, 1979.
34. Smith, H. W., Engel, C., Averbrook, B., and Longmire, W. P., Jr.: Problems of retained and recurrent common bile duct stones. Surgery 66:291, 1969.
35. Warren, K. W., and Whitcomb, F. F., Jr.: Diagnosis and treatment of benign biliary tract stricture. J. Hosp. Pract. Feb.: 62, 1971.
36. Way, L. W.: Retained common duct stones. Surg. Clin. North Am. 53:1139, 1973.

PEDIATRIC DISEASES OF THE GALLBLADDER AND BILE DUCTS

by Edward B. Singleton, M.D.

14

EMBRYOLOGY

An understanding of the formation of the biliary tree is necessary for an appreciation of the congenital defects that may involve this structure. The liver arises as a bud or diverticulum from the caudal portion of the foregut at approximately four weeks of intrauterine life. Growth of the diverticulum into the septum transversum occurs rapidly and is accompanied by its division into two parts. The large cranial part is the primordium of the liver and with growth becomes the glandular structures and ducts of the liver. This hepatic portion rapidly elongates and divides into the right and left lobes of the liver. The connective tissue framework and vascular structures as well as the biliary structures and mesenteric connection derive from the mesoderm of the septum transversum and vitelline veins. This hepatic mass expands rapidly and by the fifth week occupies almost the entire abdominal cavity (Fig. 14–1).

The second division of the hepatic diverticulum is a small caudal portion, which forms the gallbladder and cystic duct. Initially the extrahepatic ductal system is occluded with endodermal cells but is later recanalized. The caudal cystic portion of the primitive hepatic diverticulum elongates into the gallbladder and cystic duct, which drains into the main biliary duct. The lumen of the biliary ductal system is established by the seventh week, and bile is secreted by the twelfth week. The pancreas develops as a ventral and dorsal pancreatic bud, and as the duodenum elongates and rotates the two pancreatic primordia fuse with the ventral mass, joining with the right side of the dorsal pancreas. The short ventral duct fuses with the dorsal duct, which then usually atrophies, leaving the single pancreatic duct emptying into the common bile duct. Although a variety of anomalies of the liver may occur, only those involving the gallbladder and ductal system will be considered in this chapter.

The majority of abnormalities of the biliary ductal system in the pediatric patient are usually secondary to intrauterine infection or congenital faults in the development of the biliary tree. In addition, acquired diseases more commonly seen in the adult patient may occasionally be encountered in infants and children. There are many complex metabolic diseases of infancy and early childhood that produce fibrosis and cirrhosis of the liver. The majority of these conditions do not lend themselves to radiologic evaluation. Only those conditions, both congenital and acquired, that can be evaluated by conventional radiographic procedures, transhepatic cholangiography, computed tomography, sonography, and nuclear imaging will be discussed.

METHODS OF VISUALIZING THE BILIARY TREE

Oral cholecystography is unpredictable in the infant, and satisfactory opacification of the gallbladder is not as dependable as in older children and adults. The usual recommended dose of iopanoic acid (Telepaque) is 0.15 gm/kg of body weight in children weighing less than 13 kg; 2 gm/kg for children 13 to 23 kg;

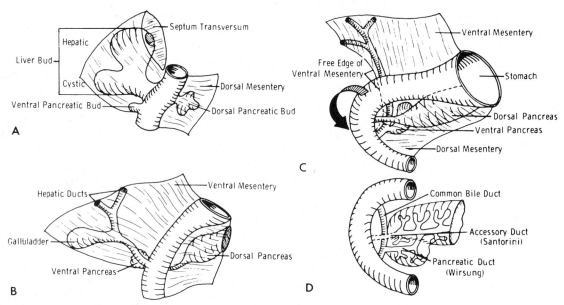

Figure 14–1. Development of the liver and pancreas. *A*, Lateral view. *B, C*, Antero-posterior view. *D*, Pancreatic and bile duct formation. (Reprinted with permission from Singleton, Wagner, and Dutton: Radiology of the Alimentary Tract in Infants and Children. Philadelphia: W. B. Saunders, 1977.)

and 3 gm/kg for children over 23 kg. Bétou-lières and coworkers advocated the use of Solu-Biloptine (known in the United States as Oragrafin) at a dosage of 0.45 gm/kg of body weight in infants under one month of age and 0.90 gm/kg in older age groups. In our institution we prescribe 0.5 gm/kg of Oragrafin for infants; 1 gm/kg for children between the ages of two and five; 1.5 gm/kg for children five to ten years old; 2 gm/kg for children 10 to 15 years old; and 3 gm/kg for children over 15 years of age. The results reported by Betou-lieres and associates[4] and Nahum, Poree, and Sauvegrain[8] are reported as superior to the results of other methods of oral cholecystography. In our own experience, all methods of oral cholecystography are unpredictable in the infant age group. Whether this is due to difficulties in introducing contrast media into the stomach of young infants, unexplained alterations of absorption of the contrast media, or interference of the normal abundance of overlying small bowel and colonic gas in this age group is speculative. It is also important to realize that the biliary tract in infants and young children is particularly small and the narrow channels are difficult to visualize.

The results of intravenous cholecystography are even more disappointing than those of oral cholecystography in visualizing the biliary system of infants and young children. Iodipamide sodium (Cholegrafin), given in a dose of 0.6 to 1.2 ml/kg of body weight, has been reported successful in intravenous cholecystography. The bound iodine content of iodipamide methylglucamine is greater with a recommended dose of 0.3 to 0.6 ml/kg of body weight. Visualization of the biliary system theoretically takes place 30 minutes to 4 hours after injection of the contrast medium, but attempts to visualize the biliary system by this method are more often unsuccessful than successful.

Operative cholangiography is used primarily in the differentiation of biliary atresia and congenital hepatitis and in demonstrating the anatomy of a choledochal cyst. At the time of laparotomy a 50 per cent solution of any of the sterile water-soluble contrast media used for excretory urography is injected into either the gallbladder or whatever portion of the ductal system can be identified. The usual amount of contrast medium varies from 5 to 15 ml.

Computed tomography in infants has not enjoyed the success in evaluating the biliary system that it has had in older children and adults. This is partially due to the need for sedation, even using a fast scan time, and the lack of perivisceral fat in this age group, making delineation of visceral structures more difficult. However, choledochal cysts and alterations in the size of the intrahepatic biliary ducts can be clearly appreciated by this method.

Sonography is an important modality in the evaluation of choledochal cysts and the intrahepatic ductal dilatation that usually accompanies this anomaly. The sonographic evaluation of the gallbladder in the pediatric patient is more accurate than cholecystography. Ultrasound scanning of the gallbladder is preferably performed in the morning prior to feeding because of the contractility of the gallbladder after ingestion of fatty foods including milk. To ensure maximum dilatation of the gallbladder, only fruit juices should be given prior to the examination. Real-time sonography of the gallbladder is especially helpful in young children, and sedation is rarely required.

Both computed tomography and sonography are rarely useful in visualizing intrahepatic bile ducts unless they are dilated, as in cases of choledochal cyst, occasionally in older children with biliary atresia, and in a variety of causes of biliary tract ectasia.

Percutaneous transhepatic cholangiography is seldom attempted in infants and children. The minute size of the intrahepatic ducts makes transhepatic injection nearly impossible, but when there is dilatation of intrahepatic ducts, particularly when ultrasound shows intrahepatic ductal dilatation, transhepatic injection may be used if clinically indicated.

Endoscopic retrograde cholangiopancreatography is not practical in the pediatric age group, again because of the limitation in size of the ductal systems.

CONGENITAL ANOMALIES OF THE BILIARY TREE

There are a variety of congenital defects of the liver including partial or complete absence, cystic lesions (frequently associated with both infantile and adult polycystic disease of the kidney), congenital hepatic fibrosis (frequently associated with renal tubular ectasia or medullary sponge kidney), and variations in position of the liver (commonly associated with anomalies of the spleen and complex congenital heart disease). However, this chapter is limited only to anomalies of the biliary tree and not the hepatic parenchyma.

The gallbladder may be in a variety of anomalous positions, but its identification in the infant and young child is frequently problematic because of the difficulties of obtaining quality oral and intravenous cholecystograms in this age group. Sonography and nuclear scintigraphy are more accurate modalities for locating the gallbladder (Fig. 14–2). Variations in position of the gallbladder accompany variations in position of the liver and may be seen in complete situs inversus, with the gallbladder in the upper left quadrant. An extremely rare anomaly is isolated left-sided liver and gallbladder without situs inversus; with this anomaly the other abdominal viscera, including the stomach, have been reported to be in their normal positions. In indeterminate abdominal solitus (heterotaxia), the liver appears in a symmetric position with the gallbladder in the midline. This anomaly is commonly accompanied by asplenia, polysplenia, or isosplenia associated with pulmonary isomerism and, frequently, complex congenital heart disease. Absence of the gallbladder is associated with biliary atresia and, frequently, polysplenia, Unusual locations of the gallbladder, including in the falciform ligament, the suprahepatic area, the abdominal wall, and the retroperitoneal area, have been reported.

Anomalous insertions of the cystic duct connecting the gallbladder to a variety of locations with the common duct and the hepatic duct and communications with both the common duct and hepatic ducts also have been described.

The most common *anomalous shape* of the gallbladder is the well-known phrygian cap, which is seen in approximately 2 to 6 per cent of all cholecystographies (Fig. 14–3). In this condition the fundus of the gallbladder is folded on itself, producing a kink in the fundus. The gallbladder may rarely appear as a diverticulum with absence of the cystic duct, simulating a diverticulum of the common bile duct. In all probability this represents a form of choledochal cyst. The septated gallbladder usually is transverse, dividing the gallbladder into two compartments (Fig. 14–4). Multiple septa also have been reported. Other anomalies of shape include siphon, fishhook, and hourglass configurations.

Absence of the gallbladder is frequently associated with infants with biliary atresia but may occur in other situations in which the intra- and extrahepatic ducts are of normal patency. The anomaly may consist of absence of only the gallbladder and cystic duct or absence of the gallbladder with a patent cystic duct. When the gallbladder is absent, anomalies of the hepatic and common ducts are frequently present, and these structures may empty separately into the duodenum. Cholecystography may be misleading because of the difficulties in visualizing the gallbladder radio-

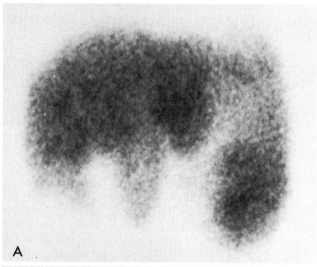

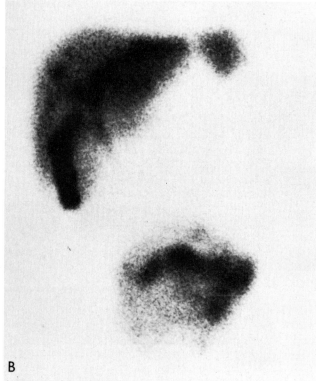

Figure 14–2. Tc-99m HIDA liver scan in a 10-year-old boy with unexplained upper right quadrant pain. *A*, Initial scan shows defect in the inferior portion of the right lobe of the liver. *B*, Delayed scan shows delineation of hepatic and common ducts and explains the lack of localized initial uptake as the result of an intrahepatic gallbladder. (Courtesy of G. E. De Puey, M.D., Dept. of Nuclear Medicine, Texas Children's Hospital.)

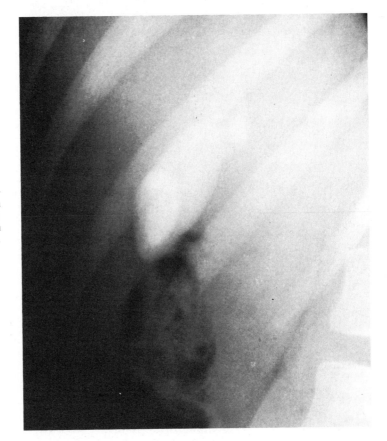

Figure 14–3. Phrygian cap in a 10-year-old girl. (Reprinted with permission from Singleton, Wagner, and Dutton: Radiology of the Alimentary Tract in Infants and Children. Philadelphia: W. B. Saunders, 1977.)

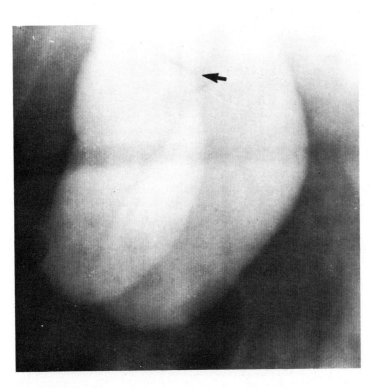

Figure 14–4. Duplication of the gallbladder in which a septum (arrow) is identified in one of the gallbladders. (Reprinted with permission from Singleton, Wagner, and Dutton: Radiology of the Alimentary Tract in Infants and Children. Philadelphia: W. B. Saunders, 1977.)

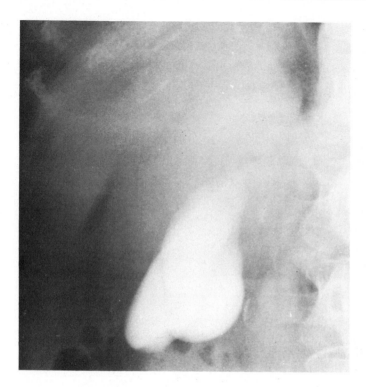

Figure 14–5. Duplication of the gallbladder. Cholecystogram shows contrast medium within two gallbladders. (Reprinted with permission from Singleton, Wagner, and Dutton: Radiology of the Alimentary Tract in Infants and Children. Philadelphia: W. B. Saunders, 1977.)

graphically in the young infant. Consequently, failure of visualization is unreliable in predicting congenital absence of the gallbladder, sonography being a more reliable method of finding the gallbladder. However, surgical exploration may be necessary to determine the presence or absence of the gallbladder if the patient is jaundiced and has signs of biliary tract obstruction.

Duplication of the gallbladder and even triplication are rare anomalies and may be incidental findings at necropsy (Fig. 14–5). Each gallbladder usually has its own cystic duct, but a single cystic duct may be present. In all of these situations, anomalous insertion of the cystic duct can occur.

A diverticulum of the gallbladder is an extremely rare anomaly and is usually located near the bladder neck. Diverticula rarely produce symptoms unless they become the site of stone formation later in life.

Congenital communications between the biliary tree and the trachea (tracheo-biliary fistulas) are very rare anomalies that produce respiratory distress in the newborn, characterized by a cough productive of green sputum.

A variety of miscellaneous anomalies of the gallbladder and cystic duct may occur. These include intramural cystic ducts, heterotopic gastrointestinal mucosa or pancreatic tissue within the gallbladder, intrahepatic gallbladder, and free-floating pendulous gallbladder, all of which are usually asymptomatic and are discovered at either laparotomy or necropsy. Congenital stenosis of the cystic duct is extremely rare and may be complicated by cholelithiasis.

HEPATIC AND COMMON DUCT

There are many causes of jaundice in the newborn, most of these being medical problems including a variety of causes of increased bilirubin production, impaired hepatic function, a variety of infections, both bacterial and nonbacterial, metabolic abnormalities, and heredofamilial disorders (Table 14–1). These cases are usually determined by appropriate laboratory tests or a combination of clinical problems and a defect in the transport of bile acids in the liver cells or bile canaliculi; radiologic studies are uninformative. Prolonged obstructive jaundice can also be associated with various anomalies of the hepatobiliary system and the gastrointestinal tract including atresia of the upper small bowel and hypertrophic pyloric stenosis. However, the great majority of newborns with prolonged jaundice have either neonatal hepatitis or biliary atresia.

Table 14–1. CAUSES OF JAUNDICE IN THE NEWBORN*

Biliary Duct Abnormalities
Extrahepatic biliary atresia
  Without associated malformations
  Associated with trisomy E
  Associated with polysplenia-heterotaxia syndrome
Intrahepatic biliary atresia
Intrahepatic atresia associated with lymphedema
Bile duct hypoplasia
Choledochal cyst
Bile plug syndrome
Fibrocystic disease
Bile duct and hepatic neoplasms
Periductal lymphadenopathy

Hepatocellular Disturbances in Biliary Excretion
Neonatal hepatitis (giant cell hepatitis)
Infectious hepatitis
  Hepatitis B (HBsAg)
  Rubella
  Cytomegalovirus
  Toxoplasmosis
  Coxsackie virus
  Syphilis
  Herpes simplex, zoster varicellosus
  Listeriosis
  Tubercle bacillus
  Systemic infectious diseases
Intestinal obstruction
Parenteral alimentation
Ischemic necrosis
Hematologic diseases
  Erythroblastosis fetalis (severe forms)
  Congenital erythropoietic porphyria
Metabolic and heredofamilial disorders
  α_1-Antitrypsin deficiency
  Galactosemia
  Tyrosinemia
  Fructosemia
  Glycogen storage disease type IV
  Lipid storage diseases
    Niemann-Pick disease
    Gaucher's disease
    Wolman's disease
  Cerebrohepatorenal syndrome (Zellweger syndrome)
  Trisomy E
  Fibrocystic disease
  Familial idiopathic cholestasis
    Byler's disease (fatal intrahepatic cholestasis)
    Hereditary cholestasis combined with peripheral
      pulmonary stenosis and other anomalies
    Arteriohepatic dysplasia

*Adapted from Morrecki, Gartner, and Lee *In* Behrman: Neonatal-Perinatal Medicine. Diseases of the Fetus and Infant. St. Louis: C. V. Mosby, 1977.

Biliary Atresia and Neonatal Hepatitis

Biliary atresia is the most common liver disease causing death in childhood in the US. Differentiation between biliary atresia and neonatal hepatitis (giant cell transformation of the liver) is extremely difficult, attested to by the large number of articles relating to these subjects in the pediatric literature. Traditionally, biliary atresia has been considered a developmental anomaly of the intra- and extrahepatic bile ducts. Currently, however, neonatal hepatitis, biliary atresia, biliary hypoplasia, and choledochal cysts are considered variations of intrauterine infection or infantile obstructive cholangiopathy. These conditions represent a spectrum of diseases, with neonatal hepatitis and biliary atresia at opposite poles and varying degrees of involvement between the two. Diminished bile flow secondary to neonatal hepatitis produces severe cholestasis, and the resulting structural damage to the bile ducts from the low flow and inflammation apparently contributes to the eventual obliteration of the biliary tree. This concept explains the difficulties in accurate differentiation of biliary atresia and neonatal hepatitis. In both conditions the clinical manifestations consist of jaundice lasting beyond three to four weeks of age, hepatomegaly, and occasionally splenomegaly. Late in the disease, malnutrition becomes obvious and biliary rickets may develop. Cirrhosis and portal hypertension develop later in life. However, differentiation is important in that if biliary atresia is present, surgical procedures may be corrective, whereas if neonatal hepatitis is present, surgery should be avoided.

Early operation (portoenterostomy) before the twelfth week of life is extremely important because the presence of patent bile ducts at the porta hepatis seems to be related to the patient's age because of the progression of the obstructive process after birth.

Methods of differentiating biliary atresia and neonatal hepatitis involving the radiologist include liver biopsy, sonography, radionuclide excretion studies, and operative cholangiography.

Histologic evaluation of needle biopsy of the liver has been reported by Hays as providing a correct diagnosis of either biliary atresia or neonatal hepatitis in 61 per cent of cases.[31] The diagnosis was uncertain in 26 per cent of 100 liver biopsies and incorrect in 13 per cent. Consequently, liver biopsy may not provide the proper diagnosis and may be misleading.

Although sonography does not consistently demonstrate normal intrahepatic biliary ducts, when the ducts are seen to be dilated they are readily detected, which is helpful in ruling out a diagnosis of intrahepatic biliary atresia. Dilated hepatic ducts suggest extrahepatic biliary atresia, stenosis, or choledochal cyst. Careful attention to the branching pattern and sonographic characteristics is important in correctly differentiating biliary channels from vascular channels of the liver.

The most common radionuclide study in differentiating biliary atresia from neonatal hepatitis has been I-131 rose bengal liver excretion studies. Recovery of less than 10 per cent of the administered dose of this radionuclide from the stool suggests biliary obstruction. Unfortunately, because approximately 20 per cent of the patients with neonatal hepatitis also fail to excrete significant amounts of I-131, the effectiveness of the test as a differential examination is limited. In addition, the relatively long half-life and resulting radiation from this isotope are disadvantages. However, if the radiopharmaceutical is excreted into the bowel, one can be confident that significant extrahepatic obstruction is not present and an operative procedure can be avoided.

Newer radiopharmaceutical products, especially the iminodiacetic acids (Tc-99m HIDA and Tc-99m PIPIDA) have largely replaced the I-131 rose bengal labeled studies because of decreased radiation, more rapid excretion, and improved hepatobiliary imaging (Fig. 14–6). The disadvantage of the short half-life of this isotope may be overcome by giving phenobarbitol before the examination. In the presence of patent extrahepatic biliary ducts, phenobarbitol enhances and accelerates biliary excretion of Tc-99m IDA and consequently is useful in differentiating biliary atresia from other causes of neonatal jaundice. The isotope naturally will not appear in the duodenum in biliary atresia. In other conditions, such as neonatal hepatitis, excretion into the duo-

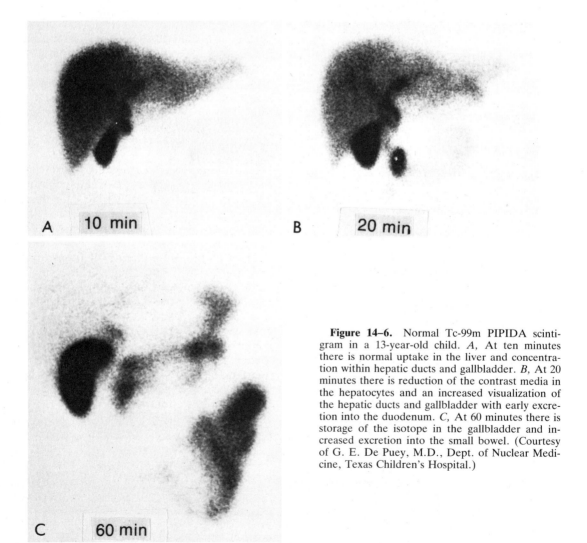

Figure 14–6. Normal Tc-99m PIPIDA scintigram in a 13-year-old child. *A,* At ten minutes there is normal uptake in the liver and concentration within hepatic ducts and gallbladder. *B,* At 20 minutes there is reduction of the contrast media in the hepatocytes and an increased visualization of the hepatic ducts and gallbladder with early excretion into the duodenum. *C,* At 60 minutes there is storage of the isotope in the gallbladder and increased excretion into the small bowel. (Courtesy of G. E. De Puey, M.D., Dept. of Nuclear Medicine, Texas Children's Hospital.)

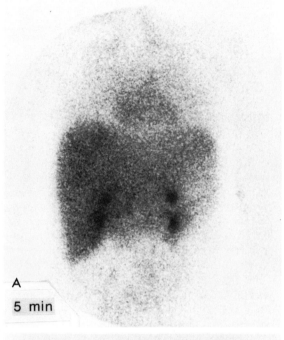

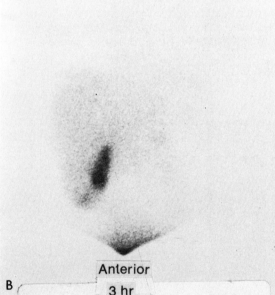

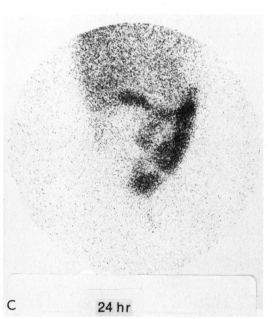

Figure 14–7. Neonatal hepatitis. *A,* At five minutes there is delayed excretion by the hepatocytes. *B,* at three hours delayed excretion is still evident but there is imaging of the gallbladder. *C,* At 24 hours delayed excretion into the small bowel has occurred. (Courtesy of G. E. De Puey, M.D., Dept. of Nuclear Medicine, Texas Children's Hospital.)

denum is expected but frequently delayed (Fig. 14–7). Although this method is more useful than I-131 rose bengal labeled excretion studies, it retains some of the disadvantages of other isotope excretion studies

Another technique for determining bile excretion is duodenal intubation with a 24-hour collection of duodenal fluid and visual inspection for biliary pigment. The predicted results are approximately the same as those found when using the I-131 rose bengal excretion test.

Laparoscopy has been used for direct visualization of the gallbladder and cholangiography through the laparoscope. Visualization of injected cholangiographic contrast media up the biliary tree and into the intestine demonstrates patency of the extrabiliary system. If the gallbladder is not visualized, the infant probably has biliary atresia, and a formal surgical procedure and operative cholangiogram are necessary. However, operative cholangiography is a difficult procedure, and direct laparotomy is performed in most cases.

Because of the difficulty in differentiating biliary atresia from neonatal hepatitis, many of the diagnostic studies are being eliminated and earlier operative intervention is being done. At the time of surgical exploration an operative cholangiogram through the gallbladder, or any visible extrahepatic duct if present, is performed. If the cholangiogram shows an intact intra- and extrahepatic biliary tract with flow of contrast media into the duodenum, a diagnosis of neonatal hepatitis is established (Fig. 14–8). Cholangiograms in the majority of infants with biliary atresia are impossible to obtain because of the inability to find a patent extrahepatic duct or gallbladder. However, injection of sterile water-soluble contrast material into a patent gallbladder or duct will demonstrate the inability of the media to pass into the common duct and the duodenum. Opacification of a common duct without demonstration of intrahepatic ducts indicates intrahepatic ductal atresia, whereas demonstration of intrahepatic ducts with an atretic common duct indicates extrahepatic ductal atresia (Fig. 14–9). If a satisfactory extrahepatic duct is

identified, anastomosis with the duodenum may be accomplished, but in the majority of cases the Kasai procedure (hepatic portoenterostomy) is carried out. This consists of careful dissection and excision of the fibrous tissue in the porta hepatis and anastomosis of the hepatic vascular bed with an intestinal segment. Unfortunately, the procedure is feasible in only 20 per cent of infants with atresia.

It is imperative that surgical correction be attempted as early as possible before significant cirrhosis has developed, i.e., before four months of age. Operative success depends on establishing bile drainage, which usually occurs one to four days after surgery. This is expected in approximately 30 to 40 per cent of cases. Unfortunately, reversal of the obliterating process may continue secondary to either the unexplained etiology or ascending cholangitis. The MacMahon-Thannhauser syndrome, or congenital absence of intralobar bile ducts, is probably part of the spectrum of infantile obstructive cholangiopathy.

Patients with biliary atresia as well as older infants and children with cirrhosis due to other causes may develop esophageal varices and rickets. These patients show severe osteoporosis as a result of the inability of the liver to manufacture the necessary amino acids and

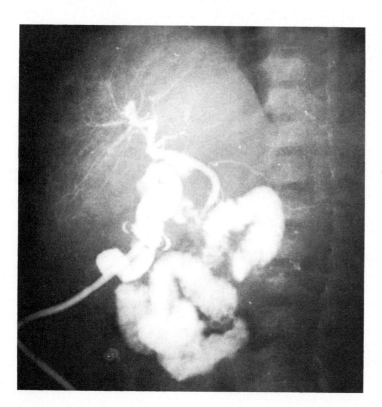

Figure 14–8. Neonatal hepatitis. Operative cholangiogram shows small compressed hepatic ducts but continuity of the ductal system with contrast media passing into the duodenum. (Reprinted with permission from Singleton, Wagner, and Dutton: Radiology of the Alimentary Tract in Infants and Children. Philadelphia: W. B. Saunders, 1977.)

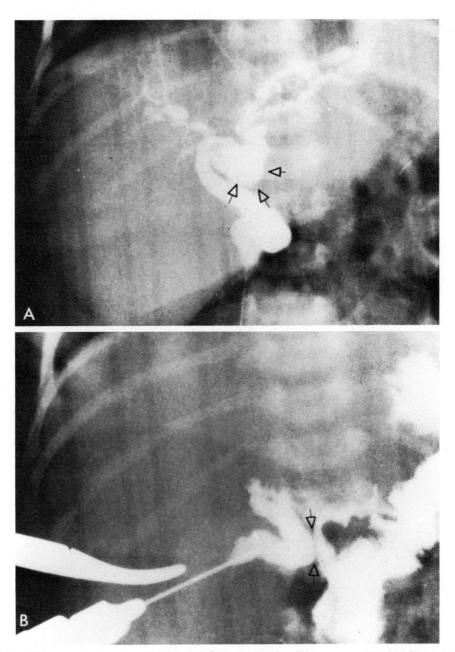

Figure 14–9. Biliary atresia in a 4-week-old male infant. *A*, Atresia of the common bile duct (arrows) is shown by the injection of the contrast medium into the gallbladder. *B*, Repeat injection after choledochoduodenostomy shows passage of contrast medium into the duodenum. (Reprinted with permission from Taybi *In* Margulis and Burhenne: Alimentary Tract Roentgenology, Vol. 2. St. Louis: C. V. Mosby, 1973.)

the resulting withdrawal of protein from the skeletal structures (Fig. 14–10). The rachitic changes are, of course, due to absence of absorption of vitamin D secondary to the absence of bile in the intestinal tract (Fig. 14–11). Osteoarthropathy is another complication of cirrhosis (Fig. 14–12) and is apparently the result of the development of vascular communications between the portal and pulmonary venous systems (Fig. 14–13).

CHOLEDOCHAL CYST

The etiology of the choledochal cyst is theoretical. One widely accepted theory holds that excessive unequal proliferation of epithelial cells in the primitive choledochus results in

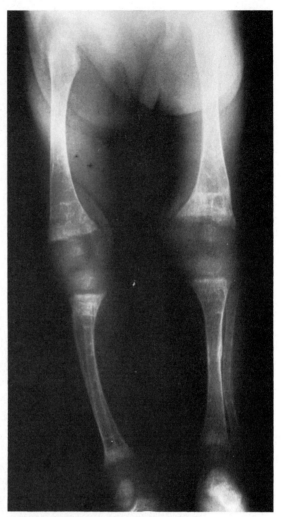

Figure 14–11. Advanced rachitic changes in an infant with biliary atresia. There is poor mineralization of the skeletal structures, and the provisional zones of calcification are indefinite, with slight widening of the growth plate. The physis is not as wide as in other causes of rickets owing to the poor cartilaginous growth.

dilatation when canalization takes place.[49] Dilatation of the common bile duct has been produced experimentally in puppies by ligation of the duct distal to curettage of the mucosa, suggesting that distal obstruction and weakening of the ductal wall are causative factors. Another theory maintains that proximal insertion of the common bile duct into the pancreatic duct results in reflux of pancreatic juice, leading to cholangitis and dilatation. However, all of these theories now seem to be taking a back seat to Landing's proposition that the choledochal cysts are part of the spectrum of viral cholangitis (infantile obstructive cholangiopathy).[47]

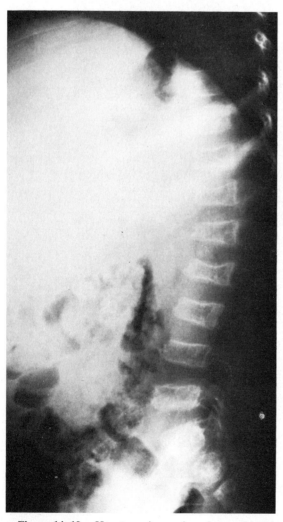

Figure 14–10. Hepatocarcinoma in a 2-year-old girl. Lateral view of the spine shows marked osteoporosis with compression fractures of many vertebrae.

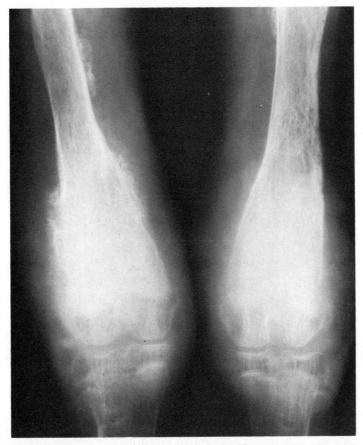

Figure 14–12.   Hepatic osteoarthropathy in patients with cirrhosis. (Courtesy of Dr. David Baker, Babies Hospital, New York, NY.)

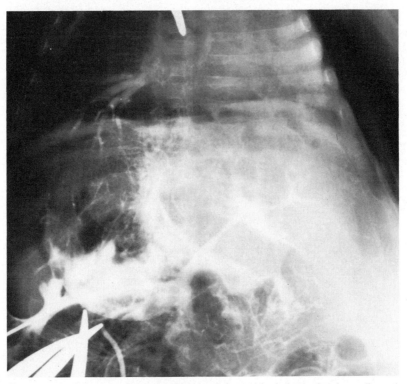

Figure 14–13.   Post-mortem injection of portal vein in an infant with cirrhosis showing collateral vessels communicating with the pulmonary veins, creating a situation comparable to arteriovenous communications and possibly explaining the osteoarthropathy that can occur in chronic liver disease.

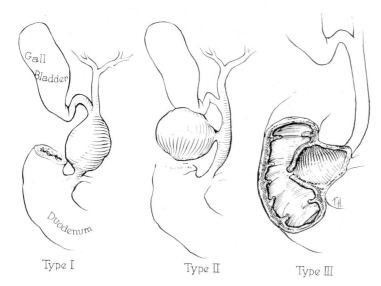

Figure 14–14. Types of choledochal cysts. Type I, cystic dilatation of the common bile duct with distal stenosis. Type II, localized diverticulum of the common bile duct. Type III, intraduodenal choledochocele. (Reprinted with permission from Singleton, Wagner, and Dutton: Radiology of the Alimentary Tract in Infants and Children. Philadelphia: W. B. Saunders, 1977.)

Although the condition is rare, hundreds of cases are reported, and a third of these are from Japan. The male to female ratio is approximately 1 to 3. The triad of abdominal pain, jaundice, and palpable mass occurs in approximately 50 per cent of the patients. In the newborn and in early infancy, obstructive jaundice is usually the presenting symptom.

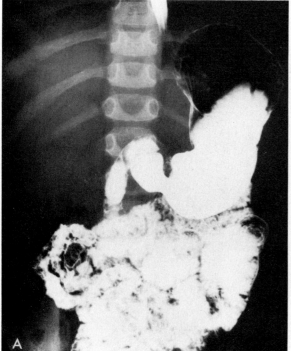

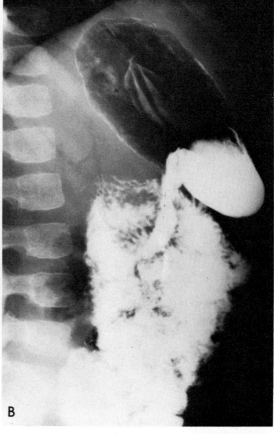

Figure 14–15. Choledochal cyst in a 4-year-old girl. A, Upper GI tract examination shows medial displacement of the second portion of the duodenum. B, Lateral view shows anterior displacement of the second portion of the duodenum. (Reprinted with permission from Singleton, Wagner, and Dutton: Radiology of the Alimentary Tract in Infants and Children. Philadelphia: W. B. Saunders, 1977.)

Most of the cases can be classified according to the three types described by Alonzo-Lej, Rever, and Pessagno (Fig. 14–14).[41] Type I is the most common and consists of localized dilatation of the common bile duct, which is frequently associated with distal narrowing. The dilatation in these cases is usually below the cystic duct but may involve the entire cystic duct and hepatic ducts. Type II is a localized diverticulum of the common bile duct and is easily corrected surgically. This is the least common of the three types. Type III is dilatation of the duodenal portion of the common bile duct and is actually a choledochocele. Authors[42] have recently extended the classification to include extrahepatic and intrahepatic biliary dilatations as well as various types of single and multiple hepatic cysts occurring without associated disease or associated with polycystic disease or congenital hepatic fibrosis. Cavernous ectasia of the intrahepatic ducts (Caroli's disease) may represent a form of choledochal cyst but is probably a separate entity.

There are a variety of methods of identifying a choledochal cyst. Conventional radiographic studies of the scout film of the abdomen and upper gastrointestinal tract examination may show the cyst displacing the duodenal loop medially and, usually, anteriorly (Fig. 14–15). Intravenous pyelography may demonstrate a choledochal cyst as a relative radiolucent mass secondary to total body opacification. Large cysts may displace the hepatic flexure of the colon and the right kidney inferiorly. This is unusual in the newborn because of the relative small size of the cyst, but in older patients the cyst is frequently large enough to be demonstrated by conventional radiography. However, in rare instances a choledochal cyst will be extremely large in young infants and will show marked displacement of the intestinal tract (Fig. 14–16). Oral cholecystography and intravenous cholangiography, in our experience, are usually unsuccessful in demonstrating a choledochal cyst. A type III choledochal cyst may be suspected from the filling defect it produces in the duodenum (Fig. 14–17). Ultrasound studies offer an excellent method of localizing the choledochal cyst and demonstrating its cystic properties (Fig. 14–18). Computed tomography is also of value in identifying the size and extent of a choledochal cyst but is a more expensive and time-consuming procedure, frequently requiring sedation in the pediatric patient. Arteriography is usually unnecessary but when used demonstrates an avascular mass with displacement of the gastro-

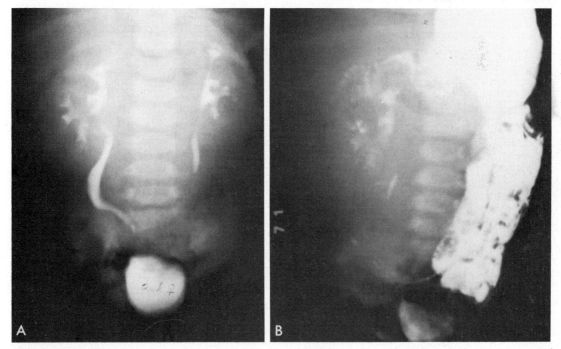

Figure 14–16. Huge choledochal cyst in 2-week-old female infant. *A,* IV pyelogram shows large mass occupying most of the abdomen and displacing the renal collecting structures and ureters. *B,* Upper GI tract examination showing displacement of bowel by a large choledochal cyst. (Courtesy of Dr. Tom Smith, Children's Mercy Hospital, Kansas City, MO.)

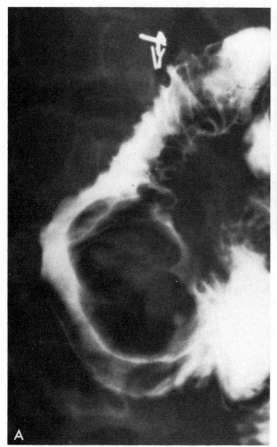

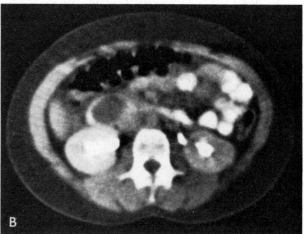

Figure 14–17. Choledochal cyst in an 11-year-old girl. *A,* Upper GI examination shows intraluminal defect of the duodenum. Surgical clips are from previous corrective procedure. *B,* Computerized tomographic study showing the intraluminal choledochal cyst.

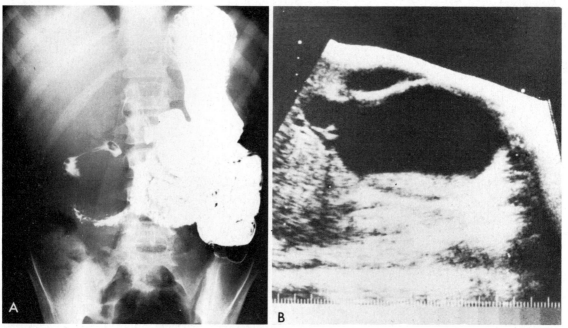

Figure 14–18. Choledochal cyst in a 10-year-old girl. *A,* Upper GI tract examination shows a mass displacing the duodenal loop. *B,* B-mode ultrasound examination shows large choledochal cyst with associated gallstones.

duodenal artery and occasionally demonstrates the rim sign of the choledochal cyst.

I-131 rose bengal scans frequently show excretion into the cyst, but the radiation using this nuclide is high. Other radiopharmaceutical products, including the iminodiacetic acids (Tc-99m IDA, Tc-99m HIDA, Tc-99m PIP-IDA) as described in the section on biliary atresia, have largely replaced I-131 rose bengal scans. The use of Tc-99m-sulphur colloid liver spleen scans will frequently show a defect in the area of the porta hepatis compatible with a choledochal cyst. Although direct percutaneous puncture and opacification of the cyst may be performed, the danger of bile peritonitis has made this unacceptable as a popular procedure.

Treatment of the lesion calls for surgical excision of the cyst, when possible, or anastomosis between the most dependent portion of the cyst and the duodenum or jejunum with a Roux-en-Y loop. The radiologist should be aware of the type of surgical correction used in any postoperative radiologic studies.

CAROLI'S DISEASE AND BILIARY DUCTAL ECTASIA

Caroli's disease, communicating cavernous ectasia, consists of segmental saccular dilatations of the intrahepatic bile ducts. The pathognomonic features of the disease include segmental saccular dilatation of the intrahepatic bile ducts, a predisposition to biliary calculi and cholangitis, and absence of portal hypertension and cirrhosis. However, because of the occasional association of this condition with choledochal cysts and hepatic fibrosis, some authors consider Caroli's disease one of the variants of cholangitis, similar to the spectrum of diseases producing biliary atresia and neonatal hepatitis. However, in the majority of textbooks and references it remains a separate entity. The malformation may be seen in the newborn, but most cases are first recognized in adulthood. Clinically there are recurrent attacks of cholangitis with upper right quadrant pain and usually no jaundice. Complications of this condition consist of stone formation within the dilated intrahepatic ducts, recurrent cholangitis, and liver abscesses. Although radiographic identification of the dilated ducts may be seen by intravenous cholangiography, the best method of demonstration is usually direct cholangiography. Sonographic studies are helpful in showing the dilated intrahepatic

ducts, and the use of radiopharmaceuticals (Tc-99m liver scan), will also show multiple filling defects. Computed tomography also may provide the imaging modality to allow one to suspect this condition, but direct opacification of the ductal system is the most helpful diagnostic procedure.

Infantile polycystic disease of the kidneys and renal tubular ectasia may be associated with hepatic ductal cysts, but sonographic demonstration is unsuccessful because of the microscopic size of the cysts. Medullary sponge kidney is usually not detected until adulthood, and consequently the cystic changes of the bile ducts have had time to attain a size that can be appreciated by sonographic studies and cholangiography (Fig. 14–19). These three conditions, infantile polycystic disease of the kidneys, renal tubular ectasia with hepatic fibrosis, and medullary cystic disease of the kidneys, are autosomal recessive abnormalities and probably represent a spectrum of the same disease process. Additional evaluation of these conditions may lead to inclusion of Caroli's disease as part of the same related spectrum.

Adult polycystic disease is an autosomal dominant condition. The renal cysts are usually not identified until adulthood but may rarely be seen in young children. Liver cysts occur in approximately one-half to one-third of adults with this condition and can be identified sonographically (Fig. 14–20).

CHOLECYSTITIS AND CHOLELITHIASIS

Although cholecystitis, especially acute acalculous cholecystitis, is uncommon in children, several large series of cases have been reported. The highest frequency of incidence is in children between the ages of 8 and 15, with an equal male to female ratio. The majority of cases appear to be of unknown etiology, but etiologic factors include infection, hereditary constitution, and metabolic diseases. Acute systemic diseases, including salmonellosis and scarlet fever, appear to be the most common predisposing factors in those cases associated with infections.

Clinically, the symptoms are similar to those seen in the adult, namely, nausea, vomiting, fat intolerance, abdominal pain, and upper right quadrant tenderness. Jaundice occurs in approximately 25 per cent of cases and is apparently due to inflammatory edema of the ductal system.

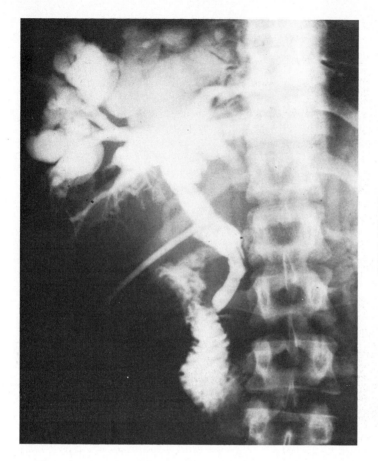

Figure 14–19. T-tube cholangiogram in a young adult male showing saccular dilatation of the hepatic ducts. Although radiographically the findings are classically those of Caroli's disease, the patient had medullary sponge kidneys, and presumably the hepatic duct saccules may be secondary to the associated intrahepatic fibrosis.

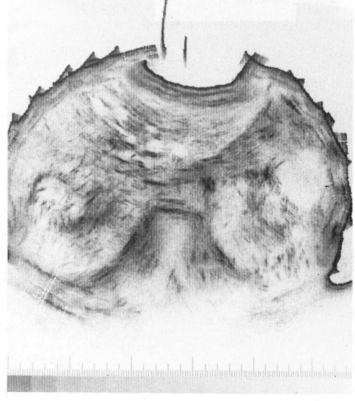

Figure 14–20. Polycystic renal disease in a young adult with associated hepatic cysts. (Courtesy of Dr. R. B. Denman, Veterans Administration Hospital, Houston, TX.)

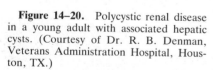

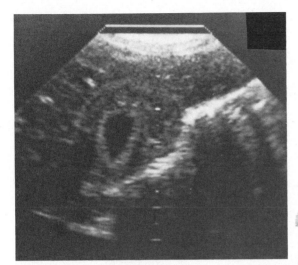

Figure 14–21. Acute cholecystitis in a 5-year-old girl. The gallbladder is dilated and the wall thickened.

Radiologic evaluation of the child is similar to that of the adult. Oral cholecystograms and intravenous cholangiograms are difficult to evaluate in the pediatric patient because of the unpredictable results. However, in cases of cholecystitis, nonvisualization of the gallbladder by these methods is to be expected. Ultrasound studies are of help in showing thickening of the gallbladder wall and, occasionally, dis-

tention of the gallbladder (Fig. 14–21). Acalculous distention of the gallbladder also has been described in children with the mucocutaneous lymph node syndrome (Kawasaki's disease), polyarteritis nodosa, leptospirosis, scarlet fever, and familial Mediterranean anemia.

Cholelithiasis is now a more common condition in children than cholecystitis, especially since scarlet fever and typhoid fever are now controlled. Girls are affected more commonly than boys, and the peak incidence is in the preadolescent and adolescent ages. Most cases of cholelithiasis are complications of chronic hemolytic anemia, including sickle cell disease, spherocytosis, and thalassemia. Biliary calculi have also been reported in patients with chronic hepatitis, leukemia, cirrhosis, cystic fibrosis, Ellis-van Creveld syndrome, and Mirizzi's syndrome (hepatic duct stenosis syndrome) and following radiotherapy for Wilms' tumor and ileal resection.

Total parenteral nutrition including the use of furosemide has been recognized as still another cause of cholelithiasis and is being reported more frequently as a causative factor owing to the increased use of hyperalimentation in the intensive care of premature and other critically ill infants. However, in our experience and in most of the reported cases,

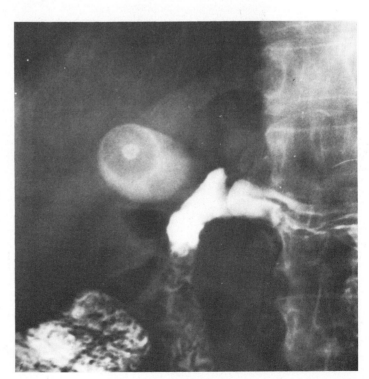

Figure 14–22. Large solitary gallstone with a calcified nidus in a 16-year-old girl.

the causes are usually unknown, as in cholelithiasis in the adult patient.[60, 61, 63, 64] The symptoms of cholelithiasis in children are similar to those found in the adult and include nausea, vomiting, epigastric pain, and tenderness.

Oral cholecystography is valuable in identifying gallstones in older children (Fig. 14–22) but is unpredictable in the infant age group. Harned and Babbitt report that opaque calculi are visualized on plain films in approximately 50 per cent of cases and stones are visualized by oral cholecystograms in 7 per cent of cases.[61] They also report nonvisualization of the gallbladder in 30 per cent of cases.

The most helpful diagnostic procedure is sonography, particularly sonography utilizing real-time techniques. The gallstones are readily identified by this modality, and the acoustic shadow is usually also present (Figs. 14–23 through 14–26).

Text continued on page 537

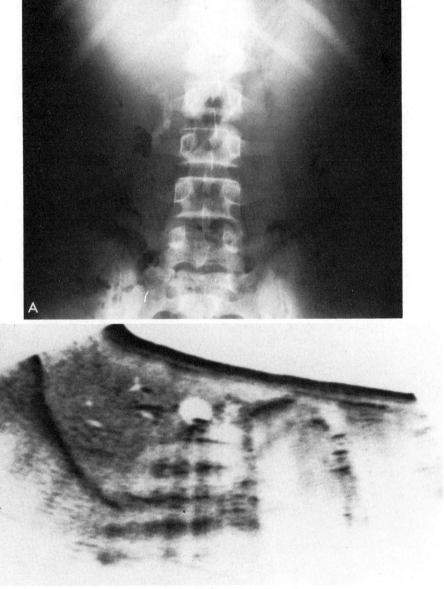

Figure 14–23. Cholelithiasis in a 15-year-old boy with hemolytic anemia. *A*, Radiograph of the abdomen shows multiple faceted gallstones in the upper right quadrant and a large spleen. *B*, B-mode ultrasound examination shows the gallstones with associated acoustic shadows.

Illustration continued on opposite page

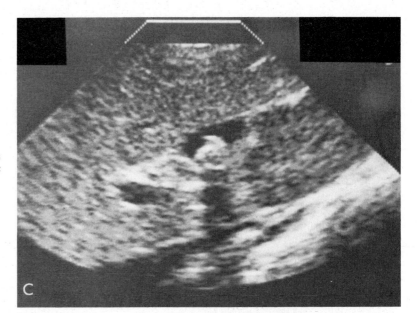

Figure 14–23. *Continued C,* Real-time sonogram also shows cholelithiasis with the acoustic shadow.

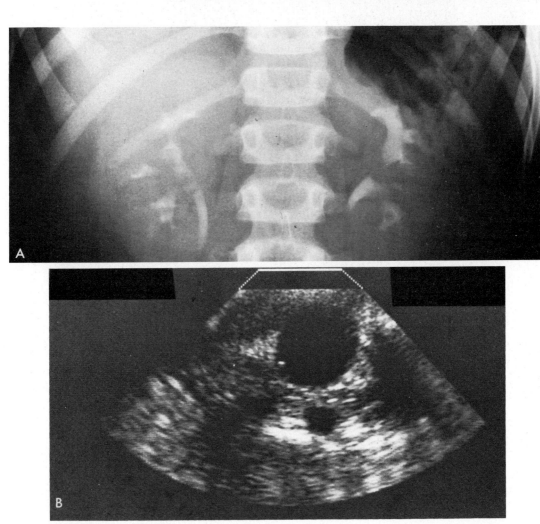

Figure 14–24. Seven-year-old boy with abdominal pain. *A,* IV pyelogram shows no abnormality of either kidney, but there is a calculus above the right transverse process of L–1. *B,*Real-time sonogram shows the solitary gallstone within the gallbladder.

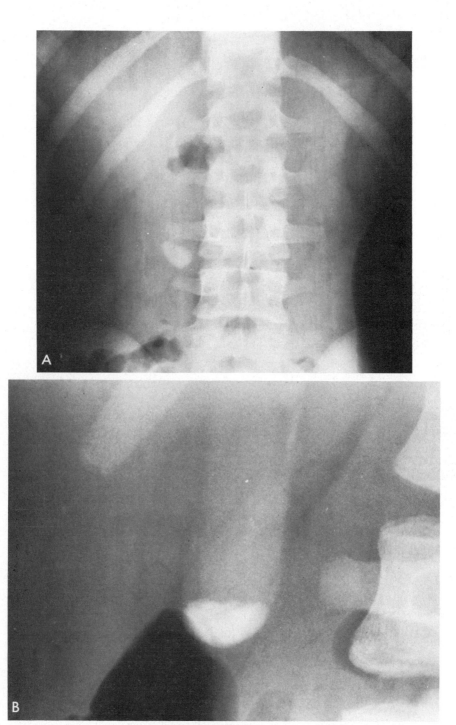

Figure 14–25. Fourteen-year-old boy with sickle cell disease. *A*, Abdominal scout film shows large calculus beneath the right transverse process of L–3. *B*, Oral cholecystogram shows poor visualization of the gallbladder and large calculus within the fundus.

Illustration continued on opposite page

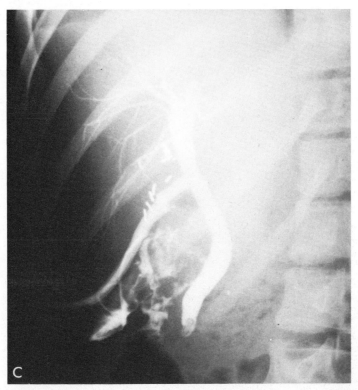

Figure 14–25. *Continued* *C,* T-tube cholangiogram made post cholecystectomy shows residual calculus in the distal end of the common duct.

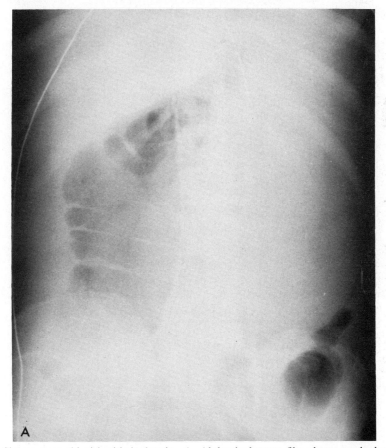

Figure 14–26. Sixteen-year-old girl with leukemia. *A,* Abdominal scout film shows marked enlargement of the spleen.

Illustration continued on following page

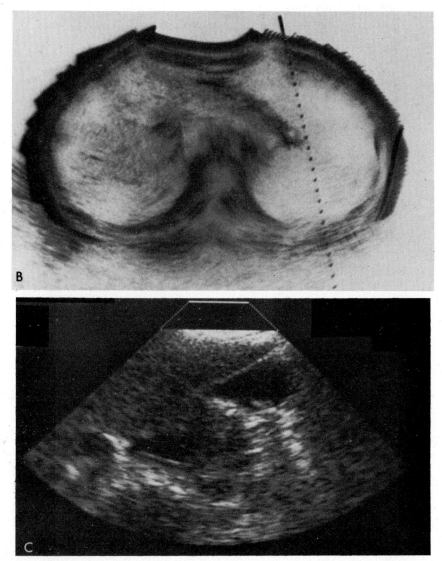

Figure 14–26. *Continued   B,* B-mode sonogram shows enlargement of the spleen and also the liver. *C,* Real-time sonographic examination shows a gallstone within the gallbladder.

The treatment of choice is cholecystectomy, and attempts to dissolve or remove stones in this age group utilizing nonoperative transcholecystic techniques are not as popular as in the adult patient.

Acute hydrops of the gallbladder is extremely rare in the pediatric patient and the cause is usually unknown, but inspissated bile, enlargement of lymph nodes with pressure on the cystic duct, scarlet fever, and amebic abcesses have been listed as possible etiologies. Sonographic studies will reveal enlargement of the gallbladder with thickening of the wall.

MISCELLANEOUS CONDITIONS

Trauma is common in children, and a history of injury may be impossible to obtain. Laceration of the liver is less common than splenic injury but should be suspected if the patient complains of upper right quadrant pain associated with a decrease in hematocrit. Ultrasound studies, computed tomography, and angiography are important diagnostic procedures that should be performed prior to surgical correction. Radiopharmaceutical uptake studies are helpful if the injury has led to extravasation of bile into the peritoneal cavity.

Spontaneous perforation of the extrahepatic bile ducts and bile peritonitis in neonates may also be detected by Tc-99m IDA cholescintigraphy.

Inspissated bile in the common duct (inspissated bile syndrome) is a rare cause of neonatal jaundice and is usually mistaken clinically for either biliary atresia or neonatal hepatitis. Operative cholangiography should demonstrate the obstructing bile plug (Fig. 14–27).

Mirizzi's syndrome is an obstruction of the common hepatic duct produced by impacted stones in the cystic duct, which cause pressure necrosis and inflammation of the common hepatic duct. Sonography will demonstrate the stones and the dilated intrahepatic ducts.

Hepatic tumors, especially rhabdomyosarcoma, arising from the bile ducts may produce a variable degree of dilatation of the ducts at the site of the neoplasm as well as proximally (Figs. 14–28 and 14–29).

In all conditions involving intrahepatic biliary duct dilations, transhepatic cholangiography would naturally be of diagnostic benefit, but this procedure is much less successful in the pediatric patient than in the adult.

Pancreatitis may produce edema and scarring of the ampulla with resulting dilatation of the proximal biliary tree including the gallbladder (Fig. 14–30).

Metachromatic leukodystrophy is a degen-

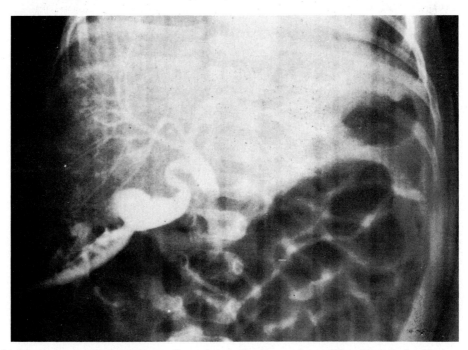

Figure 14–27. Inspissated bile syndrome. Operative cholangiogram shows filling defect in the distal common duct, which was found to be inspissated bile.

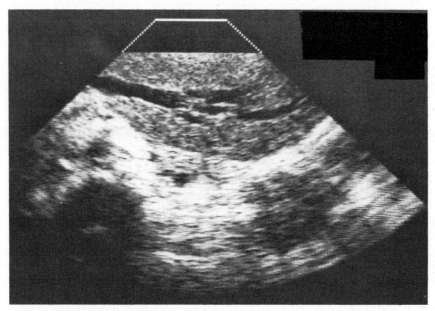

Figure 14–28. Dilated hepatic ducts in a child with hepatic carcinoma.

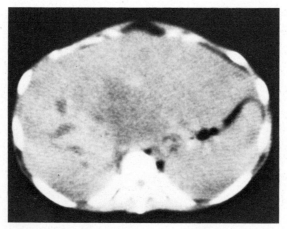

Figure 14–29. Fourteen-year-old female with hepatocellular carcinoma. Computed tomogram shows the central portion of the liver replaced by neoplasm and mild dilatation of the hepatic ducts.

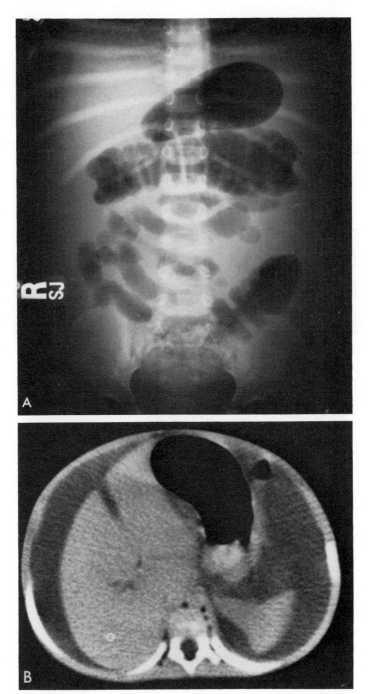

Figure 14–30. Pancreatitis with obstruction of the ampulla of Vater in a 2½-year-old female. *A,* Scout film of the abdomen shows ascites. *B,* Computed tomogram shows to better advantage the extensive ascites.

Illustration continued on following page

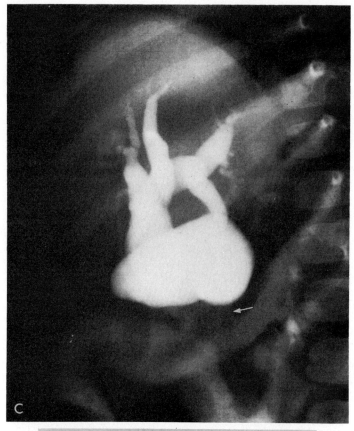

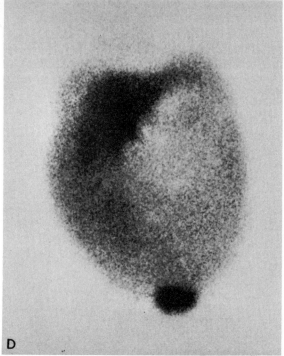

Figure 14–30. *Continued   C,* Transhepatic cholangiogram shows marked dilatation of the hepatic and common ducts with faint opacification of the obstruction at the ampulla of Vater (arrow). Some contrast medium has entered the duodenum. *D,* Tc-99m HIDA scintigram shows evidence of bile peritonitis, although its origin could not be identified at laparotomy.

erative disease of the central nervous system in which there is an accumulation of metachromatic deposits (sulfatides) in different organs (brain, kidneys, gallbladder, and so on) owing to a deficiency of the enzyme cerebroside sulfatase. In this condition there is also a progressive inability of the gallbladder to concentrate bile, and biliary stones may develop (Fig. 14–31).

Fibrocystic disease may occasionally affect the liver, producing inspissated mucus within the biliary system. Fibrocystic disease is the most common genetic disorder causing death in childhood. Intestinal obstruction due to meconium ileus may be the presenting problem at birth, but the pulmonary complications of air trapping, chronic pneumonia, and bronchiectasis; pulmonary fibrosis; hypertension; and eventually cor pulmonale are the usual pathogenic events causing death later in life.

Cystic duct obstruction resulting in a small atrophic gallbladder is a common complication in older children with cystic fibrosis. This is readily detectable by ultrasound studies (Fig. 14–32). Focal biliary cirrhosis with bile duct proliferation and distention of bile ducts by mucus are additional hepatic complications of this disease seen in older children (Fig. 14–33). Obstruction of the common bile duct and the major hepatic ducts is extremely unusual.

Sonographic studies may show dilatation of the intrahepatic ducts proximal to the inspissated plugs.

Hereditary cholestasis associated with pulmonary branch stenoses, characteristic facies (broad forehead, hypertelorism, deep-set eyes), growth retardation, vertebral anomalies, and neonatal jaundice is a condition apparently similar or identical to arteriohepatic dysplasia. There are no imaging abnormalities of the bile ducts.

Mucocutaneous lymph node syndrome (Kawasaki's disease) was first described in 1967 in Japanese children, and approximately 2 per cent of the affected patients die, usually from vasculitis involving the coronary arteries and producing cardiac arrhythmias. Gastrointestinal symptoms may be present and consist mainly of diarrhea and abdominal pain. Hydrops of the gallbladder is now a well-known complication of this syndrome, and the children with gallbladder hydrops usually can be managed with conservative therapy. Pain, tenderness, and an upper right quadrant mass are the clinical findings in these patients, and ultrasonography is the procedure of choice in making the diagnosis of hydrops of the gallbladder. The gallbladder is enlarged and the wall thickened (Fig. 14–34). Whether the hydrops is due to compression of enlarged lymph

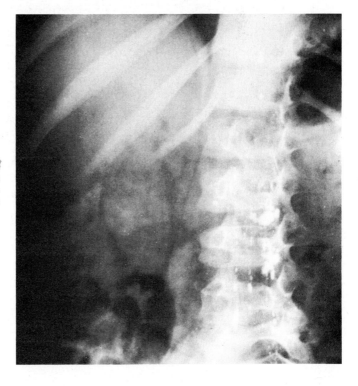

Figure 14–31. Metachromatic leukodystrophy in a young infant. The gallbladder is very faintly opacified. The faint areas of density within the gallbladder were found to be multiple small gallstones.

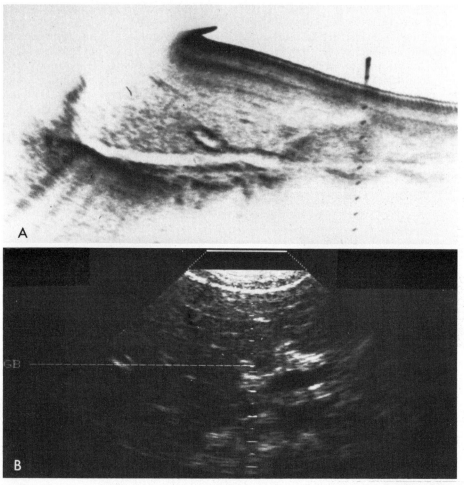

Figure 14–32. Fibrocystic disease in an 18-year-old boy. *A*, B-mode sonogram shows the gallbladder to be abnormally small. *B*, Real-time sonogram also demonstrates the small contracted gallbladder.

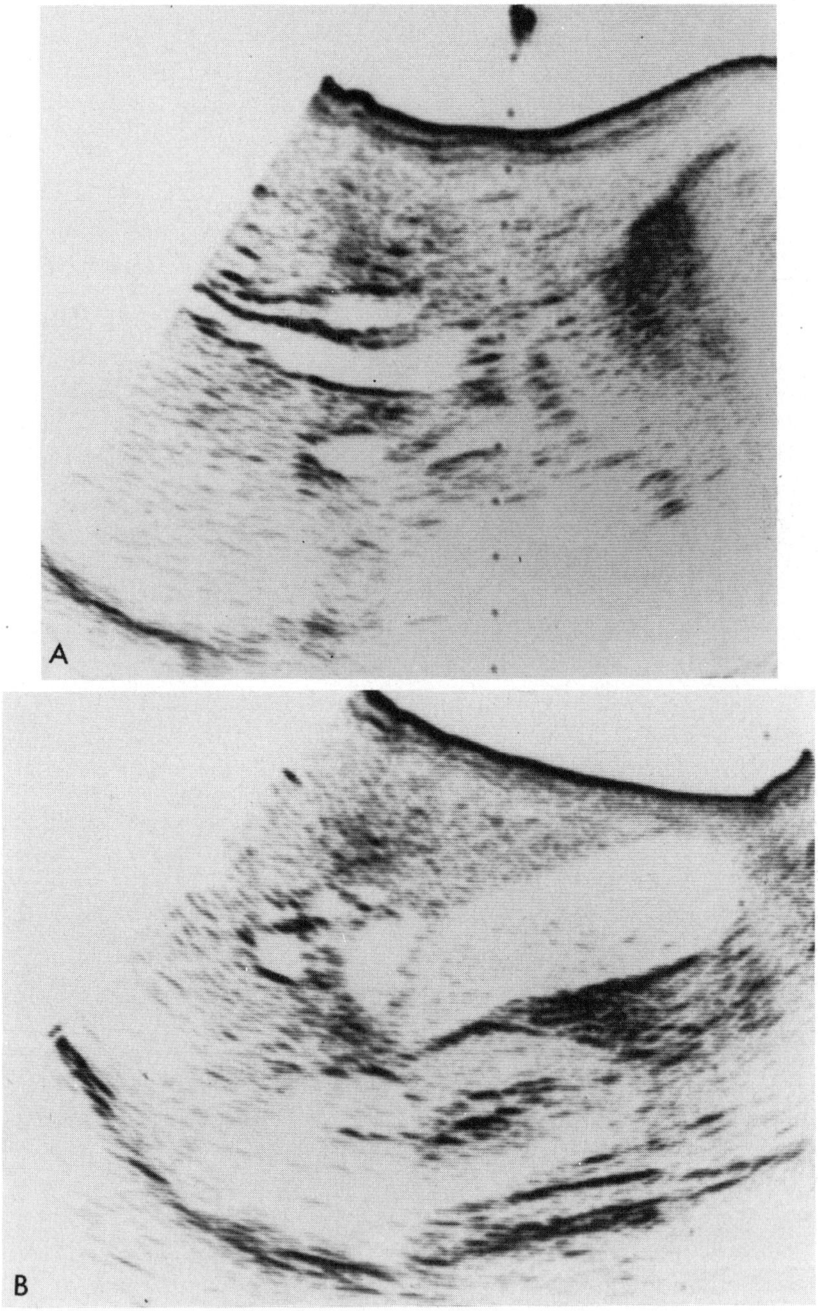

Figure 14–33. Fibrocystic disease in a 7½-year-old boy. *A,* B-mode sonogram shows the parallel channel sign of the portal vein and dilated hepatic duct. *B,* The gallbladder is dilated, and the echogenic material represents biliary sludge. (Courtesy of Dr. Rita Teele, Children's Hospital Medical Center, Boston, MA.)

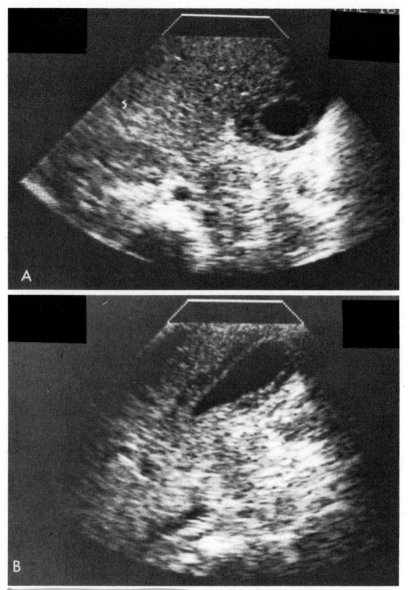

Figure 14–34. Mucocutaneous lymph node syndrome in a 2-year-old child. *A*, Transverse real-time sonogram shows dilatation of the gallbladder with thickening of the wall. *B*, Longitudinal scan again emphasizes the hydrops and thick wall.

nodes around the cystic duct or a nonspecific serositis or vasculitis is speculative.

Congenital tracheo-biliary fistula is a rare anomaly characterized clinically by the expectoration of bile. The fistula extends from the carinal angle, traverses the diaphragm, and usually invades the left hepatic duct. Abdominal scout films may show air within the biliary tree, and bronchography will demonstrate the fistulous communication between the carina and the biliary ducts.

SUMMARY

Diseases affecting the liver and bile ducts in infants are numerous, and a variety of laboratory tests, biopsies, and histologic interpretations are necessary. The radiologist's role in the diagnosis of neonatal jaundice is essentially limited to the information gained using specific radiopharmaceutical scintigraphy and the evaluation of operative cholangiograms. Sonography and computed tomography are frequently uninformative in this young age group except for the identification of a choledochal cyst.

Anomalies of the gallbladder are usually seen in the older age group and are detected by oral cholangiography. Cholecystitis and cholelithiasis present diagnostic sonographic and CT images similar to those found in the adult and are usually readily detected.

Gallbladder and ductal defects found in a variety of pediatric syndromes usually go undetected unless specifically evaluated by cholecystography or sonography after the syndrome is recognized.

References

Embryology
 1. Allan, F. D.: Essentials of Human Embryology. New York: Oxford University Press, 1969.
 2. Bremer, J. L.: Congenital Anomalies of the Viscera. Cambridge: Harvard University Press, 1957.
 3. Merten, D. F.: Formation and development of the alimentary tract. *In* Singleton, E. B., Wagner, M. L., and Dutton, R. V. (eds.): Radiology of the Alimentary Tract in Infants and Children. Philadelphia: W. B. Saunders, 1977.

Methods of Visualizing the Biliary Tree
 4. Bétoulières, P., Balmes, J., Loustanu, J. A., and Balmes, J. L.: La cholécystographie chez le nourrisson et l'enfant en bas age. J. Radiol. Electr. *45*:364, 1964.
 5. Gates, G. F.: Atlas of Abdominal Ultrasonography in Children. New York: Churchill Livingstone, 1978.
 6. Haaga, J., and Reich, N. E.: Computed Tomography of Abdominal Abnormalities. St. Louis: C. V. Mosby, 1978.
 7. Haller, J. O., and Schneider, M.: Pediatric Ultrasound. Chicago: Year Book Medical Publishers, 1980.
 8. Nahum, H., Poree, C., and Sauvegrain, J.: The study of the gallbladder and biliary ducts. Progr. Pediatr. Radiol. *2*:65, 1969.
 9. Sauvegrain, J.: The technique of upper gastrointestinal investigation in infants and children. Progr. Pediatr. Radiol. *2*:26, 1969.
10. Taybi, H.: The biliary tract in children. *In* Margulis, A. R., and Burhenne, H. J., (eds.): Alimentary Tract Roentgenology, 2nd ed. St. Louis: C. V. Mosby, 1973.

Congenital Anomalies of the Biliary Tree
11. Alderson, P. O., Gilday, D. L., and Wagner, H. N., Jr.: Atlas of Pediatric Nuclear Medicine. St. Louis: C. V. Mosby, 1978.
12. Anderson, R. D., Connell, T. H., and Lowman, R. M.: Inversion of the liver and suprahepatic gallbladder associated with eventration of the diaphragm. Radiology *97*:87, 1970.
13. Anderson, R. E., and Ross, W. T.: Congenital bilobed gallbladder. Arch. Surg. *76*:7, 1958.
14. Arcomano, J. P., and Barnett, J. C.: Diverticulum of the gallbladder; report of three cases and a review of the literature. Am. J. Digest. Dis. *4*:556, 1959.

15. Baker, D. H., and Harris, R. C.: Congenital absence of the intrahepatic bile ducts. A.J.R. *91*:875, 1964.
16. Bartone, N. F., and Grieco, R. V.: Absent gallbladder and cystic duct. A.J.R. *110*:252, 1970.
17. Boyden, E. A.: "Phrygian cap" in cholecystography; a congenital anomaly of gallbladder. A.J.R. *33*:589, 1953.
18. Brasch, J. W.: Congenital anomalies of the gallbladder and bile ducts. Surg. Clin. North Am. *38*:627, 1958.
19. Carnevali, J. F., and Kunath, C. A.: Congenital absence of the gallbladder. Arch. Surg. *78*:440, 1959.
20. Ferris, D. O., and Glazer, I. M.: Congenital absence of gallbladder: four surgical cases. Arch. Surg. *91*:359, 1965.
21. Flannery, M. G., and Caster, M. P.: Collective reviews; congenital abnormalities of gallbladder; 101 cases. Surg. Gynecol. Obstet. *103*:439, 1956.
22. Glay, A.: Double gallbladder. Report of one asymptomatic case demonstrated roentgenologically. J. Can. Assoc. Radiol. *10*:1, 1959.
23. Grossman, H., and Seed, W.: Congenital hepatic fibrosis, bile duct dilatation, and renal lesions resembling medullary sponge kidney (congenital "cystic" disease of the liver and kidneys). Radiology *87*:46, 1966.
24. Large, A. M.: Left-sided gallbladder and liver without situs inversus. Arch. Surg. *87*:982, 1963.
25. Lee, C. M., Jr.: Duplication of the cystic and common hepatic ducts, lined with gastric mucosa: a rare congenital anomaly. N. Engl. J. Med. *256*:927, 1957.
26. Ross, R. J., and Sachs, M. D.: Triplication of the gallbladder. A.J.R. *104*:656, 1968.
27. Singleton, E. B., Wagner, M. L., and Dutton, R. V. (eds.): Radiology of the Alimentary Tract in Infants and Children. Philadelphia: W. B. Saunders, 1977.

Biliary Atresia and Neonatal Hepatitis
28. Altman, R. P.: The portoenterostomy procedure for biliary atresia: a 5-year experience. Ann. Surg. *188*:351, 1978.
29. Gates, G. F., Sinatra, F. R., and Thomas, D. W.: Cholestatic syndromes in infancy and childhood. A.J.R. *134*:1141, 1980.
30. Hayden, P. W., Rudd, T. G., and Christie, D. L.: Rose bengal sodium ^{131}I studies in infants with suspected biliary atresia. Am. J. Dis. Child. *133*:834, 1979.
31. Hays, D. M.: Biliary tract and liver. *In* Holder, T. M., and Ashcraft, K. W. (eds.): Pediatric Surgery. Philadelphia: W. B. Saunders, 1980.
32. Hitch, D. C., Shikes, R. H., and Lilly, J. R.: Determinants of survival after Kasai's operation for biliary atresia using actuarial analysis. J. Pediatr. Surg. *14*:310, 1979.
33. Kasai, M.: Treatment of biliary atresia with special reference to hepatic porto-enterostomy and its modifications. *In* Bill, A. H., and Kasai, M. (eds.): Progress in Pediatric Surgery, Vol. VI. Baltimore: University Park Press, 1974.
34. Kasai, M.: Hepatic portoenterostomy and its modifications for "noncorrectible" biliary atresia. Paediatrician *3*:204, 1974.
35. Landing, B.: Considerations on the pathogenesis of neonatal hepatitis, biliary atresia, and choledochal cyst—the concept of infantile obstructive cholangiopathy. *In* Bill, A. H., and Kasai, M. (eds.): Progress in Pediatric Surgery, Vol. VI. Baltimore: University Park Press, 1974.
36. Landing, B., Wells, T., Reed, G., and Harayan, M.: Disease of the bile ducts. *In*; Gall, E., and Mostofi,

F., (eds.): The Liver. Baltimore: Williams & Wilkins, 1973.

37. Majd, M., Reba, R. C., and Altman, R. P.: Hepatobiliary scintigraphy with ^{99m}Tc-PIPIDA in the evaluation of neonatal jaundice. Pediatrics 67:140, 1981.

38. Morrecki, R., Gartner, L. M., and Lee, K.-S.: Jaundice and liver disease: II. Conjugated hyperbilirubinemia. In Behrman, R. E. (ed.): Neonatal-Perinatal Medicine. Diseases of the Fetus and Infant. St. Louis: C. V. Mosby, 1977.

39. Strauss, L., and Bernstein, J.: Neonatal hepatitis in congenital rubella. A histopathologic study. Arch. Pathol. 86:317, 1968.

40. Teng, C. T., Daeschner, C. W., Jr., Singleton, E. B., Rosenberg, H. S., Cole, V. W., Hill, L. L., and Brennan, J. C.: Liver diseases and osteoporosis in children. I. Clinical observations. II. Etiological considerations. J. Pediatr. 59:684, 1961.

Choledochal Cyst

41. Alonso-Lej, F., Rever, W. B., and Pessagno, D. J.: Congenital choledochal cysts, with a report of 2, and an analysis of 94 cases. Int. Abstr. Surg. 108:1, 1959.

42. Berk, R. N., and Clemett, A. R.: Radiology of the Gallbladder and Bile Ducts. Philadelphia: W. B. Saunders, 1977.

43. Haller, J. O., and Schneider, M.: Pediatric Ultrasound. Chicago: Year Book Medical Publishers, 1980.

44. Han, B. K., Babcock, D. S., and Gelfand, M. H.: Choledochal cyst with bile duct dilatation: Sonography and ^{99m}Tc IDA cholescintigraphy. A.J.R. 136:1075, 1981.

45. Haubek, A., Pedersen, J. H., Burcharth, F., Gammelgaard, J., Hancke, S., and Willumsen, L.: Dynamic sonography in the evaluation of jaundice. A.J.R. 136:1071, 1981.

46. Holder, T. M., Stuber, J. L., and Templeton, A. W.: Sonography as a diagnostic aid in the evaluation of abdominal masses in infants and children. J. Pediatr. Surg. 7:532, 1972.

47. Landing, B. H.: Considerations of the pathogenesis of neonatal hepatitis, biliary atresia and choledochal cyst—the concept of infantile obstructive cholangiopathy. Progr. Pediatr. Surg. 6:113, 1974.

48. Rosenfield, N., and Griscom, N. T.: Choledochal cysts: Roentgenographic techniques. Radiology 114:113, 1975.

49. Yotuyanagi, S.: Contributions to aetiology and pathology of idiopathic cystic dilatation of common bile duct, with report of three cases. Gan 30:601, 1936.

Caroli's Disease and Biliary Duct Ectasia

50. Blyth, H., and Ockenden, B. G.: Polycystic disease of kidneys and liver presenting in childhood. J. Med. Genet. 8:257, 1971.

51. Mujahed, A., Glenn, G., and Evans, J.: Communicating cavernous ectasia of the intrahepatic ducts (Caroli's disease). A.J.R. 113:21, 1971.

52. Murray-Lyon, I. M., Ockenden, B. G., and Williams, R.: Congenital hepatic fibrosis—Is it a single clinical entity. Editorial. Gastroenterology 64:653, 1973.

53. Rosewarne, M. D.: Cystic dilatation of the intrahepatic bile ducts. Br. J. Radiol. 45:825, 1972.

54. Singleton, E. B.: Radiologic evaluation of renal cystic disease in children. Curr. Probl. Diagn. Radiol. 10:1, 1981.

Cholecystitis and Cholelithiasis

55. Beale, E. F., Nelson, R. M., Bucciarelli, R. L., Donnelly, W. H., and Eitzman, D. V.: Intrahepatic cholestasis associated with parenteral nutrition in premature infants. Pediatrics 64:342, 1979.

56. Bloom, R. A., and Swain, V. A. J.: Non-calculous distention of the gallbladder in children. Arch. Dis. Child. 41:503, 1966.

57. Brenner, R. W., and Stewart, C. F.: Cholecystitis in children. Rev. Surg. 21:327, 1964.

58. Callahan, J., Haller, J. O., Cacciarelli, A. A., Slovis, T. L., and Friedman, A. P.: Cholelithiasis in infants: Association with total parenteral nutrition and furosemide. Radiology 143:437, 1982.

59. Dickinson, S. J., Corley, G., and Santulli, T. V.: Acute cholecystitis as a sequel to scarlet fever. Am. J. Dis. Child. 121:331, 1971.

60. Hanson, B. A., Mahour, G. H., and Wolley, M. M.: Diseases of the gallbladder in infancy and childhood. J. Pediatr. Surg. 6:277, 1971.

61. Harned, R. K., and Babbitt, D. P.: Cholelithiasis in children. Radiology 117:391, 1975.

62. Kieswetter, W. B.: Cholecystitis and cholelithiasis. In Mustard, W. T., Ravitch, M. M., Snyder, W. H., Jr., Welch, K. J., and Benson, C. D. (eds.): Pediatric Surgery, 2nd ed. Chicago: Year Book Medical Publishers, 1969.

63. Newman, D. E.: Gallstones in children. Pediatr. Radiol. 1:100, 1973.

64. Strauss, R. G.: Cholelithiasis in childhood. Am. J. Dis. Child. 117:689, 1969.

Miscellaneous Conditions

65. Alagille, D., Odievre, M., Gautier, M., and Dommergues, J.: Hepatic ductular hypoplasia associated with characteristic facies, vertebral malformations, retarded physical, mental and sexual development, and cardiac murmur. J. Pediatr. 86:63, 1975.

66. Gray, O. P., and Saunders, R. A.: Familial intrahepatic cholestatic jaundice in infancy. Arch. Dis. Child. 41:320, 1966.

67. Henriksen, N. T., Langmark, F., Sørland, S. J., Fausa, O., Landaas, S., and Aagenaes, Ø.: Hereditary cholestasis combined with peripheral pulmonary stenosis and other anomalies. Acta Paediatr. Scand. 66:7, 1977.

68. Holmes, L. B., Moser, H. W., Halldorsson, S., Mack, C., Pant, S. S., and Matzilevich, B.: Mental Retardation. New York: Macmillan Co., 1972.

69. Levin, S. E., Zarvos, P., Milner, S., and Schmaman, A.: Arteriohepatic dysplasia: Association of liver disease with pulmonary arterial stenosis as well as facial and skeletal abnormalities. Pediatrics 66:876, 1980.

70. Linarelli, L. G., Williams, C. N., and Phillips, M. J.: Byler's disease: fatal intrahepatic cholestasis. J. Pediatr. 81:484, 1972.

71. Magilavy, D. B., Speert, D. P., and Silver, T. M.: Mucocutaneous lymph node syndrome: report of 2 cases complicated by gallbladder hydrops and diagnosed by ultrasound. Pediatrics 61:699, 1978.

72. Neuhauser, E. B. D., Elkin, M., and Landing, B. H.: Congenital direct communication between biliary system and respiratory tract. Am. J. Dis. Child. 83:654, 1952.

73. Rosenfeld, N. S., Kelley, M. J., Jensen, P. S., Cotlier, E., Rosenfield, A. T., and Riely, C. A.: Arteriohepatic dysplasia: radiologic feature of a new syndrome. A.J.R. 135:1217, 1980.

74. Singleton, E. B., Wagner, M. L., and Dutton, R. V. (eds.): Radiology of the Alimentary Tract in Infants and Children. Philadelphia: W. B. Saunders, 1977.

CLINICAL-RADIOLOGIC PERSPECTIVES ON GALLBLADDER AND BILE DUCT IMAGING

by Howard M. Spiro, M.D.
Morton I. Burrell, M.D.
Robert K. Zeman, M.D.

15

The dramatic progress in radiologic technology has paralyzed the clinician. Once jaundice was the high point of the diagnostic week, an occasion for circling the patient to see whether his jaundice was orange or green in hue, poking at the upper right quadrant to feel for the gallbladder, and sitting around the table poring over endless lists of liver function studies trying to deduce from all of this whether jaundice was the result of an intrahepatic process or an extrahepatic obstruction. Finally, the clinician and radiologist would peer at films of the upper right quadrant to see what could be found in those dim, gray shadows. Then, the most important diagnostic decisions were whether the bilirubin level was low enough to permit an oral cholecystogram and whether a liver biopsy might be helpful in the differential diagnosis. Indeed, histologic examination of the liver sometimes seemed the best guide as to whether inflammation was present or whether the small bile ducts showed evidence of obstruction. No wonder physicians held to that old aphorism, "No living man understands jaundice," and no doubt that was the reason why exploratory laparotomy was often the only convincing diagnostic maneuver.

How far physicians have come today has been celebrated meticulously in the foregoing pages of this book. The physiologic information provided by radionuclides, the anatomic detail of computerized tomography, the real-time observations of ultrasound, and the diagnostic and therapeutic implications of endoscopic and catheter studies all make the scene as wondrous as the moon when the astronauts first landed. The clinician has had to completely change his approach to the analysis of the gallbladder and bile ducts over the past decade.[1] Undoubtedly, such rapid progress will continue to astound us as future developments uncover much more. In the near future we will know much more about tissue texture, tumor signature, and early metabolic abnormalities, aided by nuclear magnetic resonance.[2-4] Radiologists will continue to change the imaging work-up and therapeutic approaches will improve, no doubt increasing still more the anxiety of clinicians who already fear that their clinical prerogatives are being eroded, if not usurped, by this parade of new technology. Too often the reality of the images proves more exciting than the sometimes lugubrious complaints of the gassy and bloated patient. It is really no surprise then that the house officer seeing a jaundiced patient orders an ultrasound study and a HIDA scan for the next day, schedules computed tomography for whenever he can get it, and sits back to fill in the blanks and await the diagnosis.

To be fair, some physical diagnostic exploits have been superseded by the readily available demonstration of abnormal anatomy: to detect ascites by rolling the patient from side to side or eliciting a "fluid wave" is a skill rendered as archaic by ultrasound as "post-tussive rales" by the chest film. As further anatomic and metabolic refinements can be displayed by imaging techniques, the role of attentive clinicians will no doubt be to place these displays in perspective and evaluate even more critically the role of all tests in improving the well-being of their patients.

There really are only two major questions

547

that clinician and radiologist are attempting to answer in the patient with suspected biliary tract disease: (1) Is there gallbladder disease? (2) Are the bile ducts obstructed? If the bile ducts are obstructed, the surgeon wants to know the answer to two more questions: (1) What is the *level* of obstruction? (2) What is its *cause*? How far to go in this endeavor before operation is what we must think about.

It seems at first glance a bit overdone to have a large multiauthored, multidisciplinary, multitechnique approach to answer such seemingly simple questions. Part of the complexity may be perpetuated by specialists attempting to carve out a niche for their own skills or technique. After all, even the most staunch subspecialty advocate realizes that oral cholecystography, intravenous cholangiography, computed tomography, ultrasound, percutaneous transhepatic cholangiography, endoscopic retrograde cholangiopancreatography, and radionuclide scintigraphy are competing in a medical as well as financial marketplace. These tests are being evaluated, compared, and utilized by physicians with varying expertise, equipment, patients, and biases.[5-11] It is not surprising, then, that the results vary. If one scientific study tells us that transhepatic cholangiography is superior to ultrasound in the evaluation of jaundice,[12] another tells us the opposite,[13] and if the clinician ordering these studies thinks that neither is essential and that the result could be accurately predicted by examining and listening to the patient,[14, 15] what are we to think? All too often radiologists recommend irrelevant or inappropriate studies because they do not understand the clinical problem. Equally as often, an inappropriate test is ordered or its significance misconstrued by clinicians who have failed to listen to or examine their patients thoroughly or who are unfamiliar with the rapidly evolving technology of another specialty. There is no one answer at present. If there were, this book would be a lot shorter and perhaps only an algorithm.

The choice of work-up for biliary tract disease should be a decision made in concert with the patient by clinician, radiologist, and surgeon, utilizing the equipment available to best advantage, remaining cost conscious, and always trying to minimize risk and discomfort for the patient. The clinician attempting to decipher the cause of the patient's complaints should function somewhat like an orchestra conductor, extracting as much as he can from the score, harmonizing the skills of those around him, but recognizing that he cannot function alone.

Too often, however, passive deference to the power of images leads to more diagnostic tests than are necessary, inattention to an obvious clinical diagnosis because it cannot be "seen," and the pursuit of incidental images that have no relation to therapy and that sometimes lead to an unnecessary operation. The clinician must always ask whether the fact that a study can be done means that it should be done and, in a time of rising costs, whether noninvasiveness is justification enough for sending the patient through a large diagnostic mill.[16-22]

During development, all new diagnostic studies, including imaging procedures, go through five stages of technological assessment to determine the following: (1) How does the machine work (i.e., can the images be reliably produced)? (2) Does it convey useful information (i.e., does it show something worth seeing)? (3) How does it compare with older techniques? (4) Does it change the diagnostic process? (5) Does it change the outcome of the disorders (does the patient fare better)? Traditionally, the emphasis in imaging evaluation has been on stages 1 through 3, notably stage 3, since the continuous evaluation of new tests requires comparison with the old. Still, the fourth and fifth stages are ultimately the most important to the clinician and his patient.[19] One of the consequences of comparing technologies in stage 3 has been the proliferation of studies, either because of discordant results that increase clinical uncertainty or because of a natural desire to assess the relative effectiveness of different studies. Either way, there is danger that such multiplicity of testing may become the norm with regard to clinical utility.[21]

We will discuss the clinical correlates of biliary tract disease in the sequence of clinical clues, laboratory assessment, and imaging aspects. As the prudent clinician uses most diagnostic studies to confirm a strong clinical impression, we will begin with a few comments on clinical clues.

CLINICAL CLUES

The clinician regards only two complaints as likely to originate in the biliary tract: abdominal pain and jaundice. Other complaints long ascribed to the gallbladder and its ducts, such as gassiness, bloating, or even fatty food intolerance, are time honored but have been repeatedly found to have little relationship to the gallbladder or biliary tree or their function.[23] The clinician knows that such nonspecific complaints will rarely be helped by biliary tract manipulations.

Increasingly, the clinician deals with the evaluation of pain. In an era when images cast such brilliant shadows and so many imaging choices are available it is more important than ever for the clinician to have some rules for evaluating abdominal pain. The very name *biliary colic* is a misnomer. Pain from the gallbladder is not ordinarily colicky; it is usually rather steady, noncrampy, and postprandial; occurs at night; and is usually located in the upper right quadrant or midepigastrium. When gallstones lodge in the common bile duct, the pain is more likely to radiate through to the back or to the angle of the right scapula. Usually an uncomplicated attack of biliary colic lasts no more than four hours; whenever such pain lasts longer, the clinician thinks of a complicating common bile duct stone or pancreatitis. Vomiting is uncommon until pain medications are given or unless a complication is present.

In the patient with acute biliary colic, therefore, the clinician wants to know whether gallstones are present and the degree of confidence that the radiologist has in their demonstration. He will be looking for any help that he can get. Evidence of "gravel" in the patient with otherwise *bona fide* biliary colic will be more important to the clinician than evidence of gravel in a patient with nonspecific abdominal pain.

The problem comes generally in the fact that *gallstones* are common and abdominal pain of nonspecific variety that does not arise from the gallbladder is also common. The clinician has to keep in mind that the finding of gallstones by any technique does not necessarily mean that the patient's pain comes from those gallstones. It has been estimated that in the United States 20 million people have gallstones,[24-27] most of whom carry them for life, unburdened by their presence.[28-33] The significance of gallstones cannot be evaluated by the images alone; clinical evaluation to determine the course of action is not diminished but is enhanced as more imaging technology becomes available. Yet many physicians have abandoned the idea that the subjective description of pain offers any guide as to what is going on; they prefer visual images, which they see as being more reproducible than a history (as indeed they may be). Gallstones are so common, however, that they are often found as innocent bystanders in a patient whose pain has another source.[24, 28, 29] This has always been the case, and every clinician can tell stories of patients whose gallstones were removed by an enthusiastic surgeon but whose symptoms resisted the removal of his gallbladder. This happened often enough when oral cholecystography was the only way to detect gallstones, but the multiplication of tests over the past decade has increased the likelihood that gallstones will be detected and then removed when they are *not* the cause of abdominal pain. This is why it is increasingly important for the clinician to have clear standards for what he will accept as abdominal pain originating from the gallbladder or biliary tree. Too often, the post-cholecystectomy syndrome is the result of ill-advised removal of the gallbladder in patients whose upper right quadrant pain stemmed from bowel dysfunction rather than gallbladder disease.

That *cholangitis,* shaking chills, and fever to 100° or more are almost always the result of a benign obstruction of the common bile duct is a good clinical rule.[34] To be sure, very rarely cholangitis can be the result of malignant obstruction of the common bile duct and, even more rarely, an accompaniment of viral hepatitis; but these latter events are so rare that the clinician should usually take his middle-aged patient with cholangitis to have a gallstone obstructing the common bile duct. The course of diagnostic action should be dictated by the best locally available diagnostic therapeutic measures. That is, it is not unreasonable to expect that in some institutions a percutaneous approach to biliary decompression will be the initial therapy; in other institutions, removal of the offending stone by endoscopic papillotomy will gain favor. The important point is to choose the most direct study. To demonstrate the level of obstruction and locate the stones directly, the choice lies between ERCP and percutaneous transhepatic cholangiography. In our institution, many surgeons prefer to see the ducts from above and believe that their surgical approach will be better planned if they can see the status of the intrahepatic ducts and their confluence, which is more difficult to assess operatively and less likely to be demonstrated by the endoscopic approach from below. As endoscopic papillotomy becomes more common, however, the ability to remove common duct stones without operation may win out over the approach from above.[35, 36]

Jaundice

Jaundice is a relatively late manifestation of biliary obstruction. It offers some clinical clues, but to review all that the clinician thinks about the jaundiced patient would involve a textbook. It is usually easy enough, given clinical circumstances and an elevated unconjugated bilirubin level, to separate out hemolytic jaundice; unconjugated bilirubin, which accumulates as the result of hemolysis, does not pass through the kidney and so the urine remains untinged. In contrast, with viral hepatitis the urine is often dark for a few days before the jaundice develops and the stools are usually clay colored. A history of taking drugs that may cause jaundice or appropriate occupational exposure often gives useful information. Abdominal pain is less common in patients with liver disease and the prodromal period less impressive in patients with biliary tract disease than in those with disease of hepatic origin. Finally, whether the jaundice is intermittent, whether there is epigastric pain radiating through the back, and so forth offer important clinical clues. In the end, ultrasonography and some liver function studies offer the most immediately useful information.

In the evaluation of jaundice the clinician has to choose increasingly between aesthetic consideration and diagnostic utility. It is satisfying for all to see the diagnostic studies laid out; to recognize that the ultrasonogram shows dilated bile ducts in sagittal, transverse, and coronal sections and even shows the gastroduodenal artery; that computed tomography shows the retroperitoneal fat planes, liver, pancreas, and dilated bile ducts; that radionuclide scintigraphy shows delayed excretion and obstruction of the common bile duct; and that direct cholangiography confirms that all of these indirect modes were correct. Nevertheless, the job of the clinician over the next years will be to familiarize himself increasingly with what diagnostic tests can offer and to decide *which* test should be done and how *few*, not how many.[16-21]

Finally, the clinician must temper the diagnostic assessment with some common sense. The temperate middle-aged man or woman who develops persistent midepigastric pain radiating through to the back, anorexia, and a 10-lb weight loss is likely to have a carcinoma of the pancreas. If the amylase or lipase level is elevated, the overwhelming likelihood is that the obstruction lies at the ampulla or the pancreatic duct. Further diagnostic maneuvers should be addressed specifically to that problem. Simply because a test is noninvasive does not justify its use except in a research protocol. To be sure, sometimes computed tomography and ultrasonography will fortuitously pick up metastases that would not otherwise have come to attention, but in patients with pancreatic carcinoma and weight loss this finding may have less bearing on therapy and outcome than we would like to think.[37]

Clinical symptoms have lost their relevance to the clinicians of the 1980s, so amazed are they at the power of images. Sometimes the clinician fails to use good clinical judgment simply because the images do not support what he thinks is going on and because the clinical story does not seem strong enough evidence to stand up against negative images. For example, a patient may have clinical biliary colic with every diagnostic imaging study unrevealing, including ERCP. In such circumstances, the clinician is afraid to suggest an operation to remove the gallstones that are so likely because of the overwhelming number of diagnostic studies arrayed against him. Twenty years ago, when the clinician's judgment was counterbalanced only by a "normal" oral cholecystogram, he realized that 5 to 10 per cent of the time the oral cholecystogram would not show stones even when they were present, and so he let his judgment outweigh that single piece of evidence. Today, however, with so many expensive diagnostic studies proving negative, the clinician very rarely has the courage of his convictions.

LABORATORY ASSESSMENT

In the evaluation of jaundice, most liver function studies have become archaic, outmoded by diagnostic imaging. The fluctuations of the alkaline phosphatase level are of much less importance than they used to be now that images can show the dilated bile ducts so readily.[38-44] In this regard, the barrage of laboratory numbers usually presented by enthusiastic clinicians seems as overwhelming to the radiologist as the display of images sometimes does to the clinician.

Only three liver function tests are currently generally important in the jaundiced patient because of these imaging studies. The transaminase level is most important of all to exclude the possibility that the jaundiced patient has primary hepatocellular disease. The clinical setting may not suggest this possibility, particularly in a middle-aged patient, but a transaminase level above 750 units may be the only clue to primary hepatocellular disease and the fact that the jaundice is secondary to viral hepatitis rather than duct obstruction.

Other liver function studies of value in the 1980s in the jaundiced patient are those that can tell something of hepatic synthetic function: the prothrombin time and its responses to vitamin K injections, and the level of serum albumin. If a prolonged prothrombin time does not rise after injection of vitamin K, the patient has primary hepatocellular disease or at least a very badly deranged liver; if the albumin level is low, liver disease has been present for more than three weeks, since the serum albumin level falls by half in that period of time.

To be sure, in the nonjaundiced patient some other liver function studies ignored here may be helpful. The alkaline phosphatase level may be the only clue to unilateral or segmental obstruction of one of the larger hepatic ducts,[45, 46] but it is of less importance and is much less frequent in the jaundiced patient in whom the crucial question must be, "Are the bile ducts dilated?" In most jaundiced patients, the clinician will always order an assessment of amylase and lipase levels simply to help him decide whether the ampulla or the pancreatic duct is obstructed.

IMAGING ASPECTS

Gallbladder Disease

Deferring to the formidable array of radiologic images, the clinician often fails to assess the precise information he needs to know. Failure to formulate specific clinical impressions and raise clear-cut questions that can be answered by imaging techniques results in unnecessary and inappropriate tests that are not clinically useful. The number of noninvasive tests performed is proportional to the clinician's lack of confidence in his clinical diagnosis. One after another indirect test is obtained until only when the diagnosis is obvious to everyone, from professor to second-year medical student, is an invasive test yielding a specific diagnosis finally acceded to. Excessive use of noninvasive tests often leads to one ambiguous study begetting another. In this era of rising medical costs, noninvasiveness should not be the *sole* justification to perform a test.

Several aspects of the diagnosis of gallbladder disease are as yet unsettled.[47] Since gallstones can be present without causing "disease" or even symptoms and since disease can be present without gallstones in the form of acalculous cholecystitis or hyperplastic cholecystopathy, a blending of clinical and radiologic information is essential for any meaningful therapeutic decision. If this decision is difficult when gallstones are incontrovertibly present on oral cholecystography or ultrasonography, it is even more so when the images are less than certain.

The strongest evidence for gallstones on ultrasound comes from the triad of opacity, shadowing from the opacity, and motion of the opacity.[48] The presence of only two of these findings, which occurs in about a third of cases,[48] makes the evidence considerably less certain. For example, a shadowing opacity that does not move and thereby does not fulfill the third criterion may be the result of fibrosis at the porta hepatis (Fig. 15–1), a gallbladder septum, a polyp, or may even represent a cystic duct in the neck of the gallbladder[49, 50] (Fig. 15–2). It should be clear that even the imager's conclusion that "a stone is impacted in the cystic duct" should be balanced by clinical input, since a shadowing opacity can be present normally in the gallbladder neck.

Another example occurs when an opacity moves but does not shadow, a phenomenon referred to as "sludge," debris, gravel, or various other names (Fig. 15–3).[51, 57] Radiologists need to agree on precise terminology and the nature and meaning of shadowing[53-59] before diagnostic significance can be ascribed to such findings. Filly has shown that the appearance of sludge is destroyed by passing bile through a millipore filter that removes calcium bilirubinate and cholesterol crystals, from which he concludes that sludge is related to the presence of these crystals.[53] What then should the radiologist make of the finding of sludge? The clinician says that it helps him in the proper clinical setting, that is, in the patient with biliary colic, but that otherwise he ignores sludge as an incidental finding. But he does the same with incontrovertible gallstones that cause no symptoms. In one surgical series, 96 per cent of patients with sludge were said to have diseased gallbladders, two-thirds stones, and one-third acalculous cholecystitis.[48] Yet most patients with this finding probably have no symptoms from their biliary tract and its very significance may have been overstated in this surgical series, since the majority of patients with sludge are unlikely to come to operation.

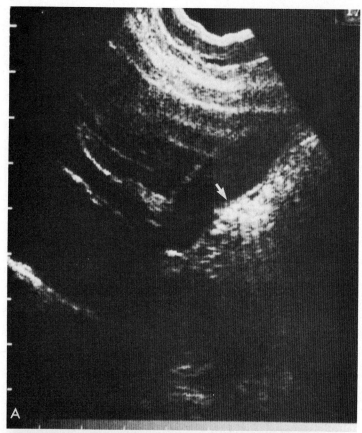

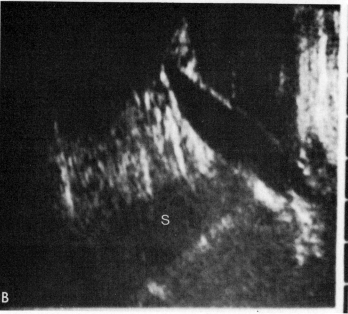

Figure 15–1. Fibrosis in gallbladder fossa. *A*, Oblique projection demonstrates a localized echogenic area (arrow) related to the wall of the gallbladder. On real-time examination this appeared distinct from bowel. *B*, A different obliquity demonstrates a broad band of shadowing (S) adjacent to the echogenic area. On multiple ultrasound examinations the echogenic opacity appeared consistently related to the gallbladder but was never seen to move within the gallbladder lumen. Oral cholecystography demonstrated a well-visualized normal gallbladder. No calcifications were seen on plain film. The patient has been asymptomatic for three years since the study. The findings were presumed to represent fibrosis adjacent to the gallbladder.

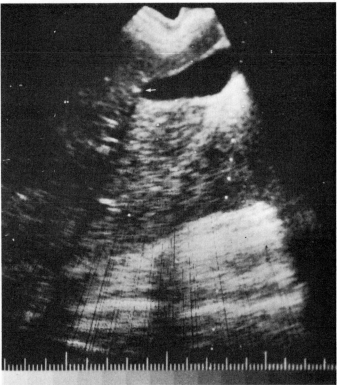

Figure 15–2. Normal shadowing of the cystic duct. Focal opacity in gallbladder neck (arrow) with well-defined area of shadowing. This opacity remained constant in position and represents a normal appearance of the cystic duct insertion into the gallbladder. If this patient were acutely ill and the clinical question one of acute cholecystitis, it might be difficult to separate out a normal shadowing opacity in this area from an impacted stone in the cystic duct neck.

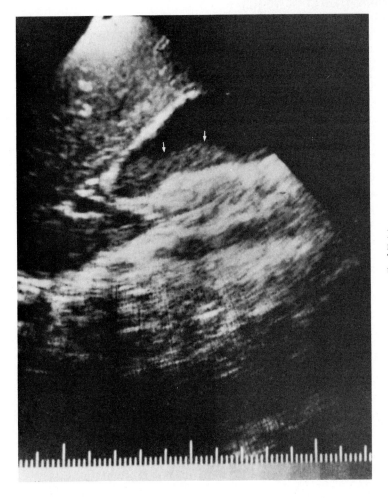

Figure 15–3. Gallbladder sludge. Nonshadowing focal opacities, which move freely in the gallbladder lumen. This patient had no symptoms referable to gallbladder disease.

If examination of the gallbladder with stones or gravel can be perplexing, the diagnosis of gallbladder disease without stones, or acalculous cholecystitis,[60-66] is even more so. Acalculous cholecystitis has achieved considerable prominence over the past few years, but removal of a normal gallbladder has not yet achieved surgical acceptability comparable with removal of a normal appendix, considered a necessary misfortune in a small percentage of patients in whom appendicitis has been questioned. We can wonder whether the degree or even incidence of inflammation in these gallbladders has been magnified by pathologists taking too seriously the degree of leukocytic infiltration normally present. The presence of leukocytes in the gallbladder as a criterion for acalculous cholecystitis is a weak one; 75 per cent of patients without a clinical history of gallbladder disease had leukocytic infiltration of the gallbladder.[67] Stronger evidence comes from hypertrophy of the gallbladder muscle in such circumstances.[68]

As for oral cholecystography, several questions still need to be answered by clinician and radiologist. We know that oral cholecystography demonstrates the concentrating ability of the gallbladder and that nonvisualization of the gallbladder is almost invariably associated with disease.[69] If so, what about the patients with nonvisualization on double-dose oral cholecystography who presumably have nonfunctional gallbladders but in whom ultrasound study does *not* demonstrate stones and who may therefore be considered to have a normal gallbladder anatomically? Obviously this question is tempered to some extent by variations in technical skill of ultrasonography, but to our knowledge such a population has not been studied and the question has not been answered. Perhaps it never will be, in view of the reluctance of clinicians in the absence of "hard copy" demonstration of stones to suggest operation; it may well be that the clinical ability to recognize cholecystitis by history and physical examination alone is less than clinicians would like to believe.[70, 71] In any event, the answers are not easy to come by.

Radiologists have searched for signs of gallbladder disease other than by direct demonstration of stones, and it is not for lack of effort that no clear answer has been forthcoming. Although oral cholecystography can clearly demonstrate stones at one end of the spectrum and, with equal certainty, failure of concentration, all of us are familiar with the litany of nongallbladder causes of nonvisuali-

zation including malabsorption, gastric outlet obstruction, and failure to take the pills.[69] Radiologists can trace pictorially the metabolic pathway of conjugated Telepaque excreted by the liver, either by demonstrating contrast in the common bile duct directly, by tomography, or by showing conjugated milky white contrast in the bowel.[72-74] In this way, radiologists infer that the fault in nonvisualization lies within the gallbladder, since the contrast got there. But what about faint visualization? Clinicians and radiologists never talk about that, particularly when the clinician thinks that in the gray world of radiology the answers to gallbladder disease are all black and white.

The ultrasonographer has as many "gray areas" in the diagnosis of gallbladder disease. In the ultrasonographic field the equivalent of faint visualization is probably increased thickness of the gallbladder wall[75-80] (Fig. 15–4). There are many causes of apparent increased wall thickness,[81-83] but it seems likely that different things are being measured, since different limits of normal are proposed. In fact, the very ability to measure the wall is variable and has been reported possible in 30 to 100 per cent of cases. It seems likely that this sign of gallbladder disease is of little value, except as an ancillary sign of gallbladder disease in conjunction with the demonstration of gallstones, when, of course, it becomes redundant. Other ultrasonographic signs, such as the size of the gallbladder or its configuration, with a tendency to roundness (Fig. 15–5) when it is under tension,[11, 84-87] or pericholecystic fluid collections[86, 88-90] (Fig. 15–6) have not proved consistent enough to be good predictors of disease.

Gallbladder "nonvisualization" also occurs on ultrasound examination as the result of purely anatomic considerations rather than the functional-anatomic failure to concentrate contrast material. It may be the result of a diseased gallbladder with an obliterated lumen, but it may also stem from a number of other causes including physiologic contraction, small volume, proximal obstruction of the biliary tree, technical error, an ectopic location of the gallbladder, or the oft-quoted but rare congenital absence of the gallbladder. One study recommended an oral cholecystogram to reduce the 12 per cent error rate of nonvisualization on ultrasound,[91] an interesting turnabout from the early contention of ultrasonographers that an ultrasound study should follow all gallbladder nonvisualizations on oral cholecystography. In the future, radiologists will attempt to separate

Text continued on page 560

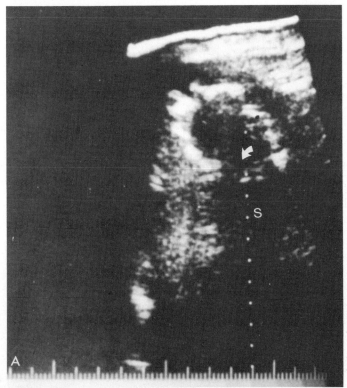

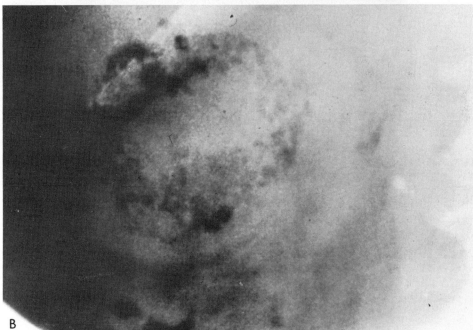

Figure 15–4. "Thick-walled gallbladder"—emphysematous cholecystitis. *A*, Ultrasound examination of the gallbladder reveals an irregular echogenic area surrounding the gallbladder, suggesting a thickened wall. On multiple projections the portion of the gallbladder farthest from the beam (arrow) could not be demonstrated. No stones were seen. *B*, Plain film of the abdomen demonstrates gas throughout the gallbladder wall, diagnostic of emphysematous cholecystitis. The echogenic area surrounding the gallbladder represents a combination of air and thickened gallbladder wall. The inability to demonstrate the posterior gallbladder wall is probably related to the attentuation and shadowing effect (S) caused by the air.

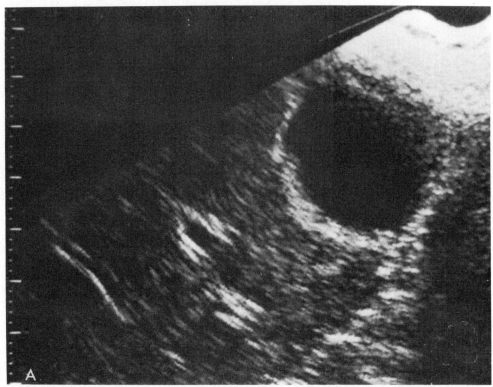

Figure 15–5. Distended gallbladder. Following a cerebrovascular accident, this 48-year-old man developed pleuritic upper right quadrant and lower thoracic pain. The gallbladder felt distended on physical examination. *A*, Sonogram demonstrates a distended gallbladder without evidence of stones.

Illustration continued on opposite page

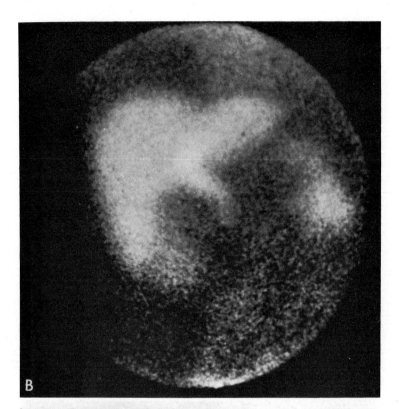

Figure 15–5. *Continued B*, Tc-HIDA scintigram at one hour demonstrates a large photon-deficient gallbladder fossa. *C*, At eight hours the gallbladder fills in, corresponding to the photon-deficient region in *B*. This case illustrates physiologic distention of the gallbladder, which mimicked acute cholecystitis on ultrasound and early HIDA studies but filled on delayed HIDA examination. A right lower lobe pneumonia was subsequently identified and treated. The gallbladder stasis might have been related to ileus from the patient's pneumonia or his cerebrovascular accident and diet. (*C* reprinted with permission from Zeman, Segal, and Caride: J. Nucl. Med. *22*:39, 1981.)

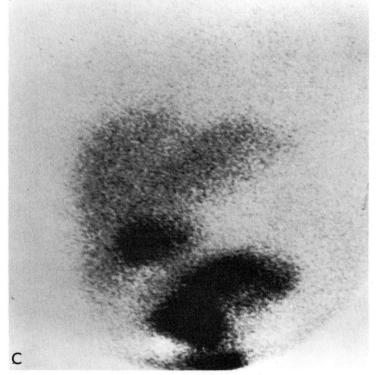

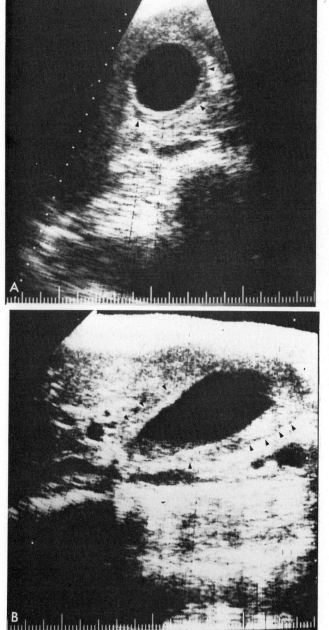

Figure 15–6. Pericholecystic fluid. *A,* A thin lucent rim (arrowheads) is seen surrounding the gallbladder. There has been some controversy as to whether this represents fluid (and has diagnostic significance for acute cholecystitis) or the outer aspect of the gallbladder wall. *B,* Similar lucency is seen in the sagittal projection (arrowheads). Sludge is seen within the gallbladder. No stones are identified.

Illustration continued on opposite page

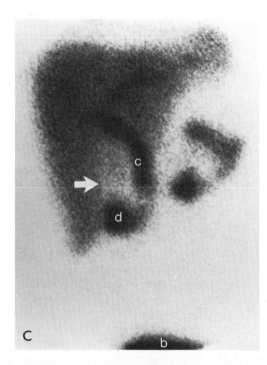

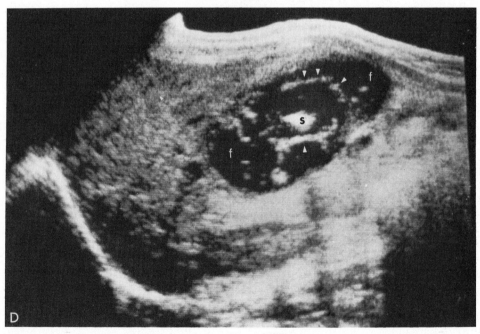

Figure 15–6. *Continued   C*, Photopenic area (arrow) represents failure to visualize the gallbladder on this HIDA scan taken at one hour. This is despite good uptake by the liver and excretion of isotope into the common duct (c) and duodenum (d). Delayed views failed to reveal any visualization of the gallbladder. Bladder activity is also seen (b). *D*, An example of a more extensive collection of fluid around the gallbladder is seen in a different patient who had a perforated gallbladder following an episode of acute cholecystitis. The pericholecystic fluid (f) represents an abscess surrounding the gallbladder. S = stone; arrowheads indicate gallbladder wall. This patient had acute cholecystitis (acalculous) confirmed at operation. The anatomic approach of ultrasound (fluid around gallbladder or thick gallbladder wall) is compared with the functional approach of scintigraphy (isotope does not enter gallbladder, therefore indicating cystic duct occlusion).(*C* reprinted with permission from Zeman et al.: Am. J. Surg. *141*:446, 1981.)

out gallbladders not seen ultrasonographically even more often into those that shadow and those that do not, in an effort to enhance the significance of this finding. The splitters will probably prevail over the lumpers, so that the clinician and radiologist must strive to maintain a broad perspective.

Hyperplastic cholecystopathy, a degenerative process of the gallbladder having a number of forms and names such as adenomyomatosis, neuromyomatosis, and cholesterolosis, has been associated with gallbladder symptoms by many observers.[92-94] The case for removal of the gallbladder in this disorder is not convincing, with internists and surgeons at opposite poles on the question of operation.[94] The radiologic demonstration by oral cholecystography of a hypercontractile, hyperconcentrating, segmented gallbladder with multiple outpouchings representing Rokitansky-Aschoff sinuses, is characteristic. Still, radiologist and clinician should be aware of the difference in language used by the pathologist who does not get nearly so excited at these sinuses, which he sees more frequently than the radiologist. Although scattered ultrasonographic reports of this disorder appear in the literature, predominantly related to wall abnormalities,[95] it has not been consistently demonstrated at ultrasonography, since no ultrasonographic feature is specific.

The recognition of acute cholecystitis by imaging techniques has come to the fore because radionuclide scans can readily confirm this disorder.[96-98] The old-fashioned clinician who felt that he could recognize acute cholecystitis by a characteristic history and positive physical findings is now surprised to read of comparisons between ultrasound and radionuclide studies in this disorder and wonders if too many studies may be carried out. In the reports of the efficacy of diagnostic techniques in acute cholecystitis, the number of patients studied to rule out acute cholecystitis who prove to have disorders other than those of the gallbladder has been impressively high, from 50 to 75 per cent.[11, 70, 71, 96, 99, 100] Does this reflect the ignorance or lack of experience of the clinician or simply his abdication in the presence of diagnostic images? Do we conclude that two-thirds of the time that the clinician considers acute cholecystitis to be present he is wrong, or are such figures merely a reflection of the laxity of diagnosis now that imaging studies are so easily available? Since a number of these studies are performed in university centers, the figures may reflect the enthusiasm of young clinicians for "objective"

data. Yet, if residents and students are taught to recognize acute cholecystitis only by positive images, this will greatly influence the way the disorder is approached and detected in the future. That is to say, if the student and resident get the idea that the only way to make the diagnosis of acute cholecystitis is to get HIDA scans and echoes, that is what they will do in practice later. Presumably ever more studies will be done for a wider and wider range of abdominal complaints as clinical discrimination decreases.

In comparing ultrasound and HIDA scans in acute cholecystitis, the basic question is whether an anatomic study to demonstrate stones, such as ultrasound, is more significant to the clinician than the functional study with a HIDA derivative, showing obstruction of the cystic duct (Fig. 15–7).[96] In the evolving comparison of these two techniques, several points emerge. (1) The demonstration that the cystic duct is patent by a normal HIDA scan with a visualized gallbladder is the most sensitive study, with a 98 per cent accuracy rate in excluding acute cholecystitis.[96] (2) The accuracy rate of ultrasonography in demonstrating stones in a patient with acute cholecystitis seems considerably less than in routine and less emergent circumstances. In one series only 66 per cent of patients with stones ultimately proved at operation were detected by ultrasound.[96] This is no doubt the result of a combination of factors, including the fact that the gallbladder is not studied in the fasting state and that ileus often leads to obscuring of the gallbladder by gas. (3) The presence of stones on ultrasound is less likely to define acute cholecystitis, since a number of patients who have stones may well have chronic cholecystitis with cholelithiasis and may not have acute cholecystitis at all.[11, 96]

Radiologists and clinicians do not always understand each other in some of these matters, and some other points have proved particularly confusing. (1) Nonvisualization of the gallbladder on HIDA scan does not guarantee acute cholecystitis; such a picture may mean acute cholecystitis, but it may also mean chronic cholecystitis or a distended gallbladder with bile so viscid that the radioisotope cannot enter the gallbladder, as sometimes happens in pancreatitis.[96] (2) Nonvisualization means simply that the gallbladder is not seen when the ducts themselves can be demonstrated. If the radionuclide is not excreted from the liver, so that the ducts themselves are not seen, nonvisualization of the gallbladder has no meaning. (3) The radionuclide study does not

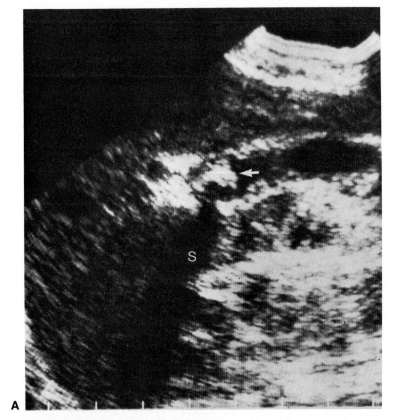

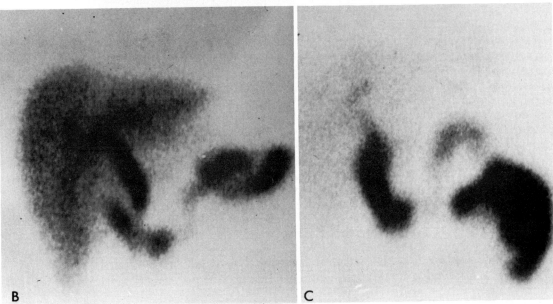

Figure 15–7. Acute cholecystitis (ultrasonography and scintigraphy). This patient with a clinical history of acute cholecystitis, which was confirmed operatively, had a stone impacted in the gallbladder neck. *A*, The shadowing opacity (arrow) remained fixed in position in the neck of the gallbladder and represented an impacted gallstone (compare with Fig. 15–2). S = shadowing. *B*, Tc-IDA scan at one hour (Tc-99m Disofenin) in the same patient shows nonvisualization of the gallbladder with normal egress of activity into the bile ducts and bowel. This represents cystic duct obstruction (see also Fig. 15–6). *C*, Delayed Tc-IDA shows good washout from the liver and bile ducts and persistent failure to opacify the gallbladder. These are the two findings one looks for in both ultrasound and Tc-IDA evaluation of patients with acute cholecystitis.

diagnose gallstones but merely shows a patent cystic duct; the presence of isotope in the gallbladder does not exclude stones.[96] Not understanding these facts, some clinicians have become disenchanted with the HIDA scan because it "misses" gallstones. (4) One ultrasonographic sign of acute cholecystitis that has evolved is the demonstration of tenderness directly over the gallbladder, the so-called "ultrasonographic Murphy sign."[11, 101] Whether this sign is to be considered an advantage for ultrasound or merely a confirmation of what is already known clinically depends on the perspective. (5) Finally, the pathologic distinction of acute cholecystitis from chronic cholecystitis is not as clear as imagers and clinicians would like.[67, 68] Moreover, we are uncertain as to what some studies refer when they "find" chronic cholecystitis by the delayed entrance of radionuclides into the gallbladder.

Other disorders of the gallbladder in which the radiologist provides visual evidence that detects disease not recognized by the clinician include hydrops with impacted stone,[102, 103] milk of calcium bile,[104, 105] porcelain gallbladder,[106, 107] and emphysematous cholecystitis (Fig. 15–4).[108-111]

Bile Duct Disease

Another major concern for the clinician is evaluation of the bile ducts, usually because of jaundice.[112] As with gallbladder disease, simple anatomic depiction of the ducts can be misleading. Patients may have ducts that are obstructed without being jaundiced (that is, segmental[113] and preicteric[114-116] obstruction or even ducts packed with stones) or they may have dilated ducts without obstruction,[117] as after operation. In addition, the extrahepatic ducts may be disproportionately dilated in obstruction without any apparent effect on the intrahepatic ducts.[118] To complicate matters even more, patients may have obstructive jaundice with nondilated ducts.[119] All of these problems make it more difficult to equate the simple presence of a dilated or nondilated biliary tree with obstructive versus nonobstructive jaundice. The ability to clinically discriminate the different causes of jaundice makes for a subtle type of "incorporation bias"[5, 20] that is difficult to eliminate completely in the objective evaluation of the accuracy of imaging tests.

In the evaluation of jaundice each study can provide different information, at times complementary, at times redundant, at times necessary, and at times gratuitous. What information is needed, such as the definition of the presence, level, and cause of obstruction, is, in fact, not absolute but depends on individual preference. Most clinicians agree that the most important aspect of imaging is to confirm that the ducts are obstructed and so avoid needless laparotomy. This can be done by many routes, but ultrasound is the current clinical favorite because of its rapid and noninvasive nature. If the presence and/or cause of obstruction is clearly evident to the clinician, as it may be when the patient is jaundiced after gallstones have been removed or in the presence of cholangitis, then simple confirmation of obstruction by demonstrating dilated ducts ultrasonographically could delay the direct demonstration of the level of obstruction by transhepatic cholangiography, which is most valuable in assessing the feasibility of an operative approach (Figs. 15–8 and 15–9). The detection of unexpected findings, such as disease in other organs, a point raised repeatedly in support of ultrasound and computed tomography in these circumstances, is relevant for the clinician only if such findings mean that operative decompression will not be carried out or that it will be carried out by the techniques of interventional radiography or endoscopic papillotomy. Such a finding may be hyperbolic if renal cysts or hemangiomas of the liver are found, discoveries of no more value than a routine screen of the general population.

What is the best approach? If the presence, location, and cause of obstruction can be documented by direct studies, they offer the most reasonable approach. Transhepatic cholangiography followed by operation or, in appropriate circumstances, ERCP followed by papillotomy should be the way to go. If "indirect" imaging, such as ultrasound, shows only dilated bile ducts without pinpointing the site of obstruction, it can be argued that this is enough for the clinician. It still seems prudent to demonstrate the nature and site of the obstruction preoperatively, since this cannot be shown with sufficient reliability on indirect studies (Figs. 15–8 and 15–9) and is not as readily obvious in many operating rooms as surgeons would like to think.[121] Multiple strictures, intrahepatic stones, high lesions, Mirizzi's syndrome,[122] unusual cystic duct insertion, and clinically significant anatomic variation of the bile duct (demonstrated in as many as 48 per

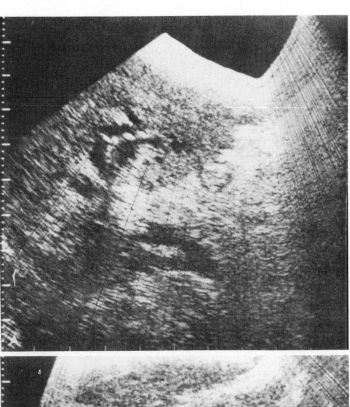

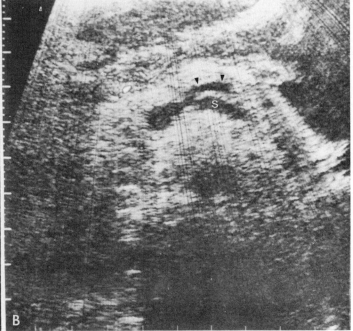

Figure 15–8. Determining location and etiology of obstruction. This elderly gentleman presented with clear-cut clinical and laboratory evidence of obstructive jaundice. He had had a cholecystectomy years ago. *A*, Sagittal ultrasound examination demonstrates multiple dilated ducts converging toward the liver hilum. The extrahepatic common duct was poorly seen (perhaps because of clips and fibrosis from previous surgery). *B*, Transverse ultrasound examination revealed a dilated pancreatic duct (arrowheads) anterior to the splenic vein (S). Combining this with the ultrasound finding of dilated bile ducts, it was inferred that the obstruction was low lying, probably at the ampulla. No gross pancreatic mass was seen on this study, but it was felt that the area was not optimally demonstrated.

Illustration continued on following page

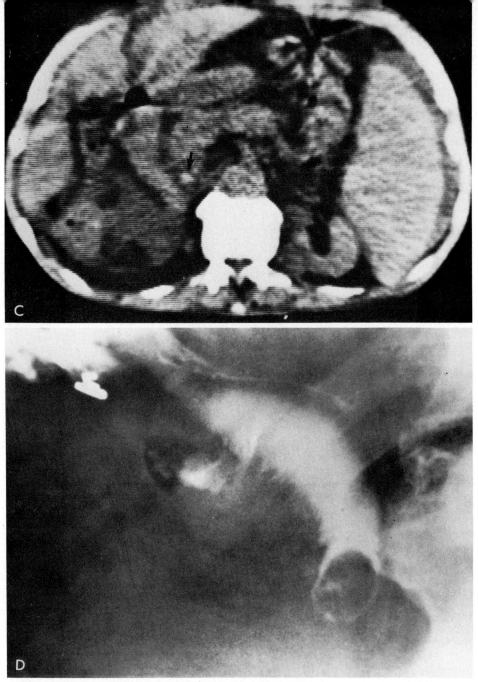

Figure 15–8. *Continued* *C*, CT scan demonstrates an opacity (arrow) for which a differential diagnosis included contrast in a duodenal diverticulum, a stone in the common duct, and calcification in the head of the pancreas. Further cuts revealed no evidence of a pancreatic mass. *D*, A transhepatic cholangiogram (skinny needle) demonstrated an impacted stone in the common duct. In this patient with suspected obstruction at the outset, all the indirect studies proved correct and provided an elegant demonstration of anatomy. However, the question is, basically, Were they the best way to obtain the desired information? The ultrasound, by combining the findings of dialted biliary ducts and a big pancreatic duct, correctly inferred a low-lying obstruction in the ampullary area, however, still leaving the question of a pancreatic lesion, an ampullary lesion, or a stone. Since a portion of the common bile duct was not visualized, a less likely possibility at this time included separate etiologies for the pancreatic and bile duct dilatation. Computerized tomographic scanning excluded a pancreatic mass and demonstrated the stone. Although clinically that appeared to fit well with the cause of obstruction, several other possible explanations for this density were raised. (At this point, it was concluded that a patient who entered with a probable obstruction of his duct had a definite obstruction of his duct due to a probable stone.) Transhepatic cholangiography demonstrated an obstructed common bile duct in the preampullary area secondary to an impacted stone. It would seem that, in this type of patient, the direct route might be the fastest and most informative method of evaluation. Since all the indirect studies were "correct" and "complementary," it is apparent that in such cases it can be difficult to sort out the relative contribution of each study from statistics alone.

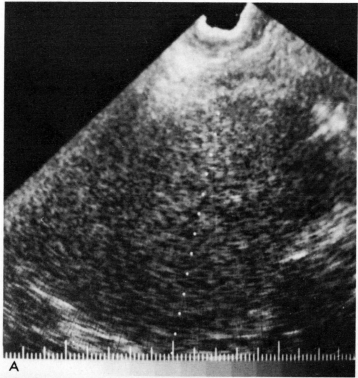

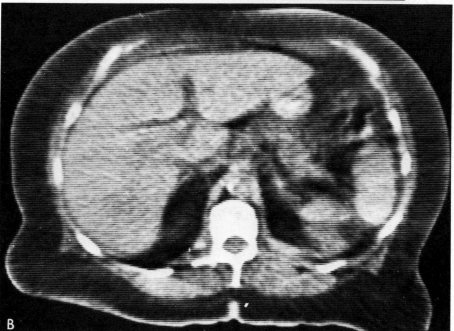

Figure 15–9. Defining anatomy. *A*, Ultrasound examination demonstrating minimal or no intrahepatic biliary dilatation (depending on one's threshold). The extrahepatic ducts were not seen. *B*, Computerized tomography did not clearly show dilated ducts on pre- and post-contrast infusion studies. There was no differential attenuation of focal areas of the liver to suggest hepatic tumor.

Illustration continued on following page

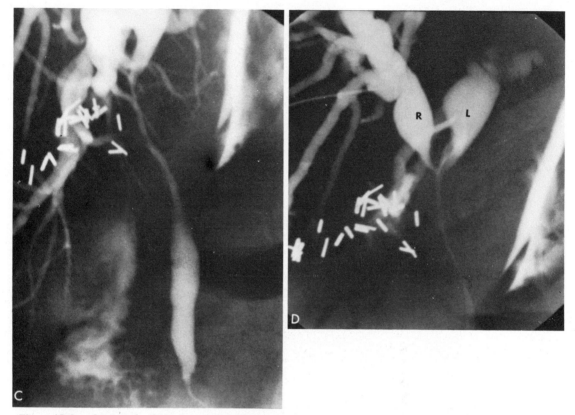

Figure 15–9. *Continued C, D,* Long infiltrating cholangiocarcinoma involving both right (R) and left (L) hepatic ducts at their junction is seen on transhepatic cholangiogram. This definition of anatomy helps the surgeon plan his operative approach and in fact determines whether operation is feasible. This patient went on to have direct cholangiography despite nonconvincing ultrasound and computed tomography studies because of a strong clinical story for obstruction. One might ask if the clinician intends to do direct cholangiography despite (1) negative screening studies (because of a strong clinical suspicion) and (2) positive screening studies to define anatomy and extent of disease. Why not go straight to the most direct demonstration in the beginning of the diagnostic evaluation?

cent of patients[123]) are invariably better demonstrated when the ducts are directly displayed. In addition, patients with stones in the common duct are the most likely group to have false-negative ultrasound studies,[86] as the ducts may be only minimally or not at all dilated. Such direct demonstration, we believe, is better done preoperatively with all the attendant advantages of radiographic-fluoroscopic control than with the limited cholangiography studies usually obtained in the operating suite. We do not enter the argument about routine operative cholangiography in all patients undergoing cholecystectomy—a nonjaundiced group—a debate continuing in surgical circles.[124, 125]

Reported opinions about the value of various techniques seem highly institutional dependent and are roughly comparable when the various techniques are used in the best of hands.[126, 127] It is reminiscent of the race "skin

to skin" or "mouth to mouth" for PTC and ERCP,[127, 128] the results not having any real bearing on the clinical situation. The ultimate question is the adaptability and usefulness in the general hospital setting of both procedures.

The imaging of bile ducts has made possible the recognition of biliary obstruction before the clinical manifestations of jaundice develop.[114] The clinician has long recognized that isolated elevation of the alkaline phosphatase level with a normal bilirubin level may be a sign of segmental obstruction of the bile ducts.[45, 46] Such conditions are not detectable in the early stages by imaging techniques,[113, 115, 116, 129] but whether therapy has improved after detection of such an early lesion in an asymptomatic patient is not clear. At Yale-New Haven Hospital an apparently healthy 59-year-old man showed an isolated increase of alkaline phosphatase level on a routine executive physical, a finding that ultimately led to the discovery of a localized obstruction of the right duct by echo and ERCP. The patient underwent lobectomy and died two weeks later of operative complications. Whether to do a major hepatic lobectomy in an asymptomatic person with a presumed cholangiocarcinoma, a tumor usually slowly progressive, or to let nature take its course, possibly allowing the patient a few more years of good health, is a question physicians have not faced many times in studying biliary tract disease. They may now face it much more frequently in view of the sophisticated imaging available.

In addition to segmental obstruction of the intrahepatic bile ducts in the patient without jaundice, the radiologist can also recognize obstruction of the common bile duct before chemical jaundice is evident.[113, 118] The common bile duct has been shown to be dilated ultrasonographically, apparently before the development of findings, but the clinician will ask why the study was done. Did the patient have some symptoms? Surely ultrasonography has not yet achieved the status of the health screening study. In the dog, obstruction of the common duct is followed by dilatation, first of the extrahepatic and then the intrahepatic ducts very shortly after the procedure, before any changes in chemistry levels take place.[130] The clinician hopes that when the images provide information that is not in keeping with his notion of the patient's ailments, the images may serendipitously detect disease in a very early, and perhaps curable, stage, but he does not know how often this will happen and whether the cost to many will be worth the benefit to a few.

On the other hand, dilated ducts can also be detected in persons in whom they have already been recognized clinically as of no significance. This may occur in the patient whose common bile duct was dilated. Once a duct has been stretched, it loses its tonicity and may not shrink back to normal; radiologic demonstration of a dilated duct after decompression may have no clinical significance; but the surgeon tends to be uncomfortable with a duct that he has worked on that does not look decompressed. In this setting, the excretion characteristics of radionuclide scans may be more helpful than anatomic studies; even though the size of the ducts does not decrease, the drainage pattern will improve.[117] A baseline ultrasonographic study in such patients may be helpful since the ducts should not *increase* in size postoperatively; unfortu-nately, such postoperative study may be impaired by air in the ducts, which obscures the ultrasound image.

It is too early for the clinician to choose between the long-term benefit of percutaneous drainage techniques of the biliary tract and operative drainage.[131-138] It would be too time consuming to review all considerations, but pancreatic cancer offers an example. Biliary duct decompression has been carried out in about 80 per cent of patients operated on for pancreatic carcinoma;[139] if percutaneous decompression can give equal relief, it will be most welcome. It should be remembered, however, that about half the patients with pancreatic cancer also require alimentary bypass to prevent gastroduodenal obstruction. In one study, of those who did not undergo such a procedure, about one-third later developed obstruction and eventually required another operation.[139] If gastroduodenal obstruction is so frequent that operation may be required, the benefit of percutaneous drainage may not be as great as it seemed at first. To be sure, the major complications of percutaneous drainage in patients with pancreatic carcinoma are infrequent, about 3 to 6 per cent, and in particular look minimal with a surgical mortality of 31 per cent.[133] The clinician recalls, however, that surgical mortality statistics are based on death within 30 days of operation; when the same strict criteria are applied to percutaneous drainage, a figure of 32 per cent can be obtained in some series. It is the cancer of the pancreas that determines the likelihood of death, not the operative approach. The clinician wonders whether what the patient gains by avoiding operation he may lose by the discomfort of the tube that must become the preoccupation of the patient, his family, and his physicians. No percutaneous tube is comfortable, and although an internal stent may solve this problem,[140, 141] one without drainage may have to be replaced at a second operation. These matters are unsettled, but the prudent clinician will not come to a judgment for several years.

When all is said and done, clearly no one paradigm, algorithm, or plan fits all instances of biliary tract disease. The approach to the patient with a stone blocking his common duct should be by endoscopic papillotomy,[35] whereas the approach to the patient with a bifurcation tumor should probably be operative or percutaneous.[138, 142] The same is true of diagnosis. If the clinician feels that he needs diagnostic studies beyond chemistries and the plain film of the abdomen, then radionuclide scintigraphy currently seems to be the wisest approach in the patient with suspected acute biliary colic. If the gallbladder is not visualized on such a study and if the clinician needs the added certainty of seeing the stones (a belt along with suspenders), then ultrasound may be added. Still, clinical judgment is always necessary because if the ultrasound does not show stones in this setting, the clinical certainty will sway the picture. On the other hand, in the patient with chronic pain and recurrent attacks, ultrasound should have more to offer than scintigraphy. The reader can imagine other approaches.

CONCLUSION

Clinicians and radiologists have all been awed by the imaging revolution. Undoubtedly, much more development will take place. Physicians must remember, however, that these tools are only as informative as the people using them and that the right answers can only come if we ask the right questions. Close cooperation between clinician and radiologist should provide direction for advances in the practical and theoretical uses of imaging. Clinician and radiologist talking together will reduce ordering of tests simply because they are available, but even more, such dialogue will remind physicians of their basic mission, of caring for patients. "No finer aim can man attain, than to alleviate another's pain" (Alexander Pope). As the frontiers of imaging continue to expand, we may come ever closer to that goal.

References

1. Berk, R. N., Ferrucci, J. T., Jr., Fordtran, J. S., Cooperberg, P. L., and Weissmann, H. S.: The radiological diagnosis of gallbladder disease—an imaging symposium. Radiology 141:49, 1981.
2. James, A. E., Jr., Portain, C. L., Holland, G. N., Gore, J. C., Rolls, F. D., Harry, S. E., and Prices, R. R.: Nuclear magnetic resonance imaging: the current state. A.J.R. 138:201, 1982.
3. Doyle, F. H., Pennock, J. M., Brouk, L. M., McDonnel, M. J., Bydder, G. M., Steiner, R. E., Young, I. R., Clarke, G. J., Pasmore, T., and Gilderdale, P. J.: Nuclear magnetic resonance imaging of the liver: initial appearance. A.J.R. 138:193, 1982.
4. Smith, F. W., Reid, A., Hutchison, J. M. S., and Mollard, J. R.: Nuclear magnetic resonance imaging of the pancreas. Radiology 142:667, 1982.
5. Ransohoff, D. F., and Feinstein, A. R.: Patterns of spectrum and bias in evaluating the efficacy of diagnostic tests. N. Engl. J. Med. 299:926, 1975.
6. McNeil, B. J., Keeler, E., and Adelstein, S. J.: Primer on certain elements of medical decision making. N. Engl. J. Med. 293:211, 1975.
7. Krook, P. M., Allen, F. H., and Bush, W. H.: Comparison of real-time cholecystosonography and oral cholecystography. Radiology 135:145, 1980.
8. Gorry, A. G., Pauker, S. G., and Shwartz, W. B.: The diagnostic importance of the normal finding. N. Engl. J. Med. 298:486, 1978.
9. Weissmann, H. S., Rosenblatt, R., Goldman, M., Freeman, L. M., and Frank, M. S.: Cholescintigraphy, ultrasonography and computerized tomography in the evaluation of biliary tract disorders. Semin. Nucl. Med. 9:22, 1979.
10. Cheng, T. H., Davis, MA. A., Seltzer, S. E., Abbruzzee, A. A., Finberg, H. J., Drum, D. E., and Jones, B.: Evaluation of hepatibiliary imaging by radionuclide scintigraphy, ultrasonography and contrast cholangiography. Radiology 133:761, 1979.
11. Freeman, L. M., Weissmann, H. S., Rosenblatt, R., Freitas, J. E., Laing, F. C., Federle, M. P., Jeffrey, R. B., and Brown, T. W.: Ultrasound versus radionuclide imaging in the evaluation of patients with acute right upper quadrant pain. Letter to the editor. Radiology 143:280, 1982.
12. Gold, J. A., Palmer, R., Cassarella, W. J., Stern, G., and Seaman, W. B.: Transhepatic cholangiography: radiological method of choice by suspected obstructive jaundice. Radiology 133:39, 1979.
13. Koenigsberg, M., Wiener, S., and Walzer, N.: Accuracy of sonography in the differential diagnosis of obstructive jaundice: comparison with cholangiography. Ann. Radiol. 133:157, 1979.
14. White, F. W.: A study of errors in the diagnosis of jaundice. N. Engl. J. Med. 229:997, 1943.
15. Shenker, S., Balint, J., and Schiff, L.: Differential diagnosis of jaundice: report of a prospective study of 61 proved cases. Am. J. Dig. Dis. 7:449, 1962.
16. Hall, F. M.: Overutilization of radiological examinations. Radiology 120:443, 1976.
17. Gregg, E. C., Rao, P. S., and Friedell, H. L.: An analysis of the value of additional diagnostic procedures. Invest. Radiol. 11:249, 1976.
18. Scheff, T. J.: Decision rules, types of errors, and their consequences in medical diagnosis. Behav. Sci. 8:97, 1963.
19. Spiro, H. M.: Images, Isaurians and internists: some reflections on medical image making. A.J.R. 136:667, 1981.
20. Schreiber, M. H.: Wilson's law of diminishing returns. A.J.R. 138:786, 1982.
21. Larson, E. B.: Promoting effective use of newer imaging techniques. A.J.R. 138:788, 1982.
22. Elkin, M.: Issues in radiology related to new technologies—President's address, RSNA. Radiology 143:1, 1982.
23. Price, W. H.: "GB complaints." Gallbladder, dyspepsia. Br. Med. J. 2:138, 1963.
24. Way, L. W., and Schleisinger, M. H.: Cholelithiasis and chronic cholecystitis. In Schleisinger, M. H., and Fordtran, J. S. (eds.): Gastrointestinal Disease, 2nd ed, Philadelphia: W. B. Saunders, 1978, p. 1294.
25. Freedman, G. D., Kannel, W. B., and Dawby, T. R.: Epidemiology of gallbladder disease: observations in the Framingham study. J. Chron. Dis. 19:273, 1966.

26. Lieber, M. M.: Incidence of gallstones and their correlation with other diseases. Ann. Surg. 135:394, 1952.
27. Ingelfinger, F.: Digestive disease as a national problem. V. Gallstones. Gastroenterology 55:102, 1968.
28. Newman, H. F., and Northrup, J. D.: The autopsy incidence of gallstones. Int. Abstr. Surg. 109:1, 1959.
29. Comfort, M. W., Gray, H. K., and Wilson, J. M.: The silent gallstone. A ten- to twenty-year follow-up of 112 cases. Ann. Surg. 128:931, 1948.
30. Newman, H. F., Northrup, J. D., Rosenblum, M., and Abrams, H.: Complications of cholelithiasis. Am. J. Gastroenterol. 50:476, 1968.
31. Weickert, A., and Robertson, B.: The natural course of gallstone disease. Gastroenterology 50:376, 1966.
32. Whitcomb, F. F., Jr.: "Should silent gallstones be removed?" Lahey Clin. Found. Bull. 20:82, 1971.
33. Robertson, H. E.: Silent gallstones. Gastroenterology 5:345, 1945.
34. Saharia, P. C., and Cameron, J. L.: Clinical management of acute cholangitis. Surg. Gynecol. Obstet. 142:369, 1976.
35. Zimmon, D. S., Falkenstein, D. B., and Kessler, R. E.: Endoscopic papillotomy for choledocholithiasis. N. Engl. J. Med. 293:1181, 1975.
36. Classen, M., and Safrany, L.: Endoscopic papillotomy and removal of gallstones. Br. Med. J. 4:371, 1975.
37. Gudjonsson, B., Livstone, E. M., and Spiro, H. M.: Cancer of the pancreas. Diagnostic accuracy and survival statistics. Cancer 42:2494, 1978.
38. Scheske, G. A., Cooperberg, P. L., Cohen, M. M., and Burhenne, H. J.: Dynamic changes in caliber of major bile ducts. Radiology 135:215, 1980.
39. Behan, M., and Kazam, E.: Sonography of the common bile duct: value of the right anterior oblique view. A.J.R. 130:701, 1978.
40. Cooperberg, P. L.: High resolution real-time ultrasound in the evaluation of the normal and obstructed biliary tract. Radiology 129:477, 1978.
41. Parulekar, S. G.: Ultrasound evaluation of common bile duct size. Radiology 133:703, 1979.
42. Graham, M. F., Cooperberg, P. L., Cohen, M. M., and Burhenne, H. J.: Size of the normal common hepatic duct following cholecystectomy: ultrasonographic study. Radiology 135:137, 1980.
43. Cooperberg, P. L., Li, D. W., Cohen, P., Max, M., Burhenne, H., and Joachim, H.: Accuracy of common hepatic duct size in the evaluation of extrahepatic biliary obstruction. Radiology 135:242, 1980.
44. Simeone, J. F., Mueller, P. R., Ferrucci, J. T., Jr., van Sonnenberg, E., Holl, D. A., Wittenberg, J., Neff, C. C., and O'Connell, R. C.: Sonography of the bile ducts after a fatty meal: an aid in detection of obstruction. Radiology 143:211, 1982.
45. Kaplan, M. M.: Alkaline phosphatase. N. Engl. J. Med. 286:200, 1972.
46. Brinsilver, H. L., and Kaplan, M. M.: Significance of elevated liver alkaline phosphatase in serum. Gastroenterology 68:1550, 1975.
47. Burhenne, H. J.: Problem areas in the biliary tract. Curr. Prob. Radiol. 5:1, 1975.
48. Crade, M., Taylor, K. J. W., Rosenfield, A. T., deGraaf, C. S., and Minihan, P.: Surgical and pathologic correlation of cholecystosonography and cholecystography. A.J.R. 131:227, 1978.
49. Sukov, R. J., Sample, W. F., Sarti, D. A., and Whitcomb, M. J.: Cholecystosonography—the junctional fold. Radiology 133:435, 1979.
50. Taylor, K. J. W., and Carpenter, D. A.: The anatomy and pathology of the porta hepatis demonstrated by gray scale ultrasonography. J.C.U. 3:117, 1975.
51. Conrad, M. R., James, J. O., and Dietchy, J.: Significance of low level echoes within the gallbladder. A.J.R. 132:967, 1979.
52. Simeone, J. F., Mueller, P. R., Ferrucci, J. T., Jr., Harbin, W. P., and Wittenberg, J.: Significance of nonshadowing focal opacities at cholecystosonography. Radiology 137:181, 1980.
53. Filly, R. A., Moss, A. A., and Way, L. W.: In vitro investigation of gallstone shadowing with ultrasound tomography. J.C.U. 7:255, 1979.
54. Grossman, M.: Cholelithiasis and acoustic shadowing. J. Clin. Ultrasound 6:182, 1978.
55. Jaffe, C. C., and Taylor, K. J. W.: The clinical impact of ultrasonic beam focusing patterns. Radiology 131:469, 1979.
56. Taylor, K. J. W., Jacobson, P., and Jaffe, C. C.: Lack of acoustic shadow on scans of gallstones. Radiology 131:463, 1979.
57. Purdom, R. C., Thomas, S. R., Kereiakes, J. G., Spitz, H. B., Goldenberg, N. J., and Krugh, K. B.: Ultrasonic properties of biliary calculi. Radiology 136:729, 1980.
58. Gonzalez, L., and MacIntyre, W. J.: Acoustic shadow formation by gallstones. Radiology 135:217, 1980.
59. Sommer, F. G., and Taylor, K. J. W.: Differentiation of acoustic shadowing due to calculi and gas collections. Radiology 135:399, 1980.
60. Adams, T. W., and Foxley, E. G.: A diagnostic technique for acalculous cholecystitis. Surg. Gynecol. Obstet. 142:168, 1976.
61. Banner, M. P., Bleshman, M. H., and Speckman, J. M.: Cholecystography: diagnostic implications for acalculous cholecystitis. A.J.R. 132:51, 1979.
62. Koehler, R. E., Stanley, R. J., and DiCroce, J.: Prolonged gallbladder opacification after oral cholecystography. Radiology 128:607, 1978.
63. Ternberg, J. L., and Keating, J. P.: Acute acalculous cholecystitis. Complication of other illnesses in childhood. Arch. Surg. 110:543, 1974.
64. Howard, R. J., and Delaney, J. P.: Acute acalculous cholecystitis. In Nagarian, J. S., and Delaney, J. P. (eds.): Surgery of the Liver, Pancreas and Biliary Tract. New York: Stratton Intercontinental Book, 1975, pp. 159–164.
65. Russell, J. G. B., Keddre, N. C., Gough, A. L., and Galland, R. B.: Radiology of acalculous gallbladder disease—a new sign. Br. J. Radiol. 49:420, 1976.
66. Glenn, F., and Becker, C. G.: Acute acalculous cholecystitis: an increasing entity. Ann. Surg. 195:131, 1982.
67. McKittry, J. P.., and McDonald, J. R.: The significance of polymorphonuclear leukocytes in gallbladders. Surgery 17:319, 1945.
68. Edlund, Y., and Zettergren, L.: Histopathology of the gallbladder in gallstone disease related to clinical data. Acta Chir. Scand. 116:450, 1958.
69. Mujahed, Z., Evans, J. H., and Whalen, J. P.: The nonopacified gallbladder on oral cholecystography. Radiology 112:1, 1974.
70. Johnson, H. C., McClaren, J. R., and Weens, H. S.: Intravenous cholangiography in the differential diagnosis of acute cholecystitis. Radiology 74:790, 1960.
71. Thorpe, C. D., Olsen, W. R., Fischer, H., Doust, V. L., and Joseph, R. R.: Emergency intravenous

cholangiography in patients with acute abdominal pain. Am. J. Surg. *125*:46, 1973.

72. Melnick, G. S., and Curcio, S. B.: The nonvisualized gallbladder: a tomographic re-evaluation. Radiology *108*:513, 1973.

73. Margulis, M., and Wohl, G. T.: Routine tomography in gallbladder nonvisualization—a method for extended positive diagnosis. A.J.R. *117*:400, 1973.

74. Pogonowska, M. J., and Collins, L. C.: Immediate repeat cholecystography with Oragrafin-calcium after initial nonvisualization of the gallbladder. Radiology *93*:179, 1969.

75. Marchal, G., and Crella, D.: Gallbladder wall thickening: a new sign of gallbladder diseases visualized by gray scale cholecystosonography. J.C.U. *6*:177, 1978.

76. Finberg, H. J., and Birnholz, J. C.: Ultrasound evaluation of the gallbladder wall. Radiology *133*:693, 1979.

77. Mindell, H. J., and Ring, A. B.: Gallbladder wall thickening. Ultrasonic findings. Radiology, *133*:699, 1979.

78. Handler, S. J.: Ultrasound of gallbladder wall thickening and its relation to cholecystitis. A.J.R. *132*:581, 1979.

79. Engel, J. M., Deitch, E. A., and Sikemma, W.: Gallbladder wall thickness: sonographic accuracy and relation to disease. A.J.R. *134*:907, 1980.

80. Saunders, R. D. C.: The significance of sonographic gallbladder wall thickening. J.C.U. *8*:143, 1980.

81. Fiske, C. E., Laing, F. C., and Brown, T. W.: Ultrasonographic evidence of gallbladder wall thickening in association with hypoalbuminemia. Radiology *135*:713, 1980.

82. Ralls, P. W., Quinn, M. F., Juttner, H. U., Halls, J. M., and Boswell, W. D.: Gallbladder wall thickening in patients without intrinsic gallbladder disease. A.J.R. *137*:65, 1981.

83. Juttner, H. V., Ralls, P. W., Quinn, M. F., and Jenney, J. M.: Thickening of the gallbladder wall in acute hepatitis. Ultrasound demonstration. Radiology *142*:465, 1982.

84. Crade, M.: Comparison of ultrasound and oral cholecystogram in the diagnosis of gallstones. Clin. Diagn. Ultrasound *1*:123, 1979.

85. Zeman, R. K., Segal, H. B., and Caride, V. J.: Tc-99m HIDA cholescintigraphy: the distended photon deficient gallbladder. J. Nucl. Med. *22*:39, 1981.

86. Taylor, K. J. W., Rosenfield, A. T., and DeGraaff, G. S.: Anatomy and pathology of the biliary tree as demonstrated. Clin. Diagn. Ultrasound *1*:103, 1979.

87. Worthen, N. J., Uszler, J. M., and Funamara, J. L.: Cholecystitis: prospective evaluation of sonography and ^{99m}Tc-HIDA cholescintigraphy. A.J.R. *137*:973, 1981.

88. Bergman, A. B., Neiman, H. L., and Kraut, B.: Ultrasonographic evaluation of pericholecystic abscesses. A.J.R. *132*:201, 1979.

89. Marchal, G. J. F., Casaer, M., Baert, A. L., Goddeeris, P. G., Kerremans, R., and Fevery, J.: Gallbladder wall sonolucency in acute cholecystitis. Radiology *133*:429, 1979.

90. Kappelman, N. O., and Saunders, R. C.: Ultrasound in the investigation of gallbladder disease. J.A.M.A. *239*:1426, 1978.

91. Harbin, W. P., Ferrucci, J. T., Jr., Wittenberg, J., and Kirkpatrick, R. H.: Nonvisualized gallbladder by cholecystosonography. A.J.R. *132*:729, 1979.

92. Jutrus, J. A., and Levisque, H. P.: Adenomyoma and adenomyomatosis of the gallbladder. Radiol. Clin. North Am. *4*:483, 1966.

93. Rain, M. D., and Midha, O.: Adenomyomatosis of the gallbladder. Surgery *78*:224, 1975.

94. Andersson, A., and Bergdahl, L.: Acalculous cholesterosis of the gallbladder. Arch. Surg. *103*:342, 1971.

95. Rice, J., Sauerbrei, E. E., Semoyas, P., Cooperberg, P. L., and Burhenne, H. J.: Sonographic appearance of adenomyomatosis of the gallbladder. J.C.U. *9*:336, 1981.

96. Zeman, R. K., Burrell, M. I., Cahow, C. E., and Caride, V.: Diagnostic utility of cholescintigraphy and ultrasonography in acute cholecystitis. Am. J. Surg. *141*:446, 1981.

97. Weissmann, H. S., Bradia, J., Sugarman, L. A., Kluger, L., Rosenblatt, R., and Freeman, L. M.: Spectrum of ^{99m}Tc IDA cholescintigraphic patterns in acute cholecystitis. Radiology *138*:167, 1981.

98. Mauro, M. A., McCartney, W. H., and Melised, J. R.: Hepatobiliary scanning—[99m]Tc PIPIDA in acute cholecystitis. Radiology *142*:193, 1982.

99. Halasz, N. A.: Counterfeit cholecystitis. A common diagnostic dilemma. Am. J. Surg. *130*:189, 1975.

100. Essenhigh, D. M.: Management of acute cholecystitis. Br. J. Surg. *53*:1032, 1966.

101. Laing, F. C., Federle, M. P., Jeffrey, R. B., and Brown, T. W.: Ultrasonic evaluation of patients with acute right upper quadrant pain. Radiology *140*:449, 1981.

102. Genereux, G. P., and Tchang, S. P. K.: Hydrops of gallbladder—unusual roentgenographic demonstration. J. Can. Assoc. Radiol. *21*:39, 1970.

103. Robinson, A. E., Erwin, J. H., Wiseman, H. J., and Kochoff, M. B.: Cholecystitis and hydrops of the gallbladder—the newborn. Radiology *122*:749, 1977.

104. Besic, L. R., Korowzoff, G., and Tiesenga, M. F.: Limy bile syndrome. J.A.M.A. *193*:145, 1965.

105. Schierholt, K. D.: Concerning the calcium-milk bile. Fortschr. Get. Roentgenstr. Nuklearmed. *127*:26, 1977.

106. Oschner, S. F., and Carrera, G. M.: Calcification of the gallbladder (porcelain gallbladder). A.J.R. *89*:847, 1963.

107. Berk, R. N., Armbuster, T. G., and Saltzstern, S. L.: Carcinoma in the porcelain gallbladder. Radiology *106*:29, 1973.

108. Campbell, E. W., and Rogers, C. L.: Submucosal gallbladder emphysema. J.A.M.A. *227*:790, 1974.

109. Poleynard, G. D., and Harris, R. D.: Diagnosis of emphysematous cholecystitis by computerized tomography. Gastrointest. Radiol. *4*:153, 1979.

110. Hunter, N. D., and Macintosh, P. K.: Acute emphysematous cholecystitis: an ultrasonic diagnosis. A.J.R. *134*:592, 1980.

111. May, R. E., and Strong, R.: Acute emphysematous cholecystitis. Br. J. Surg. *58*:483, 1971.

112. Menuck, L., and Amberg, J.: The bile ducts. Radiol. Clin. North Am. *14*:499, 1976.

113. Zeman, R. K., Gold, J. A., Gluck, L., Caride, V. J., Burrell, M., and Hoffer, P. B.: Tc[99m] HIDA scintigraphy in segmental biliary obstruction. J. Nucl. Med. *22*:456, 1981.

114. Zeman, R., Taylor, K. J. W., and Burrell, M., and Gold, J.: Ultrasound demonstration of anicteric dilatation of the biliary tree. Radiology *134*:689, 1980.

115. Weinstein, D. P., Weinstein, B. J., and Brodmerkel,

G. J.: Ultrasonography of biliary tract dilatation without jaundice. A.J.R. *132*:729, 1979.

116. Weinstein, B. J., and Weinstein, D. P.: Biliary tract dilatation in the nonjaundiced patient. A.J.R. *134*:899, 1980.

117. Zeman, R. K., Lee, C., Stahl, R. S., Cahow, C. E., Viscomi, G., Neumann, R., Gold, J. A., and Burrell, M. I.: Ultrasonography and hepatobiliary scintigraphy in the assessment of biliary enteric anastomosis. (In press.)

118. Zeman, R. K., Dorfman, G. S., Burrell, M., Stern, S., Berg, G. R., and Gold, J. A.: Disparate dilatation of the intrahepatic and extrahepatic bile ducts in surgical jaundice. Radiology *138*:129, 1981.

119. Muhletaler, C. A., Gerlock, A. J., Fleischer, A. C., and James, A. E., Jr.: Diagnosis of obstructive jaundice with nondilated bile ducts. A.J.R. *134*:1149, 1980.

120. Shanser, J. O., Korobkin, M., Goldberg, H. I., and Rohlfing, B. M.: Computed tomographic diagnosis of obstructive jaundice in the absence of intrahepatic ductal dilatation. A.J.R. *131*:389, 1978.

121. Clemett, A. R.: The interpretation of the direct cholangiogram. *In* Berk, R. N., and Clemett, A. R. (eds.): Radiology of the Gallbladder and Bile Ducts. Philadelphia: W. B. Saunders, 1977, p. 287.

122. Koehler, R. E., Melson, G., Leland, L., Joseph, K. T., and Lang, J.: Common hepatic duct obstruction by cystic duct stone: Mirizzi syndrome. A.J.R. *132*:1007, 1979.

123. Hayes, M., Goldenberg, I., and Bishop, C.: The developmental basis for bile duct anomalies. Surg. Gynecol. Obstet. *107*:447, 1958.

124. Skillings, J. C., Williams, J. S., and Henshaw, J. R.: Cost-effectiveness of operative cholangiography. Am. J. Surg. *137*:26, 1979.

125. Pagana, T. J., and Stahlgren, L. H.: Indications and accuracy of operative cholangiography. Arch. Surg. *115*:1214, 1980.

126. Harbin, W. P., Mueller, P. R., and Ferrucci, J. T., Jr.: Transhepatic cholangiography: complications and use patterns of the fine-needle technique: multi-institutional survey. Radiology *135*:15, 1980.

127. Elias, E., Hamlyn, N., Jain, S., Long, R. G., Summerfield, J. A., Dick, R., and Sherlock, S.: A randomized trial of percutaneous transhepatic cholangiography with the Chiba needle versus endoscopic retrograde cholangiography for bile duct visualization in jaundice. Gastroenterology *71*:439, 1976.

128. Conn, H. O., Redeker, A. G., and Zimmon, D. S.: PTC versus ERC—an editor's dream. Gastroenterology *71*:520, 1976.

129. Araki, T., Itai, Y., and Tasaka, A.: Computed tomography of localized dilatation of the intrahepatic bile ducts. Radiology *141*:733, 1981.

130. Zeman, R. K., Taylor, K. J. W., Rosenfield, A. T., Schwartz, A., and Gold, J. A.: Acute experimental biliary obstruction in the dog: sonographic findings and clinical implications. Radiology *136*:965, 1981.

131. Burcharth, F., and Nielbo, N.: Percutaneous transhepatic cholangiography with selective catheterization of the common bile duct. A.J.R. *127*:409, 1976.

132. Ring, E. J., Oleaga, J. A., Freiman, D. B., Husted, J. W., and Lunderquist, A.: Therapeutic applications of catheter cholangiography. Radiology *128*:333, 1978.

133. Ferrucci, J. T., Jr., Mueller, P. R., and Harbin, W. P.: Percutaneous transhepatic biliary drainage technique, results, and applications. Radiology *135*:1, 1980.

134. Pollock, T. W., Ring, E. R., Oleaga, J. A., Freiman, D. B., Mullen, J. L., and Rosato, E. F.: Percutaneous decompression of benign and malignant biliary obstruction. Arch. Surg. *114*:148, 1979.

135. Pereiras, R. V., Rheingold, O. J., Hutson, D., Mejia, J., Viamonte, M., Chiprut, R. O., and Schoff, E. R.: Relief of malignant obstructive jaundice by percutaneous insertion of a permanent prosthesis in the biliary tree. Ann. Intern. Med. *89*:589, 1978.

136. Longmire, W. P., Lippman, H. N.: Intrahepatic cholangiojejunostomy—an operation for biliary obstruction. Surg. Clin. North Am. *36*:849, 1956.

137. Cameron, J. L., Cayler, B. W., and Harrington, D. P.: Modification of the Longmire procedure. Ann. Surg. *187*:379, 1978.

138. Cahow, C. E.: Intrahepatic cholangiojejunostomy. A new simplified approach. Am. J. Surg. *137*:443, 1979.

139. Gudjonsson, B.: Pancreatic carcinoma: diagnostic and therapeutic approach—a word of caution. J. Clin. Gastroenterol. *3*:301, 1981.

140. Hellekant, C., Jonsson, K., and Genell, S.: Percutaneous internal drainage in obstructive jaundice. A.J.R. *134*:661, 1980.

141. Houevels, J., and Ihse, I.: Percutaneous transhepatic insertion of a permanent endoprosthesis in obstructive lesions of the extrahepatic bile ducts. Gastrointest. Radiol. *4*:367, 1979.

142. Bismuth, H., Franko, D., Corlette, M., and Hepp, J.: Long-term results of Roux-en-Y hepaticojejunostomy. Surg. Gynecol. Obstet. *146*:161, 1978.

INDEX

Page numbers in *italic* type indicate illustrations; (t) indicates table.